ACCP Updates in Therapeutics®:

Pharmacotherapy Preparatory Review and Recertification Course

ACCP Updates in Therapeutics:

Pharmacotherapy Preparatory Review and Recertification Course

2016 Edition

Volume I

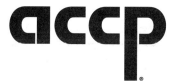

American College of Clinical Pharmacy
Lenexa, Kansas

Director of Professional Development: Nancy M. Perrin, M.A., CAE
Project Manager, Education: Zangi Miti, B.S.
Medical Editors: Carol Anne Penske and Kimma Sheldon, Ph.D.
Graphic Designer/Desktop Publisher: Steven M. Brooker

For order information or questions, contact:
American College of Clinical Pharmacy
13000 W. 87th St. Parkway
Lenexa, KS 66215-4530
Telephone: (913) 492-3311
Fax: (913) 492-0088
accp@accp.com
http://www.accp.com

To properly cite this book:
Author(s). Chapter name. In: Burke J, Cauffield J, El-Ibiary S, et al., eds. Updates in Therapeutics®: Pharmacotherapy Preparatory Review and Recertification Course, 2016 ed. Lenexa, KS: American College of Clinical Pharmacy, year:pages.

Note: The authors and publisher of the Pharmacotherapy Preparatory Review and Recertification Course recognize that the development of this material offers many opportunities for error. Despite our very best efforts, some errors may persist into print. Drug dosage schedules are, we believe, accurate and in accordance with current standards. Readers are advised, however, to check other published sources to be certain that recommended dosages and contraindications are in agreement with those listed in this book. This is especially important in new, infrequently used, or highly toxic drugs.

Library of Congress Control Number: 2016931375
ISBN: 978-1-939862-24-2

Errata: The errata for the Pharmacotherapy Preparatory Review and Recertification Course, 2016 edition, can be found at www.accp.com/media/ppc16/errata.pdf.

Continuing Pharmacy Education:

The American College of Clinical Pharmacy is accredited by the Accreditation Council for Pharmacy Education as a provider of continuing pharmacy education. The Universal Activity Numbers are as follows: Pharmacotherapy Preparatory Review and Recertification Course for home study, 2016 Edition: Pediatrics, Geriatrics, Neurology, and General Psychiatry, Activity No. 0217-0000-16-030-H01-P, 3.25 contact hours; Endocrine and Metabolic Disorders, Nephrology, and Fluids, Electrolytes, and Nutrition, Activity No. 0217-0000-16-031-H01-P, 3.5 contact hours; Biostatistics, Study Designs: Fundamentals, Interpretation, and Research Topics, and Oncology Supportive Care, Activity No. 0217-0000-16-032-H01-P, 4.0 contact hours; Critical Care, Pharmacokinetics, and Pulmonary Disorders, Gout and Immunizations, Activity No. 0217-0000-16-033-H01-P, 3.5 contact hours; Cardiology I, Cardiology II, and Men's and Women's Health, Activity No. 0217-0000-16-034-H01-P, 3.5 contact hours; Gastrointestinal Disorders, Infectious Diseases, and HIV/Infectious Diseases, Activity No. 0217-0000-16-035-H01-P, 3.0 contact hours; Policy, Practice, and Regulatory Issues, and Economic and Patient-Reported Outcomes Assessment, Activity No. 0217-0000-16-036-H04-P, 2.25 contact hours.

To earn continuing pharmacy education credit for the home-study version of the 2016 Pharmacotherapy Preparatory Review and Recertification Course, you must successfully complete and submit the web-based posttest associated with each activity within the course by October 31, 2017. Statements of continuing pharmacy education credit will be available at CPE Monitor within 2–3 business days after the successfully completed web-based posttest is submitted.

The American College of Clinical Pharmacy (ACCP) has compiled the materials in this course book for pharmacists to use in preparing for the Board of Pharmacy Specialties (BPS) Pharmacotherapy Specialty Certification Examination. There is no intent or assurance that all of the knowledge on the examination will be covered in the ACCP process. Although ACCP does use the BPS Content Outline in creating the material for this course, ACCP does not know the specific content of any particular BPS examination. BPS guidelines prohibit any overlap of individuals writing the examination and developing preparatory materials.

Board Certified Pharmacotherapy Specialist (BCPS) Recertification Credit
The Pharmacotherapy Preparatory Review and Recertification Course is part of a Board of Pharmacy Specialties (BPS)-approved professional development program for BCPS recertification credit. To be eligible to earn the 26.0 contact hours of pharmacotherapy recertification credit for the Pharmacotherapy Preparatory Review and Recertification Course, you must purchase and successfully submit the completed web-based posttest(s) by 11:59 p.m. (CDT) on September 1, 2016.

PROGRAM GOALS AND TARGET AUDIENCE

The Updates in Therapeutics®: Pharmacotherapy Preparatory Review and Recertification Course is designed to help pharmacists who are preparing for the Board of Pharmacy Specialties certification examination in pharmacotherapy as well as those seeking a general review and refresher on disease states and therapeutics. The program goals are as follows:

1. To present a high-quality, up-to-date overview of disease states and therapeutics;
2. To provide a framework to help attendees prepare for the specialty certification examination in pharmacotherapy; and
3. To offer participants an effective learning experience using a case-based approach with a strong focus on the thought processes needed to solve patient care problems in each therapeutic area.

FACULTY

John M. Burke, Pharm.D., FCCP, BCPS
Professor of Pharmacy Practice
Associate Dean for Postgraduate Education
St. Louis College of Pharmacy
St. Louis, Missouri

Jacintha S. Cauffield, Pharm.D., BCPS
Associate Professor of Pharmacy Practice
The Lloyd L. Gregory School of Pharmacy
Palm Beach Atlantic University
West Palm Beach, Florida

Anna Legreid Dopp, Pharm.D.
Clinical Pharmacist
Drug Policy Program
University of Wisconsin Hospital and Clinics
Madison, Wisconsin

Shareen El-Ibiary, Pharm.D., BCPS
Associate Professor of Pharmacy Practice
Department of Pharmacy Practice
Midwestern University College of Pharmacy-Glendale
Glendale, Arizona

Shannon W. Finks, Pharm.D., FCCP, BCPS
Associate Professor
University of Tennessee College of Pharmacy
Clinical Pharmacy Specialist, Cardiology
Veterans Affairs Medical Center
Memphis, Tennessee

Linda Gore Martin, Pharm.D., MBA, BCPS
Dean
Professor, Social and Administrative Pharmacy
University of Wyoming School of Pharmacy
Laramie, Wyoming

Leslie A. Hamilton, Pharm.D., BCPS, BCCCP
University of Tennessee Health Science Center
College of Pharmacy
Knoxville, Tennessee

Dana Hammer, Ph.D., Pharm.D.
Senior Lecturer and Director of Teaching Certificate
Program in Pharmacy Education
Department of Pharmacy
University of Washington
Seattle, Washington

Ila M. Harris, Pharm.D., FCCP, BCPS
Associate Professor
University of Minnesota Medical School
Minneapolis, Minnesota

Lisa C. Hutchison, Pharm.D., MPH, FCCP, BCPS
Professor
Department of Pharmacy Practice
University of Arkansas for Medical Sciences
College of Pharmacy
Little Rock, Arkansas

Brian K. Irons, Pharm.D., FCCP, BCPS, BCACP, BC-ADM
Associate Professor of Pharmacy Practice
Division Head – Ambulatory Care
Texas Tech University Health Sciences Center
Lubbock, Texas

Mary Ann Kliethermes, Pharm.D.
Associate Professor
Chicago College of Pharmacy
Midwestern University
Downers Grove, Illinois

Jamie L. McConaha, Pharm.D., BCACP
Assistant Professor of Pharmacy Practice
Duquesne University Mylan School of Pharmacy
Pittsburgh, Pennsylvania

Karen J. McConnell, Pharm.D., FCCP, BCPS-AQ Cardiology
Clinical Pharmacy Specialist
Cardinal Health
Clinical Associate Professor
University of Colorado Skaggs School of Pharmacy
Denver, Colorado

LeAnn B. Norris, Pharm.D., BCPS, BCOP
Clinical Assistant Professor
Department of Clinical Pharmacy and Outcomes
   Sciences
South Carolina College of Pharmacy
Columbia, South Carolina

Kirsten H. Ohler, Pharm.D., BCPS, BCPPS
Clinical Assistant Professor
University of Illinois Hospital and Health Sciences
   System
Chicago, Illinois

Christopher A. Paciullo, Pharm.D., FCCM, BCPS, BCCCP
Clinical Specialist, Cardiothoracic Surgery/Critical
   Care
Emory University Hospital
Atlanta, Georgia

Melody Ryan, Pharm.D., FCCP, BCPS
Associate Professor
University of Kentucky
Lexington, Kentucky

Curtis L. Smith, Pharm.D., BCPS
Professor
Ferris State University
Grand Ledge, Michigan

Kevin M. Sowinski, Pharm.D., FCCP
Professor of Pharmacy Practice
Purdue University College of Pharmacy
Adjunct Professor of Medicine
Indiana University School of Medicine
Indianapolis, Indiana

Jessica Tilton, Pharm.D., BCACP
Clinical Assistant Professor
University of Illinois at Chicago
Chicago, Illinois

Sheila M. Wilhelm, Pharm.D., FCCP, BCPS
Associate Professor of Pharmacy Practice
Wayne State University, Eugene Applebaum College
   of Pharmacy;
Clinical Pharmacy Specialist of Internal Medicine
Harper University Hospital
Detroit, Michigan

FACULTY DISCLOSURES

Consultancies: LeAnn Norris (Amgen)
Nothing to Disclose: John Burke, Jacintha Cauffield, Anna Legreid Dopp, Shareen El-Ibiary, Shannon Finks, Linda Gore Martin, Leslie Hamilton, Dana Hammer, Ila Harris, Lisa Hutchison, Brian Irons, Karen McConnell, Kirsten Ohler, Christopher Paciullo, Melody Ryan, Curtis Smith, Kevin Sowinski, Sheila Wilhelm

REVIEWER DISCLOSURES

The following reviewers have indicated conflicts of interest:

Consultancies: Douglas Fish (Bayer HealthCare, Cempra)
Received Grand Funding/Research Support: William L. Baker (Pfizer), Douglas Fish (Merck)
Speakers Bureau: William L. Baker (Boehringer Ingelheim)

Acknowledgments

Teresa M. Bailey, Pharm.D., BCPS
Professor
College of Pharmacy
Ferris State University
Big Rapids, Michigan

Debra J. Barnette, Pharm.D., BCPS
Assistant Professor of Clinical Pharmacy
Pharmacy Practice and Administration
The Ohio State University College of Pharmacy
Columbus, Ohio

Lisa Anne Boothby, Pharm.D., BCPS
Clinical Research Pharmacist
Drug Information Coordinator
Pharmacy Administration
Columbus Regional Healthcare System
Columbus, Georgia

Linda R. Bressler, Pharm.D., BCOP
Clinical Associate Professor
Department of Pharmacy Practice
College of Pharmacy
Director of Regulatory Affairs
Cancer and Leukemia Group B
University of Illinois
Chicago, Illinois

John M. Burke, Pharm.D., FCCP, BCPS
Professor of Pharmacy Practice
Associate Dean for Postgraduate Education
St. Louis College of Pharmacy
St. Louis, Missouri

Sheryl Chow, Pharm.D., FCCP, BCPS-AQ Cardiology
Associate Professor of Pharmacy Practice and Administration
College of Pharmacy Western University of Health Sciences
Los Angeles, California

G. Robert DeYoung, Pharm.D., BCPS
PGY1 Residency Program Director
Mercy Health Saint Mary's Campus
Clinical Pharmacist
Mercy Health Physician Partners
Grand Rapids, Michigan

Anna Legreid Dopp, Pharm.D.
Clinical Pharmacist
Drug Policy Program
University of Wisconsin Hospital and Clinics
Madison, Wisconsin

Jennifer M. Dugan, Pharm.D., BCPS
Primary Care Clinical Pharmacy Specialist
Kaiser Permanente Colorado
Evergreen, Colorado

Shareen El-Ibiary, Pharm.D., BCPS
Associate Professor of Pharmacy Practice
Department of Pharmacy Practice
Midwestern University College of Pharmacy-Glendale
Glendale, Arizona

Shannon W. Finks, Pharm.D., FCCP, BCPS
Associate Professor
University of Tennessee College of Pharmacy;
Clinical Pharmacy Specialist, Cardiology
Veterans Affairs Medical Center
Memphis, Tennessee

Edward F. Foote, Pharm.D., FCCP, BCPS
Professor
Wilkes University
Wilkes-Barre, Pennsylvania

Linda Gore Martin, Pharm.D., MBA, BCPS
Dean
Professor, Social and Administrative Pharmacy
University of Wyoming School of Pharmacy
Laramie, Wyoming

Leslie A. Hamilton, Pharm.D., BCPS
University of Tennessee Health Science Center
College of Pharmacy
Knoxville, Tennessee

Dana Hammer, Ph.D., Pharm.D.
Senior Lecturer and Director of Teaching Certificate
Program in Pharmacy Education
Department of Pharmacy
University of Washington
Seattle, Washington

Ila M. Harris, Pharm.D., FCCP, BCPS
Associate Professor
Department of Family Medicine and Community Health
University of Minnesota;
Bethesda Family Medicine
St. Paul, Minnesota

Brian A. Hemstreet, Pharm.D., FCCP, BCPS
Assistant Dean for Student Affairs
Associate Professor
Regis University School of Pharmacy
Rueckert-Hartman College for Health Professions
Denver, Colorado

Lisa C. Hutchison, Pharm.D., MPH, FCCP, BCPS
Professor
Department of Pharmacy Practice
University of Arkansas for Medical Sciences
College of Pharmacy
Little Rock, Arkansas

Trudy M.R. Hodgman, Pharm.D., FCCM, BCPS
Associate Professor of Pharmacy Practice
Clinical Coordinator/Critical Care Specialist
Northwest Community Hospital
Arlington Heights, Illinois

Brian K. Irons, Pharm.D., FCCP, BCPS, BCACP, BC-ADM
Associate Professor of Pharmacy Practice
Division Head – Ambulatory Care
Texas Tech University Health Sciences Center
Lubbock, Texas

William A. Kehoe, Pharm.D., M.A., FCCP, BCPS
Professor, Department of Pharmacy Practice
Director of Student Academic Success
T.J. Long School of Pharmacy and Health Sciences
Stockton, California

Judith Kristeller, Pharm.D., BCPS
Associate Professor
Wilkes University
Wilkes-Barre, Pennsylvania

Kelly C. Lee, Pharm.D., M.A.S., BCPP
Associate Professor of Clinical Pharmacy
Associate Dean for Assessment and Accreditation
Skaggs School of Pharmacy and Pharmaceutical Sciences
University of California San Diego
La Jolla, California

John McGlew, M.A.
Director, Government Affairs
American College of Clinical Pharmacy
Washington, D.C.

LeAnn Norris, Pharm.D., BCPS, BCOP
Clinical Assistant Professor
Department of Clinical Pharmacy and Outcomes Sciences
South Carolina College of Pharmacy
Columbia, South Carolina

Kirsten H. Ohler, Pharm.D., BCPS
Pediatric Clinical Specialist
Florida Children's Hospital
Orlando, Florida

Norma J. Owens, Pharm.D., FCCP, BCPS
Professor and Chair
Pharmacy Department
University of Rhode Island
Providence, Rhode Island

Christopher A. Paciullo, Pharm.D., FCCM, BCPS
Clinical Specialist, Cardiothoracic Surgery/
Critical Care
Emory University Hospital
Atlanta, Georgia

Robert Lee Page II, Pharm.D., FCCP, FAHA, BCPS
Associate Professor of Clinical Pharmacy and Physical
    Medicine
Schools of Pharmacy and Medicine
University of Colorado
Aurora, Colorado

Jo Ellen Rodgers, Pharm.D., BCPS
Clinical Assistant Professor
Division of Pharmacotherapy and Experimental
    Therapeutics
School of Pharmacy
University of North Carolina
Chapel Hill, North Carolina

Melody Ryan, Pharm.D., BCPS
Associate Professor
Department of Pharmacy Practice and Science
College of Pharmacy, University of Kentucky
Lexington, Kentucky

Gordan S. Sacks, Pharm.D., FCCP, BCNSP
Department Head
Professor, Pharmacy Practice
Auburn University Harrison School of Pharmacy
Auburn, Alabama

Lisa A. Sanchez, Pharm.D.
President
PE Applications
Highlands Ranch, Colorado

Curtis L. Smith, Pharm.D., BCPS
Professor
Ferris State University
Lansing, Michigan

Kevin M. Sowinski, Pharm.D., FCCP
Professor of Pharmacy Practice
Purdue University College of Pharmacy;
Adjunct Professor of Medicine
Indiana University School of Medicine
Indianapolis, Indiana

Anne P. Spencer, Pharm.D., FCCP, BCPS-AQ
Cardiology
Associate Professor of Pharmacy and Clinical Sciences
College of Pharmacy
Medical University of South Carolina
Charleston, South Carolina

Ceressa T. Ward, Pharm.D., BCPS
Clinical Coordinator
Emory Crawford Long Hospital
Atlanta, Georgia

Barbara S. Wiggins, Pharm.D., FCCP, FNLA, FAHA,
BCPS, CLS, AACC
Clinical Pharmacy Specialist – Cardiology
Department of Pharmacy Services
Medical University of South Carolina
Adjunct Associate Professor
South Carolina College of Pharmacy
Charleston, South Carolina

Sheila M. Wilhelm, Pharm.D., FCCP, BCPS
Associate Professor of Pharmacy Practice
Wayne State University, Eugene Applebaum College of
    Pharmacy;
Clinical Pharmacy Specialist of Internal Medicine
Harper University Hospital
Detroit, Michigan

Eric T. Wittbrodt, Pharm.D., FCCP, BCPS
Principal Health Outcomes Liaison
Daiichi Sankyo, Inc.
Parsippany, New Jersey

REVIEWERS

The American College of Clinical Pharmacy and the authors would like to thank the following individuals for their reviews of the Updates of Therapeutics®: Pharmacotherapy Preparatory Review and Recertification Course.

Sara Al-Dahir, Pharm.D., B.Sc., BCPS-AQ ID
Clinical Associate Professor
Xavier University of Louisiana
New Orleans, Louisiana

Lindsay M. Arnold, Pharm.D., BCPS
Cardiology & Anticoagulation Clinical Specialist
Boston Medical Center
Department of Pharmacy
Boston, Massachusetts

Jennifer Baggs, Pharm.D., BCPS, BCNSP
Clinical Pharmacist
Banner University Medical Center - Tucson
Tucson, Arizona

William L. Baker, Pharm.D., FCCP, FACC
Assistant Professor of Pharmacy Practice
University of Connecticut School of Pharmacy
Storrs, Connecticut

Kim Benner, Pharm.D., FASHP, FPPAG, BCPS
Professor of Pharmacy Practice
Samford University McWhorter School of Pharmacy
Birmingham, Alabama

John B. Bossaer, Pharm.D., BCPS, BCOP
Associate Professor of Pharmacy Practice
East Tennessee St. University, Gatton College of Pharmacy
Johnson City, Tennessee

Sheila Botts, Pharm.D., FCCP, BCPP
Chief - Clinical Pharmacy Research and Academic Affairs
Kaiser Permanente Colorado
Aurora, Colorado

Todd W. Brackins, Pharm.D., BCPP
Assistant Professor of Pharmacy Practice
Harding University College of Pharmacy
Searcy, Arkansas

Wayne E. Bradley, Pharm.D., MBA, BCPS
Predictive Therapeutica Consulting, LLC
Johns Creek, Georgia

Beth Briand, Pharm.D., BCPS-AQ ID
Clinical Pharmacy Practitioner
Baptist Medical Center Jacksonville
Jacksonville, Florida

Mary M. Bridgeman, Pharm.D., FASCP, BCPS, CGP
Clinical Associate Professor
Department of Pharmacy Practice and Administration
Ernest Mario School of Pharmacy
Rutgers, The State University of New Jersey
Piscataway, New Jersey

Sara K. Butler, Pharm.D., BCPS, BCOP
Clinical Pharmacy Specialist, Medical Oncology
Clinical Oncology Supervisor
PGY2 Oncology Residency Program Director
Department of Pharmacy
Barnes-Jewish Hospital
St. Louis, Missouri

Lisa M. Chastain, Pharm.D., BCACP
Assistant Professor of Pharmacy Practice - Ambulatory Care Division
Director PGY2 - Ambulatory Care Specialty Residency Program
Texas Tech School of Pharmacy - Dallas/Fort Worth Campus
Dallas, Texas

Jennifer N. Clements, Pharm.D., BCPS, BCACP, CDE
Chair and Associate Professor
Department of Pharmacy Practice
Presbyterian College School of Pharmacy
Clinton, South Carolina

Kristen Cook, Pharm.D., BCPS
Assistant Professor of Pharmacy Practice
University of Nebraska Medical Center, College of Pharmacy
Omaha, Nebraska

Elizabeth Farrington, Pharm.D., FCCP, FCCM, FPPAG, BCPS
Pharmacist III – Pediatrics
New Hanover Regional Medical Center
Department of Pharmacy
Wilmington, North Carolina

Douglas N. Fish, Pharm.D., FCCP, FCCM, BCPS-AQ ID
Professor
University of Colorado Skaggs School of Pharmacy and Pharmaceutical Sciences
Aurora, Colorado

Lori A. Gordon, Pharm.D., BCPS, AAHIVP
Clinical Assistant Professor
Xavier University of Louisiana, College of Pharmacy
New Orleans, Louisiana

Olga Hilas, Pharm.D., MPH, BCPS, CGP
Associate Professor
Department of Clinical Health Professions
St. John's University
College of Pharmacy & Health Sciences
Queens, New York

Lucas G. Hill, Pharm.D., BCPS
Clinical Assistant Professor
The University of Texas at Austin
Austin, Texas

Jill T. Johnson, Pharm.D., BCPS
Professor of Pharmacy Practice
University of Arkansas for Medical Sciences,
College of Pharmacy
Little Rock, Arkansas

Tyree H. Kiser, Pharm.D., FCCP, FCCM, BCPS
Associate Professor, Department of Clinical Pharmacy
University of Colorado Skaggs School of Pharmacy and
    Pharmaceutical Sciences
Aurora, Colorado

Audrey Kostrzewa, Pharm.D., MPH, BCPS
Assistant Professor of Pharmacy Practice
Concordia University Wisconsin School of Pharmacy
Mequon, Wisconsin

John McGlew, M.A.
Director, Government Affairs
American College of Clinical Pharmacy
Washington, D.C.

Nicole L. Metzger, Pharm.D., BCPS
Clinical Associate Professor
Mercer University College of Pharmacy
Atlanta, Georgia

Molly G. Minze, Pharm.D., BCACP
Associate Professor of Pharmacy Practice
Texas Tech University Health Sciences Center School of
    Pharmacy
Abilene, Texas

Jessica Njoku, Pharm.D., MPH, BCPS
Clinical Director, Pharmacy Services
Good Shepherd Health System
Longview, Texas

Carrie S. Oliphant, Pharm.D., FCCP, BCPS-AQ Cardiology
Clinical Pharmacy Specialist, Cardiology/Anticoagulation
Methodist University Hospital
Associate Professor
University of Tennessee College of Pharmacy
Memphis, Tennessee

Erin Raney, Pharm.D., BCPS, BC-ADM
Professor of Pharmacy Practice
Midwestern University College of Pharmacy-Glendale
Glendale, Arizona

Karen L. Rascati, BSPharm, Ph.D.
Professor of Health Outcomes and Pharmacy Practice
The University of Texas College of Pharmacy
Austin, Texas

Shannon L. Reidt, Pharm.D., MPH, BCPS
Assistant Professor
University of Minnesota College of Pharmacy
Minneapolis, Minnesota

Brea O. Rowan, Pharm.D., BCPS
Clinical Pharmacy Specialist
Princeton Baptist Medical Center
Birmingham, Alabama

Tracy A. Rupp, Pharm.D., RD, MPH, BCPS
Director of Public Health Policy Initiatives
National Center for Health Research
Washington, D.C.

Cynthia A. Sanoski, Pharm.D., FCCP, BCPS
Chair and Associate Professor
Jefferson College of Pharmacy
Philadelphia, Pennsylvania

Marina Suzuki, Pharm.D., Ph.D., BCPS, BCACP
Assistant Professor
Pacific University School of Pharmacy
Hillsboro, Oregon

Cheryl L. Szabo, Pharm.D., BCPS
Clinical Pharmacy Specialist, Neurology
Detroit Medical Center
Adjunct Assistant Professor of Pharmacy Practice
Wayne State University
Detroit, Michigan

Ashley H. Vincent, Pharm.D., BCPS, BCACP
Clinical Associate Professor of Pharmacy Practice
Purdue University College of Pharmacy
West Lafayette, Indiana

Kristina E. Ward, Pharm.D., BCPS
Clinical Associate Professor
Director, Drug Information Services
University of Rhode Island, College of Pharmacy
Kingston, Rhode Island

Montgomery F. Williams, Pharm.D., BCPS
Assistant Professor of Pharmacy Practice
Belmont University College of Pharmacy
Nashville, Tennessee

Elizabeth Wilpula, Pharm.D., BCPS
Clinical Pharmacy Specialist
Nephrology/Transplant
Harper University Hospital
Detroit, Michigan

Susan R. Winkler, Pharm.D., FCCP, BCPS
Professor and Chair, Pharmacy Practice
Midwestern University Chicago College of Pharmacy
Downers Grove, Illinois

Abigail M. Yancey, Pharm.D., BCPS
Associate Professor Pharmacy Practice
St. Louis College of Pharmacy
St. Louis, Missouri

TABLE OF CONTENTS

ACCP Updates in Therapeutics®:

Pharmacotherapy Preparatory Review and Recertification Course

Pediatrics

Kirsten H. Ohler, Pharm.D., BCPS, BCPPS

University of Illinois Hospital & Health Sciences System
Chicago, Illinois

Pediatrics

Kirsten H. Ohler, Pharm.D., BCPS, BCPPS

University of Illinois Hospital & Health Sciences System
Chicago, Illinois

Learning Objectives

1. Describe the most common pathogens associated with neonatal and pediatric sepsis and meningitis.
2. Describe current therapeutic options for the management of neonatal and pediatric sepsis and meningitis.
3. Identify the drugs available for preventing and treating respiratory syncytial virus.
4. Describe the most common causative organisms of otitis media and potential treatment options.
5. Identify the recommended pediatric immunization schedule and barriers to routine immunization.
6. Discuss the differences in anticonvulsant pharmacokinetics and adverse effects between children and adults.
7. Describe the current drug therapy for treating patients with attention-deficit/hyperactivity disorder.

Self-Assessment Questions

Answers and explanations to these questions can be found at the end of this chapter.

1. A 15-year-old boy with a history of exercise-induced asthma presents with fever, tachypnea, headache, and myalgia. Which is most likely to be isolated from this patient?

    A. Respiratory syncytial virus (RSV).

    B. *Streptococcus pneumoniae.*

    C. Group B *Streptococcus.*

    D. *Pseudomonas aeruginosa.*

2. Which is the best assessment of the risk of severe RSV infection and subsequent need for prophylaxis in a 3-month-old girl born at 30 weeks' gestation?

    A. This patient should receive prophylaxis if she is 6 months or younger at the beginning of RSV season.

    B. This patient is at risk only if she has chronic lung disease (i.e., necessitating more than 21% oxygen for at least the first 28 days of life).

    C. All neonates born during RSV season should receive prophylaxis.

    D. This patient should receive prophylaxis only if she has additional risk factors such as day care attendance or school-aged siblings.

3. Which is the most accurate statement about prophylaxis of bacterial meningitis?

    A. Close contacts of patients with pneumococcal meningitis should receive prophylaxis.

    B. Close contacts of patients with *Haemophilus influenzae* meningitis need prophylaxis only if their immunizations are not up to date.

    C. Rifampin is a first-line agent for prophylaxis against meningococcal meningitis.

    D. Prophylaxis against bacterial meningitis is no longer recommended regardless of the causative organism.

4. A 6-month-old baby who was born at 24 weeks' gestation is brought to the clinic in October for a routine checkup and immunizations. Which is the best recommendation to make for this patient's immunization schedule?

    A. Only two of the five immunizations due should be given at the same time; schedule another appointment for the next week to administer the rest.

    B. Oral polio vaccine should be used to reduce the number of injections needed to complete the schedule.

    C. Vaccines should be based on his corrected gestational age rather than on his chronologic age because he was born prematurely.

    D. Influenza vaccine should be administered with all other scheduled vaccinations.

5. A physician asks for your recommendation for treating a 5-year-old child with his first case of acute otitis media (AOM). Which statement is the best advice?

    A. A blood culture should be obtained to identify the causative organism.

    B. Antibiotics may not be warranted at this time.

    C. Initiate azithromycin to treat atypical organisms (e.g., mycoplasma).

    D. Administer intramuscular ceftriaxone.

6. A 16-year-old girl with asthma, a history of ventricular septal defect, and attention-deficit/hyperactivity disorder (ADHD) was initially treated with methylphenidate immediate release, but her

ADHD symptoms persisted at home and at school. Her therapy was then changed to methylphenidate OROS (Concerta). The dose was maximized during the next several weeks; however, her symptoms were still not well controlled throughout the day. She and her family report adherence to the treatment regimen. Which is the best recommendation to make for treating her ADHD?

A. Switch to clonidine.

B. Switch to extended-release mixed amphetamine salts (i.e., Adderall XR).

C. Switch to methylphenidate transdermal system (i.e., Daytrana).

D. Switch to atomoxetine.

7. A 7-year-old child with absence seizures is having breakthrough episodes on ethosuximide. Which is the most appropriate alternative therapy?

A. Valproic acid.

B. Phenytoin.

C. Phenobarbital.

D. Gabapentin.

8. In a retrospective study of the risk of appetite loss in adolescents taking a specific stimulant agent for ADHD management, 7 of 200 patients exposed to the stimulant showed appetite loss, compared with 1 of 198 control subjects (unexposed). Which choice best reflects the correct odds ratio of developing loss of appetite for the case subjects compared with the control subjects?

A. 3.

B. 6.

C. 7.

D. 8.

9. An investigator wants to establish a causal relationship between the use of ceftriaxone in premature neonates and the incidence of kernicterus. Which study design is best to use?

A. Case series.

B. Randomized controlled.

C. Retrospective cohort.

D. Crossover.

10. An 8-month-old, former 36-week gestational-age infant with hypoplastic left heart disease is admitted during RSV season for stage II (of III) repair of his heart defect. Which statement is most accurate about the use of palivizumab for RSV prophylaxis in this patient?

A. He is not at significant risk of severe RSV infection; therefore, palivizumab is not indicated.

 B. Palivizumab is indicated to reduce nosocomial transmission of RSV in high-risk patients.

C. Palivizumab is not indicated because he has undergone surgical repair of his heart defect.

 D. A dose of palivizumab should be administered postoperatively and continued throughout the RSV season.

BPS Pharmacotherapy Specialty Examination Content Outline

This chapter covers the following sections of the Pharmacotherapy Specialty Examination Content Outline:

1. Domain 1: Patient-specific Pharmacotherapy
   a. Tasks 1, 2, 3, 5, and 6
   b. Systems and Patient Care Problems
      i. Sepsis/Meningitis
      ii. Respiratory Syncytial Virus (RSV) Infection
      iii. Otitis Media
      iv. Immunizations
      v. Pediatric Seizure Disorders
      vi. Attention-Deficit/Hyperactivity Disorder
2. Domain 2: Retrieval, Generation, Interpretation and Dissemination of Knowledge in Pharmacotherapy, Task 2

I. SEPSIS AND MENINGITIS

A. Clinical Presentation
   1. Signs and symptoms
      a. Neonates
         i. General: Temperature instability, feeding intolerance, lethargy, grunting, flaring, retractions, apnea
         ii. More likely to be associated with meningitis: Bulging fontanelle and seizures
      b. Children
         i. General: Fever, loss of appetite, emesis, myalgias, arthralgias, cutaneous manifestations (e.g., petechiae, purpura, rash)
         ii. More likely to be associated with meningitis: Nuchal rigidity, back pain, Kernig sign, Brudzinski sign, headache, photophobia, altered mental status, and seizures
   2. Early versus late neonatal sepsis
      a. Onset
         i. Early: Within 3 days of birth
         ii. Late: After the first 3 days of life
      b. Risk factors
         i. Early: Very low birth weight, prolonged rupture of amniotic membranes, prolonged labor, maternal endometritis, or chorioamnionitis
         ii. Late
            (a) Unrelated to obstetric risk factors
            (b) Usually related to iatrogenic factors (e.g., endotracheal tubes, central venous catheters)
      c. Incidence
         i. Early
            (a) 0.7–3.7 of 1000 live births (8 of 1000 very-low-birth-weight infants)
            (b) Meningitis occurs in less than 10% of cases.
         ii. Late
            (a) 0.5–1.8 of 1000 live births
            (b) Meningitis occurs in 60% of cases.
   3. Cerebrospinal fluid findings (Table 1)

Table 1. Cerebrospinal Fluid Findings

Laboratory Value	Normal Child	Normal Newborn	Bacterial Meningitis	Viral Meningitis
WBC (cells/mL)	0–6	0–30	>1000	100–500
Neutrophils (%)	0	2–3	>50	<40
Glucose (mg/dL)	40–80	32–121	<30	>30
Protein (mg/dL)	20–30	19–149	>100	50–100
RBC (cells/mL)	0–2	0–2	0–10	0–2

RBC = red blood cell count; WBC = white blood cell count.

Adapted with permission from the American Academy of Pediatrics. Wubbel L, McCracken GH. Management of bacterial meningitis: 1998. Pediatr Rev 1998;19:78-84.

Patient Case

1. A baby born at 36 weeks' gestation develops respiratory distress, hypotension, and mottling at 5 hours of life. The baby is transported to the neonatal intensive care unit, where he has a witnessed seizure, and cultures are drawn. Maternal vaginal cultures are positive for group B *Streptococcus,* and three doses of penicillin were given to the mother before delivery. Which is the best empiric antibiotic regimen?

    A. Vancomycin.

    B. Ampicillin plus gentamicin.

    C. Ampicillin plus ceftriaxone.

    D. Ceftazidime plus gentamicin.

    B.   Common Pathogens for Sepsis and Meningitis (Table 2)

Table 2. Common Pathogens

Age	Organism
0–1 month	Group B *Streptococcus* *Escherichia coli* *Listeria monocytogenes* Viral (e.g., herpes simplex virus) Coagulase-negative staphylococcus (nosocomial) Gram-negative bacteria (e.g., *Pseudomonas* spp., *Enterobacter* spp.; nosocomial)
1–3 months	Neonatal pathogens (see above) *Haemophilus influenzae* type B *Neisseria meningitidis* *Streptococcus pneumoniae*
3 months–12 years	*H. influenzae* type B[a] *N. meningitidis* *S. pneumoniae*
>12 years	*N. meningitidis* *S. pneumoniae*

[a]*H. influenzae* is no longer a common pathogen in areas where the vaccine is routinely used.

    C.   Potential Empiric Antibiotic Regimens for Sepsis and Meningitis (Table 3)

Table 3. Potential Antibiotic Regimens

Age	Regimen
0–1 month	Ampicillin + gentamicin or ampicillin + cefotaxime
1–3 months	Ampicillin + cefotaxime/ceftriaxone
3 months–12 years	Ceftriaxone ± vancomycin[a]
>12 years	Ceftriaxone ± vancomycin[a]

[a]Addition of vancomycin should be based on the regional incidence of resistant *Streptococcus pneumoniae*.

Patient Cases

2. Culture results for the patient in question 1 reveal gram-negative rods in the cerebrospinal fluid. Which recommendation regarding antibiotic prophylaxis is best?

   A. The patient's 5-month-old stepsister is at high risk because she is not fully immunized; the patient should therefore receive rifampin.

   B. The patient should receive rifampin to eliminate nasal carriage of the pathogen.

   C. Antibiotic prophylaxis is not indicated in this case.

   D. All close contacts should receive rifampin for prophylaxis.

3. A 6-year-old boy presents to the emergency department with a temperature of 104°F, altered mental status, and petechiae. There is no history of trauma. A toxicology screen is negative. A complete blood cell count reveals 32×10^3 cells/mm^3 with 20% bands. Culture results are pending. The patient has no known drug allergies. Which antibiotic regimen provides the best empiric coverage?

   A. Ampicillin plus gentamicin.

   B. Cefuroxime.

   C. Ceftriaxone plus vancomycin.

   D. Rifampin.

D. Sequelae of Meningitis
   1. Hearing loss
   2. Mental retardation and learning deficits
   3. Visual impairment
   4. Seizures
   5. Hydrocephalus

E. Chemoprophylaxis of Bacterial Meningitis
   1. Purpose: Prevent the spread of *H. influenzae* and *Neisseria meningitidis*
   2. High-risk groups
      a. Household contacts
      b. Nursery or day care center contacts
      c. Direct contact with index patient's secretions
   3. Regimens (Table 4)

Table 4. Regimens for Chemoprophylaxis[a]

Drug	*Neisseria meningitidis*	*Haemophilus influenzae*
Rifampin	<1 month old: 5 mg/kg/dose PO every 12 hours × 2 days ≥1 month old: 10 mg/kg/dose PO every 12 hours × 2 days Adults: 600 mg PO every 12 hours × 2 days	20 mg/kg/dose (maximum 600 mg) PO daily × 4 days
Ceftriaxone	<15 years old: 125 mg IM × 1 dose ≥15 years old: 250 mg IM × 1 dose	Not indicated

[a]Ciprofloxacin and azithromycin are possible alternatives but not routinely recommended.

IM = intramuscularly; PO = orally.

II. RESPIRATORY SYNCYTIAL VIRUS INFECTION

A. Clinical Presentation
1. Seasonal occurrence: Typically November through April, depending on geographic location
2. Signs and symptoms
   a. Neonates and infants: Lower respiratory tract symptoms (e.g., bronchiolitis and pneumonia), wheezing, lethargy, irritability, poor feeding, and apnea
   b. Older children: Upper respiratory tract symptoms (e.g., rhinorrhea, cough)

B. Risk Factors for Severe Disease
1. Premature birth
2. Chronic lung disease or bronchopulmonary dysplasia
3. Cyanotic or complicated congenital heart disease
4. Immunodeficiency
5. Airway abnormalities or neuromuscular conditions compromising the handling of respiratory secretions
6. Other
   a. Lower socioeconomic status
   b. Passive smoking
   c. Day care attendance
   d. Siblings younger than 5 years

Patient Case

4. You are screening babies during the current respiratory syncytial virus (RSV) season for risk factors associated with the development of severe RSV infection. Which is the best recommendation about the use of palivizumab for RSV prophylaxis?

    A. Palivizumab should be prescribed for an 18-month-old, former 26-week premature infant with a history of chronic lung disease who has not received oxygen or medications during the past 8 months.

    B. Palivizumab should be prescribed for a 5-month-old, former 28-week premature infant with a history of chronic lung disease who was discharged from the hospital without oxygen or medications.

    C. Palivizumab should be prescribed for a 41-day-old baby, born at 31 weeks' gestation, without a history of chronic lung disease who will attend day care.

    D. Palivizumab should be prescribed for a 10-month-old baby, born at 37 weeks' gestation, with a surgically repaired congenital heart defect.

C. Prophylaxis
1. Nonpharmacologic: Avoid crowds during RSV season and conscientiously use good handwashing practice.
2. Palivizumab (Synagis)
   a. Dosing: 15 mg/kg/dose intramuscularly, given monthly during RSV season
   b. Effects on outcomes
      i. A 55% reduction in hospitalizations for RSV
      ii. Safe in patients with cyanotic congenital heart disease. There is a 58% decrease in palivizumab serum concentration after cardiopulmonary bypass; therefore, a postoperative dose of palivizumab is recommended as soon as the patient is medically stable.
      iii. No reduction in overall mortality
      iv. Does not interfere with the response to vaccines
      v. Not recommended for the prevention of nosocomial transmission of RSV

   c. American Academy of Pediatrics (AAP) recommendations for use were updated in 2014 (Table 5) and contain several significant changes from their 2009 policy statement.

       i. Routine prophylaxis is no longer recommended for neonates born at 29 weeks' gestation or later; previously all neonates born at less than 32 weeks' gestation were recommended to receive routine prophylaxis.

      ii. Risk factors for RSV infection such as day care attendance or siblings younger than 5 years of age are no longer considered when determining the need for prophylaxis.

     iii. Prophylaxis is not recommended in the second year of life based on a history of prematurity alone; previously neonates born at less than 28 weeks' gestation could be considered for prophylaxis during their second RSV season.

     iv. Prophylaxis should be discontinued if an RSV hospitalization occurs; previously palivizumab was continued to complete five monthly doses regardless of hospitalization.

Table 5. AAP Guidelines for Palivizumab Use

Gestational Age (weeks)	Age at Start of RSV Season (months)	Other Required Criteria	Maximal Doses
<29 + 0 days	<12		5
29–32 + 0 days	<12	Chronic lung disease necessitating more than 21% oxygen for at least the first 28 days of life	5
<32 + 0 days	<24	Consider prophylaxis for a second RSV season if chronic lung disease necessitating medical therapy within the 6 months preceding the start of RSV season	5
Any	<12	Patient with hemodynamically significant acyanotic[a] congenital heart disease receiving medication for congestive heart failure *and* will need cardiac surgery	5
Any	<12	Moderate to severe pulmonary hypertension	5
Any	<12	Congenital abnormalities of airway or neuromuscular disease	5
Any	<24	Profound immunocompromise	5

[a]Infants with cyanotic heart defects may be considered for prophylaxis after consultation with a pediatric cardiologist.

AAP = American Academy of Pediatrics; RSV = respiratory syncytial virus.

Patient Case

5. An 18-month-old baby with a history of premature birth and chronic lung disease is admitted to the pediatric intensive care unit with fever, respiratory distress necessitating intubation, and a 3-day history of cold-like symptoms. A nasal swab is positive for RSV. Which is the best intervention?

   A. Palivizumab.

   B. Dexamethasone.

   C. Cefuroxime.

   D. Intravenous fluids and supportive care.

D. Treatment
   1. Supportive care
      a. Hydration
      b. Supplemental oxygen
      c. Mechanical ventilation as needed
   2. Ribavirin
      a. Active against RSV replication
      b. Not shown to reduce mortality in immunocompetent patients
      c. Not shown to reduce ventilator days, stay in the intensive care unit or hospital, or hospital cost
      d. The AAP states that ribavirin "may be considered" in a select group of high-risk patients (e.g., those with complicated congenital heart disease, chronic lung disease or bronchopulmonary dysplasia, immunocompromise).
   3. β_2-Agonists, racemic epinephrine
      a. Not shown to improve outcome measures
      b. Some practitioners may give a trial of these therapies, but this is not considered the standard of care, nor is it recommended by the current AAP guideline.
   4. Corticosteroids
      a. Not shown to improve outcome measures
      b. Use is not recommended.
   5. Hypertonic saline
      a. Should not be administered in the emergency department
      b. May be considered for hospitalized patients; however, the evidence supporting use is weak.
   6. Antibiotics: Not indicated unless secondary bacterial infection develops

III. OTITIS MEDIA

A. Clinical Presentation
   1. Definitions
      a. Acute otitis media (AOM): Presence of middle ear effusion and evidence of middle ear inflammation
         i. Middle ear effusion may be indicated by bulging tympanic membrane, decreased or no mobility of the tympanic membrane, purulent fluid in the middle ear.
         ii. Inflammation of the middle ear may be indicated by erythema of the tympanic membrane or otalgia.
      b. Otitis media with effusion (OME): Fluid in the middle ear without evidence of local or systemic illness
      c. Recurrent AOM: Three or more episodes of acute otitis within 6 months or four episodes within 1 year
   2. Risk factors
      a. Day care attendance
      b. Family history of AOM
      c. Positioning during feeding (e.g., supine position during bottle-feeding allows reflux into eustachian tubes)
      d. Lower socioeconomic status
      e. Smokers in the household
      f. Craniofacial abnormalities or cleft palate

B. Common Pathogens
1. Viral
2. *S. pneumoniae*
3. Nontypeable *H. influenzae*
4. *Moraxella catarrhalis*

C. Treatment
1. General principles
    a. Clinical resolution will occur in a significant number of cases without antibiotic therapy.
    b. Immediate antibiotic therapy is warranted for AOM with bulging tympanic membrane, perforation, or otorrhea.
    c. Delayed antibiotic prescribing (i.e., treatment only if otalgia persists for more than 48–72 hours or temperature greater than 39°C in past 48 hours) is an acceptable strategy in children older than 2 years with AOM without severe systemic symptoms.
        i. Analgesics are more beneficial than antibiotics for relieving otalgia within the first 24 hours and are recommended regardless of antibiotic use.
        ii. Antibiotics also may be deferred in otherwise healthy children between 6 months and 2 years of age if their symptoms are mild and otitis media is unilateral (as opposed to bilateral).
        iii. Caregiver must be reliable to recognize worsening of condition and gain immediate access to medical care, if needed.
        iv. Not recommended for infants younger than 6 months
    d. Persistence of middle ear fluid is likely after treatment for AOM and does not warrant repeated treatment.
    e. Antibiotics are not generally warranted for OME because of the high rate of spontaneous resolution.
        i. Antibiotics are recommended only if bilateral effusions persist for more than 3 months.
        ii. Corticosteroids, antihistamines, and decongestants are not recommended.

2. Suggested treatment algorithm (Figure 1)

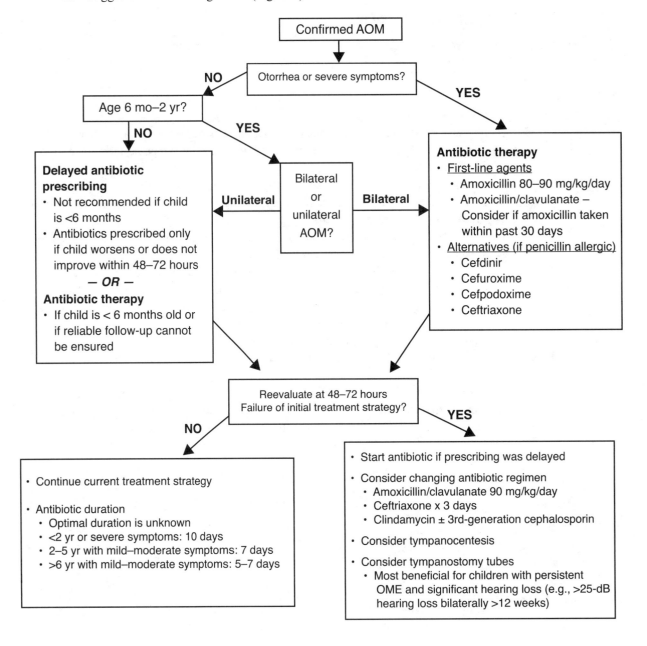

Figure 1. AOM suggested treatment algorithm.

D. Prevention Strategies
1. Antibiotic prophylaxis
    a. Reduces occurrence by about one episode per year
    b. The risk of promoting bacterial resistance may outweigh the slight benefit.
    c. AAP recommends against routine use for children with recurrent AOM.
2. Immunization: Pneumococcal and influenza vaccines should be administered according to the AAP and Advisory Committee on Immunization Practices (ACIP) recommendations.

Patient Cases

6. A 5-month-old infant who was born at term and is otherwise healthy was treated for her first case of otitis media with amoxicillin 45 mg/kg/day for 7 days. On follow-up examination, her pediatrician noticed fullness in the middle ear and a cloudy tympanic membrane with decreased mobility. She is now afebrile and eating well. Which is the best recommendation for her treatment?

    A. No antibiotics at this time.

    B. High-dose (90 mg/kg/day) amoxicillin for 7 days.

    C. Decongestant and antihistamine daily until resolution.

    D. Azithromycin.

7. A 4-year-old boy receives a diagnosis of his fourth case of otitis media within 12 months. He has not shown evidence of hearing loss or delay in language skills. Which is the best intervention at this point?

    A. Giving long-term antibiotic prophylaxis.

    B. Inserting tympanostomy tubes.

    C. Administering high-dose amoxicillin and ensuring that he is up to date on his pneumococcal and influenza vaccines.

    D. No antibiotic therapy is warranted.

IV. IMMUNIZATIONS

A. Recommended Schedule
    1. Few major changes have been made to the routine childhood schedule since 2009.
        a. Replacement of 7-valent conjugated pneumococcal vaccine with 13-valent conjugated pneumococcal vaccine (PCV13, Prevnar 13) for all children younger than 6 years
        b. Human papillomavirus vaccine (HPV4, Gardasil) received a U.S. Food and Drug Administration (FDA) label-approved indication in males 9–26 years old for prevention of genital warts. Now recommended for routine vaccination of adolescent males.
        c. For children and adolescents who have a delayed start to immunizations, a catch-up schedule exists.
        d. Refer to the National Immunization Program Web site (www.cdc.gov/vaccines).

Patient Case

8. A 1-year-old boy with a history of Kawasaki disease treated 4 months ago with intravenous immunoglobulin (IVIG) is being seen by his pediatrician for a well-child checkup. He is due for the measles, mumps, and rubella (MMR) and varicella vaccines. He has no known drug allergies, but he has many food allergies, including peanuts, eggs, and shellfish. His mother has several concerns about administering these vaccines. Which concern is the best reason to defer administering vaccines in this patient?

    A. Association between MMR vaccine administration and the development of autism.

    B. Allergic reaction after MMR administration in a patient with an egg allergy.

    C. Many concurrent vaccines can overload the patient's immune system.

    D. Decreased vaccine efficacy because of previous IVIG administration.

2. Combination vaccines
   a. Main advantage: Reduction in the number of injections needed to complete recommended schedule
   b. The FDA mandates that the safety and efficacy of combination products not be less than those of the individual components.
   c. The measles, mumps, and rubella (MMR) and varicella combination vaccine (ProQuad)
      i. Research from the Centers for Disease Control and Prevention and manufacturer indicated a higher incidence of febrile seizures in children 12–23 months of age who received the combination product compared with those who received the separate MMR and varicella vaccines.
      ii. Since June 2009, ACIP has expressed a preference for separate MMR and varicella vaccines as the first dose given to children 12–47 months of age. The combination product may be used for the second dose at any age and for the first dose in children 48 months or older.
   d. Adding hepatitis B vaccine (HepB) to combination products may result in an extra dose being provided (e.g., monovalent HepB given at birth and then combination products at 2, 4, and 6 months); however, ACIP states that this is a safe practice.
3. Interchangeability of products
   a. ACIP recommends that the same product be used throughout the primary series; however, if the previous product's identity is not known or is no longer available, any product may be used.
   b. For diphtheria, tetanus, and pertussis vaccine (DTaP): The current standard of care is to use the same product for at least the first three doses of the five-dose series; however, if the product used previously is not known or is unavailable, any product may be used.
   c. For tetanus, diphtheria, and pertussis vaccine (Tdap): Boostrix or Adacel may be used for the booster dose, regardless of the manufacturer of the DTaP product administered during the primary immunization series.
   d. For HepB: It is acceptable to use ENGERIX-B and RECOMBIVAX HB interchangeably.
   e. For polio: Oral polio vaccine and inactivated poliovirus vaccine provide equivalent protection against paralytic poliomyelitis; however, because the only cases of polio in the United States since 1979 have been vaccine associated (i.e., from the live virus in oral polio vaccine), oral polio vaccine is no longer recommended.
   f. For *Haemophilus influenzae* type b vaccine (Hib): These products may be used interchangeably; however, if the regimen is completed using PedvaxHIB exclusively, only three doses are needed; regimens using HibTITER or ActHIB include four doses.
   g. For HPV: The products differ in the HPV types against which they provide protection. HPV4 (Gardasil) protects against types 6, 11, 16, and 18. HPV2 (Cervarix) protects against types 16 and 18. HPV types 6 and 11 are associated with genital warts; types 16 and 18 are associated with gynecologic, anal, and penile cancers.

B. Barriers to Routine Immunization
   1. Contraindications
      a. Anaphylactic reaction to vaccine or any of its components
         i. Inactivated poliovirus vaccine, MMR, and varicella contain neomycin.
         ii. Influenza vaccine: Live attenuated influenza vaccine (LAIV) should be avoided in patients with severe egg allergy; inactivated influenza vaccine may be administered with close monitoring.
         iii. Severe egg allergy is not considered a contraindication to MMR, which is grown in chick embryo tissue.
      b. Acute moderate to severe febrile illness
      c. Immunodeficiency: Oral polio vaccine, MMR, varicella
      d. Pregnancy: MMR, varicella

    e. Recent administration of immune globulin: MMR, varicella

        i. Delay administration of vaccine product.

        ii. Interval between immune globulin dose and administration of vaccine depends on indication for and dose of immune globulin.

    f. Encephalopathy within 7 days after administration of a previous dose of DTaP

    g. History of intussusception: Rotavirus vaccine

2. Misconceptions about contraindications (i.e., these are *not* contraindications)

    a. Mild acute illness

    b. Current antimicrobial therapy

    c. Reaction to DTaP involving only soreness, redness, or swelling at the site

    d. Pregnancy of the mother of the vaccine recipient

    e. Breastfeeding

    f. Allergies to antibiotics other than neomycin or streptomycin

    g. Family history of an adverse effect after vaccine administration

3. Other factors associated with underimmunization

    a. Low socioeconomic status

    b. Late start of vaccination series

    c. Missed opportunities

        i. Provider unaware that vaccination is due

        ii. Failure to provide simultaneous vaccines

        iii. Inappropriate contraindications (see previous discussion)

    d. Concern about potential adverse reactions

        i. Autism: The association with MMR vaccine has not been proven.

        ii. Guillain-Barré syndrome: The association with meningococcal conjugate vaccine has not been proven.

           (a) 15 reported cases in adolescents after receiving meningococcal vaccine

           (b) ACIP continues to recommend the routine use of meningococcal vaccine.

        iii. Intussusception: An association with rotavirus vaccine led to the market withdrawal of RotaShield; two products are currently available.

           (a) Live, oral human-bovine reassortant rotavirus vaccine (RotaTeq, licensed in 2006)

           (b) Live, attenuated human rotavirus vaccine (Rotarix, licensed in 2008)

           (c) Neither product has been associated with intussusception.

        iv. Safety concerns about any vaccine product should be reported through the Vaccine Adverse Events Reporting System (VAERS).

Patient Case

9. The following patients are seeing their pediatrician today and are due for immunizations according to the routine schedule. For which patient would it be best to recommend deferring immunizations until later?

    A. A 12-month-old boy who recently completed a cycle of chemotherapy for acute lymphocytic leukemia.

    B. A 6-month-old girl receiving amoxicillin for otitis media.

    C. A 12-month-old HIV-positive boy whose most recent CD4 count was greater than 1000.

    D. A 12-year-old girl completing a prednisone "burst" (1 mg/kg/day for 5 days) for asthma exacerbation.

C. Considerations in Special Populations
    1. Preterm infants
        a. Immunize according to chronologic age.
        b. Do not lower vaccine doses.
        c. If birth weight is less than 2 kg, delay HepB vaccine because of reduced immune response until the patient is 30 days old or at hospital discharge if it occurs before 30 days of age (unless the mother is positive for HepB surface antigen).
    2. Children who are immunocompromised
        a. Should not receive live vaccines
        b. Inactivated vaccines and immune globulins are appropriate.
        c. Household contacts should not receive oral polio vaccine; however, MMR, influenza, varicella, and rotavirus vaccines are recommended.
    3. Patients receiving corticosteroids
        a. Live vaccines may be administered to patients receiving the following:
            i. Topical corticosteroids
            ii. Physiologic maintenance doses
            iii. Low or moderate doses (less than 2 mg/kg/day of prednisone equivalent)
        b. Live vaccines may be given immediately after discontinuation of high doses (2 mg/kg/day or more of prednisone equivalent) of systemic steroids given for less than 14 days.
        c. Live vaccines should be delayed at least 1 month after discontinuing high doses (2 mg/kg/day or more of prednisone equivalent) of systemic steroids given for more than 14 days.
    4. Patients with HIV infection
        a. MMR should be administered unless patient is severely immunocompromised.
        b. Varicella should be considered for asymptomatic or mildly symptomatic patients.
        c. Inactivated vaccines should be administered routinely.

Vaccine	Birth	1 mo	2 mos	4 mos	6 mos	9 mos	12 mos	15 mos	18 mos	19–23 mos	2–3 yrs	4–6 yrs	7–10 yrs	11–12 yrs	13–15 yrs	16–18 yrs
Hepatitis B[1] (HepB)	1st dose	←2nd dose→			←———— 3rd dose ————→											
Rotavirus[2] (RV) RV1 (2-dose series); RV5 (3-dose series)			1st dose	2nd dose	See footnote 2											
Diphtheria, tetanus, & acellular pertussis[3] (DTaP: <7 yrs)			1st dose	2nd dose	3rd dose			←——— 4th dose ———→				5th dose				
Haemophilus influenzae type b[4] (Hib)			1st dose	2nd dose	See footnote 4		←— 3rd or 4th dose, See footnote 4 —→									
Pneumococcal conjugate[5] (PCV13)			1st dose	2nd dose	3rd dose		←— 4th dose —→									
Inactivated poliovirus[6] (IPV: <18 yrs)			1st dose	2nd dose	←———— 3rd dose ————→							4th dose				
Influenza[7] (IIV; LAIV)						Annual vaccination (IIV only) 1 or 2 doses					Annual vaccination (LAIV or IIV) 1 or 2 doses			Annual vaccination (LAIV or IIV) 1 dose only		
Measles, mumps, rubella[8] (MMR)							←— 1st dose —→					2nd dose				
Varicella[9] (VAR)							←— 1st dose —→					2nd dose				
Hepatitis A[10] (HepA)							←———— 2-dose series, See footnote 10 ————→									
Meningococcal[11] (Hib-MenCY ≥6 weeks; MenACWY-D ≥9 mos; MenACWY-CRM ≥2 mos)							See footnote 11							1st dose		Booster
Tetanus, diphtheria, & acellular pertussis[12] (Tdap: ≥7 yrs)														(Tdap)		
Human papillomavirus[13] (2vHPV: females only; 4vHPV, 9vHPV: males and females)														(3-dose series)		
Meningococcal B[11]														See footnote 11		
Pneumococcal polysaccharide[5] (PPSV23)												See footnote 5				

Legend:
- Range of recommended ages for all children
- Range of recommended ages for catch-up immunization
- Range of recommended ages for certain high-risk groups
- Range of recommended ages for non-high-risk groups that may receive vaccine, subject to individual clinical decision making
- No recommendation

This schedule includes recommendations in effect as of January 1, 2016. Any dose not administered at the recommended age should be administered at a subsequent visit, when indicated and feasible. The use of a combination vaccine generally is preferred over separate injections of its equivalent component vaccines. Vaccination providers should consult the relevant Advisory Committee on Immunization Practices (ACIP) statement for detailed recommendations, available online at http://www.cdc.gov/vaccines/hcp/acip-recs/index.html. Clinically significant adverse events that follow vaccination should be reported to the Vaccine Adverse Event Reporting System (VAERS) online (http://www.vaers.hhs.gov) or by telephone (800-822-7967). Suspected cases of vaccine-preventable diseases should be reported to the state or local health department. Additional information, including precautions and contraindications for vaccination, is available from CDC online (http://www.cdc.gov/vaccines/recs/vac-admin/contraindications.htm) or by telephone (800-CDC-INFO [800-232-4636]).

This schedule is approved by the Advisory Committee on Immunization Practices (http://www.cdc.gov/vaccines/acip), the American Academy of Pediatrics (http://www.aap.org), the American Academy of Family Physicians (http://www.aafp.org), and the American College of Obstetricians and Gynecologists (http://www.acog.org).

NOTE: The above recommendations must be read along with the footnotes of this schedule.

Figure 2. Recommended immunization schedule for people aged 0–18 years, 2016.
For those who fall behind or start late, see the catch-up schedule at www.cdc.gov/vaccines/schedules/hcp/imz/catchup.html.

Footnotes — Recommended immunization schedule for persons aged 0 through 18 years—United States, 2016

For further guidance on the use of the vaccines mentioned below, see: http://www.cdc.gov/vaccines/hcp/acip-recs/index.html.
For vaccine recommendations for persons 19 years of age and older, see the Adult Immunization Schedule.

Additional Information

- For contraindications and precautions to use of a vaccine and for additional information regarding that vaccine, vaccination providers should consult the relevant ACIP statement available online at http://www.cdc.gov/vaccines/hcp/acip-recs/index.html.
- For purposes of calculating intervals between doses, 4 weeks = 28 days. Intervals of 4 months or greater are determined by calendar months.
- Vaccine doses administered ≤4 days or less before the minimum interval are considered valid. Doses of any vaccine administered ≥5 days earlier than the minimum interval or minimum age should not be counted as valid doses and should be repeated as age-appropriate. The repeat dose should be spaced after the invalid dose by the recommended minimum interval. For further details, see *MMWR, General Recommendations on Immunization and Reports / Vol. 60 / No. 2; Table 1. Recommended and minimum ages and intervals between vaccine doses available online at* http://www.cdc.gov/mmwr/pdf/rr/rr6002.pdf.
- Information on travel vaccine requirements and recommendations is available at http://wwwnc.cdc.gov/travel/destinations/list.
- For vaccination of persons with primary and secondary immunodeficiencies, see Table 13, "Vaccination of persons with primary and secondary immunodeficiencies," in *General Recommendations on Immunization* (ACIP), available at http://www.cdc.gov/mmwr/pdf/rr/rr6002.pdf.; and American Academy of Pediatrics. "Immunization in Special Clinical Circumstances," in Kimberlin DW, Brady MT, Jackson MA, Long SS eds. *Red Book: 2015 report of the Committee on Infectious Diseases. 30th ed. Elk Grove Village, IL: American Academy of Pediatrics.*

1. **Hepatitis B (HepB) vaccine. (Minimum age: birth)**
   Routine vaccination:
   At birth:
   - Administer monovalent HepB vaccine to all newborns before hospital discharge.
   - For infants born to hepatitis B surface antigen (HBsAg)-positive mothers, administer HepB vaccine and 0.5 mL of hepatitis B immune globulin (HBIG) within 12 hours of birth. These infants should be tested for HBsAg and antibody to HBsAg (anti-HBs) at age 9 through 18 months (preferably at the next well-child visit) or 1 to 2 months after completion of the HepB series if the series was delayed; CDC recently recommended testing occur at age 9 through 12 months; see http://www.cdc.gov/mmwr/preview/mmwrhtml/mm6439a6.htm.
   - If mother's HBsAg status is unknown, within 12 hours of birth administer HepB vaccine regardless of birth weight. For infants weighing less than 2,000 grams, administer HBIG in addition to HepB vaccine within 12 hours of birth. Determine mother's HBsAg status as soon as possible and, if mother is HBsAg-positive, also administer HBIG for infants weighing 2,000 grams or more as soon as possible, but no later than age 7 days.

   Doses following the birth dose:
   - The second dose should be administered at age 1 or 2 months. Monovalent HepB vaccine should be used for doses administered before age 6 weeks.
   - Infants who did not receive a birth dose should receive 3 doses of a HepB-containing vaccine on a schedule of 0, 1 to 2 months, and 6 months starting as soon as feasible. See Figure 2.
   - Administer the second dose 1 to 2 months after the first dose (minimum interval of 4 weeks), administer the third dose at least 8 weeks after the second dose AND at least 16 weeks after the **first** dose. The final (third or fourth) dose in the HepB vaccine series should be administered **no earlier than age 24 weeks.**
   - Administration of a total of 4 doses of HepB vaccine is permitted when a combination vaccine containing HepB is administered after the birth dose.

   Catch-up vaccination:
   - Unvaccinated persons should complete a 3-dose series.
   - A 2-dose series (doses separated by at least 4 months) of adult formulation Recombivax HB is licensed for use in children aged 11 through 15 years.
   - For other catch-up guidance, see Figure 2.

2. **Rotavirus (RV) vaccines. (Minimum age: 6 weeks for both RV1 [Rotarix] and RV5 [RotaTeq])**
   Routine vaccination:
   Administer a series of RV vaccine to all infants as follows:
   1. If Rotarix is used, administer a 2-dose series at 2 and 4 months of age.
   2. If RotaTeq is used, administer a 3-dose series at ages 2, 4, and 6 months.
   3. If any dose in the series was RotaTeq or vaccine product is unknown for any dose in the series, a total of 3 doses of RV vaccine should be administered.

   Catch-up vaccination:
   - The maximum age for the first dose in the series is 14 weeks, 6 days; vaccination should not be initiated for infants aged 15 weeks, 0 days or older.
   - The maximum age for the final dose in the series is 8 months, 0 days.
   - For other catch-up guidance, see Figure 2.

3. **Diphtheria and tetanus toxoids and acellular pertussis (DTaP) vaccine. (Minimum age: 6 weeks.**
   Exception: DTaP-IPV [Kinrix, Quadracel]: 4 years)
   Routine vaccination:
   - Administer a 5-dose series of DTaP vaccine at ages 2, 4, 6, 15 through 18 months, and 4 through 6 years. The fourth dose may be administered as early as age 12 months, provided at least 6 months have elapsed since the third dose.
   - Inadvertent administration of 4th DTaP dose early: If the fourth dose of DTaP was administered at least 4 months, but less than 6 months, after the third dose of DTaP, it need not be repeated.

3. **Diphtheria and tetanus toxoids and acellular pertussis (DTaP) vaccine (cont'd)**
   Catch-up vaccination:
   - The fifth dose of DTaP vaccine is not necessary if the fourth dose was administered at age 4 years or older.
   - For other catch-up guidance, see Figure 2.

4. **Haemophilus influenzae type b (Hib) conjugate vaccine. (Minimum age: 6 weeks for PRP-T [AC-THIB, DTaP-IPV/Hib (Pentacel) and Hib-MenCY (MenHibrix)], PRP-OMP [PedvaxHIB or COMVAX], 12 months for PRP-T [Hiberix])**
   Routine vaccination:
   - Administer a 2- or 3-dose Hib vaccine primary series and a booster dose (dose 3 or 4 depending on vaccine used in primary series) at age 12 through 15 months to complete a full Hib vaccine series.
   - The primary series with ActHIB, MenHibrix, or Pentacel consists of 3 doses and should be administered at 2, 4, and 6 months of age. The primary series with PedvaxHib or COMVAX consists of 2 doses and should be administered at 2 and 4 months of age; a dose at age 6 months is not indicated.
   - One booster dose (dose 3 or 4 depending on vaccine used in primary series) of any Hib vaccine should be administered at age 12 through 15 months. An exception is Hiberix vaccine. Hiberix should only be used for the booster (final) dose in children aged 12 months through 4 years who have received at least 1 prior dose of Hib-containing vaccine.
   - For recommendations on the use of MenHibrix in patients at increased risk for meningococcal disease, please refer to the meningococcal vaccine footnotes and also to *MMWR* February 28, 2014 / 63(RR01):1-13, available at http://www.cdc.gov/mmwr/PDF/rr/rr6301.pdf.

   Catch-up vaccination:
   - If dose 1 was administered at ages 12 through 14 months, administer a second (final) dose at least 8 weeks after dose 1, regardless of Hib vaccine used in the primary series.
   - If both doses were PRP-OMP (PedvaxHIB or COMVAX), and were administered before the first birthday, the third (and final) dose should be administered at age 12 through 59 months and at least 8 weeks after the second dose.
   - If the first dose was administered at age 7 through 11 months, administer the second dose at least 4 weeks later and a third (and final) dose at age 12 through 15 months or 8 weeks after second dose, whichever is later.
   - If first dose is administered before the first birthday and second dose administered at younger than 15 months, a third (and final) dose should be administered 8 weeks later.
   - For unvaccinated children aged 15 months or older, administer only 1 dose.
   - For other catch-up guidance, see Figure 2. For catch-up guidance related to MenHibrix, please see the meningococcal vaccine footnotes and also *MMWR* February 28, 2014 / 63(RR01):1-13, available at http://www.cdc.gov/mmwr/PDF/rr/rr6301.pdf.

   Vaccination of persons with high-risk conditions:
   - Children aged 12 through 59 months who are at increased risk for Hib disease, including chemotherapy recipients and those with anatomic or functional asplenia (including sickle cell disease), human immunodeficiency virus (HIV) infection, immunoglobulin deficiency, or early component complement deficiency, who have received either no doses or only 1 dose of Hib vaccine before 12 months of age, should receive 2 additional doses of Hib vaccine 8 weeks apart; children who received 2 or more doses of Hib vaccine before 12 months of age should receive 1 additional dose.
   - For patients younger than 5 years of age undergoing chemotherapy or radiation treatment who received a Hib vaccine dose(s) within 14 days of starting therapy or during therapy, repeat the dose(s) at least 3 months following therapy completion.
   - Recipients of hematopoietic stem cell transplant (HSCT) should be revaccinated with a 3-dose regimen of Hib vaccine starting 6 to 12 months after successful transplant, regardless of vaccination history; doses should be administered at least 4 weeks apart.
   - A single dose of any Hib-containing vaccine should be administered to unimmunized* children and adolescents 15 months of age and older undergoing an elective splenectomy; if possible, vaccine should be administered at least 14 days before procedure.

For further guidance on the use of the vaccines mentioned below, see: http://www.cdc.gov/vaccines/hcp/acip-recs/index.html.

4. **Haemophilus influenzae type b (Hib) conjugate vaccine (cont'd)**
- Hib vaccine is not routinely recommended for patients 5 years or older. However, 1 dose of Hib vaccine should be administered to unimmunized* persons aged 5 years or older who have anatomic or functional asplenia (including sickle cell disease) and unvaccinated persons 5 through 18 years of age with HIV infection.
  - *Patients who have not received a primary series and booster dose or at least 1 dose of Hib vaccine after 14 months of age are considered unimmunized.

5. **Pneumococcal vaccines. (Minimum age: 6 weeks for PCV13, 2 years for PPSV23)**
Routine vaccination with PCV13:
- Administer a 4-dose series of PCV13 vaccine at ages 2, 4, and 6 months and at age 12 through 15 months.
- For children aged 14 through 59 months who have received an age-appropriate series of 7-valent PCV (PCV7), administer a single supplemental dose of 13-valent PCV (PCV13).
Catch-up vaccination with PCV13:
- Administer 1 dose of PCV13 to all healthy children aged 24 through 59 months who are not completely vaccinated for their age.
- For other catch-up guidance, see Figure 2.
Vaccination of persons with high-risk conditions with PCV13 and PPSV23:
- All recommended PCV13 doses should be administered prior to PPSV23 vaccination if possible.
- For children 2 through 5 years of age with any of the following conditions: chronic heart disease (particularly cyanotic congenital heart disease and cardiac failure); chronic lung disease (including asthma if treated with high-dose oral corticosteroid therapy); diabetes mellitus; cerebrospinal fluid leak; cochlear implant; sickle cell disease and other hemoglobinopathies; anatomic or functional asplenia; HIV infection; chronic renal failure; nephrotic syndrome; diseases associated with treatment with immunosuppressive drugs or radiation therapy, including malignant neoplasms, leukemias, lymphomas, and Hodgkin disease; solid organ transplantation; or congenital immunodeficiency:
  1. Administer 1 dose of PCV13 if any incomplete schedule of 3 doses of PCV (PCV7 and/or PCV13) were received previously.
  2. Administer 2 doses of PCV13 at least 8 weeks apart if unvaccinated or any incomplete schedule of fewer than 3 doses of PCV (PCV7 and/or PCV13) were received previously.
  3. Administer 1 supplemental dose of PCV13 if 4 doses of PCV7 or other age-appropriate complete PCV7 series was received previously.
  4. The minimum interval between doses of PCV (PCV7 or PCV13) is 8 weeks.
  5. For children with no history of PPSV23 vaccination, administer PPSV23 at least 8 weeks after the most recent dose of PCV13.
- For children aged 6 through 18 years who have cerebrospinal fluid leak; cochlear implant; sickle cell disease and other hemoglobinopathies; anatomic or functional asplenia; congenital or acquired immunodeficiencies; HIV infection; chronic renal failure; nephrotic syndrome; diseases associated with treatment with immunosuppressive drugs or radiation therapy, including malignant neoplasms, leukemias, lymphomas, and Hodgkin disease; generalized malignancy; solid organ transplantation; or multiple myeloma:
  1. If neither PCV13 nor PPSV23 has been received previously, administer 1 dose of PCV13 now and 1 dose of PPSV23 at least 8 weeks later.
  2. If PCV13 has been received previously but PPSV23 has not, administer 1 dose of PPSV23 at least 8 weeks after the most recent dose of PCV13.
  3. If PPSV23 has been received but PCV13 has not, administer 1 dose of PCV13 at least 8 weeks after the most recent dose of PPSV23.
- For children aged 6 through 18 years with chronic heart disease (particularly cyanotic congenital heart disease and cardiac failure), chronic lung disease (including asthma if treated with high-dose oral corticosteroid therapy), diabetes mellitus, alcoholism, or chronic liver disease, who have not received PPSV23, administer 1 dose of PPSV23. If PCV13 has been received previously, then PPSV23 should be administered at least 8 weeks after any prior PCV13 dose.
- A single revaccination with PPSV23 should be administered 5 years after the first dose to children with sickle cell disease or other hemoglobinopathies; anatomic or functional asplenia; congenital or acquired immunodeficiencies; HIV infection; chronic renal failure; nephrotic syndrome; diseases associated with treatment with immunosuppressive drugs or radiation therapy, including malignant neoplasms, leukemias, lymphomas, and Hodgkin disease; generalized malignancy; solid organ transplantation; or multiple myeloma.

6. **Inactivated poliovirus vaccine (IPV). (Minimum age: 6 weeks)**
Routine vaccination:
- Administer a 4-dose series of IPV at ages 2, 4, 6 through 18 months, and 4 through 6 years. The final dose in the series should be administered on or after the fourth birthday and at least 6 months after the previous dose.
Catch-up vaccination:
- In the first 6 months of life, minimum age and minimum intervals are only recommended if the person is at risk of imminent exposure to circulating poliovirus (i.e., travel to a polio-endemic region or during an outbreak).
- If 4 or more doses are administered before age 4 years, an additional dose should be administered at age 4 through 6 years and at least 6 months after the previous dose.
- A fourth dose is not necessary if the third dose was administered at age 4 years or older and at least 6 months after the previous dose.

6. **Inactivated poliovirus vaccine (IPV). (Minimum age: 6 weeks) (cont'd)**
- If both OPV and IPV were administered as part of a series, a total of 4 doses should be administered, regardless of the child's current age. If only OPV were administered, and all doses were given prior to 4 years of age, one dose of IPV should be given at 4 years or older, at least 4 weeks after the last OPV dose.
- IPV is not routinely recommended for U.S. residents aged 18 years or older.
- For other catch-up guidance, see Figure 2.

7. **Influenza vaccines. (Minimum age: 6 months for inactivated influenza vaccine [IIV], 2 years for live, attenuated influenza vaccine [LAIV])**
Routine vaccination:
- Administer influenza vaccine annually to all children beginning at age 6 months. For most healthy, nonpregnant persons aged 2 through 49 years, either LAIV or IIV may be used. However, LAIV should NOT be administered to some persons, including 1) persons who have experienced severe allergic reactions to LAIV, any of its components, or to a previous dose of any other influenza vaccine; 2) children 2 through 17 years receiving aspirin or aspirin-containing products; 3) persons who are allergic to eggs; 4) pregnant women; 5) immunosuppressed persons; 6) children 2 through 4 years of age with asthma or who had wheezing in the past 12 months; or 7) persons who have taken influenza antiviral medications in the previous 48 hours. For all other contraindications and precautions to use of LAIV, see MMWR August 7, 2015 / 64(30):818-25 available at http://www.cdc.gov/mmwr/pdf/wk/mm6430.pdf.

For children aged 6 months through 8 years:
- For the 2015-16 season, administer 2 doses (separated by at least 4 weeks) to children who are receiving influenza vaccine for the first time. Some children in this age group who have been vaccinated previously will also need 2 doses. For additional guidance, follow dosing guidelines in the 2015-16 ACIP influenza vaccine recommendations. MMWR August 7, 2015 / 64(30):818-25, available at http://www.cdc.gov/mmwr/pdf/wk/mm6430.pdf.
- For the 2016-17 season, follow dosing guidelines in the 2016 ACIP influenza vaccine recommendations.
For persons aged 9 years and older:
- Administer 1 dose.

8. **Measles, mumps, and rubella (MMR) vaccine. (Minimum age: 12 months for routine vaccination)**
Routine vaccination:
- Administer a 2-dose series of MMR vaccine at ages 12 through 15 months and 4 through 6 years. The second dose may be administered before age 4 years, provided at least 4 weeks have elapsed since the first dose.
- Administer 1 dose of MMR vaccine to infants aged 6 through 11 months before departure from the United States for international travel. These children should be revaccinated with 2 doses of MMR vaccine, the first at age 12 through 15 months (12 months if the child remains in an area where disease risk is high), and the second dose at least 4 weeks later.
- Administer 2 doses of MMR vaccine to children aged 12 months and older before departure from the United States for international travel. The first dose should be administered on or after age 12 months and the second dose at least 4 weeks later.
Catch-up vaccination:
- Ensure that all school-aged children and adolescents have had 2 doses of MMR vaccine; the minimum interval between the 2 doses is 4 weeks.

9. **Varicella (VAR) vaccine. (Minimum age: 12 months)**
Routine vaccination:
- Administer a 2-dose series of VAR vaccine at ages 12 through 15 months and 4 through 6 years. The second dose may be administered before age 4 years, provided at least 3 months have elapsed since the first dose. If the second dose was administered at least 4 weeks after the first dose, it can be accepted as valid.
Catch-up vaccination:
- Ensure that all persons aged 7 through 18 years without evidence of immunity (see MMWR 2007 / 56 [No. RR-4], available at http://www.cdc.gov/mmwr/pdf/rr/rr5604.pdf) have 2 doses of varicella vaccine. For children aged 7 through 12 years, the recommended minimum interval between doses is 3 months (if the second dose was administered at least 4 weeks after the first dose, it can be accepted as valid); for persons aged 13 years and older, the minimum interval between doses is 4 weeks.

10. **Hepatitis A (HepA) vaccine. (Minimum age: 12 months)**
Routine vaccination:
- Initiate the 2-dose HepA vaccine series at 12 through 23 months; separate the 2 doses by 6 to 18 months.
- Children who have received 1 dose of HepA vaccine before age 24 months should receive a second dose 6 to 18 months after the first dose.
- For any person aged 2 years and older who has not already received the HepA vaccine series, 2 doses of HepA vaccine separated by 6 to 18 months may be administered if immunity against hepatitis A virus infection is desired.
Catch-up vaccination:
- The minimum interval between the 2 doses is 6 months.

For further guidance on the use of the vaccines mentioned below, see: http://www.cdc.gov/vaccines/hcp/acip-recs/index.html.

10. **Hepatitis A (HepA) vaccine (cont'd)**

Special populations:
- Administer 2 doses of HepA vaccine at least 6 months apart to previously unvaccinated persons who live in areas where vaccination programs target older children, or who are at increased risk for infection. This includes persons traveling to or working in countries that have high or intermediate endemicity of infection; men having sex with men; users of injection and non-injection illicit drugs; persons who work with HAV-infected primates or with HAV in a research laboratory; persons with clotting-factor disorders; persons with chronic liver disease; and persons who anticipate close personal contact (e.g., household or regular babysitting) with an international adoptee during the first 60 days after arrival in the United States from a country with high or intermediate endemicity. The first dose should be administered as soon as the adoption is planned, ideally 2 or more weeks before the arrival of the adoptee.

11. **Meningococcal vaccines. (Minimum age: 6 weeks for Hib-MenCY [MenHibrix], 9 months for MenACWY-D [Menactra], 2 months for MenACWY-CRM [Menveo], 10 years for serogroup B meningococcal [MenB] vaccines: MenB-4C [Bexsero] and MenB-FHbp [Trumenba])**

Routine vaccination:
- Administer a single dose of Menactra or Menveo vaccine at age 11 through 12 years, with a booster dose at age 16 years.
- Adolescents aged 11 through 18 years with human immunodeficiency virus (HIV) infection should receive a 2-dose primary series of Menactra or Menveo with at least 8 weeks between doses.
- For children aged 2 months through 18 years with high-risk conditions, see below.

Catch-up vaccination:
- Administer Menactra or Menveo vaccine at age 13 through 18 years if not previously vaccinated.
- If the first dose is administered at age 13 through 15 years, a booster dose should be administered at age 16 through 18 years with a minimum interval of at least 8 weeks between doses.
- If the first dose is administered at age 16 years or older, a booster dose is not needed.
- For catch-up guidance, see Figure 2.

Clinical discretion:
- Young adults aged 16 through 23 years (preferred age range is 16 through 18 years) may be vaccinated with either a 2-dose series of Bexsero or a 3-dose series of Trumenba vaccine to provide short-term protection against most strains of serogroup B meningococcal disease. The two MenB vaccines are not interchangeable; the same vaccine product must be used for all doses.

Vaccination of persons with high-risk conditions and other persons at increased risk of disease:

Children with anatomic or functional asplenia (including sickle cell disease):

Meningococcal conjugate ACWY vaccines:
1. Menveo
   o *Children who initiate vaccination at 8 weeks:* Administer doses at 2, 4, 6, and 12 months of age.
   o *Unvaccinated children who initiate vaccination at 7 through 23 months:* Administer 2 doses, with the second dose at least 12 weeks after the first dose AND after the first birthday.
   o *Children 24 months and older who have not received a complete series:* Administer 2 primary doses at least 8 weeks apart.
2. MenHibrix
   o *Children who initiate vaccination at 6 weeks:* Administer doses at 2, 4, 6, and 12 through 15 months of age.
   o If the first dose of MenHibrix is given at or after 12 months of age, a total of 2 doses should be given at least 8 weeks apart to ensure protection against serogroups C and Y meningococcal disease.
3. Menactra
   o *Children 24 months and older who have not received a complete series:* Administer 2 primary doses at least 8 weeks apart. If Menactra is administered to a child with asplenia (including sickle cell disease), do not administer Menactra until 2 years of age and at least 4 weeks after the completion of all PCV13 doses.

Meningococcal B vaccines:
1. Bexsero or Trumenba
2. MenHibrix

Children with persistent complement component deficiency (includes persons with inherited or chronic deficiencies in C3, C5-9, properidin, factor D, factor H, or taking eculizumab [Soliris]):

Meningococcal conjugate ACWY vaccines:
1. Menveo
   o *Children who initiate vaccination at 8 weeks:* Administer doses at 2, 4, 6, and 12 months of age.
   o *Unvaccinated children who initiate vaccination at 7 through 23 months:* Administer 2 doses, with the second dose at least 12 weeks after the first dose AND after the first birthday.
   o *Children 24 months and older who have not received a complete series:* Administer 2 primary doses at least 8 weeks apart.
2. MenHibrix
   o *Children who initiate vaccination 6 weeks:* Administer doses at 2, 4, 6, and 12 through 15 months of age.
   o If the first dose of MenHibrix is given at or after 12 months of age, a total of 2 doses should be given at least 8 weeks apart to ensure protection against serogroups C and Y meningococcal disease.

11. **Meningococcal vaccines (cont'd)**

3. Menactra
   o *Children 9 through 23 months:* Administer 2 primary doses at least 12 weeks apart.
   o *Children 24 months and older who have not received a complete series:* Administer 2 primary doses at least 8 weeks apart.

Meningococcal B vaccines:
1. Bexsero or Trumenba
   o *Persons 10 years or older who have not received a complete series.* Administer a 2-dose series of Bexsero, at least 1 month apart. Or a 3-dose series of Trumenba, with the second dose at least 2 months after the first and the third dose at least 6 months after the first. The two MenB vaccines are not interchangeable; the same vaccine product must be used for all doses.

For children who travel to or reside in countries in which meningococcal disease is hyperendemic or epidemic, including countries in the African meningitis belt or the Hajj
- administer an age-appropriate formulation and series of Menactra or Menveo for protection against serogroups A and W meningococcal disease. Prior receipt of MenHibrix is not sufficient for children traveling to the meningitis belt or the Hajj because it does not contain serogroups A or W.

For children at risk during a community outbreak attributable to a vaccine serogroup
- administer or complete an age- and formulation-appropriate series of MenHibrix, Menactra, or Menveo, Bexsero or Trumenba.

For booster doses among persons with high-risk conditions, refer to *MMWR* 2013 / 62(RR02);1-22, available at http://www.cdc.gov/mmwr/preview/mmwrhtml/rr6202a1.htm.

For other catch-up recommendations for these persons, and complete information on use of meningococcal vaccines, including guidance related to vaccination of persons at increased risk of infection, see *MMWR* March 22, 2013 / 62(RR02);1-22, and *MMWR* October 23, 2015 / 64(41); 1171-1176 available at http://www.cdc.gov/mmwr/pdf/rr/rr6202.pdf, and http://www.cdc.gov/mmwr/pdf/wk/mm6441.pdf.

12. **Tetanus and diphtheria toxoids and acellular pertussis (Tdap) vaccine. (Minimum age: 10 years for both Boostrix and Adacel)**

Routine vaccination:
- Administer 1 dose of Tdap vaccine to all adolescents aged 11 through 12 years.
- Tdap may be administered regardless of the interval since the last tetanus and diphtheria toxoid-containing vaccine.
- Administer 1 dose of Tdap vaccine to pregnant adolescents during each pregnancy (preferred during 27 through 36 weeks gestation) regardless of time since prior Td or Tdap vaccination.

Catch-up vaccination:
- Persons aged 7 years and older who are not fully immunized with DTaP vaccine should receive Tdap vaccine as 1 (preferably the first) dose in the catch-up series; if additional doses are needed, use Td vaccine. For children 7 through 10 years who receive a dose of Tdap as part of the catch-up series, an adolescent Tdap vaccine dose at age 11 through 12 years should NOT be administered. Td should be administered instead 10 years after the Tdap dose.
- Persons aged 11 through 18 years who have not received Tdap vaccine should receive a dose followed by tetanus and diphtheria toxoids (Td) booster doses every 10 years thereafter.
- Inadvertent doses of DTaP vaccine:
  - If administered inadvertently to a child aged 7 through 10 years may count as part of the catch-up series. This dose may count as the adolescent Tdap dose, or the child can later receive a Tdap booster dose at age 11 through 12 years.
  - If administered inadvertently to an adolescent aged 11 through 18 years, the dose should be counted as the adolescent Tdap booster.
- For other catch-up guidance, see Figure 2.

13. **Human papillomavirus (HPV) vaccines. (Minimum age: 9 years for 2vHPV [Cervarix], 4vHPV [Gardasil] and 9vHPV [Gardasil 9])**

Routine vaccination:
- Administer a 3-dose series of HPV vaccine on a schedule of 0, 1-2, and 6 months to all adolescents aged 11 through 12 years. 9vHPV, 4vHPV or 2vHPV may be used for females, and only 9vHPV or 4vHPV may be used for males.
- The vaccine series may be started at age 9 years.
- Administer the second dose 1 to 2 months after the first dose (minimum interval of 4 weeks); administer the third dose 16 weeks after the second dose (minimum interval of 12 weeks) and 24 weeks after the first dose.

Catch-up vaccination:
- Administer the vaccine series to females (2vHPV or 4vHPV or 9vHPV) and males (4vHPV or 9vHPV) at age 13 through 18 years if not previously vaccinated.
- Use recommended routine dosing intervals (see Routine vaccination above) for vaccine series catch-up.

CS260933-A

V. PEDIATRIC SEIZURE DISORDERS

A. Treatment Options Based on Seizure Type (Table 6)

Table 6. Treatment Options Based on Seizure Type

Seizure Type	Drugs of Choice	Alternatives
Focal (formerly "partial")	VPA, CBZ, PHT	PB, gabapentin, lamotrigine, tiagabine, topiramate, oxcarbazepine, zonisamide, levetiracetam, lacosamide
Generalized		
Tonic-clonic	VPA, CBZ, PHT	Lamotrigine, topiramate, zonisamide, levetiracetam
Myoclonic	VPA	Topiramate, zonisamide, levetiracetam
Absence	Ethosuximide, VPA	Lamotrigine, zonisamide, levetiracetam
Lennox-Gastaut	VPA, topiramate, lamotrigine	Rufinamide, clobazam, felbamate, zonisamide
Infantile spasms	ACTH	Vigabatrin, lamotrigine, tiagabine, topiramate, VPA, zonisamide

ACTH = adrenocorticotropic hormone; CBZ = carbamazepine; PB = phenobarbital; PHT = phenytoin; VPA = valproic acid.

B. Comparison of Available Antiepileptic Drugs (Table 7)

Table 7. Comparison of Available Antiepileptic Drugs

Drug	Adverse Effects	Pharmacokinetic Considerations	Other Comments
Carbamazepine	Rash Hyponatremia ↓ Bone density Teratogenic	Autoinduction ↓ Effectiveness of OCs	Significant drug interactions
Clobazam	Somnolence	Dose adjustment needed in hepatic impairment Dose adjustment needed in CYP2C19 poor metabolizers	
Felbamate	Anorexia, nausea, weight loss Insomnia, somnolence Aplastic anemia Hepatic failure	Clearance ~50:50 renal/hepatic	Significant drug interactions Aplastic anemia: Adults > children Requires signed informed consent
Gabapentin	Somnolence Weight gain	↑ Clearance in children <6 years old Dose adjustment needed in renal insufficiency Nonlinear pharmacokinetics	Minimal drug interactions Minimal cognitive effects May worsen Lennox-Gastaut
Lacosamide	Prolonged PR interval Dizziness Headache Diplopia	Dose adjustment needed in severe renal insufficiency	Use with caution if severe cardiac disease or conduction problems No clinically significant drug interactions
Lamotrigine	Rash Stevens-Johnson syndrome	Autoinduction	Rash: Children > adults Minimal cognitive effects

Table 7. Comparison of Available Antiepileptic Drugs *(continued)*

Drug	Adverse Effects	Pharmacokinetic Considerations	Other Comments
Levetiracetam	Headache Somnolence	Linear pharmacokinetics Renal excretion Clearance 40% ↑ in children No effect on CYP system	Minimal drug interactions
Oxcarbazepine	Hyponatremia (>CBZ) Rash (<CBZ)	Linear pharmacokinetics Clearance 40% ↑ in children <6 years old Induces CYP3A4 Inhibits CYP2C19	Hyponatremia more common in adults than in children Minimal cognitive effects
Phenobarbital	Cognitive dysfunction Sedation Rash ↓ Bone density	Linear pharmacokinetics ↓ Effectiveness of OCs	Significant drug interactions
Phenytoin	Rash Gingival hyperplasia Hirsutism ↓ Bone density Teratogenic	Nonlinear pharmacokinetics ↓ Effectiveness of OCs	Significant drug interactions
Rufinamide	Somnolence Rash QT interval shortening	↑ Level with concurrent VPA	Somnolence: Minimized with slow dose titration Rash: All reported cases are in children
Tiagabine	Dizziness Nonconvulsive status epilepticus (case reports)	Clearance 50% ↑ in children	Minimal cognitive effects
Topiramate	Cognitive dysfunction Weight loss Glaucoma Oligohidrosis	↑ Clearance in children Dose adjustment needed in renal insufficiency	Weight loss more common in obese patients Children at higher risk of oligohidrosis than adults
Valproic acid	Weight gain Menstrual irregularities Polycystic ovarian syndrome Hyperandrogenism Hepatotoxicity Teratogenic Thrombocytopenia	CYP induction > in children	Significant drug interactions Most cases of hepatotoxicity in children <2 years old
Vigabatrin	Vision loss Weight gain		Available only through restricted distribution program
Zonisamide	Weight loss Rash Oligohidrosis Somnolence Agitation Hallucinations	Linear pharmacokinetics Primarily renal excretion No effect on CYP system	Better tolerated by children than by adults

CBZ = carbamazepine; CYP = cytochrome P450; OC = oral contraceptive; PHT = phenytoin; VPA = valproic acid.

Patient Case

10. A 14-year-old moderately obese girl comes to the clinic with an erythematous pruritic rash. She was initiated on oxcarbazepine about 3 weeks ago for the management of partial seizures. Her medical history is significant only for seizures. She recently became sexually active with a male and admits inconsistent contraceptive use. Which intervention is best for her?

    A. Change to carbamazepine.

    B. Change to levetiracetam.

    C. Change to valproic acid.

    D. No change in therapy is necessary.

VI. ATTENTION-DEFICIT/HYPERACTIVITY DISORDER

A. Clinical Presentation

1. *Diagnostic and Statistical Manual for Mental Disorders (DSM-V)* criteria

   a. Either (i) or (ii)

      i. Six or more of the following symptoms of inattention have been present for at least 6 months to a point that is disruptive and inappropriate:

         Inattention

         (a) Often does not give close attention to detail/makes careless mistakes

         (b) Often has trouble keeping attention on tasks/activities

         (c) Often does not seem to listen

         (d) Often does not follow instructions

         (e) Often has trouble organizing activities

         (f) Often avoids or dislikes things that require long periods of mental effort

         (g) Often loses things needed for tasks or activities

         (h) Often is easily distracted

         (i) Often is forgetful

      ii. Six or more of the following symptoms of hyperactivity-impulsivity have been present for at least 6 months to a point that is disruptive and inappropriate:

         Hyperactivity

         (a) Often fidgets or squirms

         (b) Often is unable to remain seated when it is expected

         (c) Often runs or climbs when and where it is not appropriate

         (d) Often has difficulty with quiet play or activities

         (e) Often is "on the go"

         (f) Often talks excessively

         Impulsivity

         (g) Often blurts out answers

         (h) Often has difficulty waiting one's turn

         (i) Often interrupts

   b. Some symptoms were present before 7 years of age.

   c. Some impairment from the symptoms is present in two or more settings.

   d. Clear evidence of significant impairment exists in social, school, or work functioning.

   e. No other mental disorder better describes the symptoms.

2. Comorbid disease states: 44%–87% of children with ADHD have at least one other disorder
   a. Oppositional defiant disorder
      i. Most common comorbid disorder in adolescents
      ii. Presence of ADHD increases the odds of oppositional defiant disorder almost 11-fold.
   b. Anxiety disorder: May exist in about 25% of children with ADHD
   c. Tics
      i. 21%–90% of children with Tourette syndrome may also have ADHD.
      ii. May not be exacerbated by stimulant agents, as once thought

---

Patient Case

11. A 9-year-old boy has a new diagnosis of ADHD. At school, he is disruptive, talks when the teacher is talking, and runs around the classroom. His parents report extreme difficulty in getting him to do his homework after school. Which is best for his initial drug therapy?
    A. Methylphenidate (OROS) (Concerta) given once daily.
    B. Methylphenidate immediate release (Ritalin) given twice daily, with doses administered 4 hours apart.
    C. Guanfacine given at bedtime.
    D. D-Methylphenidate (Focalin) given twice daily, with doses administered 4 hours apart.

B. Classification: Based on *DSM-V* Criteria (see pages 1–17)
   1. ADHD, Combined Type: Criteria (i) and (ii) both are met.
   2. ADHD, Predominantly Inattentive Type: Criterion (i) is met, but (ii) is not met.
   3. ADHD, Predominantly Hyperactive-Impulsive Type: Criterion (ii) is met, but (i) is not met.

C. Treatment Options: Combination of pharmacotherapy and behavioral therapy is more beneficial than either intervention alone.
   1. Factors affecting choice of pharmacologic agent
      a. Desired length of coverage time for symptoms
         i. Consider time of day when symptoms occur.
         ii. Consider time of day when child's activities occur (e.g., when is homework done, at what time are teenagers driving, when is child's bedtime).
      b. Child's ability to swallow pills or capsules
      c. Concomitant disease states (e.g., tic disorders)
      d. Adverse effect profile
      e. Concerns about abuse or diversion potential
         i. Children with ADHD are more likely to have a concurrent substance use disorder than those without ADHD.
         ii. Treatment with stimulant medication may reduce the risk of developing a substance use disorder.
         iii. Children treated with stimulants at a younger age are less likely to misuse or abuse substances than those in whom treatment is delayed.
      f. Expense

2. Available pharmacologic agents
   a. Stimulant medications: Some children with ADHD respond better to one stimulant type than another; therefore, both methylphenidate- and amphetamine-containing products should be tried before stimulant treatment is deemed a failure.
      i. Methylphenidate-containing products
         (a) Ramp effect: Behavioral effects are proportional to the rate of methylphenidate absorption into the central nervous system.
         (b) See Table 8 for a comparison of available products.
         (c) Adverse effects and precautions
            (1) Headache, stomachache, loss of appetite, and insomnia
            (2) Use with caution in patients with glaucoma, tics, psychosis, and concomitant monoamine oxidase inhibitor use.
            (3) Insomnia, anorexia, and tics occur more often with transdermal patch, also mild skin reactions.
      ii. Amphetamine-containing products
         (a) See Table 8 for a comparison of available products.
         (b) Adverse effects and precautions
            (1) Loss of appetite, insomnia, abdominal pain, and nervousness
            (2) May exacerbate preexisting hypertension and tic disorders
            (3) Labeling change warns of potential association with sudden cardiac death (SCD); therefore, not recommended for patients with known structural heart defects.
      iii. Potential association with SCD
         (a) No established evidence of causative relationship between stimulants and SCD
         (b) The frequency of SCD is no higher in children taking stimulants than in the general pediatric population.
         (c) The AAP recommends targeted cardiac history and careful physical examination before initiating stimulant therapy.
            (1) Routine electrocardiography is not recommended unless history and physical examination suggest cardiac disease.
            (2) For otherwise healthy children, stimulant therapy should not be withheld because of the inability to obtain an electrocardiogram or assessment by a pediatric cardiologist.
   b. Nonstimulant medications
      i. Norepinephrine reuptake inhibitors (see Table 9)
         (a) Adverse effects: Dyspepsia, decreased appetite, weight loss, and fatigue
         (b) Labeling change warns of potential for severe liver injury, although routine monitoring of hepatic function is not necessary.
         (c) Black box warning about increased risk of suicidal ideation in children and adolescents
         (d) Does not exacerbate tics
      ii. α-Adrenergic receptor agonists: See Table 9 for a comparison of available products.
      iii. Antidepressants: Non-FDA label approved for the treatment of ADHD
         (a) Noradrenergic antidepressant (e.g., bupropion [Wellbutrin])
            (1) May use immediate- or extended-release product given in two or three doses
            (2) Contraindicated for children with active seizure disorder
         (b) Tricyclic antidepressants (e.g., imipramine, nortriptyline)
            (1) Baseline electrocardiogram is recommended before therapy initiation and after each dose increase.
            (2) Desipramine should be used with extreme caution because of reports of sudden death.

Table 8. Stimulant Agents for the Treatment of ADHD

Methylphenidate-Containing Products			
Medication	**Doses per Day**	**Onset of Effect**	**Duration of Effect (hours)**	**Other Comments**
---	---	---	---	---
Methylphenidate immediate release (Ritalin)	2 or 3	20–60 minutes	3–5	50:50 racemic mixture of L-threo and D-threo isomers
Dexmethylphenidate (Focalin)	2 or 3	20–60 minutes	3–5	Only D-threo isomer, thought to be pharmacologically active enantiomer D-Threo isomer has not been shown to hinder effectiveness or increase adverse effects Recommended doses are half those of methylphenidate immediate release Offers no proven pharmacoeconomic benefit over methylphenidate immediate-release products
Methylphenidate sustained release (Ritalin SR)	1 or 2	1–3 hours	2–6	
Methylphenidate extended release (Ritalin LA)	1	20–60 minutes	6–8	Contains 50% immediate-release and 50% extended-release beads Capsule may be opened and sprinkled on applesauce Efficacy may wane in after-school or late-afternoon hours, necessitating addition of methylphenidate immediate release for later-day coverage
Methylphenidate modified release (Metadate CD)	1	20–60 minutes	6–8	Capsule contains 30% immediate-release and 70% extended-release beads (slowly released about 4 hours after ingestion) Capsule may be opened and sprinkled on applesauce Efficacy may wane in after-school or late-afternoon hours, necessitating addition of methylphenidate immediate release for later-day coverage
Methylphenidate extended release (Methylin ER)	1	20–60 minutes	8	
Dexmethylphenidate extended release (Focalin XR)	1	20–60 minutes	8–12	Bimodal drug release results in peak serum concentrations at 1½ and 6½ hours after dose administration Shorter duration of action than methylphenidate OROS, so afternoon symptom control is not as good
Methylphenidate OROS (Concerta)	1	20–60 minutes	12	Outer capsule contains ~22% of the drug, allowing immediate release; tablet core contains remainder of drug, which is released over 10 hours, minimizing peak to trough fluctuations Swallow whole; do NOT chew, crush, or divide
Methylphenidate transdermal system (Daytrana)	1	60 minutes	11–12	Apply to hip 2 hours before effect is needed Recommended to remove 9 hours after application; may be worn up to 16 hours Duration of effect is ~3 hours after patch removal May be worn while swimming or exercising

Table 8. Stimulant Agents for the Treatment of ADHD *(continued)*

Amphetamine-Containing Products				
Medication	**Doses per Day**	**Onset of Effect**	**Duration of Effect (hours)**	**Other Comments**
Mixed amphetamine salts immediate release (Adderall)	1 or 2	20–60 minutes	6	
Mixed amphetamine salts extended release (Adderall XR)	1	20–60 minutes	10	Contains 50% immediate-release and 50% extended-release beads (released 4 hours after ingestion) May be sprinkled on applesauce
Lisdexamfetamine dimesylate (Vyvanse)	1	60 minutes	10–12	Prodrug with D-amphetamine covalently bound to L-lysine Designed for less abuse potential than amphetamine No clinical evidence of superiority over other amphetamine products

ADHD = attention-deficit/hyperactivity disorder.

Table 9. Nonstimulant Agents for the Treatment of ADHD

Norepinephrine Reuptake Inhibitor				
Medication	**Doses per Day**	**Onset of Effect (weeks)**	**Duration of Effect (hours)**	**Other Comments**
Atomoxetine (Strattera)	1 or 2	2–4	10–12	May be considered first-line therapy for children with active substance abuse problem, comorbid anxiety, or tics Metabolized through cytochrome P450 2D6
α-Adrenergic Receptor Agonists				
Clonidine extended release (Kapvay)	1 or 2	1–2	10–12	May be more effective for hyperactivity than for inattention symptoms Lessens severity of tics, especially when used in combination with methylphenidate Primary adverse effect is sedation
Guanfacine extended release (Intuniv)	1	1–2	10–12	Improves comorbid tic disorder Less sedating than clonidine Abrupt discontinuation may cause rebound hypertension

ADHD = attention-deficit/hyperactivity disorder.

Patient Case

12. The patient in question 11 has been doing well in school since methylphenidate (OROS) (Concerta) was initiated 6 months ago. His late-afternoon symptoms are well controlled; however, he has had insomnia since drug therapy initiation. Which is the best modification to his treatment regimen?

    A. Administer the Concerta dose later in the day.

    B. Change to methylphenidate modified release (Metadate CD) once a day.

    C. Change to methylphenidate transdermal patch (Daytrana).

    D. Change to atomoxetine at bedtime.

REFERENCES

Sepsis and Meningitis

1. American Academy of Pediatrics (AAP). Meningococcal infections. In: Pickering LK, ed. 2012 Red Book: Report of the Committee on Infectious Diseases, 29th ed. Elk Grove Village, IL: American Academy of Pediatrics, 2012:500-9.

2. Brierly J, Carcillo JA, Choong K, et al. Clinical practice parameters for hemodynamic support of pediatric and neonatal septic shock: 2007 update from the American College of Critical Care Medicine. Crit Care Med 2009;37:666-88.

3. Dellinger RP, Levy MM, Rhodes A, et al. Surviving sepsis campaign: international guidelines for management of severe sepsis and septic shock: 2012. Crit Care Med 2013;41:580-637.

4. Polin RA; Committee on Fetus and Newborn. Sepsis management of neonates with suspected or proven early onset bacterial sepsis. Pediatrics 2012;129:1006-15.

5. Wubbel L, McCracken GH. Management of bacterial meningitis: 1998. Pediatr Rev 1998;19:78-84.

Respiratory Syncytial Virus Infection

1. American Academy of Pediatrics Committee on Infectious Diseases and Bronchiolitis Guidelines Committee. Policy statement: updated guidance for palivizumab prophylaxis among infants and young children at increased risk of hospitalization for respiratory syncytial virus infection. Pediatrics 2014;134:415-20.

2. American Academy of Pediatrics Committee on Infectious Diseases and Bronchiolitis Guidelines Committee. Technical report: updated guidance for palivizumab prophylaxis among infants and young children at increased risk of hospitalization for respiratory syncytial virus infection. Pediatrics 2014;134:e620-e638.

3. American Academy of Pediatrics (AAP). Respiratory syncytial virus. In: Pickering LK, ed. 2012 Red Book: Report of the Committee on Infectious Diseases, 29th ed. Elk Grove Village, IL: American Academy of Pediatrics, 2012:609-18.

4. Mendonca EA, Phelan KJ, Zorc JJ, et al. Clinical practice guideline: the diagnosis, management, and prevention of bronchiolitis. Pediatrics 2014;134:e1474-e1502.

Otitis Media

1. American Academy of Pediatrics (AAP). Principles of appropriate use for upper respiratory tract infections. In: Pickering LK, ed. 2012 Red Book: Report of the Committee on Infectious Diseases, 29th ed. Elk Grove Village, IL: American Academy of Pediatrics, 2012:802-5.

2. Lieberthal AS, Carrol AE, Chonmaitree T, et al. Clinical practice guideline: diagnosis and management of acute otitis media. Pediatrics 2013;131:e964-e999.

3. Rettig E, Tunkel DE. Contemporary concepts in management of acute otitis media in children. Otolaryngol Clin N Am 2014;47:651-72.

Immunizations

1. American Academy of Pediatrics (AAP). Active and passive immunization. In: Pickering LK, ed. 2012 Red Book: Report of the Committee on Infectious Diseases, 29th ed. Elk Grove Village, IL: American Academy of Pediatrics, 2012:1-109.

2. Wiley CC. Immunizations: vaccinations in general. Pediatr Rev 2015;36:249-59.

3. Smith M. Vaccine safety: medical contraindications, myths, and risk communication. Pediatr Rev 2015;36:227-238.

Pediatric Seizure Disorders

1. Anderson GD. Children versus adults: pharmacokinetic and adverse-effect differences. Epilepsia 2002;43(suppl 3):53-9.

2. Asconape JJ. Some common issues in the use of antiepileptic drugs. Semin Neurol 2002;22:27-39.

3. Sarco DP, Bourgeois BFD. The safety and tolerability of newer antiepileptic drugs in children and adolescents. CNS Drugs 2010;24:399-430.

4. Sheth R, Gidel B. Optimizing epilepsy management in teenagers. J Child Neurol 2006;21:273-9.

Attention-Deficit/Hyperactivity Disorder

1. American Academy of Pediatrics (AAP). Subcommittee on attention-deficit/hyperactivity disorder. ADHD: clinical practice guideline for the diagnosis, evaluation, and treatment of attention-deficit/hyperactivity disorder in children and adolescents. Pediatrics 2011;128:1007-22.

2. American Psychiatric Association. Diagnostic and Statistical Manual of Mental Disorders, 5th ed. Arlington, VA: American Psychiatric Association, 2013.

3. Cortese S, Holtmann M, Banaschewski T, et al. Practitioner review: current best practice in the management of adverse events during treatment with ADHD medications in children and adolescents. J Child Psychol Psychiatry 2013;54:227-46.

4. Harstad E, Levy S, and Committee on Substance Abuse. Attention-deficit/hyperactivity disorder and substance abuse. Pediatrics 2014;134:e293-301.

5. Kaplan G, Newcorn JH. Pharmacotherapy for child and adolescent attention-deficit hyperactivity disorder. Pediatr Clin North Am 2011;58:99-120.

ANSWERS AND EXPLANATIONS TO PATIENT CASES

1. Answer: B

Group B *Streptococcus, Escherichia coli, Klebsiella* spp., and *Listeria* are the most likely pathogens of neonatal sepsis or meningitis. Ampicillin plus gentamicin administered in meningitic doses would provide reasonable empiric coverage. Although coagulase-negative *Staphylococcus* is the most likely cause of nosocomial neonatal sepsis, this patient's early presentation makes a hospital-acquired pathogen extremely unlikely. Therefore, vancomycin is unnecessary. Ampicillin plus ceftriaxone would provide adequate empiric antimicrobial coverage for the most likely pathogens. However, ceftriaxone use can result in biliary sludging, leading to reduced elimination of bilirubin and a potential risk of kernicterus in neonates. Ceftazidime plus gentamicin lacks coverage for *Listeria* and group B *Streptococcus,* which is still necessary empirically even though the mother received penicillin before delivery. In addition, empiric double-coverage of gram-negative organisms is not necessary for early neonatal sepsis.

2. Answer: C

Given this patient's age and culture results, the most likely infecting organism is *E. coli* or *Klebsiella* spp. (gram-negative rods), for which antimicrobial prophylaxis is not indicated. The most common pathogens causing meningitis in neonates do not warrant antimicrobial prophylaxis. If this patient had been older and infected with *N. meningitidis* or *H. influenzae,* antibiotic prophylaxis with rifampin would have been indicated for all close contacts, regardless of age or immunization status. Rifampin prophylaxis to eliminate nasal carriage is also indicated for people who receive index diagnoses of *N. meningitidis* and treatment with an antibiotic other than ceftriaxone.

3. Answer: C

The most likely causative organisms of sepsis or meningitis in this age group are *S. pneumoniae* and *N. meningitidis.* Therefore, a regimen of ceftriaxone plus vancomycin would provide appropriate empiric coverage. Depending on the regional incidence of resistant *S. pneumoniae,* empiric vancomycin may not be necessary. Ampicillin plus gentamicin would not provide adequate coverage. Cefuroxime does not provide reliable penetration into the cerebrospinal fluid, so it would not be appropriate empiric coverage because this patient's presentation suggests he has meningitis. Rifampin would be the drug of choice for the prophylaxis of close contacts if this patient receives a diagnosis of meningococcal meningitis; however, it is inadequate for treatment.

4. Answer: B

Palivizumab is the drug of choice for prophylaxis against RSV infection in high-risk patient populations, including those born before 29 weeks' gestation, regardless of risk factors, who are 12 months or younger during RSV season. Patients born between 29 weeks' gestation and 32 weeks' gestation are no longer considered high risk based solely on their gestational age. To be considered as candidates for palivizumab prophylaxis, these infants must have a disease state (e.g., chronic lung disease, hemodynamically significant heart disease, airway anomalies, neuromuscular disease, or profound immunodeficiency) that puts them at risk for severe RSV infection. Other potential risk factors (e.g., siblings younger than 5 years or day care attenders) are no longer considered when determining the appropriateness of palivizumab prophylaxis. Patients with complex heart defects needing surgical repair are at high risk of developing severe RSV infections; however, after the repair is complete, palivizumab is no longer warranted. Patients with a history of chronic lung disease who are 24 months or younger and who are receiving, or have received in the past 6 months, oxygen or medical management for chronic lung disease are also at risk of severe RSV infection.

5. Answer: D

There is no specific treatment of RSV infection. Intravenous fluids, oxygen, and mechanical ventilation, if needed, are indicated. Palivizumab is the drug of choice for RSV prophylaxis, but it has no role in treatment. Corticosteroids have not been shown to be of benefit and are therefore not indicated. Secondary bacterial infection with *H. influenzae* or *M. catarrhalis* may occur; however, empiric antibiotic therapy is not indicated.

6. Answer: A

Persistence of middle ear fluid after an episode of AOM is common. If these findings are not associated with signs and symptoms of infection, a diagnosis of OME is made. The AAP practice guideline for the management of OME recommends watchful waiting. A watch-and-wait approach would not be appropriate for this patient if she were given a diagnosis of AOM rather than OME because she is younger than 6 months. Spontaneous resolution of OME occurs within 3 months in 75%–90% of cases after AOM without residual morbidities. Children at high risk of speech and learning problems (e.g., craniofacial anomalies, Down syndrome, severe visual impairment) may need earlier, more aggressive intervention (e.g., tympanostomy tubes). Decongestants and antihistamines do not promote resolution or improve symptoms. Antibiotics are not effective in treating OME. However, high-dose amoxicillin (80–100 mg/kg/day) is considered first-line therapy for AOM, so if this patient's treatment with the initial course of lower-dose amoxicillin fails (which is not a recommended regimen) or if she develops new signs of infection, then high-dose amoxicillin will be an appropriate treatment choice. Up to 74% of streptococcal strains have been reported to be resistant to azithromycin, which also has poor activity against *H. influenzae*, so this would not be the best antibiotic option if an infection developed.

7. Answer: C

Four cases of otitis media in 12 months is considered recurrent otitis media, for which the watch-and-wait approach is not recommended. Previously, this patient would have been a candidate for antibiotic prophylaxis; however, this practice has fallen out of favor because of the significant risk of antimicrobial resistance compared with the minor reduction in the occurrence of otitis media. Tympanostomy tubes are typically reserved for patients in whom aggressive antibiotic therapy fails and may be effective only in otitis with bulging tympanic membrane. In addition, the greatest benefit of tympanostomy tubes may be in patients with persistent OMEs resulting in significant hearing loss. As long as this patient continues to respond to high-dose amoxicillin, this will be considered a first-line regimen. In addition, the pneumococcal and influenza vaccines should be administered according to the recommended schedule because these organisms are common causes of AOM.

8. Answer: D

Vaccines are often deferred for inappropriate reasons, leading to missed opportunities for immunization. Previous administration of IVIG can decrease the efficacy of live vaccines such as MMR and varicella, but it does not affect the efficacy of inactivated products. The suggested interval between an IVIG dose and the administration of live vaccines depends on the immune globulin product and indication. Concerns about an association between MMR vaccine and the development of autism and immunizations overwhelming the immune system have been disproven by scientific evaluation. The MMR vaccine is grown in chick embryo tissue; however, an egg allergy is not a contraindication to its administration.

9. Answer: A

Immunocompromised patients should not receive live vaccines; therefore, the MMR and varicella vaccines should be deferred in these patients. Mild cold-like symptoms, or administration of antibiotics for mild illnesses such as otitis media, are not a contraindication to vaccination, and deferring immunizations for such reasons is considered a missed opportunity. Patients with HIV, especially those with asymptomatic disease, should be considered candidates for all age-appropriate vaccines, including those containing live virus and the pneumococcal vaccine. Corticosteroid administration is an indication for deferral of live vaccines only if the patient is receiving high doses (more than 2 mg/kg/day of prednisone equivalent) for more than 14 days.

10. Answer: B

Rash associated with antiepileptic drugs is a common adverse effect and generally resolves within a few days after discontinuation. There is no reliable method to determine whether the rash will remain benign or progress to a more severe skin reaction, so discontinuation of the offending drug is warranted. Carbamazepine has a higher incidence of rash than oxcarbazepine, and cross-reactivity has been noted. Valproic acid is a good choice for managing partial seizures and has a low incidence of rash. However, the principal adverse effects of valproic acid include weight gain and menstrual irregularities, both of which would be undesirable in this overweight teenage girl. In addition, valproic acid is a known teratogen (pregnancy category D) that should be avoided if other options are available in girls of reproductive age who are unreliable in their use of con- traception. Levetiracetam (pregnancy category C) has a low incidence of rash and minimal drug interactions.

11. Answer: A

Stimulants, especially methylphenidate, are gener- ally considered first-line therapy for treating ADHD. Because this patient shows symptoms at school and at home, the short duration of action (about 3-5 hours) of a twice-daily methylphenidate immediate-release regimen will probably not provide adequate symp- tom relief. Likewise, D-methylphenidate has a short duration of action. In addition, D-methylphenidate is no more effective and has no fewer adverse effects than methylphenidate immediate release. Therefore, D-methylphenidate is generally not considered cost- effective. Extended-release guanfacine was recently FDA label approved for the treatment of ADHD, but it should be reserved for patients with ADHD and tic disorders or those who have not responded to stimu- lant agents. Methylphenidate (OROS) with its longer duration of action (10–12 hours) would provide the best coverage. Therapy with this drug may be initiated with- out previous titration using methylphenidate immediate release.

12. Answer: C

Changing to a methylphenidate transdermal patch allows flexibility in the duration of drug effect. Wearing the patch for 9 hours results in about 12 hours of ther- apeutic effect; however, the patch may be removed sooner, thus reducing the duration of effect and allow- ing serum concentrations to decrease before bedtime. Response rates to atomoxetine are lower than to meth- ylphenidate (OROS) in children with ADHD. In addi- tion, the onset of therapeutic effect for atomoxetine is delayed (typically 2–4 weeks). Atomoxetine does not have the adverse effect of insomnia. Rather, fatigue and drowsiness are more common, the tolerability of which is improved with the initiation of atomoxetine at low doses with a gradual titration. The dose may also be administered in the evening to improve tolerabil- ity. Because this patient responded well to stimulant therapy with methylphenidate and there are disadvan- tages to atomoxetine (i.e., lower response rates and delayed onset), it would be best to manage the adverse effect of insomnia by altering the stimulant regimen.

Administering methylphenidate OROS later in the day would probably worsen the insomnia. A better recom- mendation would be to administer methylphenidate OROS earlier in the morning, which would allow more time in the late afternoon and evening for the serum concentration to decrease before bedtime. Changing to a shorter-acting methylphenidate product (e.g., meth- ylphenidate CD or LA) might improve the insomnia, but because of its shorter duration of action, it might compromise late-afternoon symptom control. In some cases, insomnia is related to rebound of ADHD symp- toms when the stimulant wears off, rather than a side effect of the stimulant. Addition of a short-acting stimulant late in the day may help in these cases. This does not seem to apply to this patient because his late afternoon ADHD symptoms are reported to be well controlled. Counseling about proper sleep hygiene can also be an effective intervention for the management of insomnia.

ANSWERS AND EXPLANATIONS TO SELF-ASSESSMENT QUESTIONS

1. Answer: B

The pathogens most likely to cause pediatric sepsis or meningitis are *S. pneumoniae, N. meningitidis,* and *H. influenzae. P. aeruginosa* is more commonly associated with nosocomial sepsis. Adolescents who develop an RSV infection typically present with mild upper respiratory tract symptoms, whereas this patient's presentation suggests meningitis.

2. Answer: B

Before the 2014 publication of the AAP's updated guidelines, infants who were born before 31 weeks', 6 days' gestation who were 6 months or younger at the beginning of RSV season were considered at high risk of severe infection; therefore, routine palivizumab prophylaxis was recommended based solely on their prematurity. The 2014 guidelines changed the prematurity-based criteria for routine palivizumab prophylaxis to include only infants born before 29 weeks' gestation who are younger than 12 months at the beginning of RSV season. According to the new guidelines, infants born between 29 and 32 weeks' gestation must have chronic lung disease, hemodynamically significant congenital heart disease, airway anomalies, neuromuscular disease, or profound immunocompromise to be considered candidates for palivizumab prophylaxis. Risk factors such as day care attendance and school-aged siblings are no longer considered when determining whether prophylaxis is warranted. Routine prophylaxis for otherwise healthy, full-term neonates is not recommended because evidence of benefit is lacking.

3. Answer: C

Prophylaxis with rifampin is recommended for close contacts of patients with *N. meningitidis* or *H. influenzae,* regardless of their immunization status. Postexposure prophylaxis against pneumococcal meningitis is not recommended.

4. Answer: D

All scheduled immunizations should be given during the same visit. Delaying some vaccines until a later date is considered a missed opportunity. Oral polio vaccine is no longer recommended as part of the routine schedule because of the risk of vaccine-associated poliomyelitis, which accounts for most newly diagnosed cases in the United States since 1979. Premature neonates should be vaccinated according to chronologic age, and doses should not be reduced. As of 2008, influenza vaccine is recommended for all children 6 months to 18 years of age during influenza season.

5. Answer: B

Otitis media is most commonly caused by *S. pneumoniae, H. influenzae, M. catarrhalis,* and viruses. Blood culture results do not predict causative organisms of otitis media. If the patient is older than 2 years and does not have severe symptoms (i.e., moderate to severe otalgia or temperature of 39°C or greater), delaying the decision to prescribe antibiotics is an acceptable strategy. If otalgia or fever persists for more than 48–72 hours, then antibiotic therapy is acceptable, but if these symptoms resolve spontaneously within this time, antibiotics are not necessary. If antibiotics are warranted and the patient does not have an allergy, high-dose amoxicillin is the treatment of choice rather than azithromycin. Broad-spectrum antibiotics such as ceftriaxone should be reserved for resistant cases.

6. Answer: D

In general, patients who do not respond to one stimulant agent should be treated with a different stimulant before they are considered not to have responded to this class of drug therapy. However, switching from a methylphenidate-containing stimulant to extended-release mixed amphetamine salts (a different stimulant) should be avoided in this patient because amphetamine-containing products have been associated with SCD in children with structural heart defects. The methylphenidate transdermal system has a duration of action and efficacy similar to those of methylphenidate OROS; therefore, it is unlikely to benefit this patient because her therapy with methylphenidate immediate release and methylphenidate OROS has already failed. If adherence or difficulty swallowing pills were a suspected cause of treatment failure in this patient, a patch might be a reasonable alternative. Clonidine may be added as an adjunctive therapy for patients whose treatment with a single stimulant agent fails; however, it should not be used as the sole agent for treating ADHD. Atomoxetine, a nonstimulant, would be a reasonable alternative to the stimulant class of agents in this patient because some patients respond better to one class of agent than another.

7. Answer: A

Valproic acid is considered a first-line therapy for treating absence seizures. If the patient is having breakthrough seizures on ethosuximide—also a first-line therapy—and the dose has been maximized, it is reasonable to switch to valproic acid. Phenytoin, phenobarbital, and gabapentin have not been shown effective in treating absence seizures.

8. Answer: C

	Adverse Event (loss of appetite)	
	Yes	No
Exposure (stimulant)		
Yes	7 (*a*)	193 (*b*)
No	1 (*c*)	197 (*d*)

Odds ratio = (*a*/*c*)/(*b*/*d*)

$\qquad$ = (7/1)/(193/197)

$\qquad$ = 7.15

9. Answer: C

A case series does not reliably establish a causal relationship but rather suggests a potential hypothesis to be further studied. Given the current knowledge about the potential risk of kernicterus related to ceftriaxone use, obtaining investigational review board approval for a randomized controlled or a crossover trial design would be difficult, given ethical considerations, although this study design is the gold standard for establishing a causal relationship. Therefore, a retrospective cohort would be best to investigate a causal relationship in this instance.

10. Answer: D

Patients with congenital heart defects, particularly those with hemodynamically significant lesions, are at high risk of severe RSV infection regardless of their gestational age. These patients are considered to be at high risk if they are younger than 12 months at the beginning of RSV season and have not undergone definitive surgical repair of their heart defect. It is not recommended that palivizumab be initiated as routine prophylaxis in hospitalized patients because it does not reduce the incidence of nosocomial-acquired RSV infection. However, patients currently receiving a course of palivizumab (one dose per month for 5 months) at the time of hospital admission should have that intervention continued.

In addition, cardiopulmonary bypass reduces palivizumab serum concentrations; therefore, patients undergoing congenital heart defect repair during RSV season should receive a postoperative dose of palivizumab as soon as they are medically stable, regardless of when their next scheduled dose is due.

Geriatrics

Lisa C. Hutchison, Pharm.D., MPH, BCPS, FCCP

University of Arkansas for Medical Sciences
College of Pharmacy
Little Rock, Arkansas

Geriatrics

Lisa C. Hutchison, Pharm.D., MPH, BCPS, FCCP

University of Arkansas for Medical Sciences
College of Pharmacy
Little Rock, Arkansas

Learning Objectives

1. Summarize common age-related pharmacokinetic and pharmacodynamic changes in older adults.
2. Evaluate the pharmacotherapeutic regimens of older adults to support optimal risk and benefit of medications.
3. Assess inappropriate medication prescribing in older adults using accepted tools.
4. Recommend appropriate pharmacotherapy for patients with dementia.
5. Evaluate the risks and benefits of antipsychotic use in older adults with dementia.
6. Recommend appropriate interventions for patients with BPSD (behavioral and psychological symptoms of dementia).
7. Differentiate between the types of urinary incontinence and recommend appropriate treatments.
8. Recommend an appropriate BPH (benign prostatic hypertrophy) treatment based on the AUASI (American Urological Association Symptom Index).
9. Recommend appropriate analgesic therapy for older adults with osteoarthritis.
10. Discuss the risks and benefits of medication classes used to treat rheumatoid arthritis and associated comorbidities.

Self-Assessment Questions

Answers and explanations to these questions can be found at the end of this chapter.

Questions 1 and 2 pertain to the following case:
An 85-year-old man presents to the primary care clinic after the death of his spouse 1 month ago. His medical history is significant for hypertension, hyperlipidemia, benign prostatic hypertrophy (BPH), and major depressive disorder. His current medications include lisinopril 10 mg daily, atorvastatin 20 mg daily, tamsulosin 0.4 mg daily, diazepam 5 mg at bedtime as needed for sleep, and escitalopram 10 mg daily. His daughter reports that he has been more lethargic and unsteady walking during the past 3 days. The patient reports trouble sleeping and taking diazepam every night this past week. His blood pressure is 135/72 mm Hg, and his heart rate is 76 beats/minute. Urinalysis was negative, thyroid-stimulating hormone (TSH) was within the reference range, and Geriatric Depression Scale (GDS) score was 6/15.

1. Which medication is contributing most to this patient's lethargy and confusion?
   A. Diazepam.
   B. Lisinopril.
   C. Atorvastatin.
   D. Escitalopram.

2. Which age-related change in pharmacokinetics is most likely to underlie this patient's medication-related problem?
   A. Delayed oral absorption.
   B. Decreased renal excretion.
   C. Slowed metabolism in the liver.
   D. Decreased volume of distribution.

Questions 3–5 pertain to the following case:
A 76-year-old woman was recently admitted to a long-term care facility for rehabilitation after multiple falls at home. Her medical history is significant for hypertension, hypothyroidism, Alzheimer disease (AD), hyperlipidemia, and osteoarthritis (OA). She currently takes metoprolol succinate 50 mg daily, levothyroxine 75 mcg daily, atorvastatin 10 mg daily, and donepezil 10 mg daily. Her BP is 126/80 mm Hg and heart rate is 66 beats/minute. Basic metabolic panel results were all within reference ranges; 25-hydroxy vitamin D level was 20 ng/mL, TSH 1.89 mU/L, total cholesterol 180 mg/dL, low-density lipoprotein cholesterol 140 mg/dL, high-density lipoprotein cholesterol 35 mg/dL, and triglycerides 176 mg/dL. Her Mini–Mental State Examination (MMSE) score was 16/30, and her GDS score was 2/15.

3. Which recommendation would be most appropriate to reduce the risk of falls in this patient?
   A. Begin memantine titration.
   B. Initiate vitamin D 1000 units daily.
   C. Decrease metoprolol succinate to 25 mg daily.
   D. Initiate calcium carbonate 500 mg twice daily.

4. Which is the best intervention for reducing the incidence of ischemic stroke in this patient?
   A. Initiate aspirin 81 mg daily.
   B. Increase atorvastatin to 20 mg daily.

C.   Initiate hydrochlorothiazide 25 mg daily.

D.   Increase metoprolol succinate to 100 mg daily.

5.   Which would be most appropriate for complaints of osteoarthritic knee pain?

A.   Ibuprofen 200 mg four times daily.

B.   Acetaminophen 650 mg three times daily.

C.   Tramadol 50 mg three times daily as needed for pain.

D.   Hydrocodone/acetaminophen 5/325 mg every 4 hours as needed for pain.

Questions 6–8 pertain to the following case:
An 80-year-old woman presents to your clinic accompanied by her daughter, who no longer feels comfortable leaving her mother alone because of her mother's "increasing forgetfulness." Her medical history is significant for type 2 diabetes, hypertension, coronary artery disease, congestive heart failure, and OA. She takes the following medications: acetaminophen 650 mg every 6 hours as needed for pain, lisinopril 20 mg daily, furosemide 20 mg daily, potassium chloride 20 mEq daily, carvedilol 12.5 mg twice daily, and glipizide 5 mg daily. Her MMSE score was 18/30. Blood tests obtained last week showed a normal basic metabolic panel, with the exception of a fasting plasma glucose reading of 65 mg/dL. Her hemoglobin A1C result was 5.6%. A urinalysis was negative. No nutritional deficiencies were noted. The patient's blood pressure is 130/80 mm Hg, and her heart rate is 60 beats/minute. She receives a diagnosis of AD.

6.   Which initial intervention would be most appropriate to help with this patient's cognitive function?

A.   Donepezil 10 mg daily.

B.   Galantamine ER 24 mg daily.

C.   Memantine 10 mg twice daily.

D.   Rivastigmine patch 4.6 mg daily.

7.   Which intervention would be most appropriate to prevent an adverse drug reaction?

A.   Discontinue glipizide.

B.   Discontinue lisinopril.

C.   Reduce carvedilol to 6.25 mg twice daily.

D.   Reduce potassium chloride to 10 mEq daily.

8.   One year later, the patient returns to the clinic. She has moved in with her daughter. Lately, she wanders around the house continuously. She often changes clothes and asks repetitive questions. Her current medication regimen includes donepezil 10 mg daily, which she has been taking for the past 6 months. Which would be most appropriate for this patient's new behavioral symptoms?

A.   Initiate olanzapine 5 mg daily.

B.   Initiate risperidone 0.5 mg twice daily.

C.   Change donepezil dosage to 23 mg daily.

D.   Change acetaminophen to 650 mg every 6 hours around the clock.

9.   An 80-year-old woman had a total right knee replacement 3 days ago after conservative strategies for OA failed. Her medical history is significant for hypothyroidism, OA, and hyperlipidemia. Her current medications include simvastatin 20 mg daily, risedronate 35 mg weekly, levothyroxine 75 mcg daily, and oxycodone/acetaminophen 5/325 mg 1 tablet every 4 hours as needed for moderate pain. She is in the hospital preparing for discharge. As the pharmacist is counseling the patient on her discharge medication, the patient reports experiencing a new onset of "losing her water" the day before and again overnight. Which intervention would be most appropriate for this patient?

A.   Urinalysis.

B.   Pelvic floor exercises.

C.   Tolterodine 2 mg daily.

D.   Duloxetine 20 mg daily.

Questions 10 and 11 pertain to the following case:
A 69-year-old man with hypertension and BPH is admitted to the hospital after being involved in a motorcycle collision. He sustained serious injuries, resulting in a left leg above-the-knee amputation, and has undergone several surgeries and rehabilitation in the past 2 weeks. His current medications include tamsulosin 0.4 mg daily, atenolol 25 mg daily, amlodipine 10 mg daily, senna/docusate 8.6/50 mg twice daily, oxycodone controlled release 10 mg every 12 hours, and hydromorphone 4 mg every 3 hours as needed for breakthrough pain (uses 1–2 daily). His current blood pressure is 155/88 mm Hg, heart rate is 84 beats/

minute, and postvoid residual (PVR) volume is 400 mL after voiding 110 mL. His chronic medical conditions are unremarkable except for hypertension, BPH, and gastroesophageal reflux disease (GERD).

10. Which intervention would be most appropriate for this patient?

    A. Increase tamsulosin to 0.8 mg.

    B. Increase atenolol to 50 mg daily.

    C. Change tamsulosin to terazosin 5 mg daily.

    D. Reduce hydromorphone to 2 mg every 3 hours as needed for breakthrough pain.

11. One year later, the patient has OA of his right knee. His current medications are amlodipine 10 mg daily, acetaminophen 1000 mg three times daily, omeprazole 40 mg daily, and aspirin 81 mg daily. Which agent would be best to initiate for this patient's knee pain?

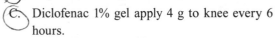

    A. Celecoxib 200 mg daily

    B. Naproxen 500 mg twice daily

    C. Diclofenac 1% gel apply 4 g to knee every 6 hours.

    D. Methylprednisolone 40 mg injected into affected joint.

Questions 12 and 13 pertain to the following case:
A 72-year-old woman, whose medical history is significant for rheumatoid arthritis, type 2 diabetes, GERD, and hypothyroidism, presents to the clinic with inflammation of the joints of the hands and stiffness lasting 1–2 hours in the morning. She is a smoker, weighs 82 kg, and is 66 inches tall. Her current medications include pantoprazole 40 mg daily, metformin 850 mg twice daily, levothyroxine 100 mcg daily, folic acid 1 mg daily, methotrexate 12.5 mg weekly, naproxen 500 mg twice daily, calcium 600 mg twice daily, and vitamin D 1000 units twice daily. Her laboratory tests show a negative rheumatoid factor but positive anti–cyclic citrullinated peptides. The physician determines that this is a flare of moderate disease.

12. Which would be the most appropriate intervention for this patient's rheumatoid arthritis?

    A. Change naproxen to prednisone 20 mg daily.

    B. Change methotrexate to 25 mg intramuscularly.

    C. Switch methotrexate to leflunomide 20 mg daily.

    D. Add sulfasalazine 500 mg twice daily and hydroxychloroquine 400 mg daily.

13. Three months later, the patient has responded to therapy. A bone mineral density T-score of –2.0 is reported from her latest scan. Her vitamin D level is 40 ng/mL. Which recommendation would be most appropriate to help reduce the risk of major osteoporotic fractures in this patient?

    A. Give raloxifene 60 mg daily.

    B. Give risedronate 35 mg weekly.

    C. Give teriparatide 20 mcg subcutaneously daily.

    D. Increase to calcium 600 mg and vitamin D 2000 mg twice daily.

BPS Pharmacotherapy Specialty Examination Content Outline

This chapter covers the following sections of the Pharmacotherapy Specialty Examination Content Outline:

1. Domain 1: Patient–specific Pharmacotherapy
    a. Tasks 1a, 1b, 2a, 2b, 2c, 3a, 3b, 3c, 3d, 4a, 4b, 4c, 4d, 6a and 6b
    b. Systems and Patient-Care Problems:
        i. Dementia
        ii. Behavioral Symptoms of Dementia
        iii. Urinary Incontinence
        iv. Benign Prostatic Hypertrophy
        v. Arthritis
        vi. Osteoarthritis and Rheumatoid Arthritis

I. OPTIMIZING PHARMACOTHERAPY IN OLDER ADULTS

A. Aging
   1. Aging is a normal process whereby the human body declines after peak growth and development. In general, aging results as the body responds to environmental stressors according to the person's health and lifestyle factors together with genetic makeup. If environmental stressors are severe enough or individual factors have too small a reserve capacity, aging causes frailty, disability, and increased vulnerability to disease and death.
   2. At present, 13.3% (2010 U.S. Census) of Americans are 65 years or older. This figure is projected to rise to 20% by 2050. Older adults constitute about 13% of the population, but they are responsible for:
      a. 34% of medication costs
      b. 36% of hospital stays
      c. 40% of medication-related hospitalizations
      d. 50% of medication-related deaths
   3. At least $30 billion/year is spent on medication-related morbidity.
   4. There is large heterogeneity in older people: Diversity is increasing, and incomes have a wide range; some people live independently into their 90s and beyond, whereas others become frail and dependent at a younger age. Measurement of aging with years of life is insensitive to the differences between older people.
      a. If an individual survives to age 65, it is likely that he or she will live an additional 13–20 years.
      b. If an individual survives to age 85, it is likely that he or she will live an additional 6–7 years.

B. Pharmacokinetic Changes Associated with Aging
   1. Common physiologic changes occur in most older adults, but they are highly variable because of differences in genetics, lifestyle, and environment.

Table 1. Common Physiologic Changes with Age That May Change Drug Pharmacokinetics

Organ System	Physiologic Change with Aging	Effect on Pharmacokinetics
GI	↑ or no change in stomach pH ↓ GI blood flow Slowed gastric emptying Slowed GI transit	↓ Absorption of some drugs and nutrients requiring acid environment Absorption rate may be prolonged
Skin	Thinning of dermis Loss of subcutaneous fat	↓ or no change to drug reservoir formation with transdermal formulation
Body composition	↓ Total body water ↓ Lean body mass ↑ Body fat ↓ or unchanged serum albumin ↑ α_1-Acid glycoprotein	↑ Volume of distribution and accumulation of lipid-soluble drugs ↓ Volume of distribution of water-soluble drugs ↑ Free fraction of highly protein-bound drugs
Liver	↓ Liver mass ↓ Blood flow to the liver ↓ or no change in CYP enzymes	↓ First-pass extraction and metabolism ↑ Half-life and ↓ clearance of drugs with a high first-pass extraction and metabolism ↓ or no change in phase I metabolism No change in phase II drug metabolism
Renal	↓ GFR ↓ Renal blood flow ↓ Tubular secretion ↓ Renal mass	↓ Renal elimination of many medications ↑ Half-life of renally eliminated drugs and metabolites

CYP = cytochrome P450; GI = gastrointestinal.

2. Absorption
    a. Iron, vitamin B_{12}, antifungals, and calcium are decreased with hypochlorhydria or achlorhydria.
    b. Slower gastric emptying may increase risk of ulceration from aspirin, nonsteroidal anti-inflammatory drugs (NSAIDs), bisphosphonates, or potassium chloride tablets.
    c. Most drugs are absorbed by passive diffusion without significant age-related changes.
    d. Transdermal formulations usually require a subcutaneous fat layer to form a drug reservoir for absorption. Use with caution in patients who are thin or cachetic.
3. Distribution
    a. Lipid-soluble benzodiazepines such as diazepam have an increased half-life in older people.
    b. Highly albumin-bound drugs such as phenytoin may have a larger fraction of free (active) drug.
    c. P-glycoprotein, an efflux transporter for several organs including the brain, decreases with aging, which may lead to higher brain concentrations of medications. One example is opioid analgesics.
4. Metabolism
    a. Morphine and propranolol clearance are substantially reduced because of a reduction in first-pass metabolism.
    b. Changes in metabolism through phase I (oxidative) and cytochrome P450 (CYP) enzymes are variable and confounded by age, sex, concomitant drugs, and genetics.
    c. Lorazepam, oxazepam, and temazepam are dependent on phase II metabolism and are less affected by age-related changes in metabolism.
5. Elimination
    a. Drugs eliminated through glomerular filtration must be dosed according to individual estimated renal function. Chronic medication examples can be found in the 2015 American Geriatrics Society (AGS) Beers Criteria.
    b. The Cockcroft-Gault equation is a validated method to estimate creatinine clearance (CrCl) for drug dosing in older adults.
    c. The National Kidney Foundation recommends using the Chronic Kidney Disease Epidemiology Collaboration (CKD-EPI) Creatinine Equation (2009) to estimate glomerular filtration rate. However, this recommendation has not been validated in older adults.

Table 2. Differences in Renal Estimation with Common Formulas

Patient: 85-year-old person with an SCr of 1 mg/dL	Cockcroft-Gault Creatinine Clearance (mL/min/1.73 m²)	MDRD Estimated Glomerular Filtration Rate (mL/min/1.73 m²)	CKD-EPI Creatinine Clearance (mL/min/1.73 m²)
64-inch-tall white woman weighing 60 kg	39	56	51 (stage 3)
64-inch-tall African American woman weighing 60 kg	39	68	60 (stage 2)
70-inch-tall white man weighing 75 kg	57	75	68 (stage 2)
70-inch-tall African American man weighing 75 kg	57	91	79 (stage 2)
Cockcroft-Gault: CrCl = [(140 − age) × weight in kg]/[(72 × SCr)] × 0.85 if female [use actual weight if it is less than ideal body weight]			
MDRD: Estimated GFR = 186 × SCr$^{1.154}$ × Age$^{-0.203}$ × 1.21 if black × 0.742 if female			
CKD-EPI Creatinine Equation 2009[a]: CKD-EPI equation expressed as a single equation: GFR = 141 × [min(SCr/κ, 1)$^{\alpha}$ × max(SCr/κ, 1)$^{-1.209}$ × Age$^{-0.993}$] × 1.018 [if female] × 1.159 [if African American]			

[a]SCr is standardized serum creatinine in milligrams per deciliter; κ is 0.7 for women and 0.9 for men, α is −0.329 for women and −0.411 for men, min indicates the minimum of SCr/κ or 1, and max indicates the maximum of SCr/κ or 1.

CKD-EPI = Chronic Kidney Disease Epidemiology Collaboration; MDRD = Modified Diet Renal Disease.

d. Some clinicians round the serum creatinine concentration (SCr) up to 1 mg/dL because older adults have lower muscle mass, which produces less creatinine, and extremely low SCr would overestimate renal function with these formulas. This rounding is not supported by evidence and remains controversial. In addition, clinicians may use adjusted weight for patients with obesity with formulas used for younger adults.

C. Pharmacodynamic Changes Common with Aging
1. Increased sensitivity
   a. Benzodiazepines
   b. Opioids
   c. Antipsychotics, metoclopramide: Extrapyramidal effects and tardive dyskinesia
   d. Tricyclic antidepressants, α-blockers, antihypertensives: Orthostatic hypotension
   e. Warfarin
   f. NSAIDs: Gastrointestinal (GI) bleeding
   g. Anticholinergic agents
2. Decreased sensitivity
   a. β-Blockers
   b. β-Agonists
3. Impaired homeostasis
   a. Diuretics, angiotensin-converting enzyme inhibitors: Sodium and electrolytes
   b. Diuretics: Hydration status

Patient Cases

Questions 1 and 2 pertain to the following case:

An 85-year-old woman (weight 65 kg) who resides at home with her daughter has a medical history significant for type 2 diabetes and hypertension, and 1 year ago, she sustained a right hip fracture after a fall. Her regularly scheduled medications include glyburide 10 mg daily, lisinopril 10 mg daily, metformin 500 mg twice daily, aspirin 81 mg daily, and a multivitamin daily. Her as-needed medications include melatonin 6 mg at bedtime as needed for sleep, meclizine 25 mg ½ tablet three times daily as needed for dizziness, and docusate 100 mg twice daily. Her laboratory results show fasting plasma glucose 90 mg/dL, sodium 138 mEq/L, potassium 4.5 mEq/L, chloride 102 mEq/L, CO_2 25 mEq/L, blood urea nitrogen (BUN) 30 mg/dL, SCr 1.8 mg/dL, and thyroid-stimulating hormone (TSH) 4.0 mU/L.

1. Considering the potential for altered pharmacokinetics, which set of medications has the highest potential to cause problems for the patient?

   A. Aspirin and melatonin.

   B. Lisinopril and meclizine.

   C. Lisinopril and metformin.

   D. Glyburide and metformin.

2. Considering the potential for increased pharmacodynamic sensitivity, which set of medications has the highest potential to cause problems for the patient?

   A. Aspirin and melatonin.

   B. Lisinopril and meclizine.

   C. Lisinopril and metformin.

   D. Glyburide and metformin.

D. Optimal Pharmacotherapy in Older People
1. An optimal pharmacotherapeutic regimen is one in which the benefit of the therapy outweighs the risk of adverse effects.
2. To reduce risk, doses of many medications must be adjusted in older people because of age-associated changes in drug pharmacokinetics and pharmacodynamics.
3. Alternate medications may be more appropriate because of these changes.
4. Therapeutic window becomes smaller even with dose and drug adjustments.

E. Drug-Related Assessment for Risk in Older Adults
1. Overuse of medications
   a. Unnecessary drugs: Use of more medications than clinically indicated and unneeded therapeutic duplication
   b. Common unnecessary drugs: GI agents, central nervous system agents, vitamins, minerals
   c. May be caused by
      i. Prescribing cascade: When drug is prescribed for treatment of another drug's adverse effects
      ii. Several prescribers
      iii. Care transitions
2. Underuse of medications
   a. Omitted but necessary or indicated drug therapy or inadequate dosing
   b. Commonly underused drugs: Anticoagulants, statins, antihypertensives
   c. Medications considered appropriate according to guidelines may be omitted because prescriber or patient is overly wary of adverse drug effects.
3. Nonadherence
   a. Unintentional nonadherence caused by complex drug regimen
   b. Dementia or other cognitive impairment increases risk.
   c. Cost of medications is another barrier.
   d. Intentional nonadherence because of patient health beliefs or concerns
4. Withdrawal syndromes
   a. Abrupt discontinuation of medication may cause rebound symptoms or delirium.
   b. Common culprits: Antihypertensives, antidepressants, anxiolytics, pain medications
5. Inappropriate medications
   a. Explicit tools commonly used to identify for quality measure. Best known is the AGS Beers Criteria for Potentially Inappropriate Medications.
      i. Evidence-based list of drugs likely to cause problems
      ii. Adopted by many federal agencies and Part D plans
      iii. Arranged as drugs and drug classes to always avoid, drugs to avoid in certain diseases or conditions, and drugs to be used with caution
      iv. Examples: Anticholinergics, long half-life benzodiazepines, sedative-hypnotics, older antipsychotics, certain opiates or pain medications, hypoglycemics, NSAIDs, and GI drugs
   b. Implicit tools are patient-centered, take more time to apply. Best studied is the Medication Appropriateness Index.
      i. 10 questions to ask about each medication regarding indication, effect, dosing, directions, interactions, duration, and cost
      ii. Indication, effectiveness, and correct dosage have most weight.
6. Choosing Wisely Campaign
   a. 10 things to question in older adults
   b. 7 of the 10 items are drug related.
      i. Antipsychotics in patients with dementia should be avoided.
      ii. Target hemoglobin A1C in diabetes management 7.5% or higher

       iii. Avoid benzodiazepines and sedative-hypnotics for insomnia, agitation, or delirium.

       iv. Do not start antimicrobials to treat bacteriuria without symptoms.

       v. Assess benefit and risk of cholinesterase inhibitors (CIs).

       vi. Appetite stimulants not helpful for anorexia or cachexia

       vii. Drug regimen review is necessary with every new prescription.

F. Function with Aging

  1. Quality of life, place of residence, and social and physical function may become more important than duration of life.

  2. Instrumental activities of daily living (IADLs)

    a. Examples: Housekeeping, using phone, managing medications, shopping, cooking, managing money

    b. Need to do these to live independently

  3. Activities of daily living (ADLs)

    a. Examples: Feeding, dressing, bathing, toileting, transferring

    b. Nursing home or home caregivers required if ADLs cannot be performed

  4. Cognitive screening: Mini–Mental State Examination (MMSE), Montreal Cognitive Assessment (MoCA), St. Louis University Mental Status (SLUMS) Examination

  5. Mood: Geriatric Depression Scale

  6. Gait and balance: Timed Up and Go, Berg Balance Scale

  7. Drugs can alter cognition, mood, and mobility.

G. Geriatric Syndromes

  1. Geriatric syndromes follow a concentric model, with multiple risk factors and numerous etiologies contributing to a clinical presentation rather than the linear model with one etiology following a defined pathogenesis.

  2. Falls

    a. Possible etiologies: Psychoactive medications, polypharmacy, orthostatic hypotension, hypoglycemia, hyponatremia, myocardial infarction, urinary tract infection

    b. Examples of contributing risk factors: Vitamin D deficiency, poor balance, deconditioning/muscle weakness, poor vision, environment

  3. Delirium

    a. Possible etiologies: Psychoactive medications, polypharmacy, hypoglycemia, hyponatremia, myocardial infarction, urinary tract infection

    b. Example of contributing risk factors: Dementia, stroke, vitamin B_{12} deficiency, poor hearing, lack of sleep

  4. Hazards of hospitalization

    a. Usual aging involves a decline in numerous organ systems, which are further compromised when an older patient is admitted to the hospital and expected to remain in bed.

      i. Immobilization leads to deconditioning. Regaining what was lost takes longer in older adults.

      ii. Immobilization and inability to obtain water lead to decreased plasma volume, which can lead to syncope, falls, and fractures.

      iii. Sensory deprivation from isolation and lack of glasses or hearing aids can lead to delirium, which may be treated with restraints or antipsychotics.

      iv. Immobilization and "tethers" (e.g., intravenous lines, oxygen lines, catheters) necessitate nursing assistance to bathroom. Unavoidable delay may lead to incontinence, catheters, infections, and pressure sores.

      v. Prescribed diets or nothing-by-mouth status lead to dehydration, malnutrition, insertion of feeding tubes, and aspiration pneumonia.

b. Preventable adverse drug events are frequent contributors to increased morbidity and mortality in older hospitalized adults.

c. Functional decline typically follows a hospitalization and is called a cascade to dependency.

d. One study showed subjects that had a loss of ADLs at discharge had a higher mortality rate (40% at 12 months), with only 30% returning to baseline function.

e. Early mobility, adequate nutrition, reduced polypharmacy, and early discharge planning may reduce functional disability and length of stay.

Patient Cases

Questions 3 and 4 pertain to the following case:

A 70-year-old woman is admitted to the hospital with a broken arm after a fall. While in the hospital, she is on bedrest most of the time, loses 2 kg (current weight 63 kg), and has trouble sleeping. She is to be discharged to a rehabilitation facility for 2–3 weeks of therapy. Her medications at discharge are glipizide 5 mg daily, lisinopril 10 mg daily, aspirin 81 mg daily, multivitamin daily, mirtazapine 15 mg at bedtime, calcium 500 mg twice daily, and tramadol 25 mg every 8 hours as needed for pain.

3. When recommending medication changes for this patient, which functional assessment is most important to evaluate?

   A. IADLs.

   B. Depression.

   C. Pressure sores.

   D. Gait and balance.

4. To maintain and improve function in this patient, which intervention is best to implement?

   A. Add simvastatin 10 mg daily.

   B. Increase lisinopril to 20 mg daily.

   C. Add vitamin D 1000 units twice daily.

   D. Change tramadol to naproxen 500 mg twice daily as needed for pain.

II. DEMENTIA

A. Epidemiology
   1. Affects 4–5 million in the United States
   2. Of people 65 years and older, 6% have dementia, increasing to 30–50% of those 85 years and older.

B. Dementia Definition: Cognitive decline in complex attention, executive function, learning and memory, language, perceptual–motor or social cognition AND interferes with work or social functions
   1. Delirium should be ruled out first.
      a. Delirium: A disturbance in attention and awareness developing over hours to days with fluctuation over the course of the day
      b. It is a geriatric syndrome, with age, underlying dementia, functional impairment, medical comorbidities as risk factors.
      c. Etiologies include medications such as sedative hypnotics, antidepressants, anticholinergics, opioids, anticonvulsants, and antiparkinson drugs.

2. *Mild cognitive impairment* (MCI) is a term used for people with some deficits in cognition that do not meet the criteria for dementia.
3. Alzheimer disease (AD) is most common type of dementia.
4. Theories of pathogenesis include cholinergic, β-amyloid plaques, tau protein (neurofibrillary tangles), genetics (apolipoprotein E4), and inflammation (cytokines, prion).
5. Several other types of dementia exist; few are reversible.

Table 3. Comparisons of Memory Impairment and Dementias with AD

Disease	Differences from AD	Treatment Notes
Common Irreversible Causes		
MCI	No interference with work or social functions 1 in 5 progress to AD	Eliminate or control risk factors for dementia May use CIs, which reduced risk of progression by 40% in one study
Vascular dementia	Includes focal neurological signs and symptoms Radiologic evidence of stroke Onset within 3–6 mo of stroke Abrupt deterioration followed by stepwise progression	Control of cardiac and vascular risk factors
Lewy body dementia	Fluctuating cognition with pronounced variation in attention and alertness Recurrent visual hallucinations Motor features of PD	Avoid typical antipsychotics, which may worsen motor symptoms
Dementia of advanced PD	PD onset predates cognitive impairment Usually at latter stages of PD	May use CIs or memantine
Frontotemporal dementia	Affects personality, behavior, self-care, and language Onset in ages 45–65 with a 2- to 10-yr course	CIs may worsen behavior and cause agitation
Reversible Causes		
Vitamin B$_{12}$ deficiency	Progressive memory loss Vitamin B$_{12}$ serum concentration < 300 pg/mL May be anemic also, but folic acid may disguise the anemia	Replace vitamin B$_{12}$ according to standard protocols
Hypothyroidism	Deficient or inadequate replacement of thyroxine	Levothyroxine replacement per standard protocols
Depression	Trouble concentrating and memory Apathy and "I don't care" responses	Treatment of depression per standard protocols
NPH	Triad of progressive memory loss, incontinence, and gait abnormality Symptoms improve after lumbar puncture	Surgical placement of ventricular shunt

AD = Alzheimer disease; CI = cholinesterase inhibitor; MCI = mild cognitive impairment; NPH = normal pressure hydrocephalus; PD = Parkinson disease.

C. Assessment Tools
   1. Folstein MMSE
      a. 30-point scale; higher is better function
      b. Untreated AD: Score usually decreases 3–4 points a year.
      c. Heavily relies on verbal and language skills so less accurate if education is poor
   2. SLUMS examination
      a. 30-point scale; higher number is better function
      b. Includes adjustment of scores for lower educational status
   3. MoCA
      a. 30-point scale; higher number is better function
      b. Less reliant on verbal or language skills
   4. Mini-Cog Assessment
      a. 5-point scale; higher number is better function
      b. Easiest to administer; takes 3 minutes

D. New Diagnostic Guidelines
   1. Recognizes three phases
      a. Preclinical, asymptomatic phase
      b. Symptomatic, predementia phase (MCI)
      c. Dementia phase
   2. Diagnosis may be identified for research purposes by:
      a. Biomarkers of increased tau or decreased β-amyloid levels in cerebrospinal fluid
      b. Reduced glucose uptake in brain on positron emission tomography scanning using florbetapir F18 or flutemetamol F18
      c. Atrophy of specific brain areas on magnetic resonance imaging
   3. Preclinical and predementia phases are targets for investigational studies to halt progression
   4. For clinicians, diagnosis usually given without these biomarkers or imaging

E. Clinical Presentation and Classification

Table 4. Stages of Alzheimer Disease

	MMSE (out of 30)	**Examples of Cognitive Loss**	**Examples of Functional Loss**
Mild	20–24	Some short-term memory loss; word-finding problems	Loss of IADLs such as laundry, housekeeping, and managing medications; may get lost in familiar places
Moderate	10–19	Disorientation to time and place, inability to engage in activities and conversation	Needs assistance with ADLs such as bathing, dressing, and toileting
Severe	< 10	Loss of speech and ambulation, incontinence of bowel and bladder	Dependency in basic ADLs such as feeding oneself; often needs around-the-clock care

ADLs = activities of daily living; IADLs = instrumental activities of daily living; MMSE = Mini–Mental State Examination.

F. Management
    1. Goals are to maintain function and cognition.
        a. Functional management and safety issues
        b. Legal considerations
    2. Nonpharmacologic therapy
        a. Education, especially with caregiver
        b. Physical exercise and mental exercise
        c. Management of comorbid conditions
        d. Avoid alcohol and medications that worsen mentation.
    3. Medical food: Caprylidene triglyceride
        a. Mechanism is to provide ketone bodies for brain to use as energy source when glucose metabolism is impaired.
        b. Not routinely used because study measures became nonsignificant

---

Patient Case

5. An 84-year-old widow lives at home alone. She can perform ADLs and most IADLs with some assistance from her daughter. Her current medications are hydrochlorothiazide 12.5 mg daily for hypertension, tolterodine LA 4 mg daily for incontinence, escitalopram 20 mg daily for depression, acetaminophen 650 mg as needed for arthritis, and calcium/vitamin D for prevention of osteoporosis. Her physician administers the MMSE, and the patient's score is 23. On physical examination, no cogwheel rigidity or tremor is noted. Which recommendation would be best at this time?

    A. Add donepezil 5 mg daily.
    B. Discontinue tolterodine and reassess the patient.
    C. Add vitamin B_{12} 1000-mg injection monthly.
    D. Switch hydrochlorothiazide to lisinopril 5 mg daily.

4. Pharmacologic therapy

Table 5. Comparison of Drugs for the Treatment of AD

Drug	Starting Dose	Maintenance Dose	Dosage Forms	Pharmacologic Properties	Comments
Cholinesterase Inhibitors					
Donepezil	5 mg daily	10 mg daily May increase to 23 mg/day	Tablets Orally disintegrating tablets	Acetylcholinesterase inhibitor; metabolized in part by CYP2D6 and CYP3A4 Protein binding 96%	Labeled for mild to moderate and moderate to severe AD
Rivastigmine	1.5 mg twice daily 4.6-mg patch daily	3–6 mg twice daily 9.5-mg patch daily; may increase to 13.3-mg patch daily	Capsules Oral solution Transdermal patch	Acetyl- and butyryl-cholinesterase inhibitor Nausea, vomiting, and diarrhea seem more intense than with other CIs	Labeled for mild to moderate and moderate to severe AD as well as mild to moderate dementia with Parkinson disease Skin reactions with patch
Galantamine	4 mg twice daily	8–12 mg twice daily 8–24 mg ER once daily	Tablets Oral solution ER capsules	Selective competitive, reversible acetylcholinesterase inhibitor and nicotine receptor modulator Metabolized in part by CYP2D6 and CYP3A4	Preferable to administer with food Renal dosing adjustment necessary
Glutamatergic Therapy					
Memantine	5 mg once daily 7 mg ER once daily	10 mg twice daily 28 mg ER once daily	Tablets Oral solution ER capsules	N-methyl-D-aspartate receptor antagonist that blocks glutamate transmission	Labeled for moderate to severe AD; may be used in combination with acetylcholinesterase inhibitors
Combination Product					
Donepezil/memantine	10/28 mg once daily in the evening	10/28 mg once daily	ER capsule	Acetylcholinesterase inhibitor and N-methyl-D-aspartate receptor antagonist	Use after stabilized on donepezil and memantine separately Renal dosing adjustment necessary

ER = extended release.

    a. Adverse effects of CIs
       i. GI: Nausea, vomiting, diarrhea, elevated risk of GI bleeding
       ii. Central nervous system: Headache, insomnia, dizziness
      iii. Cardiac: Bradycardia, orthostatic hypotension, syncope (AGS Beers Criteria note CIs as inappropriate drugs in patients with syncope)
      iv. Genitourinary: Incontinence
    b. Adverse effects of memantine: Agitation, urinary incontinence, insomnia, diarrhea, dizziness, confusion, headache

5. Consensus treatment guidelines in United States, 2001 (partly outdated)
   a. Initiate CI in patients with mild to moderate AD.
   b. No evidence one agent is superior to others
   c. Titrate to recommended maintenance dose as tolerated.
   d. May increase to maximum dose if tolerated and maintenance dose no longer effective
   e. In moderate to severe disease may use CI, or memantine, or both CI and memantine
   f. Study in 2012 found no benefit with combination therapy.
   g. Study in 2011 found no benefit of memantine in mild AD.
6. Controversy over clinical significance of responses

Table 6. Evidence for Response to Drugs for AD

Drug	Test	Testing Range	Response Difference Compared with Placebo	
			Mean	**Range**
CI	AD Assessment Scale–Cognitive	0–70	−2.7	−2.73 to −2.01
Memantine	Severe Impairment Battery	0–100	2.97	1.68 to 4.26

7. Therapy duration
   a. In general, need 3–6 months to evaluate for objective benefit with tools
   b. Longest study was for 52 weeks, but many are maintained for years.
   c. Choosing Wisely Campaign recommends evaluating at 12 weeks and considering discontinuation if goals of therapy not obtained.
   d. In general, discontinue at advanced stages of disease. Recommend tapering if on high dose.
   e. May see some rebound agitation
8. Herbals and dietary supplements
   a. Vitamin E was not shown effective in most large prospective trials. Recent randomized controlled trial of 613 veterans with mild to moderate AD over 2 years showed delay in clinical progression of 19% per year.
   b. Gingko biloba was not shown effective in prevention or treatment in randomized controlled trials.
   c. Observational studies support effect of the Mediterranean diet, exercise, and curcumin (turmeric).

Patient Cases

6. An 87-year-old man with AD is receiving rivastigmine 6 mg twice daily. His family notes improvement in his functional ability but reports that he is experiencing nausea and vomiting that appear to be related to rivastigmine. Which recommendation is best for the patient at this time?
   A. Advise the patient to take rivastigmine with an antacid.
   B. Change rivastigmine to the patch that delivers 9.5 mg daily.
   C. Discontinue rivastigmine and initiate memantine 5 mg twice daily.
   D. Add prochlorperazine 25 mg by rectal suppository with each rivastigmine dose.

Patient Cases (*continued*)

7. A 75-year-old woman with AD who lives at home with her husband has been treated with donepezil 10 mg daily for about 3 years. When she began therapy, her MMSE was 21/30; her present MMSE is 17/30. The patient cannot perform most IADLs but can perform most ADLs with cueing. About 2 months ago, her done-pezil dose was increased to 23 mg, but she could not tolerate it, and it was reduced back to 10 mg daily. Her husband asks about changing her drug treatment to help maintain her function. Which is the next best course of action?

   A. Retry donepezil 23 mg daily.

   B. Initiate memantine 5 mg daily.

   C. Add vitamin E 400 units twice daily.

   D. Switch donepezil to rivastigmine 9.5-mg patch daily.

III. BEHAVIORAL AND PSYCHOLOGICAL SYMPTOMS OF DEMENTIA

   A. Epidemiology
   1. As disease progresses from mild to moderate, behavioral and psychological symptoms of dementia (BPSD) occur. They tend to wane as disease progresses to severe.
   2. Up to 90% of patients with dementia have BPSD at some point in disease progression.
   3. Associated with high rate of disability, functional decline, poor health outcomes, physical injury, nursing home placement, and emergency services
   4. Behaviors commonly peak during late afternoon or early evening, so called "sundowning"

Table 7. Symptoms Seen During Disease Progression

MMSE Score	Stage	Symptoms
25 20	Mild	Memory loss Apathy Poor drawing Mood swings[a] Mild executive function Mild personality changes[a]
15 10	Moderate	Unable to learn Aphasia, apraxia Wandering, agitation[a] Aggression, psychosis[a] Confusion, insomnia[a] Need ADL assistance
5 0	Severe	Gait changes[a] Incontinence Loss of ADLs Bed bound

[a]Noncognitive symptoms.

ADLs = activities of daily living; MMSE = Mini–Mental State Examination.

B. Assessment
    1. Scales are rarely used in nursing home or clinical practice, but it is important to identify the target behavior, how often it is occurring, and how severe it is in order to assess the response to treatment.
    2. Assess for medical reason that may precipitate and treat, if found
        a. Pain is common issue that patient cannot communicate. Treat with scheduled acetaminophen.
        b. Delirium precipitated by medical illness or medication should be ruled out.

C. Nonpharmacologic Treatment: Cornerstone of Therapy
    1. Theory is that behavior is communication of unmet need.
    2. Eliminate antecedents and triggers.
    3. Person-centered interventions: Consider long-standing habits, values, and beliefs of patient; use distraction, music, aromatherapy.
    4. Symptoms likely to respond: Wandering, hoarding, hiding objects, repetitive questioning, withdrawal, social inappropriateness, apathy

D. Pharmacologic Treatment: None of these are U.S. Food and Drug Administration (FDA)-labeled indications.
    1. Agency for Healthcare Research and Quality has published a summary on the use of atypical antipsychotic agents for off-label indications. Atypical antipsychotics improve behavioral symptoms of dementia, but effect sizes are small (number needed to treat 5–14), and adverse effects are significant (number needed to harm [NNH] 100).
    2. Retrospective case-control study of older veterans with dementia during a 180-day period indicates haloperidol NNH = 8, compared with atypical antipsychotics with NNH = 14–31 for risk of death

Table 8. Drug Treatment for BPSD

Symptom	Presentation	Treatment Options After Nonpharmacologic Efforts Ineffective
Anxiety	Part of this is caused by the fact that they cannot remember things	Buspirone or SSRI/SNRI or gabapentin Limit benzodiazepines
Apathy	One of earliest symptoms Nonpharmacologic, tailored to patient's activities	CIs Methylphenidate, modafinil effective in small, short-term studies
Depression	Up to 80% of patients with AD have depression	SSRI or mirtazapine
Insomnia	Sleep/wake cycle is disrupted	Melatonin
Wandering	Walk so much they begin to lose weight	No drug will stop wandering
Paranoia Hallucinations Sundowning	They may think because they cannot find something, you stole it Often accuse spouse of infidelity If psychosis and delusions do not bother anyone, do not use drugs	Risperidone, olanzapine, or quetiapine. Use very low doses. ADEs may offset any benefit
Aggression, resistance to care	Most difficult and best response is to nonpharmacologic treatment	Drugs under investigation for agitation include prazosin, dextromethorphan/quinidine, and citalopram

ADE = adverse drug effect; BPSD = behavioral and psychological symptoms of dementia; SNRI = serotonin-norepinephrine reuptake inhibitor; SSRI = selective serotonin reuptake inhibitor.

Patient Cases

Questions 8 and 9 pertain to the following case:

You are evaluating the medication profile of an 87-year-old woman who resides in a secure advanced dementia unit. Her medical history includes dementia (likely AD), Parkinson disease, and osteoarthritis (OA). She needs assistance with all ADLs, including total assistance with bathing and dressing, as well as help with feeding. She transfers with minimal help to a wheelchair. Her medication regimen includes donepezil 10 mg daily, memantine 10 mg twice daily, carbidopa/levodopa 25/100 mg four times daily, and a multivitamin supplement daily. The patient's most recent MMSE score is 5/30. When reviewing the nursing notes, you note several references to the patient's continuously crying out, "Help me, help me," beginning around 5 p.m. She is medically evaluated, and reversible causes of her hypervocalization are ruled out.

8. Which initial approach is most appropriate for this patient?

    A. Begin ibuprofen 400 mg every 8 hours.

    B. Order haloperidol 1 mg every 6 hours as needed for agitation.

    C. Begin music therapy with songs the patient enjoyed when younger.

    D. Move the patient to a private room to minimize social contacts after 3 p.m.

9. After 2 months, the patient's agitation increases such that the nursing staff cannot bathe or feed her. Assuming nonpharmacologic approaches are ineffective, which is the best pharmacologic approach to treat her behavioral symptoms?

    A. Increase donepezil to 23 mg daily.

    B. Begin melatonin 6 mg at bedtime.

    C. Add quetiapine 25 mg at 4 p.m. daily.

    D. Add citalopram 10 mg daily.

IV. URINARY INCONTINENCE

A. Epidemiology
   1. Prevalence in community-dwelling older adult women is 38%.
   2. Less common in older adult men: 17%.
   3. Up to 75% of nursing home residents have urinary incontinence (UI).
   4. Transient incontinence can occur because of DRIP:
      D = Drugs, Delirium
      R = Retention, Restricted Mobility
      I = Impaction, Infection, Inflammation
      P = Polyuria, Prostatitis

B. Physiology
   1. During filling, β_3-adrenergic stimulation relaxes detrusor to increase capacity.
   2. α-Adrenergic stimulation tightens the internal bladder sphincter.
   3. Acetylcholine (M_3) mediates involuntary and volitional bladder contractions.
   4. Normal bladder emptying occurs with a decrease in urethral resistance and contraction of the bladder muscle.

5. Aging effects include decreased bladder elasticity and capacity, more frequent voiding, decline in bladder outlet and urethral resistance in women with loss of estrogen, and decrease in flow rate in men with prostatic enlargement.

C. Types of UI

Table 9. Common Types of UI and Drug-Induced Causes

Type of Incontinence	Description	Drug-Induced Causes
Urge or overactive bladder	Loss of a moderate amount of urine with an increased need to void Detrusor instability can be caused by central nervous system damage from a stroke	Cholinergic agents that stimulate the bladder such as bethanechol and CIs
Stress incontinence	Loss of small amounts of urine with increased abdominal pressure (e.g., sneezing, coughing) Stress UI is more common in postmenopausal women	α-Blockers such as prazosin decrease urethral sphincter tone
Overflow incontinence	Loss of urine because of excessive bladder volume caused by outlet obstruction or an acontractile detrusor PVR is often high (> 300 mL), indicating incomplete emptying	Anticholinergic agents, calcium channel blockers, and opioids decrease detrusor muscle contractions
Functional incontinence	Inability to reach the toilet because of mobility constraints	Sedating drugs that cause confusion Diuretics increase voiding
Mixed incontinence	UI that has more than one cause, usually stress and overactive bladder	

PVR = postvoid residual; UI = urinary incontinence.

D. Nonpharmacologic Interventions
1. Exercise and weight loss for patients with a body mass index greater than 25–30 kg/m^2
2. Stress
   a. Pelvic floor exercises (Kegel exercises) are first line for stress.
   b. Biofeedback may be needed to teach pelvic floor exercises.
   c. Stress incontinence usually responds to surgical repair.
   d. Pessaries or bulking agent injections also help stress incontinence.
3. Urge
   a. Pelvic floor exercises in combination with medication for urge or mixed UI
   b. Bladder training to increase time between voiding in urge incontinence
   c. Peripheral tibial nerve stimulation or sacral neuromodulation techniques are third line after lifestyle and pharmacologic treatments.
4. Scheduled and timed voiding may be helpful for patients with dementia.
5. Prostatectomy in men or self-catheterization for severe overflow incontinence

E. Drug Treatment

Table 10. Recommended Drug Treatment by Type of Incontinence

Type of Incontinence	Drug Treatment	Comments
Urge or overactive bladder	**Antimuscarinic and anticholinergic agents** Oxybutynin, tolterodine, fesoterodine, trospium, solifenacin, darifenacin	Magnitude of clinical efficacy is modest Differences in adverse reactions exist, but clinical differences in efficacy between these agents have not been shown Longer-acting formulations may be better tolerated
	β₃-Agonist Mirabegron	Appears well tolerated but has not been compared with antimuscarinics
	OnabotulinumtoxinA intradetrusor injections	Prevents stimulation of detrusor muscle Pre-procedure antibiotic recommended May cause urinary retention; must be able to perform self-catheterization
Stress	**α-Adrenergic agonists** Pseudoephedrine, phenylephrine	Efficacy evidence is limited
	Topical estrogens Conjugated estrogen vaginal cream or estradiol vaginal insert or ring	Use if other symptoms of estrogen deficiency Vaginal estrogens may improve severity of stress incontinence
	Serotonin/norepinephrine reuptake inhibitor Duloxetine	Not FDA labeled for stress UI; may reduce the severity of incontinence Not significantly different from placebo for symptoms Adverse effects may limit its usefulness
Overflow	**α-Adrenergic antagonists** Alfuzosin, tamsulosin, silodosin, doxazosin, terazosin, prazosin	Adverse effects vary depending on selectivity to receptors in the bladder or prostate (alfuzosin, silodosin, and tamsulosin are more specific and preferred in older adults)
	5-α-reductase inhibitors Finasteride, dutasteride	To slow progression
	Cholinomimetics Bethanechol	Stimulates the detrusor muscle but also systemic cholinomimetic effects
	Phosphodiesterase-5 inhibitors Tadalafil	5 mg once daily approved for BPH
Functional	No drug treatments	Consider interventions to remove any potential cause, barriers or obstacles; provide schedules or prompted toileting; assistance may be required to transfer on and off commode
Mixed	Focus on symptoms that dominate	Consider treatments for individual components (i.e., stress and urge)

BPH = benign prostatic hypertrophy; UI = urinary incontinence.

Table 11. Comparison of Adverse Effects from Urinary Antimuscarinic Agents[a]

Drug	Dry Mouth (%)	Constipation (%)	Dizziness (%)
Oxybutynin	88	32	38
Oxybutynin ER/XL	68	9	11
Oxybutynin TDS	10	5	4
Oxybutynin gel	8	1	3
Tolterodine IR, ER	50, 39	10, 10	4, 3
Fesoterodine	99	14	2
Trospium	33	11	?
Solifenacin	34	19	1
Darifenacin	59	28	0

[a]Treatment of Overactive Bladder in Women. Agency for Healthcare Research and Quality publication no. 09-E017. August 2009. Mirabegron is not available for comparison.

ER/XL = extended release; IR = immediate release; TDS = transdermal delivery system.

Patient Case

10. A 75-year-old woman reports urinary urgency, frequency, and loss of urine when she cannot make it to the bathroom in time. She also wears a pad at night that she changes two or three times because of incontinence. Her medical history is significant for mild cognitive impairment (MMSE = 25), OA, and hypothyroidism. A urinalysis is negative. Physical examination is normal, and her postvoid residual (PVR) is normal (less than 100 mL). Which therapy would be best to initiate in this patient at this time?

    A. Mirabegron.

    B. Darifenacin.

    C. Pelvic floor exercises and solifenacin.

    D. Pelvic floor exercises and tolterodine IR.

V. BENIGN PROSTATIC HYPERTROPHY

A. Epidemiology
   1. BPH usually develops after age 40.
   2. By age 60, 50% of all men have BPH; by age 85, 90% have BPH.

B. Pathophysiology and Clinical Presentation
   1. Type II 5-α-reductase facilitates conversion of testosterone to dihydrotestosterone (DHT), resulting in prostate growth.
   2. Lower urinary tract symptoms (LUTS) are seen in 25% of men.
      a. Voiding (obstructive) symptoms: Decreased force, hesitancy, dribbling
      b. Storage (irritative) symptoms: Urinary urgency, frequency, nocturia, dysuria
   3. The American Urological Association Symptom Index (AUASI) can help determine severity and appropriate treatment. The index consists of seven questions evaluating the severity of LUTS on a 0–5 scale. Higher numbers indicate more severe symptoms.

C. Evaluation
   1. Medical history, digital rectal examination, BUN, SCr, and urinalysis
   2. If suspect prostate cancer, plan treatment with 5-α reductase inhibitor, prostate-specific antigen (PSA)

3. If suspect significant urinary retention, need to assess PVR. If PVR is greater than 50 mL, patients have an elevated risk of infection.

4. Assess for medications that may exacerbate BPH symptoms.

    a. α-Adrenergic agonists (decongestants) can stimulate smooth muscle contraction in the prostate and urethra, obstructing urinary flow through the urethra.

    b. Anticholinergic drugs (urinary and GI antispasmodics, antihistamines, tricyclic antidepressants, phenothiazines) can reduce the ability of the bladder detrusor muscle to contract and empty the bladder.

    c. Diuretics can increase urinary frequency and volume.

    d. Testosterone replacement can stimulate prostate growth.

5. If AUASI score is 0–7 (mild), then watchful waiting.

6. Patients with high AUASI scores of 20 and up (severe disease) should be assessed for prostatectomy.

7. Patients with moderate disease (scores 8–19) are candidates for medical treatment.

D. Drug Treatment

  1. α-Adrenergic blockers: Relieve LUTS in men with moderate or severe AUASI scores by reducing smooth muscle contractions in the urethra and surrounding tissues

    a. Nonspecific α-adrenergic blockers such as doxazosin and terazosin also lower blood pressure significantly.

    b. Newer agents are uroselective antagonists of α_1-adrenergic receptors (tamsulosin, silodosin) and selective antagonists of postsynaptic α_1-adrenergic receptors (alfuzosin) in the prostate and bladder. They may have less associated hypotension.

    c. All α-blockers can cause hypotension.

    d. Compared with placebo, the α-blockers lower the AUASI by 4–6 points in patients with LUTS and BPH.

    e. All α-blockers are metabolized through the CYP3A4 pathway and have drug interactions with strong CYP3A4 inhibitors and inducers.

    f. Intraoperative floppy iris syndrome is a concern with α-blockers, especially tamsulosin. Men with LUTS being offered α-blockers should be asked about planned cataract surgery. Men with planned cataract surgery should avoid the initiation of α-blockers until their cataract surgery is completed. If already taking an α-blocker, the patient needs to inform his surgeon so that precautions can be taken.

  2. α-Reductase inhibitors

    a. These agents prevent the conversion of testosterone to DHT, modify the disease course, and may reduce the risk of urinary retention and surgical interventions.

      i. Finasteride competitively inhibits type II 5-α-reductase and lowers prostatic DHT by 80%–90%.

      ii. Dutasteride is a nonselective inhibitor of both type I and II 5-α-reductase. Prostatic DHT production is quickly suppressed with this agent.

      iii. Despite these pharmacologic differences, no differences between these two agents were observed in trials; both reduce prostate size.

    b. α-Reductase inhibitors do not immediately reduce LUTS and should be reserved for use in men with large prostate volume (more than 40 g). At least 6 months of therapy is usually needed to achieve clinical benefit. Prostate size may be reduced by about 25% during this interval.

    c. PSA concentrations are used to monitor for prostate cancer. Because these agents lower PSA concentrations, a baseline PSA test is recommended before initiating treatment with α-reductase inhibitors.

    d. Long-term therapy with an α-reductase inhibitor can increase the risk of high-grade tumors of the prostate in healthy men without a history of prostate cancer.

3.   Phosphodiesterase type-5 inhibitors
     a.   Tadalafil 5 mg once daily is approved for use in BPH.
     b.   Mechanism is thought to be caused by phosphodiesterase-induced smooth muscle relaxation in the bladder, urethra, and prostate.
     c.   Studied as monotherapy; the FDA does not recommend in combination with α-blockers because the combination has not been adequately studied for the treatment of BPH, and there is a risk of lowering blood pressure. May be used in practice to treat both BPH and erectile dysfunction with a 4-hour separation of doses.
4.   Combination therapy
     a.   May be needed in men with LUTS, a larger prostate size, and an elevated PSA
     b.   Finasteride and doxazosin most studied; dutasteride is FDA label approved for use with tamsulosin in symptomatic men having an enlarged prostate.
     c.   Two large clinical trials [Medical Therapy of Prostatic Symptoms (MTOPS) and the Combination of Avodart and Tamsulosin studies (CombAT)] evaluated monotherapy versus combination therapy and concluded that in men with LUTS and an enlarged prostate, further benefit can be achieved by using the two drugs in combination.
5.   Supplements
     a.   Saw palmetto plant extract (*Serenoa repens*)
          i.   Conflicting evidence about the efficacy of saw palmetto in relieving LUTS; 2012 systematic review suggested no benefit over placebo
          ii.   Use of this agent with 5-α-reductase inhibitors may reduce the efficacy of the reductase inhibitors.
     b.   β-Sitosterol, *Pygeum africanum* show some benefit, but short-term studies
6.   Surgery is preferred in men with severe symptoms and in those with moderate symptoms who have not adequately responded to medical options.
7.   Anticholinergic agents can be appropriate and effective treatment alternatives in men without an elevated PVR when LUTS are predominantly storage (irritative) symptoms.

Table 12. Comparison of Drugs for the Treatment of Benign Prostatic Hypertrophy

Medication	Dose Range	Adverse Effects	Comments
Terazosin Doxazosin	1–10 mg daily 1–8 mg daily	Orthostatic hypotension	Initiate at low dose; can titrate every 2–7 days Start at bedtime
Alfuzosin ER	10 mg daily	Orthostatic hypotension	No need to titrate Take after a meal
Tamsulosin modified release	0.4–0.8 mg daily	May cause less orthostasis Causes ejaculatory dysfunction	Start at bedtime
Silodosin	8 mg daily 4 mg daily if CrCl 30–50 mL/min/1.73 m^2	Causes ejaculatory dysfunction; appears less sedating	Contraindicated if CrCl < 30 mL/min/1.73 m^2 Take with food
Finasteride Dutasteride Dutasteride/ tamsulosin	5 mg daily 0.5 mg daily 0.5/0.4 mg daily	Decreased libido Pregnancy category X	Onset of action is usually 6 mo Monitor PSA
Tadalafil	5 mg daily	Orthostatic hypotension	Avoid use with α-blockers No data in combination or with long-term use

CrCl = creatinine clearance; PSA = prostate-specific antigen.

Patient Case

11. An 85-year-old man with LUTS visits his physician, who determines his AUASI score is 15. His blood pressure is 118/70 mm Hg sitting. A digital rectal examination confirms the diagnosis of BPH, and the physician schedules a further workup including a prostate ultrasound, which shows a prostate volume of 31 g. Which therapy is best at this time?

    A. Terazosin.

    B. Finasteride plus saw palmetto.

    C. Tamsulosin.

    D. Finasteride plus tamsulosin.

VI. OSTEOARTHRITIS

A. Epidemiology
1. OA is the most prevalent form of arthritis, affecting more than 46 million Americans.
2. Highly associated with aging
3. Women are afflicted more often than men.
4. Large weight-bearing joints (e.g., hip and knee) are commonly affected.

B. Etiology and Pathophysiology
1. Risk factors include age, female sex, obesity, genetics, sports activities, occupation, previous injury, acromegaly
2. Loss of cartilage occurs in the joint as the balance of chondrocyte function shifts from formation to destruction. Secondary inflammation and production of cytokines play a role.
3. Subchondral bone and the synovium are damaged, and the joint space narrows.
4. Single injuries or repeated micro-injuries may initiate or accelerate process.
5. Symptoms of pain result from activation of nociceptive nerve endings in the damaged joint.
6. Therapy goals: To relieve pain and swelling, maintain or improve joint function, prevent loss of function, and maintain or improve quality of life

C. Nonpharmacologic Treatment
1. Patient education: Lifestyle, expectations, when to seek care
2. Weight loss decreases the biomechanical load on large weight-bearing joints; even a small amount of weight loss helps decrease pain and disability.
3. Exercise
4. Physical and occupational therapy
5. Surgery

D. Drug Therapy
1. Acetaminophen is first line, with as-needed doses followed by scheduled dosing to maximum of 3 g daily in divided doses (over-the-counter dose). Maximum of 4 g daily may be allowed for healthy older adults with closer monitoring by health care team.
    a. 1000 mg every 6 hours for up to three times daily or 650 mg every 6 hours
    b. Ensure that patient knows to watch for "hidden" acetaminophen in other products.
    c. Monitor for hepatotoxicity in patients with elevated risk of liver disease (previous liver problems, heavy alcohol consumption) with periodic liver function tests.

2. NSAIDs are used if acetaminophen response inadequate in select patients.
   a. Avoid chronic use or, if necessary, use a COX-2 selective NSAID, or add a proton pump inhibitor to reduce the risk of GI bleeding.
   b. If one NSAID is not effective, switch to others.
   c. Monitor for adverse effects: Rash, abdominal pain, GI bleeding, renal impairment, hypertension, heart failure, and drug-drug interactions
   d. For patients taking aspirin (for cardiac disease), a proton pump inhibitor may be recommended for gastric protection. Patients should be educated to take aspirin at least 30 minutes before their first daily dose of NSAID in the morning to avoid any interactions or reductions in aspirin efficacy. Naproxen appears to be safest with respect to cardiac risk.
   e. Monitor in chronic users: Complete blood cell count, BUN, SCr, and aspartate aminotransferase at least annually
3. Topical agents: Helpful for knees or smaller joints near surface of skin. Limited efficacy for widespread joint pain
   a. Capsaicin difficult to administer: Wear gloves, avoid contact with eyes, and do not skip doses. Local irritation occurs in 40%.
   b. Diclofenac 1% gel (or patch is FDA labeled for minor trauma): Four short-term trials showed a 50% reduction in pain in 40% of subjects (number needed to treat = 5); longer-term trials had number needed to treat = 10. Comparative trials with oral administration showed no difference in proportion who received pain relief.
4. Intra-articular glucocorticoid injections
   a. Methylprednisolone or triamcinolone 10- to 40-mg injection depending on size of joint; may be repeated every 3 months
   b. Primary adverse effects are risk of septic arthritis, synovitis
5. Intra-articular hyaluronans may be used if glucocorticoid injections are ineffective.
   a. Meta-analysis indicates effects last up to 30 weeks.
   b. Frequency of injection undetermined: Annual or more often?
6. Alternative dietary supplements: Glucosamine sulfate, 400–500 mg taken three times daily, with or without chondroitin, may be considered for chronic therapy to prevent joint degradation and relieve pain.
   a. Evidence to support treatment is contradictory
   b. The adverse effect profile of glucosamine/chondroitin is similar to that of placebo.
7. Opioids
   a. Patients with persistent, moderate to severe pain from OA who do not respond to more conservative strategies are candidates for treatment with opioids. AGS recommends treatment with opioids for OA when older patients do not respond to initial acetaminophen therapy rather than chronic use of NSAIDs.
   b. Hydrocodone/acetaminophen combination now Schedule II.
   c. Tramadol alone or in combination with acetaminophen is an alternative when NSAIDs are ineffective or contraindicated.
   d. Stronger opioids can be more effective but can incur more significant adverse effects.
   e. Monitor and anticipate opioid adverse effects and treat accordingly.

Patient Case

12. An 85-year-old man presents with pain from hip OA. He has hypertension, coronary artery disease, and BPH. For his OA, he has been taking acetaminophen 650 mg three times daily. He reports that acetaminophen helps but that the pain persists and limits his ability to walk. Which is the best next step for this patient?

    A. Change acetaminophen to celecoxib.

    B. Add hydrocodone.

    C. Change acetaminophen to ibuprofen.

    D. Add glucosamine.

VII. RHEUMATOID ARTHRITIS

A. Epidemiology
   1. A systemic disease characterized by a bilateral inflammatory arthritis that usually affects the small joints of the hands, wrists, and feet
   2. The prevalence is estimated to be between 1% and 2%, with women predominating until after age 60, when it becomes equal.
   3. Rheumatoid arthritis (RA) can occur at any age but has an increasing prevalence up to age 70.
   4. RA is an autoimmune disease with a strong genetic predisposition.

B. Pathophysiology and Clinical Presentation
   1. Chronic inflammation of the synovium leads to proliferation and development of a pannus.
   2. The pannus invades joint cartilage and eventually causes erosion of the bone and joint destruction.
   3. The cause of the initial inflammatory activation is unknown, but once activated, the immune system produces antibodies and cytokines that accelerate cartilage and joint destruction.
   4. Patients present with joint pain and stiffness, fatigue, and other inflammatory symptoms. Symptoms also include warmth, redness, and swelling of the joints, usually with symmetrical distribution.
   5. Laboratory tests often reveal a positive rheumatoid factor (RF), elevated sedimentation rate, C-reactive protein, anti–cyclic citrullinated peptide antibodies, and normochromic normocytic anemia.
   6. RA can also affect other organs, causing pulmonary fibrosis, vasculitis, and dry eyes.

C. Treatment
   1. The treatment goal is to control the inflammatory process so that disease remission occurs. This leads to relief of pain, maintenance of function, and improved quality of life. Treatment response can be measured by:
      a. Reduction in the number of affected joints and in joint tenderness and swelling
      b. Improvement in pain
      c. Decreased amount of morning stiffness
      d. Reduction in serologic markers such as RF
      e. Improvement in quality-of-life scales
   2. Nonpharmacologic treatment: Concurrent with pharmacologic treatment
      a. Rest during periods of disease exacerbation
      b. Occupational and physical therapy to support mobility and maintain function
      c. Maintenance of a normal weight (avoid overweight and obesity) to reduce biomechanical stress on joints
      d. Assistive devices if needed
      e. Surgery for tendons or joints

3. Disease-modifying antirheumatic drugs (DMARDs)
    a. Start DMARD within 3 months of diagnosis.
    b. Step-down approach: Start with DMARD (1 or more depending on disease severity) together with anti-inflammatory drug (NSAID, steroid). As pain is controlled, reduce anti-inflammatory agent. As joint damage and inflammation is controlled, reduce DMARD.
    c. Nonbiologic DMARDs are first line.
        i. Methotrexate has most long-term data and better outcomes.
        ii. Hydroxychloroquine has slow onset of action.
        iii. Sulfasalazine is drug of choice in pregnancy but has slow onset too.
        iv. Leflunomide substitutes with comparable efficacy to methotrexate.
        v. Some patients with poor prognostic indicators such as functional limitation, extra-articular disease, positive RF, anti–cyclic citrullinated peptide antibodies, or bony erosions on radiography may be candidates for combination DMARD therapy.
    d. Biologic DMARDs are used in combination for severe disease or as alternatives if nonbiologic DMARDs are ineffective or contraindicated. Etanercept, infliximab, abatacept, or rituximab are most often used.
4. NSAIDs, glucocorticosteroids, or both can be used to provide immediate treatment of pain and inflammation.
    a. NSAIDs do not affect disease progression in RA; their anti-inflammatory effect occurs within 1–2 weeks of daily dosing, whereas the analgesic effect begins within several hours of administration.
    b. Glucocorticosteroids (dosed at 10 mg daily or less) are not recommended for long-term use because of their many adverse effects and long-term complications. They are often used as bridge therapy to provide anti-inflammatory effects while waiting for the DMARDs to take effect.

Table 13. Selected DMARDs for Rheumatoid Arthritis

Drug	Customary Dose	Comments
Nonbiologic DMARDs		
Methotrexate	7.5–15 mg every week	Probably first-line DMARD; monitor for myelosuppression, liver dysfunction, and pulmonary fibrosis; a teratogen
Leflunomide (Arava)	10–20 mg/day	Similar to methotrexate; an initial loading dose may give therapeutic response within the first month
Hydroxychloroquine (Plaquenil)	200–300 mg twice daily	Must routinely monitor for ocular toxicity; however, this agent has a better adverse effect profile overall
Sulfasalazine	500–1000 mg twice daily	GI adverse effects often limit the use of this agent
Biologic DMARDs		
Etanercept (Enbrel)	50 mg SC weekly	Binds to TNF, inactivating this cytokine; generally well tolerated; usually used in those whose methotrexate therapy fails; monitor for infection; check baseline PPD
Infliximab (Remicade)	3 mg/kg IV at 0, 2, and 6 wk; then every 8 wk thereafter	A mouse/human chimeric antibody to TNF; used in combination with methotrexate to prevent formation of antibodies to this protein; monitor for infection; check baseline PPD
Adalimumab (Humira)	40 mg SC every 2 wk	Human antibody to TNF; less antigenic than other TNF antibodies; monitor for infection; check baseline PPD
Anakinra (Kineret)	100 mg SC daily	IL-1 receptor antagonist; avoid combination therapy with TNF agents because of elevated risk of infection
Rituximab (Rituxan)	Two infusions of 1000 mg given 2 wk apart	Chimeric antibody to CD20 protein on B lymphocytes; corticosteroid infusions help reduce infusion reactions; used in combination with methotrexate to improve response
Abatacept (Orencia)	Weight-based dose every 2 wk for two doses and then monthly (i.e., 750 mg for those weighing 60–100 kg)	Inhibits interactions between antigens and T cells; may be useful in those who do not respond to TNF inhibitors; monitor for infusion reactions
Golimumab (Simponi)	50 mg SC every month	Monoclonal antibody against TNF Intended for use in combination with methotrexate Monitor for infections
Certolizumab pegol (Cimzia)	400 mg SC at 0, 2, and 4 wk; then 200 mg every other week	Monoclonal antibody against TNF; may have best response when used in combination with methotrexate Monitor for infections
Tocilizumab (Actemra)	4 mg/kg IV infusion every 4 wk; can increase to 8 mg/kg on the basis of clinical response	Anti–human IL-6 receptor monoclonal antibody; indicated for patients who have not responded to TNF inhibitors Monitor for infections
Tofacitinib (Xeljanz)	5 mg twice daily	Oral Janus kinase inhibitor; intended as second-line therapy Can be used as monotherapy or in combination with methotrexate

DMARD = disease-modifying antirheumatic drug; IL = interleukin; IV = intravenous(ly); NSAID = nonsteroidal anti-inflammatory drug; PPD = purified protein derivative; SC = subcutaneously; SSRI = selective serotonin reuptake inhibitor; TNF = tumor necrosis factor.

D. Comorbid Conditions
1. Patients with RA are more likely to develop other chronic diseases either from the effects of RA or from medications used to treat RA.
2. Cardiovascular disease (myocarditis and heart failure) causes 40% of all deaths in patients with RA. Low-dose aspirin, omega-3 fatty acids, statins, or combination therapy should be considered.
   a. Follow standard guidelines to lower cardiovascular risk factors.
   b. European guidelines recommend multiplying risk score by 1.5 for patients with RA who have disease of 10 years or more, are positive for RF or anti–cyclic citrullinated peptide, or have severe extra-articular disease manifestations (two of the three should be present).
3. Infection risk is elevated, particularly pulmonary infections and sepsis. A history of tuberculosis or hepatitis B calls for extra vigilance. Tuberculosis screening is required for patients who are considered for therapy with biologic DMARDs.
4. Malignancy is more common, particularly GI cancers and lymphoproliferative disorders. In addition, melanoma and lung cancer rates were elevated in one cohort study.
5. Osteoporosis is more common in patients with RA. Calcium and vitamin D are recommended. In addition, bisphosphonates should be considered for prevention if prednisone 5 mg or more daily is prescribed.

Patient Case

13. A 65-year-old woman received a diagnosis of RA 1 year ago. At the time of her diagnosis, her RF titer was 1:64; she presented with joint inflammation in both hands and about 45 minutes of morning stiffness. She began therapy with oral methotrexate and currently receives 15 mg weekly, folic acid 2 mg daily, ibuprofen 800 mg three times daily, and omeprazole 20 mg daily. At today's clinic visit, the patient reports the recurrence of her symptoms. Radiographic evaluation of her hand joints shows progression of joint space narrowing and bone erosion. Which is the next best step for this patient's RA treatment?

    A. Administer etanercept.

    B. Change to leflunomide.

    C. Add prednisone bridge therapy.

    D. Switch to hydroxychloroquine.

Acknowledgment: The contributions of the previous authors, Drs. Norma Owens, Jennifer Dugan, and Dominick Trombetta, are acknowledged.

REFERENCES

Principles to Promote Optimal Medication Use in Older People

1. AGS Expert Panel on the Care of Older Adults with Multimorbidity. Patient-centered care for older adults with multiple chronic conditions: a stepwise approach from the American Geriatrics Society. J Am Geriatr Soc 2012;60:1957-68.

2. American Geriatrics Society. 2015 updated Beers Criteria for potentially inappropriate medication use in older adults. American Geriatrics Society 2015 Beers Criteria Update Expert Panel. J Am Geriatr Soc 2015;63:2227-46.

3. American Geriatrics Society. Ten Things Physicians and Patients Should Question. Released February 21, 2013 (1–5) and February 27, 2014 (6–10). Available at www.choosingwisely.org/doctor-patient-lists/american-geriatrics-society/. Accessed November 19, 2015.

4. Dowling TC, Wang ES, Ferrucci L, et al. Glomerular filtration rate equations overestimate creatinine clearance in older individuals enrolled in the Baltimore Longitudinal Study on aging: impact on renal drug dosing. Pharmacotherapy 2013;33:912-21.

5. Elliott DP. Pharmacokinetics and pharmacodynamics in the elderly. In: Schumock G, Brundage D, Chapman M, et al., eds. Pharmacotherapy Self-Assessment Program, 5th ed. Lenexa, KS: American College of Clinical Pharmacy, 2004:115-30.

6. Hajjar ER, Gray SL, Slattum PW, et al. Chapter e8. Geriatrics. In: DiPiro JT, Talbert RL, Yee GC, et al., eds. Pharmacotherapy: A Pathophysiologic Approach, 9th ed. Available at http://accesspharmacy.mhmedical.com/content.aspx?bookid=689&sectionid=48811433. Accessed November 25, 2014.

7. Handler SM, Wright RM, Ruby CM, et al. Epidemiology of medication-related adverse events in nursing homes. Am J Geriatr Pharmacother 2006;4:264-72.

8. Higashi T, Shekelle PG, Solomon DH, et al. The quality of pharmacologic care for vulnerable older patients. Ann Intern Med 2004;140:714-20.

9. Hutchison LC, O'Brien CE. Changes in pharmacokinetics and pharmacodynamics in the elderly patient. J Pharm Pract 2007;20:4-12.

10. Inouye SK, Studenski S, Tinetti ME, et al. Geriatric syndromes: clinical, research and policy implications of a core geriatric concept. J Am Geriatr Soc 2007;55:780-91.

11. Labella AM, Merel SE, Phelan EA. Ten ways to improve the care of elderly patients in the hospital. J Hosp Med 2011;6:351-7.

12. Moore TJ, Cohen MR, Furberg CD. Serious adverse drug events reported to the Food and Drug Administration, 1998–2005. Arch Intern Med 2007;167:1752-9.

13. National Kidney Foundation. Glomerular Filtration Rate. Available at https://www.kidney.org/sites/default/files/docs/12-10-4004_abe_faqs_aboutgfrrev1b_singleb.pdf. Accessed November 19, 2015.

14. Onder G, van der Cammen TJM, Petrovic M, et al. Strategies to reduce the risk of iatrogenesis in complex older adults. Age Ageing 2013;42:284-91.

15. Schwartz JB. The current state of knowledge on age, sex, and their interactions on clinical pharmacology. Clin Pharmacol Ther 2007;82:87-96.

Dementia

1. Alzheimer's Association. Health Care Professionals and Alzheimer's. 2015. Available at www.alz.org/health-care-professionals/health-care-clinical-medical-resources.asp. Accessed November 19, 2015.

2. Birks J. Cholinesterase inhibitors for Alzheimer's disease. Cochrane Database Syst Rev 2006;1:CD005593.

3. Dubois B, Feldman HH, Jacova C, et al. Research criteria for the diagnosis of Alzheimer's disease: revising the NINCDS-ADRDA criteria. Lancet Neurol 2007;6:734-46.

4. Dysken MW, Sano M, Asthana S, et al. Effect of vitamin E and memantine on functional decline in Alzheimer disease: the TEAM-AD VA Cooperative randomized trial. JAMA 2014;311:33-44.

5. Gill SS, Anderson GM, Fischer HD, et al. Syncope and its consequences in patients with dementia receiving cholinesterase inhibitors. Arch Intern Med 2009;169:867-73.

6. Grimmer T, Kurz A. Effects of cholinesterase inhibitors on behavioural disturbances in Alzheimer's disease: a systematic review. Drugs Aging 2006;23:957-67.

7. Hilas O, Ezzo DC. Dementias and related neuropsychiatric issues. In: Richardson M, Chant C, Cheng JWM, et al., eds. Pharmacotherapy Self-Assessment Program, 7th ed. Neurology and psychiatry. Lenexa, KS: American College of Clinical Pharmacy, 2012:91-110.

8. Howard R, Lindesay J, Ritchie C, et al. Donepezil and memantine for moderate-to-severe Alzheimer's disease. N Engl J Med 2012;366:893-903.

9. Inouye SK, Westendorp RG, Saczynski JS. Delirium in elderly people. Lancet 2014;383:911-22.

10. Linnebur SA. Geriatric assessment, chapter 4 In: Hutchison LC, Sleeper RB, eds. Fundamentals of Geriatric Pharmacotherapy. Bethesda, MD: American Society of Health-System Pharmacists, 2010:71-90.

11. National Institute on Aging. Alzheimer's Diagnostic Guidelines. Available at www.nia.nih.gov/research/dn/alzheimers-diagnostic-guidelines. Accessed November 19, 2015.

12. Qaseam A, Snow V, Cross JT, et al. Current pharmacologic treatment of dementia: a clinical practice guideline from the American College of Physicians and the American Academy of Family Physicians. Ann Intern Med 2008;148:370-8.

13. Rubin CD. The primary care of Alzheimer disease. Am J Med Sci 2006;332:314-33.

14. Slattum PW, Peron EP, Hill AM. Chapter 38. Alzheimer's disease. In: DiPiro JT, Talbert RL, Yee GC, et al., eds. Pharmacotherapy: A Pathophysiologic Approach, 9th ed. Available at http://accesspharmacy.mhmedical.com/content.aspx?bookid=689&sectionid=45310488.

Behavioral Symptoms of Dementia

1. Agency for Health Care Research and Quality. Off-label use of atypical antipsychotics: an update. Aug 1, 2012. Available at http://effectivehealthcare.ahrq.gov/ehc/products/150/1193/off_lab_ant_psy_clin_fin_to_post.pdf. Accessed November 19, 2015.

2. Ballard C, Hanney ML, Theodoulou M, et al. The dementia antipsychotic withdrawal trial (DART-AD): long-term follow-up of a randomized placebo-controlled trial. Lancet Neurol 2009;8:151-7.

3. Ballard C, Sharp S, Corbett A. Dextromethorphan and quinidine for treating agitation in patients with Alzheimer disease dementia. JAMA 2015;314:1233-5.

4. Ballard CG, Waite J, Birks J. Atypical antipsychotics for aggression and psychosis in Alzheimer's disease. Cochrane Database Syst Rev 2006;1:CD003476.

5. Banerjee S, Hellier J, Romeo R, et al. Study of the use of antidepressant for depression in dementia: the HTA-SADD trial—a multicentre, randomized, double-blind, placebo-controlled trial of the clinical effectiveness and cost effectiveness of sertraline and mirtazapine. Health Technol Assess 2013;17:1-166.

6. Howard RJ, Juszczak E, Ballard CG, et al. Donepezil for the treatment of agitation in Alzheimer's disease. N Engl J Med 2007;357:1382-92.

7. Maher AR, Maglione M, Bagley S, et al. Efficacy and comparative effectiveness of atypical antipsychotic medications for off-label uses in adults. JAMA 2011;306:1359-69.

8. Maust DT, Kim HM, Seyfried LS, et al. Antipsychotics, other psychotropics, and the risk of death in patients with dementia. Number needed to harm. JAMA Psychiatry 2015;72:438-45.

9. Sadowsky CH, Galvin JE. Guidelines for the management of cognitive and behavioral problems in dementia. JABFM 2012;25:350-66.

10. Schneider LS, Dagerman KS, Insel P. Risk of death with atypical antipsychotic drug treatment for dementia. Meta-analysis of randomized placebo-controlled trials. JAMA 2005;294:1934-43.

11. Schneider LS, Tariot PN, Dagerman KS, et al. Effectiveness of atypical antipsychotic drugs in patients with Alzheimer's disease. N Engl J Med 2006;355:1525-38.

12. Sink KM, Holden KF, Yaffe K. Pharmacological treatment of neuropsychiatric symptoms of dementia. A review of the evidence. JAMA 2005;293:596-8.

13. Sutor B, Rummans TA, Smith GE. Assessment and management of behavioral disturbances in nursing home patients with dementia. Mayo Clin Proc 2001;76:540-50.

14. Yury CA, Fisher JE. Meta-analysis of the effectiveness of atypical antipsychotics for the treatment of behavioural problems in persons with dementia. Psychother Psychosom 2007;76:213-8.

Urinary Incontinence and Benign Prostatic Hypertrophy

1. American Urological Association. Clinical Guidelines. Management of Benign Prostatic Hyperplasia. 2010. Available at www.auanet.org/content/guidelines-and-quality-care/clinical-guidelines.cfm?sub=bph. Accessed November 19, 2015.

2. Edwards JL. Diagnosis and management of benign prostatic hyperplasia. Am Fam Physician 2008;77:1403-10.

3. Filson CP, Hollingsworth JM, Clemens JQ, Wei JT. The efficacy and safety of combined therapy with α-blockers and anticholinergics for men with benign prostatic hyperplasia: a meta-analysis. J Urol 2013;190:2153-65.

4. Gormley EA, Lightner DJ, Burglio KL, et al. Diagnosis and Treatment of Overactive Bladder (non-neurogenic) in Adults: AUA/SUFU Guideline. American Urological Association, May 2012, updated 2014. Available at www.auanet.org/common/pdf/education/clinical-guidance/Overactive-Bladder.pdf. Accessed November 19, 2015.

5. Gormley EA, Lightner DJ, Faraday M, et al. Diagnosis and treatment of overactive bladder (non-neurogenic) in adults: AIA/SUFU guideline amendment. J Urol 2015;193:1572-80.

6. Huang A. Nonsurgical treatments for urinary incontinence in women. Summary of primary findings and conclusions. JAMA 2013;173:1463-4.

7. Kaplan SA, Roehrborn CG, McConnell JD, et al. Long-term treatment with finasteride results in a clinically significant reduction in total prostate volume compared to placebo over the full range of baseline prostate sizes in men enrolled in the MTOPS trial. J Urol 2008;180:1030-3.

8. Porst H, Oelke M, Goldfischer ER, et al. Efficacy and safety of tadalafil 5 mg once daily for lower urinary tract symptoms suggestive of benign prostatic hyperplasia: subgroup analyses of pooled data from 4 multinational, randomized, placebo-controlled clinical studies. Urology 2013; 82:667-73.

9. Rees J, Bultitude M, Challacombe B. The management of lower urinary tract symptoms in men. BMJ 2014;348:g3861.

10. Roehrborn CG, Siami P, Barkin J, et al. The effects of dutasteride, tamsulosin and combination therapy on lower urinary tract symptoms in men with benign prostatic hyperplasia and prostatic enlargement: 2-year results from the CombAT study. J Urol 2008;179:616-21.

11. Rogers R. Urinary stress incontinence in women. N Engl J Med 2008;358:1029-36.

12. Sherman JJ. Health issues in older men. In: Dunsworth T, Richardson M, Chant C, et al., eds. Pharmacotherapy Self-Assessment Program, 6th ed. Women's and Men's Health. Lenexa, KS: American College of Clinical Pharmacy, 2008:163-80.

13. Tacklind J, MacDonald R, Rutks I, et al. *Serenoa repens* for benign prostatic hyperplasia. Cochrane Database Syst Rev 2012;12:CD001423.

14. Wood LN, Anger JT. Urinary incontinence in women. BMJ 2014;349:g4531.

15. Yamaguchi O, Nishizawa O, Takeda M, et al. Clinical guidelines for overactive bladder. Int J Urol 2009;16:126-42.

Osteoarthritis and Rheumatoid Arthritis

1. American Geriatrics Society. Pharmacological management of persistent pain in older persons. J Am Geriatr Soc 2009;57:1331-46.

2. Bruce SP. Rheumatoid arthritis. In: Richardson M, Chant C, Cheng JWM, et al., eds. Pharmacotherapy Self-Assessment Program, 6th ed. Chronic Illness II. Lenexa, KS: American College of Clinical Pharmacy, 2009:73-90.

3. Clegg DO, Reda DJ, Harris CL, et al. Glucosamine, chondroitin sulfate, and the two in combination for painful knee osteoarthritis. N Engl J Med 2006;354:795-808.

4. Eriksson J, Neovius M, Bratt J, et al. Biological vs conventional combination treatment and work loss in early rheumatoid arthritis. A randomized trial. JAMA Intern Med 2013;173:1407-14.

5. Fosbol E, Folke F, Jacobsen S, et al. Cause-specific cardiovascular risk associated with nonsteroidal antiinflammatory drugs among healthy individuals. Circ Cardiovasc Qual Outcomes 2010;3:395-405.

6. Hochberg MC, Altman RD, April KT, et al. American College of Rheumatology 2012 recommendations for the use of nonpharmacologic and pharmacologic therapies in osteoarthritis of the hand, hip, and knee. Arthritis Care Res 2012;64:465-74.

7. McAlindon TE, LaValley MP, Gulin JP, et al. Glucosamine and chondroitin for treatment of osteoarthritis: a systematic quality assessment and meta-analysis. JAMA 2000;283:1469-75.

8. O'Dell JR, Curtis JR, Mikuls TR, et al. Validation of the methotrexate-first strategy in patients with early, poor-prognosis rheumatoid arthritis: results from a two-year randomized, double-blind trial. Arthritis Rheum 2013;65:1985.

9. Peters MJL, Symmons DPM, McCarey D, et al. EULAR evidence-based recommendations for cardiovascular risk management in patients with rheumatoid arthritis and other forms of inflammatory arthritis. Ann Rheum Dis 2010;69:325-31.

10. Singh JA, Furst DE, Bharat A, et al. 2012 update of the 2008 American College of Rheumatology recommendations for the use of disease-modifying antirheumatic drugs and biologic agents in the treatment of rheumatoid arthritis. Arthritis Care Res 2012;64:625-39.

11. Smolen JS, Landewe R, Breedveld FC, et al. EULAR recommendations for the management of rheumatoid arthritis with synthetic and biological disease-modifying antirheumatic drugs: 2013 update. Ann Rheum Dis 2014;72:492-509.

12. Stoffer MA, Schoels MM, Smole JS, et al. Evidence for treating rheumatoid arthritis to target: results of a systematic literature search update. Ann Rheum Dis 2016;75:16-22.

ANSWERS AND EXPLANATIONS TO PATIENT CASES

1. Answer: D

Renal elimination is usually the most significantly changed pharmacokinetic value in older people. This patient's advanced age and diseases will add to her loss of renal function. Using the Cockcroft-Gault equation, this patient's estimated CrCl is 24 mL/minute/1.73 m². Creatinine clearance = [(140 − 85)65/(72 × 1.8)] × 0.85. At this level of function, glyburide elimination would be prolonged, and metformin use is contraindicated (Answer D is correct). The aspirin is low dose, and melatonin is safe even at very high doses (Answer A is incorrect). Although lisinopril is renally eliminated, dosing is based on response, and meclizine has mostly hepatic metabolism with no dosage adjustment in renal insufficiency (Answer B is incorrect). Answer C is incorrect because lisinopril is not considered potentially inappropriate in older adults like glyburide has been identified.

2. Answer: B

Common pharmacodynamic changes associated with aging include impaired homeostasis for electrolytes with angiotensin-converting enzyme inhibitors such as lisinopril and increased sensitivity to anticholinergic adverse effects from drugs such as meclizine (Answer B is correct). Lisinopril, metformin, and glyburide have primarily pharmacokinetic problems because of renal excretion changes when used in older adults (Answers C and D are incorrect). Melatonin is extremely safe without pharmacodynamic or pharmacokinetic issues in older adults, and the aspirin is low dose, so there is less problem with GI bleeding than with higher doses (Answer A is incorrect).

3. Answer: D

This patient experienced a geriatric syndrome (a fall) and hazards of hospitalization (decline in organ systems and function) seen with many older adult patients. At this time, she has several risk factors for another fall, including a history of falls, diseases such as diabetes and hypertension, dizziness, and use of several drugs. An assessment of gait and balance would help determine the severity of her risk (Answer D is correct). Although IADL assessment gives a good overall functional assessment, it does not focus on the risks associated with increased falls (Answer A is incorrect).

Evaluating the presence or severity of depression or of pressure sores would not be functional assessments, although they do affect functional abilities (Answers B and C are incorrect).

4. Answer: C

Efforts to maintain bone and muscle strength are more important for this patient than primary prevention of cardiovascular disease with simvastatin or lisinopril. Most older people do not consume a diet rich in vitamin D; moreover, most older people have less sun exposure and are more likely to be deficient in vitamin D, which is a risk factor for falls and reduced muscle strength. Furthermore, naproxen is not a good alternative for the patient because of increased risk of GI bleeding and worsening renal function (Answer C is correct). Although simvastatin and lisinopril can prevent complications caused by cardiovascular disease after extended use, they have not been shown to improve functional abilities in the short term (Answers A and B are incorrect). Pain management is important for functional status, but use of opioids compared with non-opioids has not been associated with differences in functional status (Answer D is incorrect).

5. Answer: B

This patient has a positive screen for mild dementia. However, when evaluating her cognitive loss, it is important to limit the use of any drug that could contribute to confusion, such as those identified on the AGS Beers Criteria, before beginning treatment for an unconfirmed condition (Answer A is incorrect). Anticholinergics such as tolterodine can cause confusion, so it would be best to discontinue this agent and reassess cognition before beginning treatment for AD (Answer B is correct). In addition, before beginning vitamin B_{12} injections, the patient should have laboratory evidence of deficiency (Answer C is incorrect). Without a serum sodium, there is no reason to anticipate that hydrochlorothiazide would cause her cognitive decline, so a switch to lisinopril is not indicated at this time (Answer D is incorrect).

6. Answer: B

Rivastigmine is a potent inhibitor of acetyl and butyryl cholinesterase, leading to significant cholinergic adverse effects such as nausea, vomiting, and diarrhea. However, use of the transdermal delivery system generates even plasma concentrations and lessens the incidence of cholinergic adverse effects. Because the maintenance dose has been achieved with rivastigmine 12 mg, this patient can switch to the patch that delivers 9.5 mg/day (Answer B is correct). Antacids will not substantially alleviate the GI effects of CI inhibitors, and prochlorperazine is anticholinergic (Answers A and D are incorrect). Because rivastigmine appears to work, it is better to continue its use, if possible, than to switch to memantine (Answer C is incorrect).

7. Answer: B

Over 3 years, this patient has declined only 4 points on her MMSE, which suggests a treatment response to donepezil. Furthermore, the patient can still live at home with her husband, and she has maintained some function in her basic ADLs. However, she has not responded to a higher donepezil dose, and there is no evidence that retrying it later is useful (Answer A is incorrect). Switching from one CI to another has not been shown effective (Answer D is incorrect). Because she has benefited from donepezil use, she should not abruptly discontinue it. Some, but not all, clinical trials with memantine show an additional treatment response when memantine is added to donepezil therapy. When the benefits, risks, and costs have been openly discussed and family preferences are to consent to therapy, a time-based trial is reasonable. Memantine should be initiated at 5 mg daily (Answer B is correct). Donepezil can be evaluated for tapering after memantine titration is achieved. Vitamin E has shown no effect in most large prospective trials of AD and is not first choice to provide benefit (Answer C is incorrect).

8. Answer: C

Patients in the late stages of dementia (as evidenced by an MMSE of 5/30) with behavior issues would benefit most from nonpharmacologic treatment such as music therapy (Answer C is correct). Social isolation would likely increase symptomatology, and haloperidol is not recommended until nonpharmacologic treatments have failed or patients have become a harm to themselves or others. In addition, the haloperidol dose is excessive, with risk outweighing benefit (Answers B and D are incorrect). Although pain control may be useful, ibuprofen is not the first drug of choice and has more

risk of harm than benefit in a frail older adult patient (Answer A is incorrect).

9. Answer: C

Increasing the dose of a CI has not been shown effective in reducing agitation with dementia (Answer A is incorrect). The patient has become a harm to self (because of refusing care), so a course of quetiapine is appropriate, assuming other nonpharmacologic treatments have been tried unsuccessfully (Answer C is correct). Citalopram has small studies showing evidence of effectiveness in the literature, but its role in therapy for agitation is unclear (Answer D is incorrect). No sleep disturbance is noted, so melatonin is unlikely to help (Answer B is incorrect).

10. Answer: C

This patient has symptoms of urge incontinence. Pelvic floor exercises in conjunction with drug therapy should be offered for initial therapy (Answer C is correct). Darifenacin alone is not the best treatment (Answer B is incorrect). There is some evidence that solifenacin, a selective muscarinic blocker, does not worsen cognition, and it would be preferred to tolterodine in this patient with MCI (Answer D is incorrect). Mirabegron is a newer agent with less evidence of its exact role in therapy, and it should not be offered without pelvic floor exercises (Answer A is incorrect).

11. Answer: C

Pharmacologic therapy targeted at reducing urethral sphincter pressure has proved effective in reducing BPH symptoms. Tamsulosin is an α-adrenergic blocker with more specific activity for the genitourinary system. Given that the patient already has low normal blood pressure, tamsulosin would be preferred to terazosin (Answer C is correct; Answer A is incorrect). Orthostatic hypotension can still occur with all α-adrenergic blockers, so patients should be monitored when therapy is initiated. Finasteride, a 5-α-reductase inhibitor, and combination therapy with these agents are recommended when there is evidence of large prostate size (Answer D is incorrect). Saw palmetto is not recommended in combination with 5-α-reductase inhibitors because it may reduce the efficacy of the reductase inhibitors (Answer B is incorrect).

12. Answer: B

The AGS recommends treatment with opioids for OA when older patients do not respond to initial therapy with acetaminophen (Answer B is correct). The NSAIDs and COX-2 inhibitors are seldom considered when a thorough assessment of the patient shows that the risk of treatment (GI bleeding and worsening renal function) does not outweigh the potential benefit (Answers A and C are incorrect). Glucosamine can be added to this patient's medication regimen; however, even if effective, it will not provide immediate pain relief (Answer D is incorrect).

13. Answer: A

This woman has indicators of a poor prognosis with rheumatoid arthritis (positive RF, many symptoms) and has not responded to methotrexate therapy. Although the next treatment step is not entirely clear, her best choices are between double or triple combination DMARD therapy and a biologic agent. Leflunomide or hydroxychloroquine would not be recommended as monotherapy for someone who has not responded to methotrexate (Answers B and D are incorrect). Etanercept has a response in 60%–75% of patients whose therapy with methotrexate has failed (Answer A is correct). Glucocorticosteroids are used as adjunctive therapy for the first several months of treatment with a disease-modifying agent and would not be adequate treatment at this time (Answer C is incorrect).

ANSWERS AND EXPLANATIONS TO SELF-ASSESSMENT QUESTIONS

1. Answer: A
Diazepam is a long-acting benzodiazepine that can accumulate in older patients, resulting in excessive lethargy, sedation, and unsteady gait, and the patient admits taking it every night during the past week (Answer A is correct). A worsening of the patient's depression is evident with the recent bereavement; however, that would not explain the unsteady gait (Answer D is incorrect). Lisinopril is not likely to cause this problem with his blood pressure at target, and atorvastatin is not a common cause of lethargy and confusion) (Answers B and C are incorrect).

2. Answer: C
In older patients, the volume of distribution of lipid-soluble drugs such as diazepam is increased, not decreased (Answer D is incorrect). In addition, changes in metabolism through phase I (oxidation) are diminished (Answer C is correct). Diazepam tends to accumulate with reduced capacity for elimination, resulting in excessive sedation and an increased risk of falls in older patients. Oral absorption is not significantly altered in older adults for chronic medications (Answer A is incorrect). Decreased renal excretion is likely but is not a significant contributor in this patient, given the drugs in his medication list (Answer B is incorrect).

3. Answer: B
The patient is not experiencing any symptoms of hypotension; therefore, no changes in her metoprolol therapy are warranted (Answer C is incorrect). Insufficient information is provided to determine the need to add memantine at this time (Answer A is incorrect). Adding vitamin D to this resident's regimen, given her deficient serum concentrations, may help reduce falls (Answer B is correct). Adding calcium carbonate may be helpful to reduce fractures but will not reduce fall risk (Answer D is incorrect).

4. Answer: A
The U.S. Preventive Services Task Force recommends aspirin use in women 55–79 years of age to prevent ischemic strokes in women with a low risk of GI bleeding. This patient, who has no history of GI bleeding, would probably benefit from low-dose aspirin (Answer A is correct). Increasing the dose of metoprolol or adding

hydrochlorothiazide might increase the risk of falls without providing additional risk reduction at her current blood pressure (Answers C and D are incorrect). Similarly, increasing her atorvastatin dose might marginally improve her low-density lipoprotein cholesterol but would not significantly change her risk of ischemic stroke. Furthermore, given that this patient is older than 75, the newest guidelines for prevention of cardiovascular disease do not recommend titration above moderate-intensity statin therapy (Answer B is incorrect).

5. Answer: B
An initial trial of acetaminophen at doses less than 3 g/day is a reasonable option for frail patients with OA pain (Answer B is correct). Ibuprofen and tramadol would be alternatives when more conservative medications have failed a trial of 1–2 weeks (Answers A and C are incorrect). As-needed hydrocodone/acetaminophen should be used cautiously in older patients who have significant osteoarthritic pain and cannot tolerate other drugs (Answer D is incorrect).

6. Answer: D
All CIs have similar efficacy. The rivastigmine transdermal patch is better tolerated than the oral dosage formulation. Donepezil tends to be better tolerated than the other oral CIs. Doses of cholinesterase medications should be titrated slowly to prevent GI upset. The initial dose of donepezil is 5 mg daily at bedtime, and for galantamine ER, the dose is 8 mg once daily (Answers A and B are incorrect). The rivastigmine patch 4.6 mg is the appropriate initial starting dose (Answer D is correct). Memantine has shown no beneficial effect in maintaining cognitive function as measured by MMSE scores (Answer C is incorrect).

7. Answer: A
This patient's current fasting blood glucose of 65 mg/dL and A1C value of 5.6% should prompt the pharmacist to request glipizide discontinuation (Answer A is correct). The recommendation for an A1C goal for older patients with several comorbid conditions is to keep it above 7.5%. The goals of therapy are to prevent hypoglycemia in older patients at greatest risk of this adverse drug reaction. There is no rationale for reducing the carvedilol dose, and given her normal basic metabolic

panel and blood pressure, reducing potassium chloride or discontinuing lisinopril is not indicated at this time (Answers B–D are incorrect).

8. Answer: D

There is no evidence at this time that would support increasing the donepezil dose to 23 mg to manage behavioral symptoms of dementia (Answer C is incorrect). The off-label use of atypical antipsychotic medications in patients with behavioral symptoms of dementia should be reserved for patients who pose a danger to themselves or others or experience hallucinations or delusions that are stressful to them (Answers A and B are incorrect). Adding acetaminophen to treat possible pain that could be causing the patient's behavior should be tried before more aggressive strategies (Answer D is correct).

9. Answer: A

Any new symptom of UI in an older adult should be thoroughly evaluated to determine whether there is a reversible cause. Infection, or the "I" in the mnemonic DRIP, may be the cause of the new symptoms in this patient. Urinalysis would be the most appropriate intervention for this reversible cause of incontinence (Answer A is correct). Tolterodine is used in urge incontinence that does not respond to an adequate pelvic floor muscle trial (Answer C is incorrect). Duloxetine has been used off-label for stress incontinence (Answer D is incorrect). Pelvic floor muscle exercises or Kegel exercises should be first-line therapy for stress, urge, or mixed incontinence in women (Answer B is incorrect).

10. Answer: C

In this patient with comorbid conditions of hypertension and BPH, the choice of α-blockers is based on the adverse effect profiles. This patient has an elevated PVR volume, so changing tamsulosin to terazosin might achieve a reduction in both blood pressure and urinary retention (Answer C is correct; Answer A is incorrect). Increasing the atenolol dose would address just the increased blood pressure, with no effect on the current problem of acute urinary retention (Answer B is incorrect). The patient is receiving moderate doses of controlled-release opioid, so reducing the hydromorphone dose for breakthrough pain is unlikely to help reduce the obstruction that may be worsened by the narcotics (Answer D is incorrect).

11. Answer: C

This patient is receiving 3 g of acetaminophen daily without adequate response, so a change in treatment is indicated. Diclofenac gel may provide adequate relief without systemic adverse effects (Answer C is correct). The patient, who has a history of GERD, is taking aspirin, so naproxen is not preferred (Answer B is incorrect). Evidence indicates that initially GI bleeding is reduced with celecoxib, but this is not maintained with chronic use (Answer A is incorrect). Methylprednisolone injection is more aggressive treatment and may be considered if topical diclofenac is ineffective (Answer D is incorrect).

12. Answer: D

In patients with recurring rheumatoid arthritis symptoms, moderate disease activity, and presence of a poor prognostic factor (anti–cyclic citrullinated peptides), adding sulfasalazine and hydroxychloroquine to methotrexate follows guidelines from the 2012 American College of Rheumatology recommendations update for the treatment of rheumatoid arthritis (Answer D is correct). Specifically, they recommend either double or triple combination DMARD therapy for patients with an inadequate response to methotrexate. Prednisone may be used as bridge therapy, but continued therapy may not be supported by a risk-benefit analysis (Answer A is incorrect). Changing the administration of methotrexate from the oral route to the intramuscular route would not confer any significant advantage in this case (Answer B is incorrect). Similarly, changing methotrexate to monotherapy with leflunomide would provide no significant benefits (Answer C is incorrect).

13. Answer: B

Patients with a low bone mass and a T-score of –2.5 or less at the femoral neck, total hip, or lumbar spine, with a 10-year probability of having a major osteoporosis-related fracture of 20% or greater on the basis of the World Health Organization Fracture Risk Assessment Tool, would benefit from an osteoporosis medication. This patient's risk fits that category, and she is already taking adequate calcium and vitamin D (Answer D is incorrect). Adding a bisphosphonate is the most appropriate intervention at this time (Answer B is correct). Adding raloxifene or teriparatide is inappropriate for the treatment of this patient right now but might be appropriate care in a different scenario (Answers A and C are incorrect).

Neurology

Melody Ryan, Pharm.D., MPH, BCPS

University of Kentucky
Lexington, Kentucky

NEUROLOGY

MELODY RYAN, PHARM.D., MPH, BCPS

UNIVERSITY OF KENTUCKY
LEXINGTON, KENTUCKY

Learning Objectives

1. Differentiate between various seizure medications on the basis of use and adverse effects.
2. Develop a treatment strategy for status epilepticus.
3. Identify appropriate treatment strategies for primary and secondary stroke prevention.
4. Determine the appropriateness of treatment with tissue plasminogen activator for acute stroke.
5. Examine common adverse effects associated with the treatment of Parkinson disease.
6. Differentiate between regimens for acute and prophylactic treatment of migraine, tension, and cluster headaches.
7. Identify common adverse effects of disease-modifying therapies for multiple sclerosis.

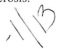

Self-Assessment Questions

Answers and explanations to these questions can be found at the end of this chapter.

1. T.L. is a 35-year-old man with complex partial seizures. He is otherwise healthy. He was placed on phenytoin after a seizure about 2 months ago. He currently takes phenytoin 100 mg 3 capsules orally every night. During his clinic visit, he tells you he has had no seizures, and he has no signs of toxicity. He is allergic to sulfa drugs. His phenytoin serum concentration is 17.7 mcg/mL. Which is the best interpretation of this concentration?

   A. It is too low.
   B. It is too high.
   C. It is just right.
   D. A serum albumin concentration is necessary to interpret this concentration.

2. B.V. is a 28-year-old woman brought to your emergency department for treatment of status epilepticus. She receives lorazepam 4 mg intravenously with subsequent seizure cessation. Which medication is the best next treatment step for B.V.?

   A. Topiramate.
   B. Phenytoin.
   C. Zonisamide.
   D. Diazepam.

3. J.H. is a 42-year-old man with complex partial seizures for which he was prescribed topiramate. He has been increasing the topiramate dose every other day according to instructions from his primary care provider. He comes to the pharmacy where you work but seems a little confused and has difficulty finding the words to have a conversation with you. Which is the best assessment of J.H.'s condition?

   A. Discontinue topiramate; he is having an allergic reaction.
   B. Increase the topiramate dose; he is having partial seizures.
   C. Slow the rate of topiramate titration; he is having psychomotor slowing.
   D. Get a topiramate serum concentration; he is probably supratherapeutic.

Questions 4 and 5 pertain to the following case:
R.H. is a 59-year-old man who presents to the emergency department for new-onset left-sided weakness that began 6 hours ago. He has a history of hypertension and coronary artery disease. His medication list includes atenolol 50 mg/day orally, hydrochlorothiazide 25 mg/day orally, and aspirin 325 mg/day orally. His vital signs include blood pressure (BP) 160/92 mm Hg, heart rate 92 beats/minute, respiratory rate 14 breaths/minute, and temperature 38°C. The treatment team assesses this patient for treatment with tissue plasminogen activator and asks for your opinion.

4. Which reply is best, given this information?

   A. R.H. should be treated with tissue plasminogen activator.
   B. R.H. should not be treated with tissue plasminogen activator because the onset of his stroke symptoms was 6 hours ago.
   C. R.H. should not be treated with tissue plasminogen activator because he has hypertension.
   D. R.H. should not be treated with tissue plasminogen activator because he takes aspirin.

5. R.H. survives his stroke. As part of his discharge treatment plan, you evaluate his risk factors for a second stroke. His aspirin therapy is discontinued. Which medication for secondary stroke prevention is best to initiate at this time?

   A. Dipyridamole.

   B. Enoxaparin.

   C. Heparin.

   D. Clopidogrel.

Questions 6 and 7 pertain to the following case:
C.P. is a 69-year-old man given a diagnosis of Parkinson disease 7 years ago. He states that he is most bothered by his bradykinesia symptoms. On examination, he also has a pronounced tremor, postural instability, and masked facial expression. He currently takes carbidopa/levodopa/entacapone 25 mg/100 mg/200 mg orally four times daily, ropinirole 1 mg orally three times daily, and selegiline 5 mg orally twice daily. He has no drug allergies. He also describes a worsening of his Parkinson disease symptoms, which fluctuate randomly during the day. He has developed a charting system for his symptoms during the day, and no relationship seems to exist with the time he is scheduled to take his carbidopa/levodopa/entacapone doses.

6. Which condition best describes C.P.'s fluctuating Parkinson disease symptoms?

   A. Wearing-off.

   B. On-off.

   C. Dyskinesia.

   D. Dystonia.

7. For his symptoms, C.P. is given a prescription for apomorphine. Which statement about this drug is most accurate?

   A. He must be trained on self-injection techniques with saline, but he can administer his first dose of apomorphine at home when he needs it.

   B. He should not take apomorphine if he is allergic to penicillin.

   C. If he does not take a dose for more than 1 week, he should begin with a loading dose with his next injection.

   D. It may cause severe nausea and vomiting.

8. W.S. is a 57-year-old man initiated on rasagiline for treatment of his newly diagnosed Parkinson disease. He develops a cough, body aches, and nasal congestion. Which medication is best to treat W.S.'s symptoms?

   A. Guaifenesin.

   B. Dextromethorphan.

   C. Tramadol.

   D. Pseudoephedrine.

Questions 9 and 10 pertain to the following case:
R.M. is a 47-year-old woman with long-standing migraine headaches. Her headache pain is easily relieved with sumatriptan 100 mg orally as needed. However, with her last dose she experienced substernal chest pain radiating to her left arm. She reported to her local emergency department, where she had a complete workup. Her final diagnoses were coronary artery disease and hypertension. For these conditions, she was placed on hydrochlorothiazide 25 mg orally every morning.

9. Which drug is best for R.M. to use for her migraine headaches?

   A. Frovatriptan.

   B. Zolmitriptan.

   C. Dihydroergotamine.

   D. Naproxen.

10. If R.M. needs a drug for migraine prophylaxis, which agent is best to recommend?

   A. Propranolol.

   B. Valproic acid.

   C. Amitriptyline.

   D. Gabapentin.

Questions 11–13 pertain to the following case:
L.M. is a 43-year-old man who received a diagnosis of progressive-relapsing multiple sclerosis 2 years ago. He has been taking glatiramer acetate since then. However, there was no discernible decrease in the number of exacerbations he has experienced. He has spasticity in his legs, which has caused several falls in the past month, and he experiences fatigue that worsens as the day progresses.

11. Which drug therapy is best for L.M.'s multiple sclerosis?

    A. Cyclophosphamide.

    B. Methylprednisolone.

    C. Azathioprine.

    D. Fingolimod.

12. Which drug is best to treat L.M.'s spasticity?

    A. Diazepam.

    B. Baclofen.

    C. Carisoprodol.

    D. Metaxalone.

13. Which drug is best to treat L.M.'s fatigue?

    A. Propranolol.

    B. Lamotrigine.

    C. Amantadine.

    D. Ropinirole.

BPS Pharmacotherapy Specialty Examination Content Outline

This chapter covers the following sections of the Pharmacotherapy Specialty Examination Content Outline:

1. Domain 1: Patient-Specific Pharmacotherapy
   a. Tasks 1:1–5, 1:7–8, 1:11–12, 3:2, 4:1–2, 4:5–7

I. EPILEPSY

A. Epidemiology
   1. Ten percent of the population will have a seizure.
   2. About 50 million people worldwide have epilepsy.
   3. About 50% of patients with a new diagnosis become seizure free on their first treatment, with up to 70% becoming seizure free after treatment adjustment.

B. Classification of Seizures: Seizures are generally classified according to the International League Against Epilepsy (ILAE) scheme, adopted in 1981, with modifications in 2001 and 2010 (Berg AT, Berkovic SF, Brodie MJ, et al. Revised terminology and concepts for organization of seizures and epilepsies: report of the ILAE Commission on Classification and Terminology, 2005-2009. Epilepsia 2010;51:676-85).
   1. Focal seizures are conceptualized as originating at some point within networks limited to one hemisphere.
      a. No specific classification within focal seizures is recommended.
      b. The terms *simple partial seizure, complex partial seizure,* and *secondarily generalized seizure* have been eliminated from classification; however, they are still used to describe seizures.
   2. Generalized seizures are conceptualized as originating at some point within and rapidly engaging bilaterally distributed neural networks.
      a. Absence: Typical absence seizures are brief and abrupt, last 10–30 seconds, and occur in clusters. Absence seizures usually result in a short loss of consciousness, or the patient may stare, be motionless, or have a distant expression on his or her face. Electroencephalograms (EEGs) performed during seizure activity usually show three Hz spike-and-wave complexes. Absence seizures can be further classified as typical, atypical, myoclonic absence, and eyelid myoclonia.
      b. Myoclonic: Consist of brief, lightning-like jerking movements of the entire body or the upper and occasionally lower extremities. Myoclonic seizures can be further classified as myoclonic, myoclonic atonic, or myoclonic tonic.
      c. Tonic-clonic: Typically, there are five phases of a primary tonic-clonic seizure: flexion, extension, tremor, clonic, and postictal. During the flexion phase, the patient's mouth may be held partly open, and the patient may experience upward eye movement, involvement of the extremities, and loss of consciousness. In the extension phase, the patient may be noted to extend his or her back and neck; experience contraction of thoracic and abdominal muscles; be apneic; and have flexion, extension, and adduction of the extremities. The patient may cry out as air is forced from the lungs in this phase. The tremor phase occurs as the patient goes from tonic rigidity to tremors and then to a clonic state. During the clonic phase, the patient will experience rhythmic jerks. The length of the entire seizure is usually 1–3 minutes. After the seizure, the patient may be postictal. During this time, the patient can be difficult to arouse or very somnolent. Before the seizure, a patient may experience a prodrome but not an aura.
      d. Clonic: Only the clonic phase of a tonic-clonic seizure; rhythmic, repetitive, jerking muscle movements
      e. Tonic: Only the flexion or extension phases of a tonic-clonic seizure
      f. Atonic: Characterized by a loss of muscle tone. Atonic seizures are often described as drop attacks, in which a patient loses tone and falls to the ground.
   3. Status epilepticus is a condition resulting either from the failure of the mechanisms responsible for seizure termination or from the initiation of mechanisms, which lead to abnormally prolonged seizures after 5 minutes. It is a condition that can have long-term consequences after 30 minutes, including neuronal death, neuronal injury, and alteration of neuronal networks, depending on the type and duration of seizures. Mortality is up to 20% for status epilepticus.

4. Nonepileptic seizures are paroxysmal nonepileptic episodes resembling epileptic seizures that can be organic or psychogenic.

5. Other associated symptoms
   a. Prodrome: Awareness of an impending seizure before it occurs. The prodrome may consist of headache, insomnia, irritability, or feeling of impending doom.
   b. Aura: A focal seizure, without loss of consciousness, consisting of sensory or autonomic symptoms that may precede evolution to a bilateral, convulsive seizure. Patients may experience feelings of fear, embarrassment, or déjà vu. Automatic behavior (automatism) and psychic symptoms may occur. Automatisms may include lip smacking, chewing, swallowing, abnormal tongue movements, scratching, thrashing of the arms or legs, fumbling with clothing, and snapping the fingers. Psychic symptoms include illusions, hallucinations, emotional changes, dysphasia, and cognitive problems.

C. Diagnosis
   1. Physical examination should be performed, with special attention to neurologic findings. The neurologic examination may include examination of the head, vision, cranial nerves, motor function, cerebellar function, and sensory function.
   2. Laboratory tests are based on the history and physical examination results; a full diagnostic onslaught is unnecessary in many patients. Because metabolic causes of seizures are common, serum glucose, electrolytes, calcium, complete blood cell counts, and renal function tests may be necessary. A toxicology screen may also be prudent.
   3. EEGs are used to help confirm the diagnosis, classify seizures, locate the site of the seizures, and select the best seizure medication. The best time to perform an EEG is while the patient is having seizures. If it is not possible to perform the EEG during seizures, it should be performed as soon after the seizure as possible. Depending on the clinical situation, an EEG may be obtained under normal conditions, when the patient is sleep deprived, or when the patient is asleep. Patients whose seizures are difficult to diagnose or control may need prolonged closed-circuit video–EEG monitoring. Keep in mind that an interictal (when the patient is not having clinical seizures) EEG may be normal but that this does not preclude the diagnosis of epilepsy.
   4. Magnetic resonance imaging is the neuroimaging technique of choice for epilepsy. Computed tomography (CT) scanning can be useful in finding brain lesions when magnetic resonance imaging cannot be performed in a timely fashion.

D. Treatment
   1. Medications (see Tables 1–5)
      a. Benzodiazepines
         i. Mechanism of action: Augment γ-aminobutyric acid–mediated chloride influx
         ii. Tolerance may develop: Usually used as adjunctive, short-term therapy
         iii. Most commonly used drugs: Chlorazepate (Tranxene), clobazam (Onfi), clonazepam (Klonopin), diazepam (Valium), and lorazepam (Ativan)
         iv. All benzodiazepines are controlled substances, scheduled as C-IV.
         v. Nonepileptic indications: Chlorazepate (anxiety disorders, anxiety), clonazepam (panic disorder with or without agoraphobia), lorazepam (anxiety disorders, anxiety)
      b. Carbamazepine (Carbatrol, Epitol, Equetro, Tegretol, Teril)
         i. Mechanism of action: Fast sodium channel blocker
         ii. Pharmacokinetics: Enzyme inducer, autoinduction
         iii. Adverse effects: Rash (occurs after a delay of 2–8 weeks), syndrome of inappropriate antidiuretic hormone release, aplastic anemia, thrombocytopenia, anemia, leukopenia

      iv. Extended-release tablets (Tegretol XR) 100, 200, and 400 mg; extended-release capsules (Carbatrol) 100, 200, and 300 mg available. Dosing is still twice daily. Do not crush or chew. Extended-release capsules (Carbatrol) can be opened and sprinkled on food. Ghost tablets can be seen in the stool with the extended-release tablets (Tegretol XR).

      v. Patients with the *HLA-B*1502* allele are at a 10-fold elevated risk of Stevens-Johnson syndrome.

        (a) Testing is recommended for Asians (including Indians).

        (b) More than 15% of populations in Hong Kong, Malaysia, the Philippines, and Thailand have this allele.

      vi. Patients with the *HLA-A*3101* allele are also at a 12-fold elevated risk of hypersensitivity syndrome and a 3-fold elevated risk of maculopapular exanthema.

        (a) The prevalence of this allele is 2%–5% in northern European populations and 9.1% of Japanese populations.

        (b) No recommendations for testing for this allele have been issued.

      vii. Nonepileptic indication: Trigeminal neuralgia

  c. Eslicarbazepine acetate (Aptiom)

      i. Mechanism of action: Fast sodium channel blocker

      ii. Prodrug for S(+)-licarbazepine, an active metabolite of oxcarbazepine

      iii. Adjust dose if creatinine clearance (CrCl) is less than 50 mL/minute.

  d. Ethosuximide (Zarontin)

      i. Mechanism of action: T-type calcium current blocker

      ii. Useful only for absence seizures

  e. Ezogabine (Potiga)

      i. Mechanism of action: Potassium channel opener

      ii. Adverse effects: Urinary retention, hallucinations, QT prolongation, pigment changes in retina, or blue discoloration of the lips, nail beds, face, legs, sclera, and conjunctiva

      iii. Monitoring recommendations: Baseline and periodic eye examinations (every 6 months) with visual acuity testing and dilated fundus photography

      iv. Ezogabine is a schedule V controlled substance

  f. Felbamate (Felbatol)

      i. Mechanism of action: Blocks glycine site on *N*-methyl-D-aspartate receptor

      ii. Serious adverse effects: Hepatotoxicity, aplastic anemia. Patient or guardian must sign consent form. Used only when seizures are severe and refractory to other medications and when the benefit clearly outweighs the potential adverse effects

  g. Fosphenytoin (Cerebyx)

      i. Mechanism of action: Prodrug for phenytoin; fast sodium channel blocker

      ii. Uses: Parenteral formulation for loading or maintenance dosing in place of phenytoin; status epilepticus

      iii. Pharmacokinetics: Enzyme inducer, nonlinear kinetics

      iv. Dosing: Phenytoin equivalents are used; 1 mg of phenytoin = 1.5 mg of fosphenytoin = 1 mg of phenytoin equivalent. Intramuscular or intravenous dosing is appropriate.

      v. Adverse effects: Hypotension, perianal itching, other adverse effects of phenytoin

      vi. Advantages over phenytoin

        (a) Intramuscular or intravenous dosing

        (b) Phlebitis is minimized.

        (c) Infusion can be up to 150 mg of phenytoin equivalents per minute.

        (d) Can deliver in normal saline solution or D_5W (5% dextrose [in water] injection)

    h. Gabapentin (Neurontin)

       i.   Mechanism of action: Inhibition of α2δ subunit of voltage-dependent calcium channels

      ii.   Pharmacokinetics: Not metabolized, eliminated renally; adjustments may be necessary for renal dysfunction and hemodialysis.

     iii.   Nonepileptic indication: Postherpetic neuralgia pain

     iv.   Doses often exceed product information maximum of 3600 mg/day.

      v.   Extended-release tablets (Gralise) 300 and 600 mg are available. Their indication is for postherpetic neuralgia, not epilepsy.

     vi.   Gabapentin enacarbil (Horizant) extended-release tablets 300 and 600 mg are available. This agent is a prodrug for gabapentin and is indicated for postherpetic neuralgia and restless legs syndrome, not epilepsy.

    i. Lacosamide (Vimpat)

       i.   Mechanism of action: Slow sodium channel blocker

      ii.   Maximal dose of 300 mg/day with a CrCl of 30 mL/minute or less or with mild to moderate hepatic impairment

     iii.   Adverse effects: PR interval prolongation or first-degree atrioventricular block; baseline and steady-state electrocardiogram recommended in patients with known cardiac conduction problems, taking medications known to induce PR interval prolongation, or with severe cardiac disease

     iv.   Controlled substance schedule V because of euphoric effects

      v.   Parenteral formulation: Has a U.S. Food and Drug Administration (FDA) indication only for replacement of oral formulation

    j. Lamotrigine (Lamictal)

       i.   Mechanism of action: Decreases glutamate and aspartate release, delays repetitive firing of neurons, blocks fast sodium channels

      ii.   Rash is a primary concern; lamotrigine must be titrated slowly to avoid a rash.

     iii.   Valproic acid decreases lamotrigine metabolism; this interaction requires even slower titration and lower final doses.

     iv.   Estrogen-containing oral contraceptives increase lamotrigine clearance, so twice the amount of lamotrigine may be necessary.

      v.   Extended-release tablets (Lamictal XR) are available (25 mg, 50 mg, 100 mg, 200 mg, 250 mg, 300 mg).

     vi.   Nonepileptic indications: Maintenance treatment of bipolar I mood disorder

    k. Levetiracetam (Keppra)

       i.   Mechanism of action: May prevent hypersynchronization of epileptiform burst firing and propagation of seizure activity

      ii.   Pharmacokinetics: Not metabolized extensively, adjust dose in renal dysfunction, no drug interactions with other seizure medications

     iii.   Parenteral use: Currently indicated by the FDA only for replacement of oral dosing; however, sometimes used for status epilepticus

     iv.   Extended-release tablets (500 mg, 750 mg) are available for once-daily dosing.

l. Oxcarbazepine (Trileptal)
   i. Mechanism of action: Fast sodium channel blocker
   ii. Pharmacokinetics: Active metabolite 10-monohydroxy oxcarbazepine; enzyme inducer, no autoinduction
   iii. Adverse effects: Hyponatremia more common than with carbamazepine (increased dose and increased age increase risk of hyponatremia); blood dyscrasias less common than with carbamazepine; 25%–30% of patients with hypersensitivity to carbamazepine will have hypersensitivity to oxcarbazepine; rash
   iv. Extended-release tablets (Oxtellar XR) are available (150 mg, 300 mg, 600 mg).
m. Perampanel (Fycompa)
   i. Mechanism of action: Noncompetitive antagonist of the inotropic α-amino-3-hydroxy-5-methyl-4-isoxazole propionic acid (AMPA) glutamate receptor
   ii. Pharmacokinetics: 95%–96% protein bound to albumin and α_1-acid glycoprotein; metabolized by cytochrome P450 (CYP) 3A4 and 3A5; 105-hour half-life
   iii. Adverse effects: Neuropsychiatric effects (irritability, aggression, anger, anxiety), dizziness, gait disturbance, weight gain
   iv. Perampanel is a schedule III controlled substance.
n. Phenobarbital (Luminal)
   i. Mechanism of action: Increases γ-aminobutyric acid–mediated chloride influx
   ii. Pharmacokinetics: Enzyme inducer
   iii. Adverse effects: Hyperactivity, cognitive impairment
   iv. Phenobarbital is a schedule IV controlled substance
   v. Nonepileptic use: Anxiety
o. Phenytoin (Dilantin, Phenytek)
   i. Mechanism of action: Fast sodium channel blocker
   ii. Pharmacokinetics: Enzyme inducer, nonlinear kinetics
   iii. Administration considerations
      (a) Intravenous formulation: Very basic product. Phlebitis and extravasation are concerns; hypotension; maximal infusion rate of 50 mg/minute. Can prepare only in normal saline solution
      (b) Oral suspension: Must be shaken well; adheres to feeding tubes and is bound by enteral nutrition products
   iv. Dose-related adverse effects: Nystagmus, ataxia, drowsiness, cognitive impairment
   v. Non–dose-related adverse effects: Gingival hyperplasia, hirsutism, acne, rash, hepatotoxicity, coarsening of facial features
p. Pregabalin (Lyrica)
   i. Mechanism of action: Inhibition of α2δ subunit of voltage-dependent calcium channels
   ii. Pharmacokinetics: Not metabolized, renally excreted, reduce dose in renal dysfunction
   iii. Adverse effects: Drowsiness, blurred vision, weight gain, edema, angioedema, creatine kinase elevations (three reports of rhabdomyolysis), rash
   iv. Schedule V controlled substance: Insomnia, nausea, headache, diarrhea reported after abrupt discontinuation
   v. Nonepileptic indications: Neuropathic pain associated with diabetic neuropathy, postherpetic neuralgia, and fibromyalgia

Table 1. Medication Selection for Various Seizure Types[a]

Drug	Focal	Generalized Tonic-Clonic	Absence	Atypical Absence	Atonic	Myoclonic	Infantile Spasms	Status Epilepticus	Lennox-Gastaut Syndrome
Acetazolamide	4	4	3	3	—	—	—	—	—
Carbamazepine	1	1	—	—	4	4	—	—	—
Clobazam	4	4	3	—	—	3	—	—	1
Clonazepam	3	3	2	2	1	2	2	—	1
Corticotropin	—	—	—	—	—	—	1	—	—
Diazepam	—	—	—	4	—	4	4	1	2
Eslicarbazepine	4	—	—	—	—	—	—	—	—
Ethosuximide	—	—	1	1	—	4	—	—	—
Ezogabine	4	—	—	—	—	—	—	—	—
Felbamate	5	5	5	—	—	5	—	—	5
Gabapentin	1	2	—	—	—	—	—	—	—
Lacosamide	1	—	—	—	—	—	—	3	—
Lamotrigine	1	1	2	4	3	3	—	—	1
Levetiracetam	1	1	4	—	—	3	—	3	—
Lorazepam	3	3	3	3	—	3	—	1	—
Oxcarbazepine	1	1	—	—	3	3	—	—	—
Perampanel	4	—	—	—	—	—	—	—	—
Phenobarbital	2	2	2	—	—	3	—	2	—
Phenytoin	2	2	—	—	—	3	—	1	—
Pregabalin	4	—	—	—	—	—	—	—	—
Primidone	2	2	2	—	—	—	—	—	—
Rufinamide	4	3	3	—	3	—	—	—	1
Tiagabine	4	—	—	—	4	4	—	—	—
Topiramate	1	1	3	—	3	1	—	—	—
Valproic acid	2	1	1	1	1	1	1	2	—
Vigabatrin	5	5	—	—	—	—	5	—	—
Zonisamide	1	3	3	—	—	4	—	—	—

[a]Not all uses are U.S. Food and Drug Administration (FDA)-approved indications. 1 = first-line drug; 2 = second-line drug; 3 = some therapeutic effect; 4 = adjunctive therapy; 5 = used only when benefits outweigh risks.

Table 2. Selected Interactions Between Seizure Medications

Antiepileptic Drug	Added Seizure Medication	Change in Serum Concentration of the Initial Seizure Medication	Mechanism
Carbamazepine	Ethosuximide	Decreased	Increased metabolism
	Felbamate	Decreased, increased epoxide (active component of carbamazepine)	Inhibits epoxide degradation
	Phenobarbital	Decreased	Increased metabolism
	Phenytoin	Decreased	Increased metabolism
	Primidone	Decreased	Increased metabolism
	Rufinamide	Decreased	Increased metabolism
Clobazam	Eslicarbazepine	Increased	Decreased metabolism
Eslicarbazepine	Carbamazepine	Decreased	Increased metabolism
	Phenobarbital	Decreased	Increased metabolism
	Phenytoin	Decreased	Increased metabolism
Ezogabine	Carbamazepine	Decreased	Probable increased metabolism
	Phenytoin	Decreased	Probable increased metabolism
Felbamate	Carbamazepine	Decreased	Increased metabolism
	Phenytoin	Decreased	Increased metabolism
Lamotrigine	Carbamazepine	Decreased	Increased metabolism
	Phenobarbital	Decreased	Increased metabolism
	Phenytoin	Decreased	Increased metabolism
	Primidone	Decreased	Increased metabolism
	Rufinamide	Decreased	Increased metabolism
	Valproic acid	Increased	Decreased metabolism
Oxcarbazepine	Carbamazepine	Decreased	Increased metabolism
	Phenobarbital	Decreased	Increased metabolism
	Phenytoin	Decreased	Increased metabolism
	Valproic acid	Decreased	Unknown
Perampanel	Carbamazepine	Decreased	Increased metabolism
	Oxcarbazepine	Decreased	Increased metabolism
	Phenytoin	Decreased	Increased metabolism
Phenobarbital	Oxcarbazepine	Increased	Decreased metabolism
	Phenytoin	Increased	Unknown
	Rufinamide	Increased	Decreased metabolism
	Valproic acid	Increased	Inhibition of metabolism

Table 2. Selected Interactions Between Seizure Medications *(continued)*

Antiepileptic Drug	Added Seizure Medication	Change in Serum Concentration of the Initial Seizure Medication	Mechanism
Phenytoin	Carbamazepine	Decreased	Increased metabolism
	Eslicarbazepine	Increased	Decreased metabolism
	Oxcarbazepine	Increased or no change	Unknown
	Phenobarbital	Increased or decreased	Decreased or increased metabolism
	Rufinamide	Increased	Unknown
	Topiramate	Increased	Decreased metabolism
	Valproic acid	Decreased total; increased free	Displacement from binding sites
	Vigabatrin	Decreased	Increased metabolism
Primidone	Carbamazepine	Increased phenobarbital concentration	Unknown
	Phenytoin	Increased phenobarbital concentration	Unknown
Rufinamide	Carbamazepine	Decreased	Increased metabolism
	Phenobarbital	Decreased	Increased metabolism
	Phenytoin	Decreased	Increased metabolism
	Primidone	Decreased	Increased metabolism
	Valproic acid	Increased	Decreased clearance
Topiramate	Carbamazepine	Decreased	Increased metabolism
	Lamotrigine	Decreased	Unknown
	Phenytoin	Decreased	Increased metabolism
	Valproic acid	Decreased	Increased metabolism
Valproic acid	Carbamazepine	Decreased	Increased metabolism
	Felbamate	Increased	Unknown
	Oxcarbazepine	Decreased	Unknown
	Phenobarbital	Decreased	Increased metabolism
	Phenytoin	Decreased	Increased metabolism
	Primidone	Decreased	Increased metabolism
	Topiramate	Decreased	Increased metabolism
Zonisamide	Carbamazepine	Decreased	Increased metabolism
	Phenobarbital	Decreased	Increased metabolism
	Phenytoin	Decreased	Increased metabolism

Table 3. Selected Interactions of Non-AEDs on Seizure Medications

Seizure Medication	Other Drug	Effect on the Seizure Medication	Mechanism
Carbamazepine	Cimetidine	Increased serum concentration	Inhibition of carbamazepine metabolism
	Diltiazem	Increased serum concentration	Inhibition of carbamazepine metabolism
	Erythromycin	Increased serum concentration	Inhibition of carbamazepine metabolism
	Isoniazid	Increased serum concentration	Inhibition of carbamazepine metabolism
	Nefazodone	Increased serum concentration	Inhibition of carbamazepine metabolism
	Theophylline	Decreased serum concentration	Increased carbamazepine metabolism
	Troleandomycin	Increased serum concentration	Inhibition of carbamazepine metabolism
	Verapamil	Increased serum concentration	Inhibition of carbamazepine metabolism
Clobazam	Fluconazole	Increased serum concentration	Inhibitor of CYP2C19
	Fluvoxamine	Increased serum concentration	Inhibitor of CYP2C19
	Omeprazole	Increased serum concentration	Inhibitor of CYP2C19
	Ticlopidine	Increased serum concentration	Inhibitor of CYP2C19
Gabapentin	Antacids	Decreased serum concentration	Decreased bioavailability
Lamotrigine	Estrogen-containing contraceptives	Decreased serum concentration	Possibly induction of glucuronidation of lamotrigine
	Rifampin	Decreased serum concentration	Possibly induction of glucuronidation of lamotrigine
Perampanel	Ethanol and other CNS depressants	CNS additive or supra-additive effects	Additive CNS depression
	Rifampin	Decreased serum concentration	Increased metabolism
	St. John's wort	Decreased serum concentration	Increased metabolism
Phenobarbital; primidone	Ethanol	Acute ethanol ingestion may cause CNS additive effects and respiratory depression; chronic ethanol ingestion may result in variable effects	Additive CNS depression and decreased barbiturate metabolism with acute ethanol ingestion

Table 3. Selected Interactions of Non-AEDs on Seizure Medications *(continued)*

Seizure Medication	Other Drug	Effect on the Seizure Medication	Mechanism
Phenytoin	Anticoagulants, oral	May increase phenytoin serum concentration; decreased or increased anticoagulant effects	Complex mechanism
	Antineoplastics (bleomycin, cisplatin, vinblastine, methotrexate, carmustine)	Decreased pharmacologic effect	Unknown, possible decreased absorption caused by antineoplastic mucosal damage
	Chloramphenicol	Increased phenytoin serum concentration; decreased or increased chloramphenicol serum concentration	Inhibition of phenytoin metabolism; effect on chloramphenicol unknown
	Cimetidine	Increased serum concentration	Inhibition of phenytoin metabolism
	Diazoxide	Decreased pharmacologic effect; decreased serum concentration	Increased phenytoin metabolism
	Diltiazem	Increased serum concentration	Inhibition of phenytoin metabolism
	Disulfiram	Increased serum concentration	Inhibition of phenytoin metabolism
	Folic acid	Decreased serum concentration	Complex mechanism
	Isoniazid	Increased serum concentration	Inhibition of phenytoin metabolism
	Phenylbutazone	Increased serum concentration	Inhibition of phenytoin metabolism; plasma protein displacement
	Rifampin	Decreased serum concentration	Increased phenytoin metabolism
	Sulfonamides	Increased serum concentration	Inhibition of phenytoin metabolism
	Trimethoprim	Increased serum concentration	Inhibition of phenytoin metabolism
Topiramate	Hydrochlorothiazide	Increased serum concentration	Unknown
Valproic acid	Estrogen-containing oral contraceptives	Decreased serum concentration	Possibly induction of glucuronidation of lamotrigine
	Meropenem	Decreased serum concentration	Increased valproic acid metabolism
	Rifampin	Decreased serum concentration	Increased valproic acid metabolism
	Salicylates	Increased pharmacologic effect	Plasma protein displacement; increased free valproic concentration

AED = antiepileptic drug; CNS = central nervous system; CYP = cytochrome P450.

Table 4. Pharmacokinetic Parameters of Seizure Medications When Used as Monotherapy

Drug	Therapeutic Serum Concentration (mcg/mL)	Bioavail-ability (%)	Plasma Protein Binding (%)	Vd (L/kg)	Eliminated Unchanged (%)	Clinically Active Metabolites	Half-life (hours)
Acetazolamide	10–14	100	>90	0.23	100	None	48–96 10–15 (children)
Carbamazepine	4–12	>70	40–90	0.8–1.9 1.5 (neonates) 1.9 (children)	Little, if any	10,11-epoxide	12–17 8–14 (children)
Clobazam	Not established	100	80–90	100	3	N-desmethyl-clobazam	36–2 71–82 (N-desmethylclobazam)
Clonazepam	20–80 ng/mL	100	47–80	3.2	Low percentage	7-amino, low activity	19–50 22–33 (children)
Eslicarbazepine	Not established	90	<40	0.87	90	R-licarbazepine, oxcarbazepine	13–20
Ethosuximide	40–100	100	0	0.6–0.7	10–20	None	52–60 24–36 (children)
Ezogabine	Not established	60	80	2–3	36	NAMR	7–11
Felbamate	30–60[a]	>90	22–36	0.74–0.85	40–50	None	11–20 13–23 (children)
Gabapentin	2–20[a]	Dose-dependent	<3	0.65–1.04	75–80	None	5–7
Lacosamide	Not established	100	<15	0.6	40	None	13
Lamotrigine	1–13	98	55	0.9–1.2	10	None	12–55 24–30 (children)
Levetiracetam	12–46[a]	100	<10	0.5–0.7	66	None	7 5 (children)
Oxcarbazepine	3–35[a]	100[b]	67	0.7	<1	10-monohydroxy	9[b]
Perampanel	Not established	100	95–96	—	20–36	None	105
Phenobarbital	15–40	80–100	40–60	0.7–1	25	None	80–100 45–173 (neonates) 37–73 (children)
Phenytoin	10–20	85–95	>90	0.6–0.8	<5	None	~20[c] 10–140 (neonates)[c] 5–18 (children)[c]
Pregabalin	Not established	≥90	0	0.5	90	None	6
Primidone	4–12 (20)[d]	90–100	80	0.6	20–40	Phenobarbital PEMA	10–15; 17 (PEMA) 4.5–18 (children) 10–36 (PEMA; children)
Rufinamide	Not established	85	34	50[e]	2	None	6–10
Tiagabine	0.02–0.2[a]	90–95	96	1.2	—	None	3.2–5.7
Topiramate	5–20[a]	80	13–17	0.6–0.8	70	None	12–21
Valproic acid	40–100 (150)[d]	100	>90[f]	0.2	<5	Unknown	8–17 4–14 (children)
Vigabatrin	Not established	100	0	1.1	80	None	7.5 5.7 (infants)
Zonisamide	10–40	50	40	1.45	35	None	63

[a]Therapeutic serum concentrations not well established.

[b]Bioavailability decreased in children <8 years and in older adults; clearance is 80% higher in children 2–4 years and 40% higher in children 4–12 years compared with adults.

[c]Michaelis-Menten pharmacokinetics; half-life varies with serum concentration; therefore, it might be better to express phenytoin elimination in the length of time it takes to clear 50% of the drug from the body, for example.

[d]Upper end of the serum concentration range is not definitely established.

[e]Depends on dose.

[f]May vary with serum concentration.

NAMR = N-acetyl metabolite of ezogabine; PEMA = phenylethylmalonamide; Vd = volume of (drug) distribution.

q. Primidone (Mysoline)
  i. Mechanism of action: Increases γ-aminobutyric–mediated chloride influx
  ii. Metabolized to phenobarbital and phenylethylmalonamide
  iii. Primidone, phenobarbital, and phenylethylmalonamide all have antiepileptic action.
  iv. Pharmacokinetics: Enzyme inducer
  v. Also used for essential tremor
r. Rufinamide (Banzel)
  i. Mechanism of action: Fast sodium channel blocker
  ii. Pharmacokinetics: Absorption increased by food (should be administered with food); metabolized by hydrolysis rather than through CYP enzymes
  iii. Decreases concentrations of ethinyl estradiol and norethindrone
  iv. Has an FDA indication only for Lennox-Gastaut syndrome
  v. Slightly shortens the QT interval and therefore should not be used in patients with familial short QT syndrome
  vi. Available as an oral solution
s. Tiagabine (Gabitril)
  i. Mechanism of action: Blocks γ-aminobutyric reuptake in the presynaptic neuron
  ii. Associated with new-onset seizures and status epilepticus in patients without epilepsy
t. Topiramate (Topamax)
  i. Mechanism of action: Fast sodium channel blocker, enhances γ-aminobutyric activity, and antagonizes AMPA/kainate activity, weak carbonic anhydrase inhibitor
  ii. Pharmacokinetics: Not extensively metabolized, eliminated in urine
  iii. Adverse effects: Drowsiness, paresthesias, psychomotor slowing (titrate slowly), weight loss, renal stones, acute angle closure glaucoma, metabolic acidosis, and hyperthermia (associated with decreased perspiration, or oligohidrosis)
  iv. Extended-release formulations (Trokendi XR, Qudexy XR)
  v. Nonepileptic indication: Prophylaxis of migraine headaches
u. Valproic acid (Depacon, Depakene, Depakote, Stavzor)
  i. Mechanism of action: Blocks T-type calcium currents, blocks sodium channels, increases γ-aminobutyric production
  ii. Pharmacokinetics: Enzyme inhibitor
  iii. Parenteral use: Has FDA indication only for replacement of oral dosing; however, sometimes used for status epilepticus, especially if absence status epilepticus
  iv. Adverse effects: Hepatotoxicity, nausea and vomiting, weight gain, interference with platelet aggregation, pancreatitis, alopecia, tremor
  v. Available in immediate-release (valproic acid [Depakene]) capsules for three- or four-times-daily dosing; delayed-release (enteric coated) (divalproex sodium [Depakote], valproic acid [Stavzor]) capsules and tablets for twice-daily dosing (if patient on enzyme inducer, drug is dosed more frequently); and extended-release (divalproex sodium [Depakote ER]) tablets for once-daily dosing
  vi. Nonepileptic indications: Manic episodes associated with bipolar disorder, prophylaxis of migraine headaches
v. Vigabatrin (Sabril)
  i. Mechanism of action: Irreversible inhibition of γ-aminobutyric acid transaminase
  ii. Pharmacokinetics: Induces CYP2C9; renal elimination
  iii. Adverse effects: Fatigue, somnolence, nystagmus, tremor, blurred vision, vision impairment, weight gain, arthralgia, abnormal coordination, and confusional state
  iv. Serious adverse effect: Vision loss; increased risk with higher total dose and duration; periodic vision testing necessary; restricted distribution program; only used for refractory complex partial seizures and infantile spasms

  v. Available as oral powder for solution

  w. Zonisamide (Zonegran)

    i. Mechanism of action: Fast sodium channel blocker, blocks T-type calcium currents, weak carbonic anhydrase inhibitor

    ii. Nonacrylamine sulfonamide: Avoid in sulfa-sensitive patients; it is sometimes used in patients with nonserious sulfa allergies, particularly when nonacrylamides (i.e., sulfonylureas) have been used successfully.

    iii. Pharmacokinetics: Long half-life

    iv. Adverse effects: Depression, rash, psychomotor slowing, paresthesias, kidney stones, blood dyscrasias, hyperthermia (associated with decreased perspiration, or oligohidrosis)

Table 5. Starting and Maximal Adult Seizure Medicine Doses

Drug	Starting Dose	Usual Maximal Dose
Carbamazepine	200 mg twice daily	1600 mg/day
Clobazam	10 mg/day	40 mg/day
Clonazepam	0.5 mg 3 times/day	20 mg/day
Eslicarbazepine	400 mg/day	1200 mg/day
Ethosuximide	250 mg twice daily	1.5 g/day
Ezogabine	100 mg 3 times/day	1200 mg/day
Felbamate	400 mg 3 times/day	3600 mg/day
Gabapentin	300 mg 3 times/day	3600 mg/day
Lacosamide	50 mg twice daily	400 mg/day
Lamotrigine	With valproic acid: 25 mg every other day Without carbamazepine, phenytoin, phenobarbital, primidone, or valproic acid: 25 mg/day With carbamazepine, phenytoin, phenobarbital, primidone, and not with valproic acid: 50 mg/day	With valproic acid: 200 mg/day Without carbamazepine, phenytoin, phenobarbital, primidone, or valproic acid: 375 mg/day With carbamazepine, phenytoin, phenobarbital, primidone, and not with valproic acid: 500 mg/day
Levetiracetam	500 mg twice daily	3000 mg/day
Oxcarbazepine	300 mg twice daily	2400 mg/day
Perampanel	With enzyme-inducing seizure medications: 4 mg/day Without enzyme-inducing seizure medications: 2 mg/day	With enzyme-inducing seizure medications: 12 mg/day Without enzyme-inducing seizure medications: 8 mg/day
Phenobarbital	1–3 mg/kg/day	300 mg/day
Phenytoin	100 mg 3 times/day	600 mg/day
Pregabalin	75 mg twice daily	600 mg/day
Primidone	100 mg at bedtime	2000 mg/day
Rufinamide	200–400 mg twice daily	3200 mg/day
Tiagabine	With carbamazepine, phenytoin, primidone, phenobarbital: 4 mg/day Without carbamazepine, phenytoin, primidone, phenobarbital: 2 mg/day	With carbamazepine, phenytoin, primidone, phenobarbital: 56 mg/day
Topiramate	25–50 mg/day	1000 mg/day
Valproic acid	10–15 mg/kg/day	60 mg/kg/day
Vigabatrin	500 mg twice daily	3000 mg/day
Zonisamide	100 mg/day	600 mg/day

2. Surgery: Surgery can sometimes drastically reduce the number of seizures; possible surgical procedures include removal of the seizure focus, corpus callosotomy, or implantation of vagus nerve stimulators.

3. Status epilepticus

    a. Treatment principles

        i. Ascertain ABCs (airway, breathing, and circulation).

        ii. Laboratory values (fingerstick blood glucose, complete blood cell count, basic metabolic panel, calcium, magnesium, and seizure medicine serum concentrations, if applicable) are sent to determine any reversible causes of status epilepticus.

        iii. Give an emergent medication to stop the seizure immediately.

        iv. Follow with an urgent medication to prevent the recurrence of seizures.

        v. In general, all drugs for status epilepticus should be given parenterally.

        vi. Neuromuscular-blocking drugs do not stop seizures; they stop only the muscular response to the brain's electrical activity.

    b. Emergency medications

        i. Lorazepam: Drug of choice

            (a) Rapid onset (2–3 minutes)

            (b) Dosage 0.1 mg/kg (up to 4 mg/dose) at rate of up to 2 mg/minute; may repeat every 5–10 minutes

        ii. Diazepam

            (a) Rapid onset, short duration

            (b) Dosage 0.15 mg/kg (up to 10 mg/dose) at rate of up to 5 mg/minute. May repeat every 5 minutes

            (c) Rectal gel formulation can be given in absence of intravenous access.

        iii. Midazolam: Preferred for intramuscular administration

            (a) Rapid onset, short duration

            (b) Dosage 0.2 mg/kg (up to 10 mg/dose). Can be given intramuscularly, intranasally, or buccally

    c. Urgent medications

        i. Phenytoin: Dosage 20 mg/kg; administration rate less than 50 mg/minute

        ii. Fosphenytoin: Administration rate less than 150 mg of phenytoin equivalent per minute

        iii. Phenobarbital: Dosage 20 mg/kg at 50–100 mg/minute

        iv. Valproic acid: Dosage 20–40 mg/kg at up to 6 mg/kg/minute; does not have FDA-labeled approval for status epilepticus

        v. Levetiracetam: 20–30 mg/kg over 15 minutes; does not have FDA-labeled approval for status epilepticus

        vi. Lacosamide: 200- to 400-mg bolus over 15 minutes; does not have FDA-labeled approval for status epilepticus

    d. Refractory status epilepticus medications

        i. Pentobarbital: Load 5–15 mg/kg up to 50 mg/minute; follow with a 0.5- to 5-mg/kg/hour infusion.

            (a) May have severe hypotension, necessitating treatment with vasopressors; should have continuous blood pressure (BP) measurement

            (b) Must be on ventilator

        ii. Thiopental: Load 2–7 mg/kg up to 50 mg/minute; follow with 0.5- to 5-mg/kg/hour infusion.

            (a) May have severe hypotension, respiratory depression, cardiac depression

            (b) Must be on ventilator

        iii. Midazolam: Load 0.2-mg/kg infused up to 2 mg/minute; follow with a 0.05- to 2-mg/kg/hour infusion.

            (a) May have hypotension, respiratory depression

            (b) May experience tachyphylaxis

      iv. Propofol: Load a 1- to 2-mg/kg intravenous bolus for 30–60 seconds; follow with a 20- to 200-mcg/kg/minute infusion.

        (a) Significant source of lipids

        (b) Some reports of seizure exacerbation with propofol

        (c) Must be on ventilator

4. Special populations

  a. Older adults: Pharmacokinetic changes in older adults that may affect seizure medications include the following:

     i. Carbamazepine: Decreased clearance

     ii. Phenytoin: Decreased protein binding if hypoalbuminemic or in renal failure

     iii. Valproic acid: Decreased protein binding

     iv. Diazepam: Increased half-life

     v. Phenylethylmalonamide (active metabolite of primidone): Decreased clearance if CrCl is decreased

     vi. Lamotrigine: Decreased clearance

     vii. Seizure medications with renal elimination must be adjusted according to the CrCl value.

  b. Women's health

     i. During their reproductive years, women with epilepsy should:

       (a) Take the best drug for their seizure type. A recent proposal from the ILAE recommends that women of childbearing age not be given valproic acid unless other therapies have failed.

       (b) Be treated with monotherapy, if possible.

       (c) Discuss the possible decrease in hormonal contraceptive effectiveness if taking enzyme-inducing medications (Table 6).

       (d) Use folic acid supplementation with no less than 0.4 mg/day.

     ii. Three practice guidelines exist regarding epilepsy during pregnancy (relevant material excerpted below).

       (a) Avoiding valproic acid monotherapy or polytherapy during the first trimester of pregnancy should be considered to decrease the risk of major congenital malformations, particularly neural tube defects, facial clefts, hypospadias, and poor cognitive outcomes. Valproic acid use has now been associated with lower IQ scores at ages 3 and 4½ (Meador KJ et al. Effects of fetal antiepileptic drug exposure: outcomes at age 4.5 years. Neurology 2012;78:1207-14).

       (b) To reduce the risk of major congenital malformations and poor cognitive outcomes, avoiding the use of seizure medication polytherapy during pregnancy, if possible, should be considered.

       (c) Limiting the dose of valproic acid or lamotrigine during the first trimester, if possible, should be considered to lessen the risk of major congenital malformations.

       (d) Avoiding the use of phenytoin, carbamazepine, and phenobarbital, if possible; may be considered to reduce the risk of cleft palate (phenytoin), posterior cleft palate (carbamazepine), cardiac malformations (phenobarbital), and poor cognitive outcomes (phenytoin, phenobarbital).

       (e) Women with epilepsy taking seizure medications during pregnancy probably have an elevated risk of small-for-gestational-age babies and 1-minute Apgar scores less than 7.

       (f) Monitoring of lamotrigine, carbamazepine, and phenytoin serum concentrations during pregnancy should be considered.

       (g) Having levetiracetam and oxcarbazepine (as the monohydroxylated derivative) serum concentrations monitored during pregnancy may be considered.

Table 6. Effect of Seizure Medications on Hormonal Contraceptives

Seizure Medication	Oral Contraceptives, Contraceptive Patch, Contraceptive Vaginal Ring, Progestogen Implant	Medroxyprogesterone Acetate Depot Injection, Levonorgestrel-Releasing Intrauterine System
Carbamazepine Clobazam Eslicarbazepine Felbamate Lamotrigine Oxcarbazepine Perampanel Phenobarbital Phenytoin Primidone Rufinamide Topiramate[a]	Decrease effectiveness	No effect
Benzodiazepines Ethosuximide Gabapentin Lacosamide Levetiracetam Pregabalin Tiagabine Valproic acid Vigabatrin Zonisamide	No effect	No effect

[a]Above doses of 200 mg/day.

E. Other Issues
1. Starting therapy after a first seizure
    a. Guidance from the American Epilepsy Society and the American Academy of Neurology
    b. Adults with an unprovoked first seizure (e.g., not meningitis, intoxication) will have a 21%–45% chance of having more seizures within the next 2 years. Higher risks are associated with prior brain insults, EEG with epileptiform abnormalities, and nocturnal seizures.
    c. Starting antiepileptic drug (AED) therapy will probably reduce recurrence risk within the first 2 years but may not increase quality of life.
    d. Starting AED therapy early does not change long-term risk of seizures.
2. Driving: All states place driving restrictions on people with epilepsy; some require mandatory physician reporting to the state department of transportation.
3. Medication discontinuation
    a. The American Academy of Neurology has a practice guideline (Practice parameter: a guideline for discontinuing antiepileptic drugs in seizure-free patients—a summary statement. Neurology 1996;47:600-2. Available at http://aan.com/professionals/practice/pdfs/gl0007.pdf) with the following criteria for withdrawal:
        i. Patient should be seizure free for 2–5 years on seizure medication.
        ii. Patient should have a single type of partial or primary generalized tonic-clonic seizures.
        iii. Patient should have a normal neurologic examination and normal IQ.
        iv. Patient's EEG should have become normalized with seizure medication treatment.

    b.   If a drug is discontinued, it is usually tapered for several months; a typical regimen would reduce the dose by one-third for 1 month, reduce it by another one-third for 1 month, and then discontinue it.

4.   Monitoring

    a.   Number of seizures: The goal number of seizures is always zero.

    b.   Signs of toxicity

    c.   Laboratory values: Specific for each drug

    d.   Blood concentrations: Available for many of the medications, commonly used for carbamazepine, phenobarbital, phenytoin, and valproic acid. The ILAE has a position paper on therapeutic drug monitoring, giving situations in which serum concentrations are most likely to be of benefit:

        i.   When a person has attained the desired clinical outcome, to establish an individual therapeutic concentration that can be used subsequently to assess potential causes for a change in drug response

        ii.   As an aid in the diagnosis of clinical toxicity

        iii.   To assess adherence, particularly in patients with uncontrolled seizure or breakthrough seizures

        iv.   To guide dosage adjustment in situations associated with increased pharmacokinetic variability (e.g., children, older adults, patients with associated diseases, drug formulation changes)

        v.   When a potentially important pharmacokinetic change is anticipated (e.g., in pregnancy, or when an interacting drug is added or removed)

        vi.   To guide dose adjustments for seizure medications with dose-dependent pharmacokinetics, particularly phenytoin

5.   Sexual dysfunction

    a.   Described in 30%–60% of men and women with epilepsy

    b.   Includes hyposexuality, orgasmic dysfunction, and erectile dysfunction

    c.   Mechanism may be induction of CYP isoenzymes to increase testosterone metabolism, increased hepatic synthesis of sex hormone–binding globulin, or induction of aromatase, which converts free testosterone to estradiol.

    d.   Sexual dysfunction has been reported with carbamazepine, phenobarbital, phenytoin, pregabalin, topiramate, and zonisamide.

    e.   Improved sexual functioning has been reported with lamotrigine and oxcarbazepine.

6.   Bone health

    a.   Osteopenia or osteoporosis is found in 38%–60% of patients in tertiary epilepsy clinics.

    b.   Increased fractures in patients with epilepsy and with seizure medication use

    c.   Risk is increased with increased treatment duration; there is a dose-response relationship; the medications most often associated with poor bone health are carbamazepine, clonazepam, phenobarbital, phenytoin, and valproic acid. However, there is now evidence that all seizure medications may contribute to osteopenia or osteoporosis.

    d.   Proposed mechanisms: Hepatic induction of CYP isoenzymes leads to increased vitamin D catabolism, impaired calcium absorption, calcitonin deficiency, vitamin K interference, and direct detrimental effect on bone cells.

    e.   Proposed treatments: High-dose vitamin D (4000 international units/day for adults and 2000 international units/day for children) improves bone mineral density compared with low doses; estrogen may be helpful for women but may also trigger seizures in some women.

7.   Suicidality

    a.   Meta-analysis of 199 placebo-controlled clinical trials of 11 drugs (n=43,892 patients older than 5 years) showed patients who received seizure medications had about twice the risk of suicidal behavior or ideation (0.43%) compared with patients receiving placebo (0.22%), and there were four completed suicides in the treatment group versus zero in the placebo group.

i. Risk increased at 1 week and continued through week 24.

ii. Patients with epilepsy (relative risk [RR] = 3.6), psychiatric disorders (RR = 1.6), or other conditions (RR = 2.3) were all at elevated risk of suicidality; no differences between drugs; no differences between age groups

b. The FDA requires a warning and a medication guide for all seizure medications.

c. Recent observational studies show mixed results. When specific AEDs are examined, the ones most associated with depression and suicidality are levetiracetam, perampanel, phenobarbital, primidone, tiagabine, topiramate, and vigabatrin.

d. An expert consensus statement was released in 2013 making the following points:

i. Although some (but not all) AEDs can be associated with treatment-emergent psychiatric problems that may lead to suicidal ideation and behavior, the actual suicidal risk is yet to be established; however, it seems to be very low. The risk of discontinuing AEDs or refusing to initiate them is significantly worse and can actually result in serious harm, including death to the patient.

ii. Suicidality in epilepsy is multifactorial. Primary operant variables include postictal suicidal ideation; a history of psychiatric disorders, particularly mood and anxiety disorders (and above all, when associated with prior suicidal attempts); and a family history of mood disorder complicated by suicide attempts.

iii. When starting or switching AEDs, patients should be advised to report any changes in mood and suicidal ideation.

Patient Cases

Questions 1–3 pertain to the following case:
T.M. is an 18-year-old new patient in the pharmacy where you work. He presents a prescription for carbamazepine 100 mg 1 orally twice daily with instructions to increase to 200 mg 1 orally three times daily. Currently, he does not take any medications and does not have any drug allergies. During your counseling session, T.M. tells you he must have blood drawn for a test in 3 weeks.

1. Which common potential adverse effect of carbamazepine is best assessed through a blood draw?

    A. Leukopenia.

    B. Renal failure.

    C. Congestive heart failure.

    D. Hypercalcemia.

2. One month later, T.M. returns to your pharmacy with a new prescription for lamotrigine 25 mg with instructions to take 1 tablet daily for 2 weeks, followed by 1 tablet twice daily for 2 weeks, followed by 2 tablets twice daily for 2 weeks, and then 3 tablets twice daily thereafter. He tells you that he is discontinuing carbamazepine because he developed a rash a few days ago. Which response is best?

    A. The rash is probably caused by carbamazepine because carbamazepine rash often has delayed development.

    B. The rash is unlikely to be caused by carbamazepine because carbamazepine rash usually presents after the first dose.

    C. The rash is probably not caused by carbamazepine; it is probably attributable to carbamazepine-induced liver failure.

    D. The rash is probably not caused by carbamazepine; it is probably attributable to carbamazepine-induced renal failure.

Patient Cases *(continued)*

3. T.M. wants to know why it is necessary to increase the dose of lamotrigine so slowly. Which reply is best?

    A. It causes dose-related psychomotor slowing.

    B. It causes dose-related renal stones.

    C. It causes dose-related paresthesias.

    D. It causes dose-related rash.

4. J.G. is a 34-year-old patient who has been maintained on carbamazepine extended release 400 mg orally twice daily for the past 2 years. She has had no seizures for the past 4 years. She presents to the emergency department in status epilepticus. Which drug is best to use first?

    A. Diazepam.

    B. Lorazepam.

    C. Phenytoin.

    D. Phenobarbital.

5. S.R. is a 37-year-old patient who began taking phenytoin 100 mg 3 capsules orally at bedtime 6 months ago. He has experienced several seizures since then, the most recent of which occurred 7 days ago. At that time, his phenytoin serum concentration was 8 mcg/mL. The treating physician increased his phenytoin dose to 100 mg 3 capsules orally twice daily. Today, which best represents his expected serum concentration?

    A. 10 mcg/mL.

    B. 14 mcg/mL.

    C. 16 mcg/mL.

    D. 20 mcg/mL.

6. S.S. is a 22-year-old woman who has always had episodes of "zoning out." Recently, one of these episodes occurred after an examination while she was driving home. She had a noninjury accident, but it prompted a visit to a neurologist. She is given a diagnosis of absence seizures. Which drug is best to treat this type of epilepsy?

    A. Phenytoin.

    B. Tiagabine.

    C. Carbamazepine.

    D. Ethosuximide.

7. J.B. is a 25-year-old man with a history of seizure disorder. He has been treated with phenytoin 200 mg orally twice daily for 6 months, and his current phenytoin concentration is 6.3 mcg/mL. His neurologist decides to increase his phenytoin dose to 300 mg twice daily. Which adverse effect is J.B. most likely to experience related to the dose increase?

    A. Drowsiness.

    B. Acne.

    C. Gingival hyperplasia.

    D. Rash.

Patient Cases (*continued*)

8. M.G., a 15-year-old boy with a diagnosis of juvenile myoclonic epilepsy, has been prescribed sodium divalproate. On which adverse effect is it best to counsel M.G.?

   A. Oligohidrosis.

   B. Renal stones.

   C. Alopecia.

   D. Word-finding difficulties.

Questions 9 and 10 pertain to the following case:

G.Z., a 26-year-old woman, presents with a 6-month history of "spells." The spells are all the same, and all start with a feeling in the abdomen that is difficult for her to describe. This feeling rises toward the head. The patient believes that she will then lose awareness. After a neurologic workup, she is given a diagnosis of focal seizures evolving to a bilateral, convulsive seizure. The neurologist is considering initiating either carbamazepine or oxcarbazepine.

9. Which is the most accurate comparison of carbamazepine and oxcarbazepine?

   A. Oxcarbazepine causes more liver enzyme induction than carbamazepine.

   B. Oxcarbazepine does not cause rash.

   C. Oxcarbazepine does not cause hyponatremia.

   D. Oxcarbazepine does not form an epoxide intermediate in its metabolism.

10. When you see G.Z. 6 months later for a follow-up, she tells you she is about 6 weeks pregnant. She has had no seizures since beginning drug therapy. Which strategy is best for G.Z.?

   A. Discontinue her seizure medication immediately.

   B. Discontinue her seizure medication immediately and give folic acid.

   C. Continue her seizure medication.

   D. Change her seizure medication to phenobarbital.

II. ISCHEMIC STROKE

A. Epidemiology
   1. Updated definitions
      a. Central nervous system (CNS) infarction: Brain, spinal cord, or retinal cell death attributable to ischemia, based on pathologic evidence, imaging, or other objective evidence of cerebral, spinal cord, or retinal focal ischemic injury in a defined vascular distribution, *or* clinical evidence of cerebral, spinal cord, or retinal focal ischemic injury, based on symptoms persisting for 24 hours or more or until death, and other etiologies excluded
      b. Ischemic stroke: An episode of neurologic dysfunction caused by focal cerebral, spinal, or retinal infarction
   2. Third or fourth most common cause of death in all developed countries
   3. More than 795,000 cases per year in the United States (128,842 deaths)
   4. Most common cause of adult disability

5. Risk factors
   a. Nonmodifiable
      i. Age: Stroke risk doubles each decade after 55 years.
      ii. Race: Risk for Native Americans is greater than for African Americans, whose risk is greater than for whites.
      iii. Sex: Risks are greater for men than for women; however, about half of strokes occur in women.
      iv. Low birth weight: Odds of stroke for those with birth weights less than 2500 g are twice has high as the odds for those weighing more than 4000 g.
      v. Family history: Parental history increases risk; some coagulopathies (e.g., protein C and S deficiencies, factor V Leiden mutations) are inherited.
   b. Somewhat modifiable: Diabetes mellitus increases risk 1.8–6 times; risk reduction has not been shown for glycemic control.
   c. Modifiable
      i. Hypertension increases risk 1.4–8 times; 32% risk reduction with control
      ii. Smoking increases risk 1.9 times; 50% risk reduction in 1 year, baseline risk at 5 years with smoking cessation; exposure to environmental cigarette smoke also increases risk.
      iii. Oral contraceptives with less than 50 mcg of estrogen double risk of stroke; those with more than 50 mcg of estrogen increase risk 4.5 times; risk increases with age; adding smoking to oral contraceptive use increases risk of stroke 7.2 times; obesity and hypertension also increase the risk with oral contraceptives.
      iv. Postmenopausal hormone therapy increases risk 1.4 times.
      v. Atrial fibrillation increases risk 2.6–4.5 times; 68% risk reduction with warfarin
      vi. Coronary heart disease increases risk 1.55 times (women) to 1.73 times (men).
      vii. Asymptomatic carotid stenosis increases risk 2 times; about a 50% risk reduction with endarterectomy
      viii. Dyslipidemia: High total cholesterol increases risk 1.5 times; low high-density lipoprotein cholesterol (less than 35 mg/dL) increases risk 2 times; 27%–32% risk reduction with statins in patients with coronary heart disease, hypertension, or diabetes. Twenty-five percent risk reduction with high-dose statins compared with low-dose statins
      ix. Obesity (especially abdominal body fat) increases risk 1.75–2.37 times; risk reduction with weight loss is unknown.
      x. Physical inactivity increases risk 2.7 times; risk reduction with increased activity is unknown.
      xi. Sickle cell disease increases risk 200–400 times; 91% risk reduction with transfusion therapy
      xii. Peripheral artery disease increases risk 3 times; impact of risk reduction strategies is unknown.
      xiii. Pregnancy increases risk 2.4 times over nonpregnant women; the risk remains elevated for the first 6 weeks postpartum.
      xiv. Patent foramen ovale increases the risk of stroke in young patients (younger than 55 years).
      xv. Depression increases the risk of stroke 1.35 times compared with nondepressed people.
   d. Less well documented: Alcohol abuse (5 or more drinks a day), hyperhomocystinemia, drug abuse (cocaine, amphetamines, and heroin), hypercoagulability, periodontal disease, inflammation and infection, sleep-disordered breathing (sleep apnea and snoring), metabolic syndrome, and migraine with aura

B. Primary Prevention
1. Reduction in risk factors (e.g., control of hypertension, smoking cessation, control of diabetes, cholesterol reduction)
2. Patient education: Patients should be educated about stroke warning signs and instructed to seek emergency care if they experience any of them. Warning signs: Sudden numbness or weakness of the face, arm, or leg, especially on one side of the body; sudden confusion; trouble speaking or understanding; sudden trouble seeing in one or both eyes; sudden trouble walking; dizziness, loss of balance or coordination; sudden, severe headache with no known cause
3. Treatment of atrial fibrillation: Up to 70% of cases are inappropriately treated.
    a. Recommendations based on Lansberg MG, O'Donnell MJ, Khatri P, et al. Antithrombotic and thrombolytic therapy for ischemic stroke: Antithrombotic Therapy and Prevention of Thrombosis, 9th ed. American College of Chest Physicians Evidence-Based Clinical Practice Guidelines. Chest 2012;141:e601S-36S. Available at http://journal.publications.chestnet.org/pdfaccess.ashx?ResourceID=6568275&PDFSource=13. Accessed September 17, 2014; You JJ, Singer DE, Howard PA, et al. Antithrombotic and thrombolytic therapy for atrial fibrillation: Antithrombotic Therapy and Prevention of Thrombosis, 9th ed. American College of Chest Physicians Evidence-Based Clinical Practice Guidelines. Chest 2012;141:e531S-75S. Available at http://journal.publications.chestnet.org/pdfaccess.ashx?ResourceID=6568280&PDFSource=13. Accessed September 17, 2014; Culebras A, Messe SR, Caturvedi S, et al. Summary of evidence-based guideline update: prevention of stroke in nonvalvular atrial fibrillation. Neurology 2014;82:716-24. Available at www.neurology.org/content/82/8/716.full. Accessed September 17, 2014; and Meschia JF, Bushnell C, Boden-Albala B., et al. Guidelines for primary prevention of stroke. A statement for healthcare professionals from the American Heart Association/American Stroke Association. Stroke 2014;45:3754-832. Available at http://stroke.ahajournals.org/content/45/12/3754. Accessed February 17, 2015.
    b. CHA_2DS_2-VASc is used for risk stratification.
        i.   Assign 1 point each for congestive heart failure, hypertension, age 65–74 years, diabetes, vascular disease, or female sex.
        ii. Assign 2 points for previous stroke or transient ischemic attack (TIA) or age 75 years or older.
        iii. Total for the CHA_2DS_2-VASc score
             (a) If 0, give no therapy.
             (b) If 1, give no therapy, aspirin, or oral anticoagulant.
             (c) If 2 or more, give oral anticoagulant.
    c. Dabigatran (Pradaxa)
        i.   When oral anticoagulation is recommended, current guidelines suggest dabigatran 150 mg twice daily over warfarin (target international normalized ratio [INR] of 2.5). Dabigatran had similar rates of hemorrhage, but intracranial hemorrhage was less likely with dabigatran, and GI hemorrhage was more likely.
        ii.   Mechanism of action: Direct thrombin inhibitor
        iii. Dose: 150 mg twice daily; dose reduction needed in severe renal dysfunction
        iv.   Dose reduction to 75 mg twice daily is recommended when administered with dronedarone or systemic ketoconazole in patients with a CrCl of 30–50 mL/minute.
        v.   Avoid the use of dabigatran and P-glycoprotein (P-gp) inhibitors in patients with a CrCl of 15–30 mL/minute.
        vi.   Avoid use in patients with a CrCl less than 15 mL/minute or advanced liver disease.
        vii. Avoid use in patients with mechanical heart valves.
        viii. The capsule should not be opened because it increases bioavailability by 75%.

ix. Idarucizumab (Praxbind) is a monoclonal antibody fragment used to reverse dabigatran anticoagulation.

    (a) Specific for dabigatran; can use other anticoagulants to anticoagulate patient, if needed

    (b) Dose is 5 g.

    (c) May restart dabigatran in 24 hours

d. Rivaroxaban (Xarelto) is probably as effective as warfarin with similar risk of major bleeding. Higher risk of GI bleeding and lower risk of intracranial hemorrhage and fatal bleeding.

    i. Mechanism of action: Direct factor Xa inhibitor

    ii. Dose: 20 mg/day with evening meal; dose reduction needed in renal dysfunction

    iii. Metabolized by CYP3A4/5, CYP2J2, P-gp, and *ABCG2;* avoid concomitant use with strong inhibitors or inducers.

e. Apixaban (Eliquis) is probably more effective than warfarin, with similar risk of stroke and less risk of bleeding and mortality.

    i. Mechanism of action: Direct, competitive factor Xa inhibitor

    ii. Dose: 5 mg twice daily; dose reduction needed in renal dysfunction

    iii. Metabolized by CYP3A4 and P-gp; reduce dose if given with inhibitors (e.g., ketoconazole, itraconazole, ritonavir, clarithromycin); avoid with strong inducers (e.g., rifampin, carbamazepine, phenytoin, St. John's wort)

f. Warfarin (Coumadin) is probably more effective than clopidogrel plus aspirin, but intracranial bleeding is more common.

    i. INR range 2–3

    ii. Give warfarin if patient has atrial fibrillation and mitral stenosis or prosthetic heart valve.

C. Treatment of Acute Event

  1. Heparin

    a. Good data on outcomes unavailable; generally not recommended for stroke treatment at therapeutic doses; increases risk of hemorrhagic transformation; heparin is often used for deep venous thrombosis prevention at a dose of 10,000–15,000 units/day given subcutaneously.

    b. Avoid in hemorrhagic stroke.

  2. Streptokinase: Should be avoided because of excess mortality

  3. Tissue plasminogen activator (Activase)

    a. Within 4½ hours of symptom onset

    b. Three-month outcome significantly improved (decreased disability)

    c. Intracerebral hemorrhage increased but no increase in mortality

    d. Dose 0.9 mg/kg intravenously (maximum is 90 mg), with 10% as a bolus and the remainder over 1 hour. The bolus should be administered within 60 minutes of hospital arrival.

    e. Antiplatelet agents should be held for 24 hours after tissue plasminogen activator administration

    f. Exclusion criteria

      i. Intracranial bleeding (or history) or subarachnoid bleeding

      ii. Other active internal bleeding

      iii. Intracranial/spinal surgery, head trauma, stroke within 3 months

      iv. Major surgery or serious trauma within 2 weeks, if risk of bleeding outweighs the anticipated benefits of reduced stroke-related neurological deficits

      v. Gastrointestinal (GI) hemorrhage within 3 weeks or structural GI malignancy

      vi. Blood pressure greater than 185/110 mm Hg. If medications are given to lower blood pressure, it should be stabilized before beginning treatment and maintained below 180/105 mm Hg for at least the first 24 hours after treatment.

      vii. Glucose less than 50 mg/dL or greater than 400 mg/dL, unless subsequently normalized

        viii. Arterial puncture at a noncompressible site within 1 week

        ix. Intracranial intra-axial neoplasm, arteriovenous malformation, or giant unruptured and unsecured aneurysm

        x. INR greater than 1.7, activated partial thromboplastin time greater than 40 seconds, prothrombin time greater than 15 seconds, platelet count less than 100,000 cells/m^3, those patients who have received a dose of low molecular weight heparin within the previous 24 hours, or those patients who have taken direct thrombin inhibitors or direct factor Xa inhibitors in the previous 48 hours

        xi. Infective endocarditis

        xii. Pregnancy, if the anticipated benefits of treating moderate to severe stroke do not outweigh the anticipated risks of uterine bleeding

        xiii. Additional criteria for the 3- to 4½-hour period have been largely abandoned. Benefit of treatment with NIH Stroke Scale greater than 25 in this time period is uncertain.

    4. Initiate aspirin (160- to 325-mg initial dose with 50- to 100-mg maintenance dose) within 48 hours of stroke onset in patients not eligible for tissue plasminogen activator.

    5. Use of a stent retriever within 6 hours may be useful in select patients who have received tissue plasminogen activator.

D. Secondary Prevention

    1. Reduction in all modifiable risk factors (specific changes below based on Kernan WN, Ovbiagele B, Black HR, et al. Guidelines for the prevention of stroke in patients with stroke and transient ischemic attack: a guideline for healthcare professionals from the American Heart Association/American Stroke Association. Stroke 2014;45:2160-236. Available at http://stroke.ahajournals.org/content/45/7/2160.full.pdf+html?sid=0efbdc13-bba8-4e90-b197-d58dd042f816. Accessed September 17, 2014.)

        a. Hypertension: Goal less than 140/less than 90 mm Hg. With lacunar stroke, may target less than 130 mm Hg systolic

        b. Hyperlipidemia: High-intensity statin therapy should be initiated or continued as first-line therapy in women and men less than 75 years of age who have had stroke or TIA.

    2. Carotid endarterectomy if 70%–99% stenosis. For 50%–69% stenosis, carotid endarterectomy recommendation depends on age, sex, and comorbidities; use aspirin 50–100 mg/day and statin therapy before and after the procedure.

    3. Carotid angioplasty and stenting may be an alternative to carotid endarterectomy in some patients, particularly younger patients.

    4. Antiplatelet therapy: Each agent has shown efficacy in reducing secondary stroke risk. Guidelines differ slightly on their recommendations. The American Stroke Association suggests that aspirin, aspirin/extended-release dipyridamole, and clopidogrel are all options after a first stroke or TIA, and the combination of aspirin and clopidogrel might be considered for initiation within 24 hours of a minor ischemic stroke or TIA or in the setting of intercranial atherosclerotic disease and continued for 90 days; however, long-term treatment increases risk of hemorrhage. The American Association of Chest Physicians recommends clopidogrel or aspirin/dipyridamole over aspirin or cilostazol.

        a. Aspirin

           i. Dose: Between 75 and 100 mg/day

           ii. If the patient has an additional stroke while taking aspirin, there is no evidence that increasing the aspirin dose will provide additional benefit.

        b. Aspirin/dipyridamole (Aggrenox)

           i. Capsule contains dipyridamole extended-release pellets (200 mg) and aspirin tablet (25 mg).

           ii. Dose: 1 capsule orally twice daily

           iii. Most common adverse effects: Headache, nausea, and dyspepsia; can increase liver enzymes

    c. Clopidogrel (Plavix)
- i. Inhibits adenosine diphosphate–induced platelet aggregation
- ii. Dose: 75 mg/day orally
- iii. Very low incidence of neutropenia (0.04% severe)
- iv. Rarely, thrombotic thrombocytopenic purpura has been reported.
- v. Partly metabolized by CYP2C19; there may be interactions with inhibitors of CYP2C19, notably proton pump inhibitors, or with genetic polymorphisms of this enzyme. The FDA has issued an alert on this topic (www.fda.gov/Drugs/DrugSafety/PostmarketDrugSafety InformationforPatientsandProviders/DrugSafetyInformationforHeathcareProfessionals/ ucm190787.htm).

    d. Cilostazol (Pletal)
- i. Inhibits cyclic adenosine monophosphate phosphodiesterase type 3–induced platelet aggregation
- ii. Dose: 100 mg orally twice daily on an empty stomach
- iii. Metabolized extensively by CYP3A4 and CYP2C19
- iv. Adverse effects: Headache, palpitation, diarrhea, and dizziness; rarely, thrombocytopenia or agranulocytosis. Contraindicated in patients with congestive heart failure
- v. Monitoring: Complete blood cell count with differential every 2 weeks for 3 months, periodically thereafter. Thus, used infrequently

5. Anticoagulation: Warfarin (Athrombin-K, Coumadin, Jantoven, Panwarfin)
    a. Prevention of second ischemic event, if patient has atrial fibrillation, rheumatic mitral valve disease, mechanical prosthetic heart valves, bioprosthetic heart valves, or left ventricular mural thrombus formation
    b. Target INR of 2.5 (3.0 for mechanical prosthetic heart valves)

Patient Cases

Questions 11–13 pertain to the following case:

L.R. is a 78-year-old man who presents to the emergency department for symptoms of right-sided paralysis. He states that these symptoms began about 5 hours ago and have not improved since then. He also has hypertension, benign prostatic hypertrophy, diabetes mellitus, erectile dysfunction, and osteoarthritis.

11. Which is the most accurate list of L.R.'s risk factors for stroke?

    A. Erectile dysfunction, age, osteoarthritis.

    B. Sex, diabetes mellitus, osteoarthritis.

    C. Benign prostatic hypertrophy, diabetes mellitus, age, sex.

    D. Age, diabetes mellitus, sex, hypertension.

12. Is L.R. a candidate for tissue plasminogen activator for treatment of stroke?

    A. Yes.

    B. No, he is too old.

    C. No, his stroke symptoms began too long ago.

    D. No, his diabetes mellitus is a contraindication for tissue plasminogen activator.

Patient Cases *(continued)*

13. L.R. was previously taking no drugs at home. Which choice is the best secondary stroke prevention therapy for this patient?
    A. Sildenafil.
    B. Celecoxib.
    C. Aspirin.
    D. Warfarin.

14. You are the pharmacist at a community pharmacy and receive a call from M.W., a 60-year-old man recently given a diagnosis of atrial fibrillation. He is concerned about his risk of having a stroke because his friend, who also has atrial fibrillation, asked him which dose of warfarin he is taking. M.W. called you because he is not taking warfarin and wants to know whether he should. He has no other medical conditions and takes atenolol 50 mg/day orally for ventricular rate control. After encouraging M.W. to discuss this with his physician, what should you tell him?
    A. You need warfarin treatment to prevent a stroke.
    B. You do not need warfarin, but you should take aspirin and clopidogrel.
    C. You do not need drug therapy at this time.
    D. Because you have atrial fibrillation, nothing can reduce your risk of stroke.

15. L.S. is a 72-year-old woman with a medical history of hypertension, type 2 diabetes mellitus, renal failure, and atrial fibrillation. She presents to the anticoagulation clinic for her initial visit. Which best reflects her target INR?
    A. 1.5.
    B. 2.0.
    C. 2.5.
    D. 3.0.

III. PARKINSON DISEASE

A. Epidemiology
   1. Prevalence is 160 in 100,000.
   2. Onset usually between 40 and 70 years of age, with peak onset in sixth decade
   3. Slightly more common in men
   4. Observed in all countries, ethnic groups, and socioeconomic classes

B. Signs and Symptoms
   1. Cardinal signs
      a. Akinesia or hypokinesia
      b. Rigidity
      c. Tremor
      d. Posture or gait abnormalities

2. Secondary signs
   a. Cognitive dysfunction
   b. Autonomic dysfunction
   c. Speech disturbances
   d. Micrographia
   e. Masked facies

C. Treatment
   1. General treatment principles
      a. No treatment has been unequivocally shown to prevent progression of Parkinson disease; therefore, treatment is based on symptoms.
      b. In patients who need the initiation of dopaminergic treatment, either levodopa or a dopamine agonist may be used. The choice depends on the relative impact of improving motor disability (better with levodopa) compared with the lessening of motor complications (better with dopamine agonists) for each individual patient.
      c. Treatment may be initiated with rasagiline as well, but the effects are not robust.
      d. Treatment with several different classes of medications simultaneously is common.

   2. Medications
      a. Monoamine oxidase type B (MAO-B) inhibitors
         i. Selegiline (Eldepryl, Zelapar)
            (a) Loses selectivity for MAO-B at doses greater than 10 mg/day
            (b) Contraindicated with meperidine because of serotonin syndrome risk
            (c) Dose: 5 mg orally twice daily (tablets; usually morning and noon); 1.25–2.5 mg/day (orally disintegrating tablets)
            (d) Adverse effects: Nausea, hallucinations, orthostatic hypotension, insomnia (metabolized to amphetamine)
            (e) Dosage forms: Tablets, orally dissolving tablets, and patches. The patches are FDA indicated for depression; they should not usually be used to treat Parkinson disease.
         ii. Rasagiline (Azilect)
            (a) Selectivity for MAO-B has not been definitively established.
               (1) Contraindicated with meperidine because of serotonin syndrome risk
               (2) Do not administer with tramadol, methadone, dextromethorphan, sympathomimetics, fluoxetine, or fluvoxamine because of serotonin syndrome risk.
               (3) Ciprofloxacin can double the concentration of rasagiline (through CYP1A2 inhibition).
            (b) Dose: 0.5–1 mg/day orally
      b. Levodopa
         i. Improvement in disability and possibly mortality
         ii. Greatest effect on bradykinesia and rigidity; less effect on tremor and postural instability
      c. Carbidopa
         i. Combined in fixed ratios with levodopa
         ii. Prevents some of the peripheral conversion of levodopa to dopamine by inhibiting peripheral dopamine decarboxylase; therefore, levodopa is available to cross the blood-brain barrier
         iii. 75 mg/day is usually needed to inhibit peripheral decarboxylase activity.
      d. Carbidopa/levodopa (Carbilev, Parcopa, Sinemet)
         i. Pharmacokinetic considerations
            (a) High-protein diets decrease absorption.
            (b) Immediate-release half-life 60–90 minutes

(c) Orally disintegrating tablet available; not absorbed sublingually

(d) Slow-release considerations: Fewer daily doses; less plasma fluctuations; delay to effect; cannot crush; can divide. No measurable effect on "freezing"

ii. Acute adverse effects: Nausea and vomiting, orthostatic hypotension, cardiac arrhythmias, confusion, agitation, hallucinations

iii. Long-term adverse effects: Wearing-off and on-off phenomena, involuntary movements (dyskinesias)

(a) Wearing-off phenomenon is the return of Parkinson disease symptoms before the next dose. Treatment of wearing-off includes adding a dopamine agonist, adding a MAO-B inhibitor, adding a catechol-O-methyl transferase inhibitor, or increasing the frequency or dose of levodopa.

(b) On-off phenomenon is a profound, unpredictable return of Parkinson disease symptoms without respect to the dosing interval. Treatment of on-off includes adding entacapone, rasagiline, pramipexole, ropinirole, apomorphine, and selegiline or redistributing dietary protein.

(c) Dyskinesias are drug-induced involuntary movements including chorea and dystonia. Treatment of dyskinesias includes decreasing the levodopa dose or adding amantadine as an antidyskinetic drug.

iv. Therapy initiation

(a) Standard formulation: 25 mg/100 mg 1 tablet orally three times daily; also available as orally disintegrating tablet

(b) Controlled-release formulation: 1 tablet orally two or three times daily

(c) Titration always necessary

(d) A combination of formulations may be needed (e.g., ½ tablet of Sinemet 25 mg/100 mg on awakening and 1 tablet of Sinemet CR 25/100 three times daily).

e. Direct dopamine agonists

i. Drugs: Apomorphine (Apokyn), bromocriptine (Parlodel), pramipexole (Mirapex), ropinirole (Requip), rotigotine (Neupro)

ii. Bromocriptine is an ergot-derived product: Very rarely, adverse effects such as retroperitoneal, pleuropulmonary, or cardiac fibrosis have been attributed to it; regular monitoring of the electrocardiogram is recommended.

iii. Rotigotine is a transdermal system. With the initial formulation, problems occurred with crystallization of the medication. The product was withdrawn from the market and has since been reformulated.

iv. Dosing: Always titrate to final dose (Table 7).

Table 7. Usual Dosage Range for Dopamine Agonists

Agent	Usual Dosage Range (mg/day)
Bromocriptine	5–40
Pramipexole	1.5–4.5
Ropinirole	0.75–24
Rotigotine	6–8

v. Adverse effects: Nausea, vomiting, postural hypotension, hallucinations, hypersexuality, compulsive behaviors, falling asleep during activities of daily living

vi. Pramipexole and ropinirole also have FDA indications for restless legs syndrome.

vii. Ropinirole and pramipexole are available as extended-release formulations.

       viii. Apomorphine: Short-acting dopamine receptor agonist

         (a) Indication: Acute, intermittent treatment of "off" episodes associated with advanced Parkinson disease

         (b) Contraindications: Its use with 5-hydroxytryptamine-3 antagonists (ondansetron, granisetron, dolasetron, palonosetron, and alosetron) causes profound hypotension; sulfite sensitivity or allergy

         (c) Pharmacokinetics: When given orally, poorly bioavailable and extensive first-pass metabolism; used as subcutaneous injection in a pen self-injector

         (d) Adverse effects

            (1) Severe nausea and vomiting

               (A) Treat with trimethobenzamide 300 mg three times daily for 3 days before initiating treatment and for at least 6 weeks during treatment.

               (B) About 50% of patients can discontinue trimethobenzamide after 2 months.

               (C) Thirty-one percent nausea and 11% vomiting with trimethobenzamide

            (2) Hypotension

            (3) Hallucinations

            (4) Injection site reactions

            (5) Dyskinesias

         (e) Dosing

            (1) Must be titrated in a setting where BP can be monitored

            (2) In the "off" state, the patient should be given a 0.2-mL (2 mg) test dose.

            (3) Supine and standing BP taken before dose; 20, 40, and 60 minutes after dose

            (4) If tolerated, begin with a 0.2-mL dose as needed; increase by 0.1 mL if necessary.

            (5) Doses greater than 0.6 mL, more than five times daily, or greater than 20 mg/day have limited experience.

            (6) If first dose is ineffective, do not redose.

            (7) If patients do not dose for more than 1 week, reinitiate at a 0.2-mL dose.

  f. Anticholinergics

    i. Drugs: Trihexyphenidyl (Artane), benztropine (Cogentin)

    ii. Most useful for tremor

    iii. Initial dosing

      (a) Trihexyphenidyl 0.5 mg 1 tablet orally twice daily

      (b) Benztropine 0.5 mg 1 tablet orally twice daily

    iv. Adverse effects: Dry mouth, urinary retention, dry eyes, constipation, confusion

  g. Amantadine (Symmetrel)

    i. Has symptomatic benefits and may reduce dyskinesias caused by levodopa or dopamine agonists

    ii. Dosing: 100 mg 1 tablet orally two or three times daily; caution in renal dysfunction

    iii. Adverse effects: Dizziness, insomnia, anxiety, livedo reticularis, nausea, nightmares

  h. Catechol-O-methyl transferase inhibitors

    i. Prevent breakdown of dopamine, more levodopa available to cross blood-brain barrier

    ii. Tolcapone (Tasmar): Severely restricted because of hepatotoxicity; must sign consent form

    iii. Entacapone (Comtan)

      (a) Increased area under the curve, increased half-life; no change in C_{max} or T_{max} of levodopa

      (b) Dosing: 1 tablet with each carbidopa/levodopa dose; maximum of eight times daily; one dosage form (Stalevo) includes carbidopa, levodopa, and entacapone 200 mg

      (c) Must use with carbidopa/levodopa

      (d) Adverse effects: Dyskinesias, nausea, diarrhea (may be delayed for up to 2 weeks after initiation or dose increase), urine discoloration (orange), hallucinations or vivid dreams

3. Surgery: Several types of surgery are performed for Parkinson disease.
    a. Thalamotomy: Ablation of portions of the thalamus to control tremor
    b. Pallidotomy: Ablation of structures in the globus pallidus for the treatment of Parkinson disease
    c. Fetal transplants: Transplantation of dopaminergic tissue into the striatum; considered experimental
    d. Trophic factors: Glial-derived nerve growth factor and neurturin have been delivered directly to the striatum or substantia nigra; considered experimental
    e. Deep brain stimulation
        i.   Most frequently performed surgery for Parkinson disease
        ii. Thought to work by stimulating areas of the basal ganglia to reversibly block the neuronal activity in the area
        iii. Patient selection focuses on patients with
             (a) Motor fluctuations or dyskinesias that are not adequately controlled with optimized medical therapy
             (b) Medication-refractory tremor
             (c) Intolerance of medical therapy
             (d) Some centers will not perform the surgery in patients older than 70 years.
        iv. Two areas are targeted.
             (a) Globus pallidum
                 (1) Reduces off-time
                 (2) Reduces dyskinesias
                 (3) Thought to have fewer cognitive adverse effects than subthalamic nucleus stimulation
             (b) Subthalamic nucleus
                 (1) Reduces off-time
                 (2) Reduces dyskinesias
                 (3) Thought to be more effective than globus pallidum stimulation
4. Special situations
    a. Hallucinations or psychosis may be caused by either Parkinson disease or treatment.
        i.   Discontinue or reduce Parkinson disease medications as tolerated.
        ii. If an antipsychotic is needed, use quetiapine or clozapine as the first choice.
        iii. Avoid typical antipsychotics, risperidone, and olanzapine because they may worsen Parkinson symptoms.
    b. Cognitive disorders
        i.   Discontinue or reduce Parkinson disease medications as tolerated.
        ii. Rivastigmine has an FDA indication for treatment; other cholinesterase inhibitors may have efficacy.
    c. Sleep disorders, depression, agitation, anxiety, constipation, orthostatic hypotension, seborrhea, and blepharitis can be seen in Parkinson disease; treat as usual.

Patient Cases

Questions 16 and 17 pertain to the following case:
L.S. is taking carbidopa/levodopa 25 mg/100 mg orally four times daily and trihexyphenidyl 2 mg orally three times daily for Parkinson disease. L.S.'s wife reports that he is often confused and experiences constipation; he has trouble talking because of his dry mouth.

16. Which change is best to resolve these symptoms?
    A. Increase carbidopa/levodopa.
    B. Increase trihexyphenidyl.
    C. Decrease carbidopa/levodopa.
    D. Decrease trihexyphenidyl.

17. Six months later, L.S. returns to the clinic concerned that his carbidopa/levodopa dose is wearing off before his next dose is due. Which recommendation is best?
    A. Increase the carbidopa/levodopa dose.
    B. Decrease the carbidopa/levodopa dose.
    C. Increase the dosing interval.
    D. Decrease the dosing interval.

18. P.J. is a 57-year-old man with an 8-year history of Parkinson disease. His current drugs include carbidopa/levodopa 50 mg/200 mg orally four times daily, entacapone 200 mg orally four times daily, and amantadine 100 mg three times daily. He presents to the clinic with a reddish blue discoloration on his lower arms and legs. Which, if any, of his drugs is the most likely cause of this condition?
    A. Carbidopa/levodopa.
    B. Entacapone.
    C. Amantadine.
    D. None; probably represents venous stasis.

19. L.L. is a 47-year-old man with Parkinson disease. He takes carbidopa/levodopa 50 mg/200 mg orally four times daily. He recently noticed an involuntary twitching movement of his left foot. Which is the best therapy for L.L.'s dyskinesia?
    A. Add ropinirole.
    B. Add selegiline.
    C. Increase the carbidopa/levodopa dose.
    D. Decrease the carbidopa/levodopa dose.

Patient Cases *(continued)*

20. C.A., a 57-year-old white man who just retired from the New York City Fire Department, has been experiencing tremors in his right hand that have become progressively worse for the past 6 months. He has difficulty walking. He also has backaches and no longer plays golf. In addition, he is losing his sense of taste. He is given a diagnosis of Parkinson disease. Which is the best treatment for this man?

    A. Trihexyphenidyl.

    B. Entacapone.

    C. Apomorphine

    D. Ropinirole.

IV. HEADACHE

A. Definitions
   1. Classic migraine: At least two attacks with at least three of the following: One or more fully reversible aura symptoms, at least one aura symptom for more than 4 minutes, or two or more symptoms occurring in succession; no single aura symptom lasts more than 60 minutes; headache follows aura within 60 minutes.
   2. Migraine without aura: At least five attacks of headache lasting 4–72 hours with at least two of the following: Unilateral location, pulsating quality, intensity moderate or severe, aggravation by walking stairs or similar routine physical activity. During headache, at least one of the following: Nausea or vomiting, photophobia, phonophobia
   3. Tension: At least 10 previous headaches, each lasting from 30 minutes to 7 days, with at least two of the following: Pressing or tightening (nonpulsating) quality, intensity mild to moderate, bilateral location, no aggravation with physical activity
   4. Cluster: Several episodes, short-lived but severe, of unilateral, orbital, supraorbital, or temporal pain. At least one of the following must occur: Conjunctival injection, lacrimation, nasal congestion, rhinorrhea, facial sweating, miosis, ptosis, or eyelid edema.
   5. Analgesic rebound headache: If patients use analgesics often (usually defined as more than three times weekly), they may develop analgesic rebound headache. Patients with this condition usually present with a chronic daily headache, for which they take simple or narcotic analgesics. Treatment consists of the withdrawal of all analgesics (but not prophylactic medications).

B. Epidemiology
   1. Migraine: 15%–17% of women, 5% of men
   2. Tension: 88% of women, 69% of men
   3. Cluster: 0.01%–1.5% of population; ratio of men to women is 6:1.

C. Treatment
   1. Migraine
      a. Prophylaxis should be considered if any of the following criteria are met: Migraines are recurrent and interfere with daily routine, migraines are frequent, patient experiences inefficacy or inability to use acute therapy, patient prefers prophylaxis as therapy, cost of acute medications is problematic, adverse effects with acute therapies occur, or migraine presentation is uncommon.

i. General principles
   (a) Use lowest effective dose.
   (b) Give adequate trial (2–3 months).
   (c) If patient has a coexisting condition, consider prophylaxis choice (e.g., β-blockers are contraindicated in patients with asthma but beneficial in hypertension).
ii. Medications with established efficacy
   (a) Frovatriptan (for menstrually associated migraine, short-term prophylaxis only)
   (b) Metoprolol
   (c) Onabotulinum toxin A
   (d) Petasites (butterbur extract)
   (e) Propranolol
   (f) Timolol
   (g) Topiramate
   (h) Valproic acid
iii. Medications with probable efficacy
   (a) Amitriptyline
   (b) Atenolol
   (c) Fenoprofen
   (d) Histamine, subcutaneous
   (e) Ibuprofen
   (f) Ketoprofen
   (g) Magnesium
   (h) MIG-99 (feverfew extract)
   (i) Nadolol
   (j) Naproxen/naproxen sodium
   (k) Naratriptan (for menstrually associated migraine, short-term prophylaxis only)
   (l) Riboflavin
   (m) Venlafaxine
   (n) Zolmitriptan (for menstrually associated migraine, short-term prophylaxis only)
iv. Medications with possible efficacy
   (a) Candesartan
   (b) Carbamazepine
   (c) Clonidine
   (d) Coenzyme Q10
   (e) Cyproheptadine
   (f) Estrogen
   (g) Flurbiprofen
   (h) Guanfacine
   (i) Lisinopril
   (j) Mefenamic acid
   (k) Nebivolol
   (l) Pindolol
v. Medications with conflicting or inadequate evidence of efficacy: Acetazolamide, aspirin, bisoprolol, fluoxetine, fluvoxamine, gabapentin, hyperbaric oxygen, indomethacin, nicardipine, nifedipine, nimodipine, omega-3, protriptyline, verapamil
vi. Medications that are possibly ineffective, probably ineffective, or ineffective: Acebutolol, botulinum toxin, clomipramine, clonazepam, lamotrigine, montelukast, nabumetone, oxcarbazepine, telmisartan

    b. Acute treatment
- i. Triptans (Table 8)
  - (a) Sumatriptan and zolmitriptan have nonoral administration routes (subcutaneous [sumatriptan], intranasal [sumatriptan and zolmitriptan], transdermal [sumatriptan]) that should be considered for patients with nausea or vomiting.
  - (b) Orally disintegrating tablets are available for zolmitriptan and rizatriptan if patients do not have access to water; however, they do not work faster than oral tablets and are not absorbed sublingually.
  - (c) All are contraindicated in patients with or at risk of coronary artery disease, stroke, uncontrolled hypertension, peripheral vascular disease, ischemic bowel disease, and pregnancy; they should not be used in patients with hemiplegic or basilar migraines.
  - (d) Drug interactions: Contraindicated within 2 weeks of MAO inhibitors; do not use within 24 hours of ergotamines; caution with other serotonin-active medications. Propranolol increases serum concentrations of rizatriptan; thus, a 5-mg dose should be used with propranolol, and the dose should not exceed 15 mg/day.
- ii. Ergots
  - (a) Dihydroergotamine has nonoral administration routes (subcutaneous, intravenous, and intranasal) that should be considered for patients with nausea or vomiting.
  - (b) All are contraindicated in patients with, or at risk of, coronary artery disease, stroke, uncontrolled hypertension, peripheral vascular disease, ischemic bowel disease, and pregnancy; they should not be used in patients with hemiplegic or basilar migraines.
- iii. Nonsteroidal anti-inflammatory drugs: Usually effective for only mild to moderate headache pain
- iv. Opioids: Butorphanol has a nonoral administration route (intranasal) that should be considered for patients with nausea or vomiting.
- v. Isometheptene combination products: Conflicting evidence about efficacy
- vi. Antiemetics: Prochlorperazine, metoclopramide, and chlorpromazine are most commonly used; there is some suggestion that they have independent antimigraine action; all are available in nonoral forms.
- vii. Status migrainosus: Attack of migraine, with headache phase lasting more than 72 hours despite treatment. Headache-free intervals of less than 4 hours (sleep not included) may occur.
  - (a) Corticosteroids: Either intravenous or oral dosing
  - (b) Dihydroergotamine: Intravenous dosing
  - (c) Sodium valproate: Intravenous loading

2. Tension
    a. Prophylaxis
- i. Tricyclic antidepressants
- ii. Botulinum toxin

    b. Acute treatment
- i. Acetaminophen
- ii. Nonsteroidal anti-inflammatory drugs

3. Cluster
    a. Prophylaxis
- i. Verapamil
- ii. Melatonin
- iii. Suboccipital injection of betamethasone
- iv. Lithium: May be efficacious at serum concentrations as low as 0.3 mmol/L

b. Treatment

    i. Triptans: Subcutaneous and intranasal sumatriptan and intranasal zolmitriptan are effective. Oral formulations usually do not act quickly enough, but oral zolmitriptan showed efficacy in one trial.

    ii. Oxygen: 100% oxygen at 6–12 L/minute relieves pain in 50%–85% of patients.

    iii. Intranasal lidocaine: 20–60 mg as a nasal drop or spray (must be compounded)

    iv. Octreotide and 10% cocaine have been used with some effect.

Table 8. Selected Agents for Migraine Headache

	Dosage Forms	Tmax	Half-life (hours)	Dose	Maximal Dose/ 24 Hours (mg)
Triptans					
Almotriptan (Axert)	Tablets 6.25 mg, 12.5 mg	1–3 hours	2–4	1 tablet, may repeat in 2 hours	25
Eletriptan (Relpax)	Tablets 20 mg, 40 mg	1 hour	4–5	1 tablet, may repeat in 2 hours	80
Frovatriptan (Frova)	Tablets 2.5 mg	2–4 hours	26	1 tablet, may repeat in 2 hours	7.5
Naratriptan (Amerge)	Tablets 1 mg, 2.5 mg	2–3 hours	6	1 tablet, may repeat in 4 hours	5
Rizatriptan (Maxalt)	Tablets 5 mg, 10 mg	1–1.5 hours	1.8	1 tablet, may repeat in 2 hours	30
	Orally disintegrating tablets 5 mg, 10 mg	1.6–2.5 hours	1.8	1 tablet, may repeat in 2 hours	30
Sumatriptan (Alsuma, Imitrex, Sumavel, Zecuity)	SC injection 4 mg, 6 mg	12 minutes	1.9	1 injection, may repeat in 1 hour	12
	Intranasal 5 mg, 20 mg	30 minutes	2	1 spray in one nostril, may repeat in 2 hours	40
	Tablets 25 mg, 50 mg, 100 mg	2 hours	2.5	1 tablet, may repeat in 2 hours	200
	Iontophoretic transdermal system 6.5 mg/4 hours	1.1 hours	3.1	1 patch, may repeat in 2 hours	13
Zolmitriptan (Zomig)	Tablets 2.5 mg, 5 mg	1.5 hours	3.75	1 tablet, may repeat in 2 hours	10
	Orally disintegrating tablets 2.5 mg, 5 mg	3 hours	3.75	1 tablet, may repeat in 2 hours	10
	Intranasal 2.5 mg, 5 mg	3 hours	3	1 spray in one nostril, may repeat in 2 hours	10
Triptan/nonsteroidal anti-inflammatory combination					
Sumatriptan/naproxen sodium (Treximet)	Tablets 85 mg/500 mg	1 hour/ 5 hours	2/19	1 tablet, may repeat in 2 hours	170/1000
Ergots					
Ergotamine tartrate (Ergomar)	Sublingual tablets 2 mg	Unknown	2	1 tablet under tongue, may repeat in 1 hour	6
Dihydroergotamine (DHE 45; Migranal)	Intranasal 4-mg ampules	0.9 hour	10	1 spray (0.5 mg) in each nostril, repeat in 15 minutes	3
	IV/IM/SC 1 mg/mL 1-mL vials	SC 15–45 minutes	9	1 mL IV/IM/SC, may repeat in 1 hour	2 mg IV; 3 mg IM/SC

IM = intramuscular; IV = intravenous; SC = subcutaneous.

Patient Cases

21. M.R., a 34-year-old woman, has throbbing right-sided headaches. She experiences nausea, sonophobia, and photophobia with these headaches but no aura. She usually has headaches twice a month. She is hypertensive and morbidly obese. She takes an ethinyl estradiol/progestin combination oral contraceptive daily and hydrochlorothiazide 25 mg/day orally. She has a diagnosis of migraine headaches. Which medication is best for prophylaxis of her headaches?
    A. Propranolol.
    B. Valproic acid.
    C. Amitriptyline.
    D. Lithium.

22. S.R. is a 54-year-old female homemaker with squeezing, bandlike headaches that occur three or four times weekly. She rates the pain of these headaches as 7/10 and finds acetaminophen, aspirin, ibuprofen, naproxen, ketoprofen, and piroxicam only partly effective. She wants to take a prophylactic drug to prevent these tension headaches. Which drug is best for prophylaxis of her headaches?
    A. Propranolol.
    B. Valproic acid.
    C. Amitriptyline.
    D. Lithium.

23. D.S. is a 49-year-old male computer programmer who describes lancinating right-eye pain and tearing several times a day for 2–3 days in a row. He will have no episodes for 2–3 weeks but then will have recurrent episodes. In the office, he receives oxygen by nasal cannula during an episode, and his pain is relieved. He has a diagnosis of cluster headaches. Which drug is best for prophylaxis of his headaches?
    A. Propranolol.
    B. Valproic acid.
    C. Amitriptyline.
    D. Lithium.

24. M.K. is a 44-year-old woman with right-sided headaches of moderate intensity that are accompanied by severe nausea and vomiting. Which triptan is best to treat M.K.'s migraine headaches?
    A. Almotriptan.
    B. Naratriptan.
    C. Rizatriptan.
    D. Sumatriptan.

Patient Cases *(continued)*

25. One of the neurologists you work with read a meta-analysis of migraine treatments (Oldman AD, Smith LA, McQuay HJ, et al. Pharmacological treatment for acute migraine: quantitative systematic review. Pain 2002;91:247-57). He is most interested in the outcome of sustained relief at 24 hours, but he is confused by the number-needed-to-treat (NNT) analyses. He shows you the following table:

Drug	NNT
Ergotamine + caffeine	6.6
Eletriptan 80 mg	2.8
Rizatriptan 10 mg	5.6
Sumatriptan 50 mg	6.0

Which statement provides the best interpretation of these data?

A. Eletriptan 80 mg is the most effective agent.

B. Ergotamine plus caffeine is the most effective agent.

C. Eletriptan has the most adverse effects.

D. Ergotamine plus caffeine has the most adverse effects.

V. MULTIPLE SCLEROSIS

A. Definitions
1. Autoimmune disorder with areas of CNS demyelination and axonal transaction
2. Clinical course
   a. Clinically isolated syndrome; first clinical presentation for which the criterion of dissemination in time has not been met to diagnose multiple sclerosis (MS)
   b. Classified as relapsing or progressive disease; subclassified according to disease activity and progression: Relapsing-remitting: 85% of patients at diagnosis, develops into progressive disease in 50% of patients within 10 years

B. Epidemiology
1. Diagnosis usually between 20 and 50 years of age
2. Twice as many women as men develop multiple sclerosis.
3. Whites and people of northern European heritage are more likely to develop MS.
4. Risk factors: Family history of MS, autoimmune disease, or migraine; personal history of autoimmune disease or migraine; cigarette smoke exposure (women only)

C. Treatment
1. Acute relapses are treated with corticosteroids.
   a. Intravenous methylprednisolone: The usual dose is 1 g/day as one dose or divided doses for 3–5 days.
   b. Oral prednisone: The usual dose is 1250 mg/day given every other day for five doses.
   c. Intravenous adrenocorticotropic hormone
   d. Neurologic recovery is the same with or without an oral prednisone taper.

2. Disease-modifying therapies (Table 9)
    a. Alemtuzumab (Lemtrada)
        i. Mechanism of action: Binds to CD52, a cell surface antigen on T cells, B cells, natural killer cells, monocytes, and macrophages; causes lysis of T and B cells
        ii. Adverse effects
            (a) Autoimmunity including thyroid disorders (34%), immune thrombocytopenia, glomerular nephropathies
            (b) Infusion reactions (e.g., anaphylaxis, angioedema, bronchospasms, nausea, urticaria) occur in up to 92% of patients and necessitate corticosteroids during treatment.
            (c) Increased infections: Screen for herpes zoster and immunize, if needed; screen for tuberculosis before initiating therapy; prophylaxis for herpes infections is necessary during treatment.
            (d) May increase risk of thyroid cancer, melanoma, and lymphoma
            (e) Administered only under a restricted distribution program
        iii. Avoid live virus vaccines during treatment; complete all vaccines 6 weeks before initiation of therapy
    b. Beta interferons (Avonex, Betaseron, Extavia, Plegridy, Rebif)
        i. Mechanism of action: Suppress T-cell activity, downregulate antigen presentation by major histocompatibility complex class II molecules, decrease adhesion molecules and matrix metalloproteinase 9, increase anti-inflammatory cytokines, and decrease inflammatory cytokines
        ii. Adding polyethylene glycol to interferon beta-1a decreases frequency of injections
        iii. Injection site reactions: More common in subcutaneously administered products. It may help to bring a drug to room temperature before injection, ice the injection site, and rotate injection sites.
        iv. Flulike symptoms: Usually dissipate in 2–3 months. It may help to inject the dose in the evening. Begin at the 0.25- to 0.5-mg dose and slowly increase, and use ibuprofen or acetaminophen.
        v. Neutralizing antibodies: Develop in some patients 6–18 months after treatment begins; frequency and administration route affect neutralizing antibody development; relapse rates are higher in patients with persistently high antibody titers; antibodies may disappear even during continued treatment; show cross-reactivity with other beta interferons.
    c. Dimethyl fumarate (Tecfidera)
        i. Mechanism of action: Antioxidant and cytoprotective; inhibits proinflammatory cytokines, increases anti-inflammatory cytokines
        ii. Adverse effects
            (a) Skin flushing: Occurs in up to 38% of patients, usually within 30–45 minutes of dosing; involves the face, chest, and neck; dissipates after 15–30 minutes; peaks within first month of therapy and decreases thereafter; aspirin may block flushing, taking with food helps prevent
            (b) GI events: Occur in up to 41% of patients; peak within first month of therapy and decrease thereafter
            (c) Lymphocytes decrease by 30% in the first year of therapy and then stabilize.
    d. Glatiramer acetate (Copaxone)
        i. Mechanism of action: Decreases type 1 helper T cells; increases type 2 helper T cells; increases production of nerve growth factors
        ii. Injection site reactions: Icing the site before and after injection may help.
        iii. Systemic reactions: May involve flushing, chest tightness, palpitations, anxiety, and shortness of breath; this is noncardiac; recurrence is infrequent.

e. Fingolimod (Gilenya)

   i. Mechanism of action: Binds to the S1P receptor 1 expressed on T cells, prevents activation of T cells

   ii. Contraindicated in patients with myocardial infarctions, unstable angina, stroke, TIAs, or decompensated heart failure necessitating hospitalization or class III/IV heart failure, history of Mobitz type II second- or third-degree atrioventricular block or sick sinus syndrome unless patient has a pacemaker, baseline QTc interval greater than or equal to 500 milliseconds, or treatment with class Ia or class III antiarrhythmic drugs

   iii. Patients must be monitored for bradycardia for 6 hours after the first dose; if therapy is discontinued for more than 2 weeks, patients must be remonitored.

   iv. Adverse effects

      (a) Bradycardia: Electrocardiogram is recommended within 6 months for patients using antiarrhythmics (including β-blockers and calcium channel blockers), those with cardiac risk factors, and those with slow or irregular heartbeat. Heart rate returns to baseline within 1 month of continued dosing.

      (b) Atrioventricular conduction delays: First- and second-degree block

      (c) Decrease in lymphocytes: A recent complete blood cell count should be available before therapy starts. Infections may be more common. Discontinue therapy for serious infections; test patients without varicella zoster vaccine or infection history for varicella zoster virus antibodies, and immunize antibody-negative patients (wait 1 month to begin fingolimod).

      (d) Macular edema: Ophthalmologic evaluation at baseline and 3–4 months after fingolimod initiation; a history of uveitis or diabetes mellitus increases risk.

      (e) Respiratory effects: Decreases in forced expiratory volume over 1 second and diffusion lung capacity for carbon monoxide can be seen.

      (f) Elevation of liver enzymes

      (g) Hypertension: Monitor during treatment.

      (h) Extended effects of drug for up to 2 months after discontinuation necessitate extended monitoring for many adverse effects.

   v. Drug interactions

      (a) Ketoconazole: Increased fingolimod

      (b) Vaccines: Less effective during and 2 months after fingolimod treatment; avoid live, attenuated vaccines.

   vi. Avoid pregnancy during treatment and for 2 months after treatment.

f. Mitoxantrone (Novantrone)

   i. Mechanism of action: Decreases monocytes and macrophages, inhibits T and B cells

   ii. Indicated for secondary progressive, progressive-relapsing, and worsening-relapsing-remitting multiple sclerosis; used infrequently because of toxicity

   iii. Because of the potential for toxicity, mitoxantrone is reserved for patients with rapidly advancing disease whose other therapies have failed.

   iv. Patients taking mitoxantrone should not receive live virus vaccines; other vaccines should be held for 4–6 weeks after dose.

   v. Cardiotoxicity: Echocardiograms or multiple-gated acquisition scans must be performed at baseline and before each infusion. Systolic dysfunction occurs in about 12% of patients; congestive heart failure occurs in about 0.4%. Cardiotoxicity is not dose-, sex-, or age-related. Cyclooxygenase 2 inhibitors should be avoided.

   vi. Therapy-related acute leukemia occurs in about 0.8% of patients.

vii. Other laboratory tests (complete blood cell count, bilirubin, aspartate aminotransferase, alanine aminotransferase, alkaline phosphatase, and pregnancy test) must be performed before each infusion.

viii. Avoid pregnancy during treatment.

g. Natalizumab (Tysabri)

   i. Mechanism of action: Block T-cell entry into the CNS

   ii. Indicated for relapsing forms of multiple sclerosis but distributed through restricted distribution program because of progressive multifocal leukoencephalopathy risk (0.24%)

   iii. Adverse effects

     (a) Hypersensitivity reactions: Itching, dizziness, fever, rash, hypotension, dyspnea, chest pain, anaphylaxis, usually within 2 hours of administration

     (b) Progressive multifocal leukoencephalopathy: Rapidly progressive viral CNS infection; usually results in death or permanent disability. Patient selection guidelines are for patients with relapsing-remitting disease whose other treatment (efficacy or intolerability) has failed or who have an aggressive initial course; it should not be used in combination with other disease-modifying therapies. On January 20, 2012, an FDA-issued drug safety communication associated positive tests for John Cunningham virus (JCV) antibodies as a risk factor for progressive multifocal leukoencephalopathy. Thus, patients with all three of the following risk factors—presence of antiJCV antibodies, longer duration of natalizumab treatment (especially beyond 2 years), and previous treatment with an immunosuppressant medication (mitoxantrone, azathioprine, methotrexate, cyclophosphamide, mycophenolate mofetil)—are at 1.1% chance of developing progressive multifocal leukoencephalopathy.

     (c) Antibodies to natalizumab, associated with increased relapses and hypersensitivity reactions, develop in 9%–12% of patients.

h. Teriflunomide (Aubagio)

   i. Mechanism of action: Prevents activation of lymphocytes

   ii. Indicated for relapsing forms of multiple sclerosis

   iii. Pharmacokinetics: Long half-life (8–19 days); takes about 3 months to reach steady-state concentrations; takes an average of 8 months to eliminate drug (serum concentrations less than 0.02 mcg/mL) and may take up to 2 years

   iv. Adverse effects

     (a) Hepatotoxicity may occur; teriflunomide should not be used in patients with preexisting liver disease or with alanine aminotransferase more than 2 times the upper limit of normal

     (b) GI effects: Diarrhea, nausea

     (c) Dermatologic effects: Alopecia, rash

     (d) Infection: Neutropenia and lymphopenia may occur; tuberculosis infections reported (negative tuberculosis skin test required at baseline); live virus vaccinations should not be administered.

     (e) Teratogenic: Pregnancy category X (based on animal studies); negative pregnancy test at baseline; adequate contraception should be ensured; if pregnancy desired for men or women, teriflunomide should be discontinued, accelerated elimination procedures should be undertaken, and two serum concentrations less than 0.02 mcg/mL taken 14 days apart should be confirmed.

   v. Accelerated elimination procedures

     (a) Cholestyramine 8 g every 8 hours for 11 days (if not tolerated, may use 4 g)

     (b) Activated charcoal powder 50 g every 12 hours for 11 days

3. Symptomatic therapies
    a. Patients may experience fatigue, spasticity, urinary incontinence, pain, depression, cognitive impairment, fecal incontinence, constipation, pseudobulbar affect, and sexual dysfunction; treatment should be with standard therapies for these symptoms.
    b. Fatigue: Treatment may be nonpharmacologic (rest, assistive devices, cooling strategies, exercise, stress management) or pharmacologic (amantadine, methylphenidate).
    c. Spasticity: Therapies must be centrally acting.
        i. First line: Baclofen, tizanidine
        ii. Second line: Dantrolene, diazepam
        iii. Third line: Intrathecal baclofen
        iv. Focal spasticity: Botulinum toxin
    d. Walking impairment: Dalfampridine (Ampyra)
        i. Indicated to improve walking in patients with multiple sclerosis by improving walking speed
        ii. Potassium channel blocker, prolongs action potentials in demyelinated neurons
        iii. Dose: 10 mg orally twice daily; extended-release tablets
        iv. Contraindicated in patients with a history of seizures or moderate or severe renal impairment
        v. Adverse effects: Seizures, urinary tract infections, insomnia
    e. Pseudobulbar affect: Dextromethorphan/quinidine
        i. Affects 10% of patients
        ii. Episodes of inappropriate laughing or crying
        iii. Dextromethorphan prevents excitatory neurotransmitter release.
        iv. Low-dose quinidine blocks first-pass metabolism of dextromethorphan, thus increasing dextromethorphan serum concentrations.

Table 9. Comparison of Disease-Modifying Therapies

Drug (Brand)	Dose	Route	Frequency	Adverse Effects
Alemtuzumab (Lemtrada)	First course: 12 mg/day over 4 hours × 5 days Second course: 12 mg/day over 4 hours × 3 days 12 months after first course	IV	Daily for 5 days, then daily for 3 days 12 months later	Infusion reaction 92% Rash 53% Thyroid disorders 34% Headache 52% Infections 13%–19%
Dimethyl fumarate (Tecfidera)	120 mg twice daily × 7 days; then 240 mg twice daily	PO	Twice daily	Skin flushing 38% GI events 41%
Fingolimod (Gilenya)	0.5 mg	PO	Daily	Increased AST/ALT 14% Infections 13% Diarrhea 12% Hypertension 6% Bradycardia 4% Blurred vision 4% Lymphopenia 4% Leukopenia 3%
Glatiramer acetate (Copaxone)	20 mg 40 mg	SC SC	Daily Three times/week	Injection site reaction 90% Systemic reaction 15%

Table 9. Comparison of Disease-Modifying Therapies *(continued)*

Drug (Brand)	Dose	Route	Frequency	Adverse Effects
Interferon beta-1a (Avonex)	30 mcg	IM	Weekly	Flulike symptoms 61% Anemia 8%
Interferon beta-1a (Rebif)	22 or 44 mcg	SC	Three times/ week	Flulike symptoms 28% Injection site reactions 66% Leukopenia 22% Increased AST/ALT 17%–27%
Interferon beta-1b (Betaseron)	0.25 mg	SC	Every other day	Flulike symptoms 60%–76% Injection site reactions 50%–85% Asthenia 49% Menstrual disorder 17% Leukopenia 10%–16% Increased AST/ALT 4%–19%
Mitoxantrone (Novantrone)	12 mg/m^2 Up to 140 mg/m^2 (lifetime dose)	IV	Every 3 months	Nausea 76% Alopecia 61% Menstrual disorders 61% Urinary tract infection 32% Amenorrhea 25% Leukopenia 19% γ-Glutamyl transpeptidase increase of 15%
Natalizumab (Tysabri)	300 mg	IV	Every 4 weeks	Headache 38% Fatigue 27% Arthralgia 19% Urinary tract infection 20% Hypersensitivity reaction <1%
Pegylated interferon beta-1a (Plegridy)	125 mcg	SC	Every 2 weeks	Injection site reactions 62% Flulike symptoms 47% Headache 44% Myalgia 19%
Teriflunomide (Aubagio)	7 mg or 14 mg	PO	Daily	Diarrhea 15%–18% Nausea 9%–14% Alopecia 10%–13% Neutropenia 10%–15% Lymphopenia 7%–10% Elevated ALT 3%–5% Hypertension 4% Peripheral neuropathy 1%–2%

ALT = alanine aminotransferase; AST = aspartate aminotransferase; GI = gastrointestinal; IM = intramuscular; IV = intravenous; PO = by mouth; SC = subcutaneous.

Patient Cases

Questions 26–28 pertain to the following case:

S.F. is a 33-year-old African American woman of Cuban descent living in the Miami area. This morning, her right leg became progressively weaker over about 3 hours. She was previously healthy except for a broken radius when she was 13 years old and a case of optic neuritis when she was 25 years old.

26. Which method is best for treating S.F.'s exacerbation?

    A. Interferon beta-1a.

    B. Glatiramer acetate.

    C. Mitoxantrone.

    D. Methylprednisolone.

27. Which therapy is best for S.F. to prevent further exacerbations?

    A. Interferon beta-1a.

    B. Interferon beta-1b.

    C. Glatiramer acetate.

    D. Any of the above.

28. S.F. elects to start interferon beta-1b and wants to know whether she can prevent or minimize some of the adverse effects. Which advice is best?

    A. Always give the injection at the same time of day.

    B. Lie down for 2 hours after the injection.

    C. Rotate injection sites.

    D. Use a heating pad on the injection sites.

29. B.B. is a 33-year-old woman with a recent diagnosis of multiple sclerosis. Her neurologist wants you to discuss with her potential medications to prevent exacerbations. During the discussion, you find that she and her husband are planning to have a baby in the next few years and that she is terrified of needles. Which choice is best for B.B.?

    A. Glatiramer acetate.

    B. Mitoxantrone.

    C. Teriflunomide.

    D. Dimethyl fumarate.

REFERENCES

Epilepsy

1. Brophy GM, Bell R, Claassen J, et al. Guidelines for the evaluation and management of status epilepticus. Neurocrit Care 2012;17:3-23. A review of emergency management of status epilepticus, including expert consensus opinion.

2. Glauser T, Ben-Manachem E, Bourgeois B, et al. Updated ILAE evidence review of antiepileptic drug therapy efficacy and effectiveness as initial monotherapy of epileptic seizures and syndromes. Epilepsia 2013;54:551-63. Available at www.ilae.org/Visitors/Documents/Guidelines-epilepsia-12074-2013.pdf. Accessed September 18, 2014. Reviews levels of evidence for all antiepileptic drugs for monotherapy of partial seizures in adults, children, and older adults, generalized seizures in adults and children.

3. Harden CL, Hopp J, Ting TY, et al. Practice parameter update: management issues for women with epilepsy. Focus on pregnancy (an evidence-based review): obstetrical complications and change in seizure frequency. Neurology 2009;73:126-32. Available at www.neurology.org/content/73/2/126.full.html. Accessed September 18, 2014. Provides conclusions about the influence of seizure medications on the risk of cesarean delivery, late pregnancy bleeding, premature contractions, and premature labor and delivery.

4. Harden CL, Meador KJ, Pennell PB, et al. Practice parameter update: management issues for women with epilepsy. Focus on pregnancy (an evidence-based review): teratogenesis and perinatal outcomes. Neurology 2009;73:133-41. Available at www.neurology.org/content/73/2/133.full.html. Accessed September 18, 2014. Provides conclusions about the effect of seizure medications on the risk of major congenital malformations, poor cognitive outcomes, and other adverse effects.

5. Harden CL, Pennell PB, Koppel BS, et al. Practice parameter update: management issues for women with epilepsy. Focus on pregnancy (an evidence-based review): vitamin K, folic acid, blood levels, and breastfeeding. Neurology 2009;73:142-9. Available at www.neurology.org/content/73/2/142.full.html. Accessed September 18, 2014. Provides conclusions about the use of preconception folic acid, the ability of seizure medications to cross the placenta, and the penetration of seizure medications into breast milk. Provides recommendations about the monitoring of seizure medication serum concentrations during pregnancy.

6. Mula M, Kanner AM, Schmitz B, et al. Antiepileptic drugs and suicidality: an expert consensus statement from the Task Force on Therapeutic Strategies of the ILAE Commission on Neuropsychobiology. Epilepsia 2013;54:199-203. Expert opinion paper reviewing available data on the risk of suicide and suicidal behavior while taking antiepileptics for epilepsy.

7. National Institute for Health and Clinical Excellence. The Epilepsies: The Diagnosis and Management of the Epilepsies in Adults and Children in Primary and Secondary Care. NICE Clinical Guideline 137. Issued January 2012. Available at www.nice.org.uk/guidance/CG137. Accessed September 18, 2014. Extensive review of diagnosis and treatment of seizures, including medical management.

8. Perucca E, Tomson T. The pharmacological treatment of epilepsy in adults. Lancet Neurol 2011;10:446-56. A solid review of current treatment issues and practices, including when treatment should be initiated, drugs of choice for initial treatment, management of drug-refractory patients, and discontinuation of seizure medications in seizure-free patients.

Stroke

1. Culebras A, Messe SR, Caturvedi S, et al. Summary of evidence-based guideline update: prevention of stroke in nonvalvular atrial fibrillation. Neurology 2014;82:716-24. Available at www.neurology.org/content/82/8/716.full. Accessed September 17, 2014. Detailed discussion of stroke prevention in patients with atrial fibrillation.

2. Goldstein LB, Bushnell CD, Adams RJ, et al. Guidelines for the primary prevention of stroke: a guideline for healthcare professionals from the American Heart Association/American Stroke Association. Stroke 2011;42:517-84. This is an extremely detailed discussion of the risk factors

for stroke and their influence on primary stroke occurrence.

3. Lansberg MG, O'Donnell MJ, Khatri P, et al. Antithrombotic and thrombolytic therapy for ischemic stroke: Antithrombotic Therapy and Prevention of Thrombosis, 9th ed. American College of Chest Physicians Evidence-Based Clinical Practice Guidelines. Chest 2012;141:e601S-36S. Comprehensive review of evidence for secondary stroke prevention.

4. You JJ, Singer DE, Howard PA, et al. Antithrombotic and thrombolytic therapy for atrial fibrillation: Antithrombotic Therapy and Prevention of Thrombosis, 9th ed. American College of Chest Physicians Evidence-Based Clinical Practice Guidelines. Chest 2012;141:e531S-75S. Gold standard for anticoagulation recommendations in atrial fibrillation.

5. Demaerschalk BM, Kleindorfer DO, Adeoye OM, et al. Scientific rationale for the inclusion and exclusion criteria or intravenous alteplase in acute ischemic stroke. A statement for healthcare professionals from the American Heart Association/American Stroke Association. Stroke 2016;47:581-641. Comprehensive, recent analysis of data to support or refute exclusion criteria for tissue plasminogen activator use in ischemic str

Parkinson Disease

1. Horstink M, Tolosa E, Bonuccelli U, et al. Review of the therapeutic management of Parkinson's disease. Report of a joint task force of the European Federation of Neurological Societies and the Movement Disorder Society—European Section. Part I. Early (uncomplicated) Parkinson's disease. Eur J Neurol 2006;13:1170-85. Guidelines for treatment of the patient who has recently received a diagnosis of Parkinson disease.

2. Horstink M, Tolosa E, Bonuccelli U, et al. Review of the therapeutic management of Parkinson's disease. Report of a joint task force of the European Federation of Neurological Societies and the Movement Disorder Society—European Section. Part II. Late (complicated) Parkinson's disease. Eur J Neurol 2006;13:1186-202. Similar to the above reference but with an emphasis on the patient with long-standing Parkinson disease. A short review of surgical treatments is also included.

3. Miyasaki JM, Shannon K, Voon V, et al. Practice parameter: evaluation and treatment of depression, psychosis, and dementia in Parkinson disease (an evidence-based review). Report of the Quality Standards Subcommittee of the American Academy of Neurology. Neurology 2006;66:996-1002. Available at www.neurology.org/cgi/reprint/66/7/983.pdf. Accessed October 15, 2013. Reviews available evidence on depression, psychosis, and dementia. Provides more in-depth reading and summarizes most clinical trials on the subject.

4. Olanow CW, Stern MB, Sethi K. The scientific and clinical basis for the treatment of Parkinson disease (2009). Neurology 2009;72(suppl 4):S1-136. An extensive treatise on pathophysiology and treatment of Parkinson disease.

5. Pahwa R, Factor SA, Lyons KE, et al. Practice parameter: treatment of Parkinson disease with motor fluctuations and dyskinesia (an evidence-based review). Report of the Quality Standards Subcommittee of the American Academy of Neurology. Neurology 2006;66:983-95. Available at www.neurology.org/cgi/reprint/66/7/983. Accessed October 15, 2013. Reviews available evidence on motor adverse effects and their treatment. Good for more in-depth reading.

6. Zesiewicz TA, Sullivan KL, Amulf I, et al. Practice parameter: treatment of nonmotor symptoms of Parkinson disease. Report of the Quality Standards Subcommittee of the American Academy of Neurology. Neurology 2010;74:924-31. Provides detailed reading on treating symptoms other than the cardinal signs of Parkinson disease.

Headaches

1. Francis GJ, Becker WJ, Pringsheim TM. Acute and preventative pharmacologic treatment of cluster headache. Neurology 2010;75:463-73. Systematic review and meta-analysis of treatment trials for cluster headache. Endorsed by the American Academy of Neurology.

2. Holland S, Silberstein SD, Freitag F, et al. Evidence-based guideline update: NSAIDs and other complementary treatments for episodic migraine prevention in adults: report of the Quality Standards Subcommittee of the American Academy of Neurology and the American Headache Society.

Neurology 2012;78:1346-53. Available at www.neurology.org/content/78/17/1346.full.pdf. Accessed October 15, 2013. Discussion of use of nonsteroidal anti-inflammatory drugs and complementary and alternative medicines for migraine prevention.

3. Silberstein SD, Holland S, Freitag F, et al. Evidence-based guideline update: pharmacologic treatment for episodic migraine prevention in adults: report of the Quality Standards Subcommittee of the American Academy of Neurology and the American Headache Society. Neurology 2012;78:1337-45. Available at www.neurology.org/content/78/17/1337.full. Accessed October 15, 2013. Discussion of prophylactic medications for migraine prevention, excluding nonsteroidal anti-inflammatory drugs, complimentary therapies, and botulinum toxin.

Multiple Sclerosis

1. Bendtzen K. Critical review: assessment of interferon-β immunogenicity in multiple sclerosis. J Interferon Cytokine Res 2010;30:759-66. Discussion of the known aspects of interferon-neutralizing antibodies.

2. Goodin DS, Cohen BA, O'Connor P, et al. Assessment: the use of natalizumab (Tysabri) for the treatment of multiple sclerosis (an evidence-based review). Neurology 2008;71:766-73. Available at www.neurology.org/content/71/10/766.full.pdf. Accessed October 15, 2013. A supplement to the primary guideline and a discussion of progressive multifocal leukoencephalopathy related to natalizumab administration.

3. Goodin DS, Frohman EM, Garmany GP, et al. Disease-modifying therapies in multiple sclerosis: subcommittee of the American Academy of Neurology and the MS Council for Clinical Practice Guidelines. Neurology 2002;58:169-78. Current guideline, reaffirmed July 19, 2008.

4. Marriott JJ, Miyasaki JM, Gronseth G, et al. Evidence report: the efficacy and safety of mitoxantrone (Novantrone) in the treatment of multiple sclerosis. Report of the Therapeutics and Technology Assessment Subcommittee of the American Academy of Neurology. Neurology 2010;74:1463-70. Available at www.neurology.org/cgi/reprint/74/18/1463. Accessed October 15, 2013. Review of evidence associating mitoxantrone with cardiac dysfunction and therapy-related acute leukemia.

ANSWERS AND EXPLANATIONS TO PATIENT CASES

1. Answer: A
Leukopenia is a common adverse effect of carbamazepine. Up to 10% of patients experience a transient decrease in their white blood cell count; however, the potential for serious hematologic abnormalities, including agranulocytosis and aplastic anemia, exists. Complete blood cell counts are recommended before initiation and periodically during therapy.

2. Answer: A
In general, dermatologic reactions to anticonvulsants occur after a delay of 2–8 weeks rather than immediately after medication initiation.

3. Answer: D
The rash that occurs with lamotrigine is often related to the speed of titration. Valproic acid inhibits the metabolism of lamotrigine; therefore, when these drugs are used together, the lamotrigine titration must be slowed even further. Psychomotor slowing, renal stones, and paresthesias are associated with topiramate and zonisamide.

4. Answer: B
Lorazepam is the drug of choice for status epilepticus. It is less lipophilic than diazepam; therefore, it does not redistribute from the CNS as quickly. After the seizures are stopped with lorazepam, a long-acting drug (phenytoin, fosphenytoin, or phenobarbital) should be administered to prevent further seizures.

5. Answer: D
Phenytoin shows nonlinear pharmacokinetics. A small increase in dose may result in a large increase in serum concentration. Therefore, without performing any calculations, we can surmise that an increase from 300 mg/day to 600 mg/day would more than double the serum concentration.

6. Answer: D
Ethosuximide is useful for absence seizures. The other listed medications are not used for absence seizures.

7. Answer: A
Drowsiness is a dose-related adverse effect of phenytoin. Acne, gingival hyperplasia, and rash can also be adverse effects, but they are not dose related.

8. Answer: C
Valproic acid and its derivatives are associated with alopecia. The hair will grow back if the drug is discontinued and sometimes even if the drug is continued. There are reports of the regrown hair being curly when patients previously had straight hair.

9. Answer: D
Carbamazepine forms an active epoxide intermediate (carbamazepine-10,11-epoxide), whereas oxcarbazepine does not. Carbamazepine induces more liver enzymes than oxcarbazepine. However, hyponatremia is more closely associated with oxcarbazepine than carbamazepine. Both drugs can cause allergic rashes.

10. Answer: C
Alterations to seizure treatment regimens can be made when patients present to the health system before pregnancy. In this case, a different drug may be chosen, or medications may be eliminated if the patient is taking more than one seizure medication. In addition, efforts should be made to maintain the patient on the lowest possible doses that control seizures. However, when the patient presents to the health system already pregnant, the current medications are usually continued to avoid the risk of an increase in seizures during a medication change. Again, the lowest possible doses that control seizures should be used.

11. Answer: D
Nonmodifiable risk factors for stroke include age, race, and male sex. Somewhat modifiable risk factors include hypercholesterolemia and diabetes mellitus. Modifiable stroke risk factors include hypertension, smoking, and atrial fibrillation. Less well-documented risk factors include obesity, physical inactivity, alcohol abuse, hyperhomocystinemia, hypercoagulability, hormone replacement therapy, and oral contraceptives. Modification of risk factors, if possible, may translate into reduced stroke risk, which should be a focus of all stroke prevention plans.

12. Answer: C

There are many contraindications to administering tissue plasminogen activator for stroke, mainly focused on bleeding risk. There is no upper limit on age. There is a strict 4½-hour limit for treating strokes.

13. Answer: C

All patients experiencing a stroke should be placed on a drug to prevent future events. Appropriate choices include aspirin, ticlopidine, cilostazol, clopidogrel, dipyridamole/aspirin, and warfarin. However, because of the risk of neutropenia, ticlopidine is usually not used first-line. If the patient has atrial fibrillation, he or she should be treated with warfarin, dabigatran, apixaban, or rivaroxaban. If the patient does not have atrial fibrillation, warfarin offers no benefit and has considerable risk compared with aspirin. Otherwise, any of these drugs are reasonable choices.

14. Answer: C

No therapy is an appropriate choice for this patient (CHA$_2$DS$_2$-VASc score of 0) because he is younger than 65 years and has no other risk factors such as hypertension or a prosthetic valve.

15. Answer: C

The target INR for a patient younger than 75 years with hypertension and diabetes mellitus is 2.5.

16. Answer: D

Anticholinergic drugs (benztropine and trihexyphenidyl) commonly cause adverse effects such as confusion, dry mouth, urinary retention, and constipation in older patients. Decreasing or eliminating these drugs may resolve the difficulties.

17. Answer: D

Wearing-off phenomenon is the return of Parkinson disease symptoms before the next dose. This problem can be resolved by giving doses more often, administering the controlled-release formulation of carbidopa/levodopa, or adding a catechol-O-methyl transferase inhibitor. The terms *increase the dosing interval* and *decrease the dosing interval* are often misinterpreted. To increase the dosing interval means to give the doses farther apart.

18. Answer: C

Amantadine can cause livedo reticularis, a condition in which the dilation of capillary blood vessels and the stagnation of blood within these vessels cause a mottled, reddish blue discoloration of the skin. This usually occurs on the trunk and extremities; it is more pronounced in cold weather. Although simple venous stasis could occur, livedo reticularis is more likely in this patient.

19. Answer: D

Treatment of dyskinesias includes decreasing the levodopa dose, removing selegiline or dopamine agonists from the drug regimen, or adding amantadine.

20. Answer: D

Ropinirole, a direct dopamine agonist, is a good choice for initial treatment in a patient with Parkinson disease. Trihexyphenidyl would control his tremor but would not improve his difficulty walking, which probably represents bradykinesia. Entacapone is a catechol-O-methyltransferase inhibitor; it should be used only in conjunction with carbidopa/levodopa. Apomorphine is for severe on-off symptoms.

21. Answer: A

A β-blocker is a good choice for a patient with the coexisting condition of hypertension. Valproic acid and amitriptyline could both increase weight gain in a morbidly obese patient. Lithium is used for prophylaxis of cluster headaches.

22. Answer: C

Amitriptyline is as effective as prophylaxis for tension headaches. β-Blockers and valproic acid are usually used for migraine headache prophylaxis, and lithium is used for prophylaxis of cluster headaches.

23. Answer: D

Lithium is a prophylactic agent for cluster headaches. β-Blockers and valproic acid are usually used for migraine headache prophylaxis. Amitriptyline is useful for migraine and tension headaches.

24. Answer: D
Sumatriptan is available as an injectable and as a nasal spray and would be more appropriate to use in a patient with severe nausea and vomiting. Zolmitriptan is available as a nasal spray. The other triptans are available only in oral preparations.

25. Answer: A
The NNT is a concept used to express the number of patients it would be necessary to treat to have one patient experience benefit (or to experience adverse effects, if looking at harm). It is calculated as NNT = 1/[(% improved on active therapy) − (% improved on placebo)]. The NNT is calculated for each treatment and is therefore treatment-specific. Low NNTs indicate high treatment efficacy. If an NNT of 1 were calculated, it would mean that every patient on active therapy improved and that no patient on placebo improved.

26. Answer: D
Methylprednisolone is the only option used for treating acute exacerbations. Other options are high-dose oral prednisone or adrenocorticotropic hormone. Interferon beta-1a, glatiramer acetate, and mitoxantrone are all used as disease-modifying therapies.

27. Answer: D
The beta interferons and glatiramer acetate are appropriate initial choices for disease-modifying therapy. Mitoxantrone and natalizumab would not be used as a first-line therapy because of their potential toxicities.

28. Answer: C
Rotating the injection sites for the self-injections is a good strategy for preventing injection site reactions. Other strategies that might help prevent these reactions are icing the injection site before injection and bringing the drug to room temperature. The injections should be administered at about the same time of day, but this is not a strategy for preventing adverse effects.

29. Answer: D
Patients unable to give self-injection because of their fear of needles should not be given glatiramer acetate, which is a subcutaneous injection. Mitoxantrone has significant toxicities, and it is infrequently used to treat multiple sclerosis. In addition, this drug is pregnancy category X. Teriflunomide may take up to 2 years for elimination or rapid elimination protocols before pregnancy; thus, it would not be a good choice in this patient. Dimethyl fumarate has no data in human pregnancy right now and is pregnancy category C. However, this patient should carefully plan her conception and can discontinue the medication before pregnancy. Of the available choices, dimethyl fumarate is the best answer.

ANSWERS AND EXPLANATIONS TO SELF-ASSESSMENT QUESTIONS

1. Answer: C

The therapeutic range for phenytoin is 10–20 mcg/mL. Although a serum concentration should never be interpreted without clinical information, this patient is having no seizures, nor is he experiencing toxicity. Because he is otherwise healthy, does not have known kidney dysfunction, and is not elderly, there is no need for an albumin concentration.

2. Answer: B

In general, medications to treat status epilepticus should be in parenteral formulation to facilitate rapid administration. Once the seizures of status epilepticus have been stopped, a second, long-acting drug should be initiated to prevent seizure recurrence. Medications typically used for this purpose include phenytoin, fosphenytoin, phenobarbital, and (sometimes) valproic acid. Another benzodiazepine need not be administered because this patient's seizure activity has ceased.

3. Answer: C

Psychomotor slowing is a very troublesome adverse effect for many patients initiated on topiramate. It usually manifests as difficulty concentrating, difficulty thinking, word-finding difficulties, and a feeling of slowness of movement. The usual dosage titration for topiramate calls for increasing the dose every week. This patient has been increasing the topiramate dose every other day. Because psychomotor slowing is related to the speed of titration, this makes slowing the titration rate the most probable answer. Partial seizures could present as confusion; however, they are unlikely to be a continuous condition.

4. Answer: B

Patients who can be treated within 4½ hours of stroke symptom onset should be considered for tissue plasminogen activator. Uncontrolled hypertension (greater than 185/100 mm Hg) is a contraindication to tissue plasminogen activator treatment. Active use of heparin (with an elevated partial thromboplastin time) or warfarin (with an elevated INR) is a contraindication, but use of aspirin is not. This patient's onset of stroke symptoms began 6 hours ago, so he is not eligible for tissue plasminogen activator treatment.

5. Answer: D

All stroke survivors need secondary stroke prevention drugs. If a patient claims to be adherent to aspirin when his first stroke occurred, a different drug is usually considered. Clopidogrel or dipyridamole/aspirin would be an acceptable choice. Heparin and enoxaparin are not suitable for long-term home use in secondary stroke prevention.

6. Answer: B

Wearing off is the return of symptoms before the next dose. It has a definite pattern, whereas on-off is unpredictable. Dyskinesias and dystonias are long-term adverse effects of carbidopa/levodopa.

7. Answer: D

The first dose of apomorphine must be given in a clinic setting. The patient should not take apomorphine if he is allergic to metabisulfite. The dose should be retitrated if he has not taken apomorphine for 1 week. Apomorphine causes severe nausea and vomiting.

8. Answer: A

Because of the MAO inhibition induced by rasagiline, patients should not take meperidine, propoxyphene, tramadol, methadone, dextromethorphan, sympathomimetics, fluoxetine, or fluvoxamine. Guaifenesin can be safely taken in this situation.

9. Answer: D

The choice of drug for acute treatment of a patient with migraines and cardiac disease presents a difficulty. All triptans and ergotamines are contraindicated in this situation. A nonsteroidal anti-inflammatory drug is a possible choice.

10. Answer: A

When possible, a drug for migraine prophylaxis should be selected to confer additional benefit to a patient for a concomitant disease state. In the patient with coronary artery disease and hypertension, propranolol would be an excellent choice for migraine prevention.

11. Answer: D

Fingolimod is the only one of the given choices with an FDA indication for the treatment of multiple sclerosis. In addition, it has the best clinical trial evidence of efficacy. Methylprednisolone is used for treating acute multiple sclerosis exacerbations. Cyclophosphamide and azathioprine have been studied in progressive forms of multiple sclerosis, but their data are not as robust as are those for fingolimod.

12. Answer: B

Treatment of spasticity in multiple sclerosis requires the use of a centrally acting agent. Of the choices given, only diazepam and baclofen are centrally acting. Because of the significant fatigue and drowsiness occurring with diazepam, baclofen is usually a first-line therapy. Another acceptable choice would be tizanidine.

13. Answer: C

Agents used to treat multiple sclerosis–related fatigue include amantadine and methylphenidate. The other choices are not used in multiple sclerosis.

General Psychiatry

Jacintha Cauffield, Pharm.D., BCPS

Palm Beach Atlantic University
Lloyd L. Gregory School of Pharmacy
West Palm Beach, Florida

GENERAL PSYCHIATRY

JACINTHA CAUFFIELD, PHARM.D., BCPS

PALM BEACH ATLANTIC UNIVERSITY
LLOYD L. GREGORY SCHOOL OF PHARMACY
WEST PALM BEACH, FLORIDA

Learning Objectives

1. Examine pharmacotherapeutic options for managing major depression, bipolar disorder, schizophrenia, anxiety disorders, insomnia, and substance use disorder.

2. Select a drug used to treat these disorders with respect to its unique pharmacologic properties, therapeutic uses, adverse effects, and cognitive and behavioral effects.

3. Formulate a pharmacotherapeutic treatment plan when presented with a patient with diagnoses of major depression, bipolar disorder, schizophrenia, anxiety disorder, insomnia, or substance use disorder.

Self-Assessment Questions

Answers and explanations to these questions can be found at the end of this chapter.

1. A.B. is a 25-year-old woman who presents to your practice with a depressed mood that has worsened during the past few weeks. She struggles to get out of bed in the morning. When she is not sleeping, she is eating. She has gained 10 lb in the past month. She is worried about her job and does not feel like she is "pulling her weight," even though she recently received a glowing evaluation. She has passive thoughts of harming herself but no definite plan. Her medical history includes anxiety, gastroesophageal reflux disease, and hypothyroidism. She currently takes levothyroxine 100 mcg daily, lansoprazole 30 mg every morning, and alprazolam 0.5 mg three times daily for anxiety. Which medication would best treat her symptoms?

    A. Desipramine.
    B. Fluoxetine.
    C. Mirtazapine.
    D. Paroxetine.

2. K.M. is a 56-year-old woman with recurrent major depression, type 2 diabetes with newly diagnosed neuropathy, obesity, and coronary artery disease. She currently takes citalopram 40 mg daily, carvedilol 25 mg twice daily, lisinopril 40 mg daily, and metformin 1000 mg twice daily. She is tearful during her appointment and continues to have symptoms of depression despite initial improvement on citalopram. She wants to switch antidepressants. Which would be most beneficial?

    A. Bupropion.
    B. Duloxetine.
    C. Nortriptyline.
    D. Sertraline.

3. L.J. is a 45-year-old man who presents agitated and sweating. His right eyelid started twitching about 1 hour ago, and he cannot get it to stop. He developed cold symptoms 2 days ago and began taking dextromethorphan and pseudoephedrine. His medical history includes depression, hypertension, and hyperlipidemia. He takes paroxetine 40 mg at bedtime, diltiazem XR 240 mg daily, and rosuvastatin 10 mg daily. Which combination of medications is most likely contributing to his current symptoms?

    A. Cetirizine and paroxetine.
    B. Dextromethorphan and pseudoephedrine.
    C. Diltiazem and pseudoephedrine.
    D. Paroxetine and dextromethorphan.

4. H.G. is a 31-year-old man with a 5-year history of type I bipolar disorder, for which he takes lithium 300 mg twice daily. His lithium serum concentration, taken yesterday before his morning dose of lithium, is 1.0 mEq/L. He has been without manic symptoms for the past few years. He was admitted for a suicide gesture using acetaminophen. For the past few weeks, he has lost interest in his job and is isolating himself from other people. Which medication would best help his acute symptoms?

    A. Aripiprazole.
    B. Lamotrigine.
    C. Quetiapine.
    D. Venlafaxine.

5. H.K. is a 28-year-old woman (height 61 inches, weight 165 lb) with a history of type I bipolar disorder. She takes lithium 450 mg twice daily. Her last serum concentration (3 months ago) was 0.7 mEq/L. She presents today for an annual examination. Her laboratory test results include sodium 138 mEq/L, potassium 4.7 mEq/L, serum creatinine 0.9 mg/dL, glucose 124 mg/dL, and

thyroid-stimulating hormone (TSH) 24 U/mL. She has gained 15 lb in the past 2 months. Additional medications include olanzapine 10 mg at bedtime (for 1 year), Yasmin daily, and a multivitamin. Which most likely accounts for these findings?

A. Hypothyroidism.

B. Lithium concentration.

C. Olanzapine.

D. Yasmin.

6. I.T. is a 43-year-old woman with rapid-cycling bipolar disorder, hypertension, obesity, and asthma. She recently switched from lithium to divalproex sodium 500 mg daily. She additionally takes lamotrigine 150 mg twice daily, aripiprazole 30 mg daily, ramipril 10 mg daily, albuterol HFA 2 puffs every 6 hours, and fluticasone/salmeterol dry powder inhaler (DPI) 250/50 twice daily, She started a prednisone taper 3 days ago for an asthma exacerbation. Today, she presents with abdominal pain with rebound tenderness, nausea, and vomiting. Laboratory test results include sodium 141 mEq/L, potassium 3.3 mEq/L, chloride 95 mEq/L, carbon dioxide 26 mmol/L, serum creatinine 1.0 mg/dL, glucose 72 mg/dL, cholesterol 165 mg/dL, triglycerides 188 mg/dL, aspartate aminotransferase (AST) 27 IU/L, alanine aminotransferase (ALT) 21 IU/L, amylase 456 U/L, and lipase 387 U/L. Which medication is most likely responsible for her current clinical picture?

A. Aripiprazole.

B. Divalproex sodium.

C. Lamotrigine.

D. Prednisone.

7. N.B. is a 36-year-old man with 16-year history of schizophrenia and alcohol use disorder. He was recently switched to aripiprazole from haloperidol because of gynecomastia and impotence. Today, he is pacing your office. He seems anxious and agitated. He has not been sleeping well and feels uncomfortable in his skin. Which medication would most help relieve his symptoms?

A. Benztropine.

B. Dantrolene.

C. Lorazepam.

D. Propranolol.

8. T.Y. is a 64-year-old woman with a 25-year history of schizophrenia. During the past year, she has developed involuntary chewing motions and abnormal blinking, which have begun interfering with her ability to eat. She currently takes haloperidol 2.5 mg twice daily. Her symptoms improved when her haloperidol dose was decreased from 5 mg twice daily but have not resolved. She wants to switch antipsychotics. She did not respond adequately to olanzapine or perphenazine. Which would offer the most improvement in her symptoms?

A. Chlorpromazine.

B. Clozapine.

C. Quetiapine.

D. Risperidone.

9. U.M. is a 38-year-old woman with a 4-year history of schizophrenia. Within the past year, she has been given diagnoses of type 2 diabetes and dyslipidemia. Her body mass index (BMI) is 32 kg/m². Her father died of a myocardial infarction (MI) at age 42. She has been treated with risperidone but developed galactorrhea. Concomitant medications include atorvastatin, metformin, and liraglutide. Which antipsychotic would be the best choice?

A. Olanzapine.

B. Paliperidone.

C. Quetiapine.

D. Ziprasidone.

10. N.Y. is a 20-year-old woman who presents to the emergency department after experiencing trembling, sweating, chest pain, and shortness of breath accompanied by intense fear. An MI has been ruled out. She has been given a diagnosis of panic disorder. Which medication regimen would most rapidly treat her acute symptoms?

A. Alprazolam.

B. Buspirone.

C. Hydroxyzine.

D. Paroxetine.

11. T.R. is a 55-year-old woman with generalized anxiety disorder (GAD). Concomitant medical conditions include history of breast cancer, dyslipidemia, osteoarthritis, vasomotor symptoms, and osteopenia. She takes tamoxifen, simvastatin, ibuprofen, lorazepam, and alendronate. Her physician would like her to have better control of her anxiety symptoms. He would also like to taper her off lorazepam. Which agent would be the best choice?

   A. Bupropion.

   B. Fluoxetine.

   C. Pregabalin.

   D. Venlafaxine.

12. O.P. is a 74-year-old woman who has difficulty getting to sleep. Once she falls asleep, she rests comfortably throughout the night. She struggles with keeping a consistent bedtime. This problem has been ongoing for the past few months. She has no identifiable contributing factors. Concomitant medical conditions include hypertension, arthritis, and mild cognitive impairment. She has tried diphenhydramine. She states it helped for only a few nights and "it made me loopy." She would like a medication with the least risk of hangover effect. Which medication is best?

   A. Eszopiclone.

   B. Ramelteon.

   C. Suvorexant.

   D. Zolpidem.

13. M.K. is a 23-year-old man with a history of heroin addiction. He has been successfully maintained on methadone 40 mg daily for 1 year. He would like an option that does not require him to go to a daily opioid treatment program to get his methadone dose. He is not taking other medication, nor does he abuse other substances. Which treatment regimen is most appropriate?

   A. Initiate supervised buprenorphine/naloxone.

   B. Switch to buprenorphine × 2 days; then take buprenorphine/naloxone.

   C. Switch to naltrexone.

   D. Taper to methadone 30 mg; then switch to buprenorphine.

14. C.H. is a 55-year-old man with a 30-year history of alcohol dependence. He drinks 1 pint of vodka daily. He has tried several times to quit without success. He has recently reconciled with his estranged son and wants to be sober so that he can be more present in his son's life. His liver function test results include AST 143 IU/L, ALT 74 IU/L, albumin 4.0 g/dL, alkaline phosphatase 75 IU/L, total bilirubin 0.3 mg/dL, prothrombin time (PT) 0.9 seconds, platelet count 370×10^3 cells/mm^3, and creatinine clearance (CrCl) 40 mL/minute/1.73 m^2. After detoxification, which maintenance treatment is most appropriate?

   A. Acamprosate 666 mg three times daily.

   B. Chlordiazepoxide 25 mg four times daily.

   C. Disulfiram 500 mg daily.

   D. Naltrexone 50 mg daily.

15. J.Z. is a 44-year-old man who is getting ready to be discharged from the hospital after an MI. He has a 25 pack-year history of smoking cigarettes and smokes 1-1/2 packs per day. He has tried twice unsuccessfully to quit. His medical history includes recurrent depression. He tried quitting cold turkey the first time about 5 years ago. He resumed smoking 6 months later when he lost his job. He tried again about 6 months ago using nicotine gum. He used the 2-mg strength. To save money, he chewed 7 pieces daily. Which regimen would be best?

   A. Bupropion SR 150 mg twice daily.

   B. Nicotine 4 mg gum.

   C. Nicotine patch 21 mg/day.

   D. Varenicline 0.5 mg once daily.

BPS Pharmacotherapy Specialty Examination Content Outline

This chapter covers the following sections of the Pharmacotherapy Specialty Examination Content Outline:

1. Domain 1: Patient-Centered Pharmacotherapy
    a. Task 1: 1-8, 10-14
    b. Task 3: 2,-4
    d. Task 4: 1-7
2. Domain 3: System-Based Standards and Population-Based Pharmacotherapy
    a. Task 3: 1,4

Abbreviations

ANC	Absolute neutrophil count
CBT	Cognitive behavioral therapy
EPS	Extrapyramidal symptoms
FGA	First-generation antipsychotic
GAD	Generalized anxiety disorder
MDD	Major depressive disorder
OCD	Obsessive-compulsive disorder
OH	Orthostatic hypotension
PTSD	Posttraumatic stress disorder
SGA	Second-generation antipsychotic
SNRI	Serotonin-norepinephrine reuptake inhibitor
SSRI	Selective serotonin reuptake inhibitor
TCA	Tricyclic antidepressant

Patient Cases

Questions 1–4 pertain to the following case:

L.M. is a 25-year-old man recently given a diagnosis of schizophrenia, paranoid type. He often hears voices telling him that he is "stupid and worthless" and that he should "just jump off his apartment building." His parents became very concerned about his isolative behavior and brought him to the hospital. He was given haloperidol in the psychiatry unit and now presents with neck stiffness and oculogyric crisis. Until now, he has not taken medications because he felt that he could control his symptoms on his own with vitamins and Red Bull drinks.

1. Which is the most appropriate treatment of L.M.'s symptoms at this time?
   A. Benztropine.
   B. Haloperidol.
   C. Propranolol.
   D. Quetiapine.

2. You and the psychiatric team decide to recommend risperidone for L.M. Which is the best rationale for this selection?
   A. Risperidone has minimal risk of causing extrapyramidal symptoms (EPS).
   B. Risperidone is available in a long-acting injection to increase adherence.
   C. Risperidone is effective for decreasing L.M.'s negative symptoms.
   D. Risperidone can be dosed once daily after titration to target dose.

3. Which is the best example of an adverse effect of risperidone that would be of concern in L.M.?
   A. Sedation.
   B. Anticholinergic effects.
   C. EPS.
   D. Corrected QT (QTc) prolongation.

4. One year later, L.M. is no longer responding to risperidone, and you decide to switch him to another medication. L.M. is only interested in oral medications. Given his history, which agent is most appropriate at this time?
   A. Clozapine.
   B. Fluphenazine.
   C. Olanzapine.
   D. Quetiapine.

I. SCHIZOPHRENIA

A. Characteristics
   1. Schizophrenia is a thought disorder involving a complex mix of symptoms. The *Diagnostic and Statistical Manual for Mental Disorders* (*DSM-5*) identifies five symptoms for diagnosis. At least two of the following symptoms must be present for at least 1 month, and at least one should be delusions, hallucinations, or disorganized speech.
      a. Delusions: These are erroneous beliefs involving misinterpretations of reality that are resistant to evidence refuting them. A fixed delusion will not change, no matter how much evidence is offered to the contrary.
      b. Hallucinations: These perceptual abnormalities can involve any sensory system. With schizophrenia, auditory hallucinations are most common. These can be persecutory (e.g., someone is going to get me), paranoid (e.g., someone is watching), or command (e.g., someone told me to do it).
      c. Disorganized speech: This manifests as frequent "derailment" of speech or incoherence. "Loose associations" refers to the person going from one topic to another as though the topics were connected. "Tangential" speech refers to answers to questions that are only slightly related or totally unrelated to the question. "Word salad" refers to speech that is almost incomprehensible and is very much like receptive aphasia.
      d. Disorganized or catatonic behavior
      e. Negative symptoms (see Table 1)
   2. Several symptom domains have been developed for schizophrenia. Usually, symptoms are divided into two categories: positive and negative. However, other domains have also been suggested. The most common scheme is shown in Table 1.

Table 1. Categories of Schizophrenia-Associated Symptoms

Positive (presence of something that should not be there)	Negative (absence of something that should be present)	Cognitive
Traditional and Atypical Antipsychotics Effective	**Atypical Antipsychotics May or May Not Be More Effective**	**No Current Medications Effectively Treat This**
Hallucinations[a,b]	Blunted or flat affect[a,b]	Poor executive function
Delusions[a,b]	Social withdrawal (passive-apathetic)[a,b]	Impaired attention
Paranoia or suspiciousness[a,b]	Lack of personal hygiene[a]	Impaired working memory (does not learn from mistakes)
Conceptual disorganization[a,b,c]	Prolonged time to respond[a,b]	
Hostility[b]	Poor rapport[b]	
Grandiosity[b]	Poor abstract thinking[b]	
Excitement[b]	Poverty of speech (lack of spontaneity and flow of conversation)[b]	
Loose associations	Emotional withdrawal[b]	
Thought broadcasting	Alogia (inability to carry on logical conversation)	

Table 1. Categories of Schizophrenia-Associated Symptoms *(continued)*

Positive (presence of something that should not be there)	Negative (absence of something that should be present)	Cognitive
Traditional and Atypical Antipsychotics Effective	**Atypical Antipsychotics May or May Not Be More Effective**	**No Current Medications Effectively Treat This**
Thought insertion	Ambivalence (simultaneous, contradictory thinking); prevents decision-making	
	Autism (internally directed)	
	Amotivation (avolition)	
	Anhedonia	

[a]These symptoms can be used as a brief clinical assessment for antipsychotic response; they are known as the 4-Item Positive Symptoms Rating Scale (PSRS) and the Brief Negative Symptom Assessment (BNSA).

[b]These symptoms are used to score the positive and negative portions of the Positive and Negative Symptom Scale (PANSS).

[c]Conceptual disorganization, according to the Brief Psychiatric Rating Scale, is the "degree to which speech is confused, disconnected, vague or disorganized." This includes tangential thinking, circumstantiality, sudden topic shifts, incoherence, derailment, blocking, neologisms, clanging, word salad, and other speech disorders.

B. Course of Illness
   1. Onset is usually between adolescence and early adulthood. It occurs earlier in men (i.e., early 20s) than in women (i.e., late 20s to early 30s). The incidence is about equal between sexes.
   2. Most patients fluctuate between acute episodes and remission. Periods between episodes may include some residual symptoms.
   3. There are four phases of schizophrenia: prodromal, acute, stabilization, and stable.
      a. Prodromal phase: This phase is characterized by the gradual development of symptoms that may go unnoticed until a major symptom occurs. It may include isolation, deterioration of hygiene, loss of interest in work or school, and dysphoria.
      b. Acute phase: This is the full-blown episode of psychotic behavior. Patients may be unable to care for themselves during this phase.
      c. Stabilization phase: The acute symptoms begin to decrease, and this phase may last for several months.
      d. Stable phase: During this phase, symptoms have markedly declined and may not be present. Nonpsychotic symptoms such as anxiety and depression may be present.
   4. Complete remission without symptoms is uncommon.

C. Causes
   1. The causes of schizophrenia are unknown. It appears to involve neurophysiological and psychological abnormalities.
   2. The primary neurotransmitters believed to be involved in the etiology are dopamine and serotonin. The exact relationship between these neurotransmitters remains unknown. It does appear that in some areas of the brain, dopamine overactivity results in some symptoms, whereas in others, underactivity may occur. Positron emission tomographic scanning shows areas of hypermetabolism and hypometabolism.
   3. Many potential risk factors for schizophrenia have been identified, including having a family history of schizophrenia, having a poor birth history, experiencing intrauterine trauma, living in an urban area, having stress, and being born during the winter.

D. Rating Scales
  1. The Brief Psychiatric Rating Scale (BPRS) is a general psychiatric rating scale that has been used to measure outcomes in clinical trials, including those involving schizophrenia.
  2. The Positive and Negative Symptom Scale (PANSS) is a 30-item, 7-point scale that was partly adapted from the BPRS. It is widely used to evaluate antipsychotic therapy in clinical trials but not in daily clinical practice. It requires a 45-minute interview with the patient. The interviewer must be specially trained to administer it.
  3. The Positive Symptoms Rating Scale (PSRS) and the Brief Negative Symptom Assessment (BNSA) are two different but complementary scales. Each consists of four items. Each of the items on the PSRS is scored from 1 (not present) to 7 (extremely severe). Each of the items on the BNSA is scored from 1 (normal) to 6 (severe). These scales were used in the Texas Algorithm Project, a large-scale clinical trial that assessed the value of algorithm-driven medication practices in the mentally ill. The PSRS and BNSA allow rapid clinical assessment.

E. Antipsychotics (Table 2)
  1. First-line agents for treating schizophrenia
  2. Two classes
     a. First-generation antipsychotics (FGAs; also called typical or conventional antipsychotics): These include all the older antipsychotics, including the phenothiazines. Chlorpromazine was the first to be used clinically.
     b. Second-generation antipsychotics (SGAs; also called atypical antipsychotics): These include the newer agents, beginning with clozapine. The adverse effect profile of these agents is more heterogeneous and differs from that of FGAs.
  3. All antipsychotics carry a black box warning against the use in older adult patients with dementia. FGAs may have a higher mortality rate than SGAs in older adults, particularly if they have dementia.

Table 2. Antipsychotic Agents for the Treatment of Schizophrenia by Chemical Class

Class	Agent	Degree of EPS[a]
First-generation antipsychotics (FGAs), selected (typical or conventional)		
Phenothiazines	Chlorpromazine	+2
	Fluphenazine	+3
	Mesoridazine	+1
	Perphenazine	+2/+3
	Thioridazine	+1
	Trifluoperazine	+3
Butyrophenone	Haloperidol	+3
Others	Loxapine	+2/+3
	Thiothixene	+3

Table 2. Antipsychotic Agents for the Treatment of Schizophrenia by Chemical Class *(continued)*

Class	Agent	Degree of EPS[a]
Second-generation antipsychotics (SGAs; atypical)		
	Aripiprazole	0/+1
	Asenapine	0/+1
	Brexpiprazole	0/+1
	Cariprazine	0/+1
	Clozapine	0
	Iloperidone	0/+1
	Lurasidone	0/+1
	Olanzapine	0/+1
	Paliperidone	0/+1
	Quetiapine	0/+1
	Risperidone	+1
	Ziprasidone	0/+1

[a]0 = none; +1 = low; +2 = moderate; +3 = high.

EPS = extrapyramidal symptoms.

4. Many antipsychotics are metabolized by the cytochrome P450 (CYP) system (Table 3). The presence of a CYP inducer or inhibitor may require antipsychotic dose adjustment. For example, tobacco dependence, particularly smoking, is common in patients with schizophrenia. A patient taking a CYP1A2 substrate antipsychotic who undergoes smoking cessation may require a reduction in antipsychotic dose. This is particularly true of clozapine and olanzapine. Many SGAs metabolized by 2D6 and/or 3A4 carry dose adjustment recommendations.

Table 3. Selected Antipsychotics and the CYP System

	1A2	2D6	3A4
Substrate	Asenapine Clozapine[a] Olanzapine Ziprasidone	Aripiprazole Brexpiprazole[a] Iloperidone[a] Perphenazine Risperidone	Aripiprazole Brexpiprazole[a] Cariprazine[a] Haloperidol Iloperidone[a] Lurasidone[a] Quetiapine[a] Ziprasidone
Inducer	Smoking		
Inhibitor		Chlorpromazine Fluphenazine	

[a]Dose adjustment required for inhibitor or inducer of that specific CYP enzyme.

5. QTc prolongation: Electrocardiographic (ECG) changes occur with antipsychotics. QTc prolongation can predispose the patient to ventricular arrhythmias including torsades de pointes syndrome. The risk appears highest with chlorpromazine, haloperidol, and thioridazine. Among the SGAs, clozapine, ziprasidone, and iloperidone appear to have the highest risk, although the other agents may cause ECG changes to a lesser extent or only when combined with other agents that prolong the QTc interval. Patients must be assessed for predisposing factors such as preexisting ECG abnormalities, electrolyte disturbances, and concurrent therapy with other drugs that prolong the QTc interval.

F. FGAs for Schizophrenia (Table 2)
    1. These agents can be categorized according to chemical class (Table 2) or potency as antagonists at the dopamine D_2 receptors (Table 4).
    2. Potency at D_2 receptors can be split into low and high potency. FGAs can be interconverted using dose equivalents.
        a. Low potency: Concomitant anticholinergic, antihistaminic, and α-adrenergic blocking properties are also present.
        b. High potency: Less potency at the other receptors; EPS tends to be the main adverse effect and is more prevalent than with low-potency agents.
        c. Adverse effect profiles also differ by potency (Table 4).

Table 4. Selected FGAs for the Treatment of Schizophrenia

Agent	Dose Equivalent (mg)	Potency[a]	Anticholinergic[b]	Sedation[b]	↓ BP[b]	EPS
Chlorpromazine	100	Low	4	5	5	Low
Fluphenazine	2	High	2	2	2	High
Haloperidol	2–3	High	1	2	1	High
Loxapine	10–15	Int.	3	3	2	Int.
Perphenazine	10	Int.	2	2	2	Int.
Thioridazine	100	Low	5	4	5	Low
Thiothixene	3–5	High	2	2	2	High

[a]Potency = D_2 receptor affinity

[b]Scale 1–5 = low to high.

BP = blood pressure; FGA = first-generation antipsychotic; Int. = intermediate.

    3. The range of adverse effects is relatively uniform across the class, depending on potency profile.
        a. Sedation: The degree of sedation depends on the drug. If sedation occurs, it is usually worse initially and is then tolerated better with time. It tends to be dose-related.
        b. Anticholinergic effects: Dry mouth, constipation, blurred vision, and urinary hesitancy can occur. Patients for whom these effects may be a problem should probably receive a high-potency agent.
        c. Antiadrenergic effects: The α-adrenergic blocking effect is seen as orthostatic hypotension (OH). Patients who are predisposed to such effects (e.g., older adults, dehydrated patients) should probably receive a high-potency agent.
        d. Extrapyramidal symptoms
            i. Parkinsonism: This is manifested by symptoms such as bradykinesia, rigidity, tremor, or akinesia. It is usually responsive to anticholinergic agents such as diphenhydramine, trihexyphenidyl, and benztropine.
            ii. Dystonia: These episodes are often acute. Examples include torticollis, laryngospasm, and oculogyric crisis. This is also treated with anticholinergics.
            iii. Akathisia: This is a somatic restlessness and inability to stay still or calm. Reducing the antipsychotic dose and switching to an agent with a lower incidence of akathisia are the best options but not always feasible. It responds poorly to anticholinergics. Lipophilic (fat soluble) β-blockers such as propranolol and nadolol have been used, but data analyses for efficacy are inconclusive. Benzodiazepines may play a role in symptom reduction.

iv. Tardive dyskinesia: Characterized by abnormal involuntary movements that occur with long-term antipsychotic therapy. It usually involves the orofacial muscles and is often insidious. If caught early, it can be reversible. With continued drug exposure, particularly at high doses, it is often irreversible. Risks are probably related to total cumulative dose. Symptoms may decrease with lowering the dose of antipsychotic or switching to an agent that is associated with less tardive dyskinesia. This dose reduction must be weighed against worsening of schizophrenic symptoms. The risk is higher with FGAs than SGAs, as well as older age. Clozapine has not been associated with tardive dyskinesia, and changing to this drug is preferred in patients with moderate to severe symptoms. The other atypical antipsychotics also appear to have a low potential to cause tardive dyskinesia. Anticholinergic agents should not be given to treat tardive dyskinesia and may actually worsen the symptoms.

e. Neuroleptic malignant syndrome: This is another serious complication. It occurs with all agents but appears more common with high-potency drugs. It is manifested by agitation, confusion, changing levels of consciousness, fever, tachycardia, labile blood pressure, and sweating. Its mortality rate is high, and it should be taken seriously. Discontinue the offending agent and give supportive therapy, including fluids and cooling. Bromocriptine and dantrolene have been used with varying success.

f. Endocrine effects: Galactorrhea and menstrual changes can occur because of hyperprolactinemia caused by antipsychotics. Prolactin secretion is blocked by dopamine. Dopamine blockers can increase prolactin concentrations (hyperprolactinemia).

g. Weight gain: This occurs in up to 40% of patients, with low-potency agents having higher risk. Important interventions include keeping the dose as low as possible and implementing dietary management. Weight gain may occur because of actions at histamine or serotonin receptors.

h. Sexual dysfunction: Erectile problems occur in 23%–54% of men. Loss of libido and anorgasmia may occur in men and women.

i. Venous thromboembolism (VTE): A published nested case-control study of older adults from the United Kingdom showed that FGAs and SGAs were associated with greater risk of deep VTE or pulmonary embolism than matched controls (BMJ 2010;341:c4245). Patients from primary care with schizophrenia, bipolar disorder, or dementia who had been prescribed antipsychotics in the past 24 months had a 32% elevated risk of VTE (odds ratio = 1.32 [95% confidence interval, 1.23–1.42]) and a 56% elevated risk if the treatment had been in the past 3 months. Second-generation antipsychotics had a higher risk of VTE than did first-generation drugs (73% vs. 28%, respectively). The study was limited by possible confounders such as smoking status and BMI, although these factors were deemed not to have considerably altered the results.

j. Miscellaneous: Low-potency agents such as thioridazine and chlorpromazine can cause pigmentary deposits on the retina and corneal opacity. Many of the typical agents can cause serious changes on the ECG (e.g., prolongation of the QTc interval). These changes can lead to arrhythmias and death.

4. Therapy initiation: In the past, acute episodes were treated very aggressively with high doses, and the process was called neuroleptization. Because neuroleptization can lead to adverse effects and is probably no more effective than starting with full therapeutic doses, it is no longer advocated. Dosing during the stabilization phase may be less aggressive, but a very low dose increases the risk of relapse.

5. Administration route: Oral therapy is most common; however, parenteral drugs can be used acutely if the patient does not adhere to therapy or is agitated and will not take oral medications. Haloperidol can be given intramuscularly. Intravenous haloperidol has been linked to toxicity including torsades de pointes and should not be given. Depot forms of haloperidol and fluphenazine are available, providing sustained concentrations for about 1 month for haloperidol and 2–3 weeks for fluphenazine. These are indicated only for chronic therapy in patients who have trouble adhering to oral therapy. Fluphenazine decanoate requires "bridging" with oral therapy when treatment is begun.

6. Therapy duration: Continuation of therapy during the stable phase is of concern because of the risk of adverse effects (e.g., the tardive dyskinesia associated with the older agents). This is of less concern with the newer drugs. Relapse rates are more than 50% during the first year or so after discontinuing these agents for both first-episode patients and patients who relapse; thus, maintaining the antipsychotic at the minimal effective dose continuously may be the best approach for most patients. Some first-episode patients may be tried off drugs after being symptom free for 2 years. Those with a history of episodes should probably be symptom free for 5 years before discontinuation is considered. Long-term therapy should include monitoring for metabolic complications such as diabetes, weight gain, and lipid abnormalities.

G. Second-Generation Antipsychotics for Schizophrenia
1. SGAs (or atypical antipsychotics) were developed to reduce EPS adverse effects and tardive dyskinesia and to improve efficacy. The characteristics that define "atypicality" are not all agreed on, but in general, they all share at least three characteristics:
   a. The risk of EPS is lower than with typical antipsychotics at usual clinical doses,
   b. the risk of tardive dyskinesia is reduced, and
   c. the ability to block serotonin-2 receptors is present. This third property may improve activity for the negative symptoms of schizophrenia and reduce the risk of EPS.
2. Many clinicians see atypical drugs as first-line agents, despite the higher acquisition costs of the brand-name agents. Atypical agents (particularly clozapine and olanzapine) have been associated with new-onset diabetes mellitus and metabolic syndrome. All patients prescribed atypical antipsychotics should be monitored for weight, blood pressure, fasting glucose, lipids, and waist circumference at baseline and periodically thereafter.
3. Agents
   a. Clozapine (Clozaril): The first "atypical" antipsychotic. It is indicated only for treatment-resistant schizophrenia (defined as lack of response to two or more adequate trials of antipsychotics, including at least one FGA and one SGA). Lack of response usually refers to positive symptoms, although negative symptoms may also be involved. Clozapine is the only antipsychotic indicated for the reduction of suicidal thinking in patients with schizophrenia or schizoaffective disorder. Clozapine is not associated with EPS or tardive dyskinesia, and it may lead to an improvement in negative symptoms more effectively than typical drugs.
      i. Several black box warnings limit its use.
         (a) Severe neutropenia (agranulocytosis): This is the most limiting adverse effect. It can lead to a dramatic drop in neutrophils that increases the risk of serious or fatal infections. It is defined as an absolute neutrophil count (ANC) less than 500/microliters. The incidence is about 1%–2% and is highest during the first 4–6 months of therapy. Previously, both the white blood cell count and the ANC were used to monitor safety. As of 2015, only the ANC is used, and lower values are allowed for therapy. Allowances are also made for patients who have benign ethnic neutropenia. Because of the severity of this adverse effect, all patients must be registered under a new centrally managed Risk Evaluation and Mitigation Strategies (REMS) program (www.clozapinerems.com), which consolidates the six previous individual programs. Prescribers and pharmacies must also be registered. Laboratory work must be submitted to the national registry before clozapine can be dispensed. Details of hematologic monitoring are presented in Table 5.

Table 5. Hematologic Monitoring for Clozapine

ANC Level	Clozapine Treatment Recommendations	ANC Monitoring
Normal range (> 1500/microliters)	• Initiate treatment • If treatment interrupted: - < 30 days, continue monitoring as before - ≥ 30 days, monitor as if new patient	• Weekly from initiation to 6 mo • Every 2 wk from 6 to 12 mo • Monthly after 12 mo
Mild neutropenia (1000–1499/microliters)[a]	• Continue treatment	• Three times weekly until ANC ≥ 1500 • Once ANC ≥ 1500/microliters, return to patient's last "normal range" ANC monitoring interval[b]
Moderate neutropenia (500–999/microliters)[a]	• Recommend hematology consult • Interrupt treatment for suspected clozapine-induced neutropenia • Resume treatment once ANC > 1000/microliters	• Daily until ANC ≥ 1000/microliters • Three times weekly until ANC ≥ 1500/microliters • Once ANC ≥ 1500/microliters, check ANC weekly for 4 wk; then return to patient's last "normal range" ANC monitoring interval[b]
Severe neutropenia (< 500/microliters)[a]	• Recommend hematology consult • Interrupt treatment for suspected clozapine-induced neutropenia • Do not rechallenge unless prescriber determines benefits outweigh risks	• Daily until ANC ≥ 1000/microliters • Three times weekly until ANC ≥ 1500/microliters • If patient rechallenged, resume treatment as a new patient under "normal range" monitoring once ANC ≥ 1500/microliters

[a]Confirm all initial reports of ANC > 1500/microliters with a repeat ANC measurement within 24 hr.
[b]If clinically appropriate.
ANC = absolute neutrophil count.
Information taken from September 2015 version of Clozaril package insert.

      (b) OH, bradycardia, syncope, and cardiac arrest: It is dose-related and at highest risk at initiation of therapy and rapid dose titration. It must be initiated at 12.5 mg once or twice daily, titrated slowly, and given in divided doses.

      (c) Seizures: Risk is dose related and can be minimized by starting low and titrating slowly.

      (d) Myocarditis and cardiomyopathy

    ii. Additional adverse effects: These include weight gain, sedation, hypersalivation, rapid heart rate, and fever. Note that the presence of fever should alert the clinician to the possibility of infection and agranulocytosis. If the drug is discontinued for 48 hours or more, retitration is required to avoid seizures or cardiac adverse effects.

  b. Aripiprazole (Abilify): This drug's pharmacology differs from that of other atypical agents. It is a dopamine D_2/serotonin-1 partial agonist and a serotonin-2 antagonist, sometimes called a dopamine-serotonin–stabilizing agent. It has a low risk of most forms of EPS, including tardive dyskinesia. It is associated with a high incidence of akathisia. It is available in a long-acting depot injectable (Abilify Maintena).

  c. Asenapine (Saphris) is available in a sublingual formulation. It appears to have a lower risk of metabolic effects and EPS; however, it has been associated with a high risk of orthostasis and sedation. There has also been a warning about the risk of hypersensitivity reactions with asenapine.

d. Brexpiprazole (Rexulti; approved in July 2015): Approved for the treatment of schizophrenia and the adjunct treatment of major depressive disorder (MDD). The most common dose-dependent adverse effects are akathisia, weight gain, and somnolence. Clinically significant weight gain (greater than 7%) occurs in 8%–12% of patients. It can also cause hyperglycemia and dyslipidemia. Must be adjusted for renal function

e. Cariprazine (Vraylar, approved in September 2015): Approved for the treatment of schizophrenia and manic or mixed episodes associated with type I bipolar disorder. It is not recommended for patients with a CrCl less than 30 mL/minute/1.73 m^2. It is associated with dose-related OH, particularly at initiation and with dose increases. It appears to have a low risk of weight gain (1%–8% incidence, with 8% of those gaining more than 7%). Additional adverse drug reactions include gastrointestinal (GI) symptoms, somnolence, dizziness, parkinsonism (13%–21%), and seizures. Leukopenia and neutropenia have occurred, but there are no current recommendations to monitor.

f. Iloperidone (Fanapt) appears to have a lower risk of metabolic effects. It also has a higher risk of orthostasis but a lower risk of EPS, anticholinergic symptoms, and sedation. Short- and long-term studies have also shown an association with QTc prolongation similar to that of haloperidol and ziprasidone.

g. Lurasidone (Latuda) has a low risk of metabolic and cardiac effects together with a low EPS risk. It has potent antagonistic activity at serotonin-7 and a high affinity to serotonin-1A receptors, which is theorized to have beneficial cognitive and anxiolytic effects. The maximal daily dose has recently been increased to 160 mg/day, and it should be taken with food. The recommended starting dose for moderate and severe renal impairment and when used with a moderate CYP3A4 inhibitor (e.g., diltiazem) is 20 mg, and the maximal dose is 80 mg. The recommended starting dose for moderate and severe hepatic impairment is 20 mg, and the maximal dose is 80 mg in moderate hepatic impairment and 40 mg in severe hepatic impairment.

h. Olanzapine (Zyprexa): This drug is structurally similar to clozapine and has a similar pharmacology. Unlike clozapine, however, it has not been associated with agranulocytosis. In one study, negative symptoms responded better than with haloperidol. Together with clozapine, olanzapine carries the highest risk of diabetes. For this reason, the PORT (Patient Outcomes Research Team) guidelines do not consider it a first-line treatment. It is also available as a depot injection (Relprevv). Because it has been associated with extreme sedation and delirium after administration, it is part of a REMS program (called the Zyprexa Relprevv Patient Care Program). Prescribers must undergo training, and it can only be administered within an approved institution where the patient has supervision postdose.

i. Paliperidone (Invega) is the major active metabolite of risperidone, Its pharmacologic profile is similar to that of the parent drug (see below). Paliperidone palmitate is also available as a monthly depot injection (Invega Sustenna).

j. Quetiapine (Seroquel): In addition to antagonism at the D$_2$ and serotonin-2 receptors, it has a high affinity for histamine (H$_1$) receptors. For this reason, it has a high incidence of anticholinergic adverse effects. It may also cause OH. Unlikely other antipsychotics, it offers a low incidence of EPS. Quetiapine is the preferred antipsychotic if psychosis occurs in a patient with Parkinson disease.

k. Risperidone (Risperdal): This drug is a potent dopamine D$_2$ antagonist and a serotonin-2 antagonist. It has limited anticholinergic activity. At doses of up to 6 mg/day, the incidence of EPS has been no higher than with placebo in clinical studies. However, EPS is a dose-related phenomenon that may occur in patients taking the drug even at usual doses. Patients often tolerate risperidone better than haloperidol. It probably has no advantage in patients requiring high doses of antipsychotics. Adverse effects include sedation, OH, weight gain, sexual dysfunction, and hyperprolactinemia. A long-acting intramuscular formulation (risperidone [Risperdal Consta]) is available that is better tolerated than the other intramuscular depot forms of antipsychotics. It is administered every 2 weeks and requires a 3-week bridge therapy with oral risperidone. It is generally used only after the patient is known to tolerate oral therapy. Like with long-acting risperidone, tolerability with oral therapy should be established before starting it.

l. Ziprasidone (Geodon): Use caution if combining it with other drugs (e.g., TCAs or antiarrhythmics) that can also increase the QTc interval. It is also available in a parenteral formulation for acute agitation. The drug must be taken with food to increase absorption. It now carries a warning for drug reaction with eosinophilia and systemic symptoms (DRESS), which can be fatal. It consists of three or more of cutaneous reactions (including rash or exfoliative dermatitis), eosinophilia, fever, and lymphadenopathy and one or more of the following systemic complications: hepatitis, nephritis, pneumonitis, myocarditis, and pericarditis.

4. Table 6 summarizes the adverse effects associated with SGAs.

Table 6. Adverse Effects of SGAs

Drug (generic/ brand)	Metabolic Syndrome			Cardiac (clinically significant)	Sedation	Misc. Clinically Significant Adverse Effects
	Weight gain	DM	Dyslipidemia			
Fast Facts		Cases: 60% occur within first 6 mo		OH: Tolerance builds over 2–3 mo	Tolerance usually develops	Hyperprolactinemia: No tolerance develops
Aripiprazole (Abilify)	Little to none	No	Little to none	None	Low	Decreases prolactin concentrations; akathisia
Asenapine (Saphris)	Little to none	Little to none	Little to none	Possible QTc prolongation, OH	Low	Dose-dependent EPS (akathisia)
Brexpiprazole (Rexulti)	Moderate	Moderate	Moderate	None	Low	Dose-dependent akathisia
Cariprazine (Vraylar)	Low	Low	Low	OH	Low	Dose-dependent EPS (akathisia, pseudoparkinsonism)
Clozapine (Clozaril)	Highest	Yes	High	OH, prolonged QTc tachycardia	High (antichol)	Seizures (dose-dependent), sialorrhea, neutropenia/ agranulocytosis
Iloperidone (Fanapt)	Moderate	Low	Low	QTc prolongation, OH	Low	QTc prolongation comparable with ziprasidone
Lurasidone (Latuda)	Low	Low	Low to none	None	Moderate	Dose-dependent EPS (akathisia, pseudo-parkinsonism)
Olanzapine (Zyprexa)	Highest	Yes	High	None	High (antichol)	
Paliperidone (Invega)	Low	Low	None	Possible QTc prolongation	Low	Hyperprolactinemia; daily doses > 9 mg can cause EPS
Quetiapine (Seroquel)	Moderate	Moderate	Moderate	OH	High (antichol)	Agent of choice in patients with Parkinson disease
Risperidone (Risperdal)	Moderate	Moderate	Less	OH	Low	Hyperprolactinemia; daily doses > 6 mg/day increase EPS risk
Ziprasidone (Geodon)	Little	No	Less	Prolonged QTc	Low	QTc prolongation ~15.9 msec[a]; QTc > 500 msec (increased risk of torsades de pointes) rare; no increase in rate of sudden cardiac death over other agents

[a]Compared with thioridazine (30 msec), an FGA that is not used often because of its potential to cause torsades de pointes.

antichol = anticholinergic; DM = diabetes mellitus; EPS = extrapyramidal symptoms; OH = orthostatic hypotension.

H. Adjunctive Medications
1. Lithium: This agent may augment antipsychotic action.
2. Anticonvulsants (carbamazepine and valproic acid): These agents may augment antipsychotics, but their role in therapy remains undetermined. They may be useful in patients with agitated or violent behavior.
3. Benzodiazepines: These may be useful during the acute phase for agitation or anxiety, but they are less effective for treatment of psychotic symptoms. These drugs must also be used with caution in patients with schizophrenia because this population is at high risk of substance use disorder.

I. Comparisons of FGAs and SGAs
1. Almost all treatment guidelines now suggest that SGAs are the preferred first-line agents to typical drugs because most clinicians believe they are better tolerated and pose less risk. However, studies have questioned this conclusion. In these trials, the older agents appeared to do as well in efficacy and tolerability; however, they were not conclusive. Some issues with the study design limit the findings. Some clinicians may wish to use typical agents. There is certainly pressure from a cost standpoint. The results of a study named the Cost Utility of the Latest Antipsychotic Drugs in Schizophrenia Study were published in the October 2006 issue of *Archives of General Psychiatry* (Arch Gen Psychiatry 2006;63:1079-87). The findings of this study suggest that the differences in the effect of FGAs and SGAs are not as much as had been thought.
2. The Clinical Antipsychotic Trials of Intervention Effectiveness study (CATIE, sponsored by NIMH) compared several SGAs with the older agent perphenazine. Here are some of the findings:
    a. Discontinuation
        i.   High in all groups: 74% of all patients discontinued before 18 months
        ii. Olanzapine = 64%
        iii. Perphenazine = 75%
        iv. Quetiapine = 82%
        v.   Risperidone = 74%
        vi. Ziprasidone = 79%
    b. Time to discontinuation
        i.   All causes: Longest for olanzapine (significantly longer than for quetiapine and risperidone, not the others)
        ii. Lack of efficacy: Longest for olanzapine (significantly longer than perphenazine, quetiapine, and risperidone, but not ziprasidone)
    c. Duration of successful treatment: Longest for olanzapine (significantly longer than for quetiapine, risperidone, and perphenazine, as well as for risperidone compared with quetiapine)
    d. Efficacy: PANSS scores
        i.   Scores improved in all groups as time progressed.
        ii. Initially, more improvement with olanzapine, but improvement diminished with time
    e. Adverse drug reactions
        i.   Olanzapine: More often associated with weight gain and metabolic adverse effects
        ii. Perphenazine: More often associated with EPS
3. Two meta-analyses of comparison trials were conducted. The first analysis of FGAs and SGAs suggested that clozapine, risperidone, and olanzapine were more effective than the FGAs evaluated. Other SGAs were not superior to FGAs. Further research is needed to resolve this issue (Lancet 2009;373:31-41). In the second meta-analysis, SGAs were compared for the change in total PANSS score (Am J Psychiatry 2009;166:152-63). Olanzapine was significantly more efficacious than aripiprazole (p=0.002), quetiapine (p<0.001), risperidone (p=0.006), and ziprasidone (p<0.001). Most of the efficacy differences were caused by improvement in positive, not negative, symptoms.

Patient Cases

Questions 5–8 pertain to the following case:

A.Z. is a 45-year-old woman with sleep apnea, hypertension, type 2 diabetes, and chronic pain. She is being seen in the clinic today for an assessment of her depressive symptoms and medication evaluation. She endorses sad mood, poor appetite (lost 15 lb), poor concentration, and feelings of hopelessness and worthlessness for the past 3 weeks. She has also stopped going to her book club because she is not motivated to get out of the house, and she has frequent nocturnal awakening. She denies suicidal or homicidal ideation. She denies any use of alcohol, tobacco, or illicit drugs. She is currently taking hydrochlorothiazide, metformin, hydrocodone/acetaminophen, and aspirin. Her current BMI is 20 kg/m², and her blood pressure today is 152/94 mm Hg. She reports adherence to her current medications.

5. Which SSRI would be most likely to interact with her current medications?

    A. Citalopram.

    B. Fluvoxamine.

    C. Paroxetine.

    D. Sertraline.

6. Which antidepressant would be most appropriate for A.Z.'s depressive symptoms?

    A. Bupropion.

    B. Fluoxetine.

    C. Mirtazapine.

    D. Venlafaxine.

7. It has been 4 weeks since A.Z.'s initial visit with you, and she has been treated with citalopram 20 mg/day in the morning. She still presents with sad mood, but her insomnia, concentration, and appetite have improved. She still has feelings of hopelessness and worthlessness, lack of motivation, and anhedonia. At this point, which is the best recommendation to optimize her therapy?

    A. Continue at current dose of 20 mg/day.

    B. Increase the current dose to 40 mg/day.

    C. Add bupropion 150 mg twice daily.

    D. Switch to a different SSRI.

8. Six months later, A.Z. reports that although her depression symptoms have resolved, she has "trouble" during intercourse, which is quite disturbing to her. You determine that she has anorgasmia caused by citalopram treatment. Which is the most appropriate recommendation at this time?

    A. Discontinue citalopram.

    B. Add bupropion to citalopram.

    C. Switch to a different SSRI.

    D. Switch to mirtazapine.

II. DEPRESSION

A. Identification of Depressive Disorders. This overview is based on the *Diagnostic and Statistical Manual for Mental Disorders (DSM-5)*; please consult the *DSM-5* for complete diagnostic criteria.
   1. MDD, otherwise called unipolar disorder. It is diagnosed when a patient has at least five of the following symptoms almost every day for at least 2 weeks:
      a. The patient must have a depressed mood or anhedonia (loss of interest in pleasurable activities).
      b. Additional symptoms include sleep disturbances, changes in weight or appetite, decreased energy, feelings of guilt or worthlessness, psychomotor retardation or agitation, decreased concentration, and suicidal ideation.
      c. The symptoms must interfere with the patient's everyday ability to function.
   2. Persistent depressive disorder (dysthymia): Chronic depressed mood occurring more days than not for at least 2 years but does not meet the criteria for MDD

B. Assessment of Patients with MDD
   1. Psychiatric history: A thorough history of symptoms is compared with the diagnostic criteria, and the diagnosis is made from the collected data.
   2. Clinician rating scales: These are psychometric instruments used to identify depression and assess its severity. Common examples include:
      a. The Hamilton Rating Scale for Depression (HAM-D) and the Quick Inventory of Depressive Symptoms Clinician Rated. A response is usually defined as at least a 50% reduction in the HAM-D score. "Remission" is a return to a normal state or a HAM-D of 7 or less. Scores from these scales are not required for the diagnosis, but the HAM-D is a standard instrument used to show efficacy in clinical trials for U.S. Food and Drug Administration (FDA) approval.
      b. The CGI (Clinical Global Impression) scale is a clinician-rated scale that evaluates the severity and improvement of patients overall.
   3. The MADRS (Montgomery-Åsberg Depression Rating Scale) is another instrument that evaluates symptoms of depression.
      a. Patient rating scales: These are patient-completed rating instruments. Answers to the questions are used to identify and assess the level of depression.
         i. The Patient Health Questionnaire-9 (PHQ-9) is based on the *DSM-5* diagnostic criteria for major depression. It is easily administered and assessed. For this reason, it is often used in the primary care setting. Patients can be screened with an abbreviated version (the PHQ-2). If they test positive, the PHQ-9 is administered. The PHQ-9 can also be used to monitor treatment response.
         ii. The Beck Depression Inventory
         iii. Quick Inventory of Depressive Symptoms Self-Rated
      b. Physical examination and laboratory tests: These are necessary to rule out physical causes (e.g., thyroid disorders, vitamin deficiencies) that may mimic symptoms of depression.
      c. Biologic testing: Depression is commonly associated with abnormalities in the dexamethasone suppression test and tests of the thyroid axis. However, these tests are not routinely used in clinical practice.
      d. Medications and substances (e.g., interferons, benzodiazepines, barbiturates, alcohol, central nervous system depressants, lipid-soluble β-blockers, withdrawal from stimulants, cocaine, amphetamines) can have depression as an adverse effect. Pharmacists should perform a medication and substance use review to identify possible causes.

C. Therapeutic Options

1. Psychotherapy and exercise: Examples include interpersonal psychotherapy and cognitive behavioral therapy (CBT). It takes longer to achieve effective results with psychotherapy than with pharmacotherapy. Psychotherapy may have broader and longer-lasting effects than pharmacotherapy monotherapy. Psychotherapy is recommended as monotherapy as initial treatment in patients with mild to moderate MDD (CBT and interpersonal therapy have the best evidence). Psychotherapy combined with pharmacotherapy is recommended for moderate to severe depression. The combination is more effective than either component alone.

2. Pharmacotherapy: Medication therapy may lead to a more rapid response than psychotherapy, but when it is discontinued, there is a risk of relapse and adverse effects.

3. Electroconvulsive therapy (ECT): Option for refractory depression, depression in pregnancy, psychotic depression, and other conditions for which medications may not be optimal or effective. The usual cycle is two or three treatments per week. Temporary memory loss is common, and medications that affect seizure threshold must be withdrawn before treatment. Electroconvulsive therapy has also been recently suggested as initial treatment if symptoms are severe or life threatening (American Psychiatric Association [APA] 2010 guidelines).

D. Pharmacotherapeutic Options: Considerations and Keys to Use

1. Selection: All antidepressants are considered equally efficacious. First-line medications include selective serotonin reuptake inhibitors (SSRIs), serotonin-norepinephrine reuptake inhibitors (SNRIs), bupropion, and mirtazapine. Consider possible drug-drug and drug-disease interactions, concurrent illnesses, prior responses, family members' prior responses, patient preference, and cost.

2. Onset: Physical symptoms (energy levels, sleep disturbances) improve before affective symptoms. Symptoms can respond as early as 2 weeks. In general, it takes 4–6 weeks to see the full effect of antidepressants, given the correct drug, dose, and adherence, but it may take as long as 8 weeks to see a response. Remission may take up to 12 weeks.

3. Adequate trial: An adequate trial includes the correct drug for the patient and a therapeutic dose for an appropriate duration. A therapeutic trial ranges from 4 to 8 weeks (2010 APA practice guideline).

4. Response and remission: A response is usually defined as a 50% reduction in symptoms. Remission is a return to normal mood (e.g., HAM-D of 7 or less; PHQ-9 less than 5). Optimizing the dose or duration is important for achieving remission.

5. Efficacy of antidepressants according to rigorous clinical trials is about 60%–70%, regardless of drug. Effectiveness, which is more reflective of clinical practice, is lower, about 50%–60%. The remission rate with one antidepressant is about 30%, as seen in the recent Sequenced Treatment Alternatives to Relieve Depression (STAR*D trial).

6. Drug interactions (Table 7): Many antidepressants are metabolized or inhibited by CYP enzymes.

Table 7. Antidepressants and the CYP System

	1A2	2C19	2D6	3A4
Substrate	Duloxetine	Citalopram Escitalopram Fluoxetine Imipramine Vilazodone	Amitriptyline Desipramine Duloxetine Fluoxetine Imipramine Nefazodone Nortriptyline Trazodone Venlafaxine Vortioxetine	Citalopram Escitalopram Levomilnacipran Nefazodone Trazodone Venlafaxine Vilazodone
Inducer		St. John's wort		St. John's wort
Inhibitor	**Fluvoxamine**	Amitriptyline Fluoxetine Fluvoxamine Imipramine	**Bupropion**[a] Desvenlafaxine Duloxetine **Fluoxetine** **Paroxetine** Sertraline	Fluvoxamine **Nefazodone**

[a]Metabolized by CYP2B6; boldface type indicates strong inhibitor.

E. Tricyclic Antidepressants
   1. Tricyclic antidepressants (TCAs) were the first antidepressants available. They are seldom used for depression, but they have several off-label uses such as treatment for pain syndromes, migraine prophylaxis, and anxiety disorders. They are effective, but adverse effects have limited their use. Now that newer agents with more tolerable adverse effect profiles are available, these agents are used less often.
   2. They block the reuptake of serotonin and norepinephrine (NE). The tertiary amines are more potent for NE uptake and are metabolized to active secondary amines.
   3. In addition to serotonin and NE reuptake, TCAs have α-adrenergic blockade, antihistaminic effects, and anticholinergic effects, leading to orthostasis, sedation, and anticholinergic symptoms, respectively. They also have cardiotoxic effects (Table 8).
   4. TCAs can be fatal in overdose. They cause seizures and torsades de pointes. An actively suicidal patient should not receive a TCA.

Table 8. Adverse Effect Profile of the Commonly Used Tricyclic Antidepressants

Drug	Anticholinergic	Sedation	Orthostatic Hypotension	Cardiotoxicity
Tertiary amines				
Amitriptyline	High	High	Moderate	High
Imipramine	Moderate	Moderate	High	High
Secondary amines				
Desipramine	Low	Low	Moderate	Moderate
Nortriptyline	Moderate	Moderate	Low	Moderate

5. These drugs must be used cautiously in patients with cardiac disease or seizure disorders. Patients at risk of OH are at elevated risk of falls if they take these agents, and appropriate caution should be taken.

6. One advantage of TCAs is that therapeutic serum concentrations can be measured. Therapeutic levels can be used to confirm adherence or toxicity. In clinical practice, this is an infrequent practice.

7. A withdrawal syndrome occurs if these drugs are discontinued too quickly. Symptoms reflect the reversal of anticholinergic effects and include lacrimation, nausea, and diarrhea, with insomnia, restlessness, and possible balance problems. Gradual dose reductions help reduce these symptoms.

F. Monoamine Oxidase Inhibitors
1. Monoamine oxidase inhibitors (MAOIs) block the enzyme responsible for the breakdown of certain neurotransmitters, such as NE. There are two forms of this enzyme (MAO-A and MAO-B), and drugs can block one or both of them. They are effective antidepressants and may be especially useful for atypical depression (hypersomnia, hyperphagia, and mood reactivity).
2. Nonselective drugs (phenelzine and tranylcypromine) are available in the United States.
3. Patients taking MAOIs must be educated and monitored to avoid foods high in tyramine (e.g., aged cheese, preserved meats) because of the potential for precipitating a hypertensive crisis. A dietary consultation can be helpful in this respect.
4. Drug interactions with MAOIs are considerable and include over-the-counter decongestants, antidepressants, stimulants, antihypertensives, and others. When switching a patient from another antidepressant to an MAOI, it is prudent to wait 2 weeks after the antidepressant is discontinued before initiating the MAOI (except for fluoxetine, in which case the waiting period should be 5–6 weeks). When a patient is changed from an MAOI to another antidepressant, a 2-week washout period is usually adequate.
5. Selegiline (MAO-B inhibitor) is available in a patch formulation called Emsam for the treatment of depression. It is available in doses of 6 mg/24 hours, 9 mg/24 hours, and 12 mg/24 hours. Once the dose reaches 9 mg/24 hours, an MAOI diet is required. How this drug compares with other antidepressants remains unknown.

G. Selective Serotonin Reuptake Inhibitors (SSRIs; Table 9)
1. SSRIs selectively inhibit the reuptake of serotonin into the presynaptic neuron. There has been speculation that they also desensitize the presynaptic serotonin autoreceptor involved in the negative feedback loop that normally inhibits serotonin release. Whichever is true, the result is increased serotonin concentrations in the synapse. The FDA has approved six SSRIs for the treatment of depression: fluoxetine, sertraline, paroxetine, fluvoxamine, citalopram, and escitalopram. Fluvoxamine is indicated only for obsessive-compulsive disorder (OCD) but is an effective antidepressant.

Table 9. Characteristics of SSRIs

Characteristic	Fluoxetine	Sertraline	Paroxetine	Fluvoxamine[a]	Citalopram	Escitalopram
Half-life	1–4 days	26 hr	21 hr	15 hr	32 hr	27–32 hr
Active metabolite	Yes[b]	No	No	No	No	No
Usual dose (mg/day)	20–60	50–200	10–60	50–300	20–40	10–20
Maximal daily dose (mg)	80	200	50 (depression) 60 (anxiety)	300	40	20

[a]Indicated only for obsessive-compulsive disorder; seldom used for depression.
[b]Norfluoxetine.
SSRI = selective serotonin reuptake inhibitor.

2. The efficacy of SSRIs is equal for treatment of depression. There are slight differences in adverse effect profiles, and patients may tolerate one better than another. The STAR*D trial showed that patients who do not respond to one SSRI may respond to another.

3. Blockade of serotonin reuptake leads to an increase in serotonin overall and may influence all subtypes of serotonin receptors. Some of these (serotonin-2A, serotonin-2C, serotonin-3, and serotonin-4) may be responsible for some of the unwanted adverse effects (e.g., insomnia, restlessness, GI complaints). Activation, agitation, anxiety, or panic may be seen in some patients, especially during the early phase of therapy. The most common adverse effects associated with this class of agents include GI complaints, insomnia, restlessness, headache, and sexual dysfunction. In general, the most activating SSRIs are fluoxetine and sertraline, whereas paroxetine and fluvoxamine are the most sedating. Citalopram and escitalopram have no appreciable sedating or activating effects. Sexual dysfunction is more common than reported in the prescribing information. Some interventions to consider for SSRI-induced sexual dysfunction include using the wait-and-see method, adding bupropion for the treatment of sexual dysfunction, lowering the dose of the SSRI, or adding an agent such as sildenafil or cyproheptadine. Of course, changing to a drug less likely to cause this problem is also reasonable.

4. Because these drugs have such potent serotonergic activity, combinations with other drugs affecting serotonin can lead to serotonin syndrome. Examples include MAOIs, dextromethorphan, meperidine, sympathomimetics, triptans, lithium, TCAs, and SNRIs. Serotonin syndrome includes symptoms from three clusters: neuromuscular hyperactivity (e.g. myoclonus, rigidity, tremors, incoordination), altered mental status (agitation, confusion, hypomania), and autonomic instability (hyperthermia, diaphoresis). It can be subtle in onset or be confused with neuroleptic malignant syndrome. Treatment includes discontinuing the offending agent, providing supportive measures such as cooling blankets and respiratory assistance, and providing clonazepam for myoclonus, anticonvulsants for seizures, and nifedipine for hypertension.

5. SSRIs have been associated with extrapyramidal symptoms (EPS), including akathisia, dystonia, and bradykinesia, but these are not common. This appears to result from an effect of serotonin on dopaminergic neurotransmission in the basal ganglia.

6. A withdrawal syndrome has been observed, especially for the drugs with shorter half-lives, so a gradual dose reduction (e.g., over 2–4 weeks) may be indicated. Symptoms include flulike symptoms, such as nausea and chills, and neurologic symptoms, such as paresthesias, insomnia, anxiety, and "electric shock"-type sensations. If the problem is severe or persists, the drug can be reinitiated and the dose gradually reduced again. It is most common with paroxetine, less so with sertraline, and even less likely with fluoxetine.

7. In 2001, the FDA ordered changes to citalopram package labeling limiting the daily dose to a maximum of 40 mg because of an elevated risk of QTc prolongation at daily doses greater than 40 mg. Patients who have risk factors for QTc prolongation (congenital long QTc syndrome, bradycardia, hypokalemia, hypomagnesemia, recent acute myocardial infarction, and uncompensated heart failure) or have concomitant medications that may increase QTc interval should not be treated with citalopram. Doses of citalopram should be lowered to 40 mg/day in patients who are receiving higher dosages unless the benefits significantly outweigh the risks. The maximal recommended dose of citalopram is 20 mg/day for patients with hepatic impairment, patients who are older than 60 years, patients who are CYP2C19 poor metabolizers, or patients who are taking concomitant cimetidine or another CYP2C19 inhibitor.

8. These drugs are not as lethal in cases of overdose as are TCAs. All SSRIs are available in generic form except for vilazodone and vortioxetine. The low cost and better tolerability of SSRIs warrant them as first-line treatment of MDD in most patients.

9. Extended dosing formulations: Fluoxetine 90 mg can be taken once weekly. It is taken only during continuation therapy rather than as initial treatment. Paroxetine controlled release may have lower rates of nausea in the first week of treatment; efficacy is comparable, and both formulations are administered once daily. The weekly and controlled release (CR) products are available generic but are higher in cost.

10. Escitalopram is the *S*-isomer of citalopram. It is the active component of the racemic mixture. At a 10-mg dose, it is as effective as citalopram 20 mg (or 40 mg as described in prescribing information), but at this dose, there are fewer adverse effects. At higher doses, this advantage is not as pronounced.

11. SSRIs appear to increase the risk of bleeding. Several mechanisms have been proposed, including the inhibition of serotonin activation of platelets. Case-control and cohort studies also suggest an elevated incidence of both vertebral and non-vertebral bone fractures. Hyponatremia is a potential adverse effect, particularly in older adults.

H. Serotonin-Norepinephrine Reuptake Inhibitors

1. Venlafaxine, desvenlafaxine, duloxetine, and levomilnacipran block the reuptake of NE and serotonin. Unlike TCAs, they have negligible effects at other receptors that cause anticholinergic or antihistaminic adverse effects, with the possible exception of duloxetine, which appears to have a slightly higher incidence of anticholinergic symptoms. Venlafaxine has a dose-related effect on NE compared with desvenlafaxine and duloxetine. At doses less than 150 mg/day, venlafaxine has primarily a serotonin effect.

2. Levomilnacipran (Fetzima) is a relatively new SNRI. It is the enantiomer of milnacipran, the latter of which is approved for the treatment of fibromyalgia but not depression. Levomilnacipran is not approved for the treatment of fibromyalgia. The dose must be adjusted in renal insufficiency, and its use is not recommended in end-stage renal disease. Levomilnacipran can cause hyponatremia and increase bleeding risk. The capsule should not be crushed or opened. It is metabolized through CYP3A4 (major pathway) and through CYP2C19 and CYP2D6, among others (minor pathways). Monitor signs and symptoms of potential toxicities if CYP3A4 inhibitors are used concomitantly. Both blood pressure elevations and OH can occur. It is a more potent inhibitor of NE than venlafaxine or duloxetine (NE slightly preferred to serotonin).

3. Whether the dual action of venlafaxine makes it more effective than SSRIs is an area of continued research. There appear to be patients (e.g., treatment nonresponders) who benefit either from agents that affect NE and serotonin or from combinations of drugs with that effect.

4. The adverse effect profile of venlafaxine is similar to that of the SSRIs, with GI complaints being common. Of note, venlafaxine can cause increases in blood pressure, which are usually mild and not clinically significant unless the patient already has hypertension that is not well controlled. This is a dose-related phenomenon, as described earlier. All the SNRIs may produce serotonin syndrome. In overdose situations, both duloxetine and venlafaxine have been associated with higher rates of death compared with SSRIs. The risk of suicide completion with SNRIs is still lower than with TCAs.

5. Duloxetine has also been approved for the treatment of diabetic peripheral neuropathy, fibromyalgia, and chronic musculoskeletal pain caused by chronic lower back pain or osteoarthritis pain. Be careful when using this drug with CYP2D6 inhibitors. Monitor blood pressure, because increases have been observed. This drug can cause liver toxicity and should not be used in patients with hepatic insufficiency, end-stage renal disease requiring dialysis, or severe renal impairment.

6. Abrupt discontinuation of venlafaxine can lead to a withdrawal syndrome similar to that with the SSRIs.

7. Desvenlafaxine (Pristiq) is an active metabolite of venlafaxine. Whether it has any advantage over the parent compound is controversial.

8. Both desvenlafaxine and levomilnacipran doses must be adjusted downward with decreased renal function.

I. Mixed Serotonergic Medications

1. Vilazodone (Viibryd) is an SSRI with partial agonist at the serotonin-1A receptor. The clinical significance of this effect is unknown. It has a half-life of 25 hours but does not have active metabolites. Both the usual and maximum doses are 40 mg daily.

2. Vortioxetine (Brintellix) inhibits serotonin reuptake, but its pharmacologic profile differs from that of other SSRIs. It has additional agonist activity at the serotonin-1A receptor, partial agonist activity at the serotonin-1B receptor, and antagonistic activity at the serotonin-3, serotonin-1D, and serotonin-7 receptors. The clinical significance of vortioxetine's effect on the serotonin receptors is currently unknown, but it also appears to improve measures of cognitive function that appear independent of its antidepressant effects. Vortioxetine has a half-life of 66 hours and no active metabolites. The starting and usual dose is 10 mg daily, with a maximum daily dose of 20 mg. It is metabolized by CYP2D6, and the maximal dose for poor metabolizers or patients taking a strong CYP2D6 inhibitor is 10 mg daily.

3. Trazodone is a serotonin reuptake inhibitor that also blocks serotonin-2A receptors. It does not cause anticholinergic or cardiotoxic effects, as the TCAs do, but it still causes OH and sedation. Because of its sedative properties, trazodone is often used for insomnia but at lower doses than those used to treat depression. It is important to be aware of the potential for priapism, even though it is rare (0.1% or less).

4. Nefazodone is a relative of trazodone with some pharmacologic differences. It, too, is a serotonin-2A antagonist, but it also blocks the reuptake of serotonin and NE. Some have referred to this class as serotonin antagonist reuptake inhibitors (serotonin-2A antagonist/reuptake inhibitors). Unlike trazodone, it causes minimal effects on sexual function and is less likely to cause OH. Some data suggest that the serotonin-2A–blocking activity makes this drug more effective for anxiety associated with depression. The short half-life makes it necessary to administer doses twice daily. The most common adverse effects of this drug include sedation, GI complaints, dry mouth, constipation, confusion, and light-headedness. Because it is a potent inhibitor of CYP3A4, caution is necessary when it is used concomitantly with drugs metabolized by this system. Because of the potential for liver toxicity and the black box warning, nefazodone is now considered a second- or third-line agent. Liver function tests must be monitored if nefazodone is used. The branded product has been withdrawn from the market. Generics remain available.

5. Mirtazapine is an antagonist of presynaptic α_2-autoreceptors and heteroreceptors, which results in an increase in NE and serotonin in the synapse. In addition, the drug blocks serotonin-2A (resulting in no sexual dysfunction, no anxiety, and sedation), serotonin-3 (no nausea and no GI disturbances), and serotonin-2C (weight gain) receptors. Although the drug is better tolerated than the TCAs, it still has a pronounced sedative effect, together with increased appetite, weight gain, constipation, and asthenia. Abnormal liver function tests may occur, and there appears to be a very small risk of neutropenia or agranulocytosis. Lower doses may be sedating, whereas higher doses may cause insomnia.

J. Bupropion
   1. This drug is primarily an inhibitor of dopamine and NE reuptake (at high doses), with minimal effects on serotonin. Its exact mechanism of action remains to be defined. The parent drug blocks dopamine reuptake, whereas the metabolite blocks NE reuptake.
   2. The most important adverse effect is increased risk of seizures. This risk can be minimized by the following:
      a. Avoid use in susceptible patients (e.g., history of seizure disorder, eating disorders).
      b. Do not give more than 150 mg/dose or 450 mg/day (immediate release), 400 mg/day (sustained release), or 450 mg/day (extended release).
      c. Avoid dosage titration any more often than every 4 days for sustained or extended release and every 3 days for immediate release.
      d. The sustained- and extended-release products may also cause fewer adverse effects; they have largely replaced the immediate-release tablets.
   3. The most common adverse effects include insomnia, anxiety, irritability, headache, and decreased appetite. The drug can also increase energy and cause psychosis. As noted previously, the drug may actually improve sexual function; thus, it may be useful in patients not tolerating other agents for this reason. Bupropion has also been used for attention-deficit/hyperactivity disorder and may help with concentration.

K. Antidepressants and Suicidality: Antidepressants have been associated with an increased risk of suicidal thinking and behaviors, particularly in children, adolescents, and young adults (up to 24 years of age), which has resulted in a black box warning for all antidepressants, both older and newer agents. It is important to monitor patients, especially children and adolescents, for treatment failure or worsening symptoms of depression when these drugs are initiated or the dose is increased. Other signs to watch for include suicidal ideation, agitation and anxiety (activation syndrome), and other symptoms that are unlike the presenting symptoms of depression in the patient. A medication guide must be distributed before antidepressants are dispensed.

L. Initiating, Adjusting, and Monitoring Therapy
    1. There are three phases of therapy:
        a. Short term (acute): The goal of this phase is remission, which may take 12 weeks. Remission is defined as at least 3 weeks with no symptoms of depressed mood and anhedonia and no more than 3 remaining symptoms of depression.
        b. Continuation: The goal of this phase is to keep the symptoms in remission by using full-dose therapy. This phase usually continues for 4–9 additional months to keep the patient in remission.
        c. Maintenance: Long-term therapy at full doses may be required in patients at high risk of relapse, which would include prior episodes of depression or a strong family history of relapse. The duration of this phase is determined on an individual basis.
    2. An adequate trial of any agent includes full therapeutic doses for at least 6 weeks, up to 12 weeks. If there is no response at this point, the drug can be considered a failure.
    3. When one drug has failed, another agent from another class is often tried. However, some patients who do not respond to one SSRI may respond to another, and this is a reasonable option. Treatment resistance can usually be considered when two or more agents from different classes have been tried. At this point, ECT, augmentation therapy, or combination therapy can be considered, if they have not been used already.
    4. Patients should be monitored for response through interviews or by repeating rating scales. In addition, patients (and their support systems, if available) should receive education about therapy and be closely monitored for adverse effects. Although most of the adverse effects are not life threatening, they do have an important effect on adherence.
    5. The FDA has required that package labels for antidepressants include a statement to monitor patients for emerging suicidal thoughts and behaviors and continuing depressed mood, especially when antidepressants are initiated.

M. Antidepressant Combination Therapy
    1. Drugs with different pharmacologic actions are available, and as more is learned about depression, it may be advantageous to treat different systems selectively. It is now possible to affect serotonin, NE, and dopamine differentially. Researchers are actively looking at specific symptoms of depression to determine whether certain presentations respond better to an agent that affects certain neurotransmitter systems. At this point, data are insufficient to guide treatment, but it can be expected that combinations will be used, especially for treatment-resistant depression.
    2. The use of combinations with lower doses of each may lead to fewer adverse effects.
    3. Using a second antidepressant may offset an adverse effect of another (e.g., using trazodone to treat SSRI-induced insomnia).
    4. Adding bupropion to existing SSRI therapy is a strategy for patients who do not fully respond to the SSRI alone.

N. Treatment-Resistant Depression (Augmentation Therapy)
   1. Second-generation antipsychotics (SGAs or atypical antipsychotics) are commonly used as adjuncts to antidepressant therapy. Almost all of them have been used, but only aripiprazole, brexpiprazole, and quetiapine extended release have received FDA approval for this indication. Olanzapine in combination with fluoxetine is also approved for treatment-resistant depression.
   2. Ketamine infusions
   3. Others: Lithium, liothyronine, modafinil, scopolamine

O. Treatment Algorithms
   1. Several algorithms for treatment exist, including the APA practice guideline on treating patients with MDD (available at www.psychiatryonline.com/pracGuide/pracGuideTopic_7.aspx. Accessed October 11, 2014).
   2. The STAR*D study is a large trial sponsored by the National Institute of Mental Health, designed to evaluate the effectiveness of a sequenced approach to therapy. A series of papers were published in 2006 in the *American Journal of Psychiatry* and *The New England Journal of Medicine* describing some of the results. Highlights include the following:
      a. All patients were initially treated with citalopram monotherapy, and only about 30% achieved remission.
      b. Patients who did not achieve remission were then allowed to select a "switch" strategy or "augmentation" strategy (level 2). Options included bupropion, sertraline, venlafaxine, or cognitive therapy. There were no significant differences between strategies, but slightly higher remission rates occurred with augmentation. Bupropion and buspirone augmentation worked similarly, and the former agent was better tolerated.
      c. Patients not responding to level 2 were then allowed to change to mirtazapine or nortriptyline or to have augmentation with lithium or thyroid. Again, there were not many differences. Thyroid augmentation worked as well as lithium.
      d. Remission rates decreased at each treatment level. The results suggest that less than one-third of patients achieve remission with initial SSRI monotherapy, and switching or augmentation strategies are viable options, with no marked increase in efficacy with either strategy. Switching antidepressants may be a good option for patients who do not respond to or do not tolerate a drug, and augmentation may be good for partial responders. However, continued monitoring of these observations is necessary to confirm these results.
      e. For a good review of the STAR*D findings, see Am J Psychiatry 2006;163:1905-17.

Patient Cases

Questions 9–11 pertain to the following case:

J.L. is a 26-year-old man with a history of type I bipolar disorder who presents to the inpatient unit. His wife caught him withdrawing their life savings from the bank. He states that he is the perfect candidate for the presidency. He is hyperverbal and has not slept in the past 48 hours. He is placed on a 72-hour hold for control of his manic symptoms. He has a history of nonadherence to medications and currently takes no medications. J.L.'s last hospitalization was 2 months ago, when he had significant depressive symptoms and suicidal ideation. He has three or four hospitalizations per year, and his history of medication trials includes carbamazepine, olanzapine, and lamotrigine (may be helpful but uncertain because of nonadherence). He has also received a diagnosis of hepatitis C.

9. Which statement is most applicable for selecting J.L.'s mood stabilizer at this time?

    A. Carbamazepine should be tried again because it is effective for preventing rehospitalization.

    B. Divalproex should be tried because it is good for maintenance treatment.

    C. Lithium should be tried because it can effectively treat the manic phase and prevent future episodes.

    D. Lamotrigine should be tried again because it is effective for bipolar maintenance.

10. Which adverse effects would be of most concern and would require immediate evaluation if J.L. were prescribed lithium?

    A. Hypothyroidism.

    B. Coarse tremor.

    C. Severe acne.

    D. Weight gain.

11. It is 3 months later, and J.L. has been stable on lithium 900 mg/day. During a clinic visit, you find that J.L. is confused and slurring his words. His other medications include lisinopril, ibuprofen, atorvastatin, and zolpidem. Which is best to recommend immediately?

    A. Discontinue lisinopril because it interacts with lithium.

    B. Discontinue zolpidem because it may increase confusion.

    C. Obtain a lithium concentration because J.L. may have supratherapeutic levels.

    D. Discontinue ibuprofen because it interacts with lithium.

III. BIPOLAR DISORDER

A. Overview of Bipolar Disorder
1. The *DSM-5* defines bipolar disorder by the experience of a manic or hypomanic episode. Mania can be thought of as the affective opposite of depression. Consult the *DSM-5* for a complete description of the diagnostic criteria. A manic episode is characterized by at least 1 week of an abnormal and persistently elevated mood accompanied by an increased amount of activity. Other symptoms include inflated self-esteem, irritability, decreased need for sleep, pressured speech, flight of ideas, poor attention, increased hyperactivity or agitation, and involvement in high-risk, pleasurable activities without respect to the consequences. A hypomanic episode is a milder form mania. It must exist for 4 days or longer. Unlike mania, it is not severe enough to warrant hospitalization, does not impair social or occupational functioning, and is not associated with psychosis.
2. The *DSM-5* includes two types of bipolar disorder:
    a. Bipolar I (BD I): Chronic disorder marked by one or more manic or mixed episodes and major depressive episodes
    b. Bipolar II (BD II): Chronic disorder marked by one or more major depressive episodes, accompanied by at least one hypomanic episode
    c. Cyclothymic disorder: Several periods of hypomania and mild depression, none of which meet the criteria for mania or major depressive episode
    d. Rapid cycling: At least four episodes of mania or depression in 1 year
3. Bipolar disorder, particularly type II bipolar disorder, is often misdiagnosed as major depression. The diagnosis is important because the two conditions are treated differently.

B. Lithium for Bipolar Disorders
1. The exact mechanism of action for lithium is unknown, but it appears to be neuroprotective.
2. Lithium continues to be the gold standard for treating type I bipolar disorder. It is effective for the manic and depressive components. Although it is not a particularly good antidepressant as monotherapy in unipolar depression, it is effective in patients with bipolar disorder. Lithium additionally has anti-suicidal effects when used to treat bipolar disorder.
3. Antimanic effects can occur in 1–2 weeks. Most clinicians use antipsychotics or benzodiazepines as adjunctive therapy during this period to cover the agitation and other symptoms. Antidepressant effects may take 6–8 weeks.
4. Pharmacokinetics: Its half-life is 20–24 hours. It is excreted 95% unchanged by glomerular filtration, and anything that alters glomerular filtration rate affects its clearance. Pharmacokinetic methods are available for early prediction of doses, but waiting 5–6 days for steady state seems to work just as well.
5. Initial dosing is in the range of 600–900 mg/day in divided doses and then titrated according to response and tolerability. Maintenance doses are based on serum concentrations, symptom relief, and the occurrence of adverse effects.
6. A pre-lithium workup includes a complete blood cell count, electrolytes, renal function, thyroid function tests, urinalysis, ECG, and pregnancy test for women of childbearing age.
7. Monitoring: Serum concentrations must be monitored. The half-life is about 1 day, so steady state occurs in about 5 days. Even if it is not steady state, it may be prudent to obtain a serum concentration 3 days after dosage changes. Most clinicians will aim for concentrations of 0.8–1.2 mEq/L in acute mania and 0.6–1.0 mEq/L during maintenance. Concentration-response data are based on 12-hour postdose concentrations, so order levels in the morning 12 hours after the last evening dose. Perform renal function tests, thyroid function tests, and a urinalysis every 6–12 months.
8. Adverse effects are common with lithium and are most common during therapy initiation or after dose changes. Some points to consider are listed in Table 10.

9. Symptoms of lithium toxicity include lethargy, coarse tremor, confusion, seizures, and coma and may even result in death. Patients who present to urgent care on lithium therapy should always be monitored for lithium toxicity before any medication adjustments are made. Lithium concentration and sodium/renal function should be drawn so that lithium concentrations can be accurately estimated.

Table 10. Adverse Effects Associated With Lithium

Problem	Potential Interventions
Rash or ↑ psoriasis	Discontinue the drug temporarily or permanently
Tremor	Reduce dose (Cp); add β-blocker
CNS toxicity (e.g., agitation, confusion)	Reduce dose (Cp)
Gastrointestinal (nausea, vomiting, diarrhea)	Reduce dose; try extended-release product
Hypothyroidism	Discontinue Li or give levothyroxine
Polydipsia or polyuria	Reduce dose, manage intake, and try amiloride or HCTZ, but know that HCTZ will ↑ Li Cp; single bedtime dosing helps
Interstitial fibrosis, glomerulosclerosis	Controversial! Keep dose at lowest effective concentration
Teratogenicity	Avoid during first trimester, if possible

CNS = central nervous system; Cp = plasma concentration; HCTZ = hydrochlorothiazide; Li = lithium.

10. Pregnancy: Lithium is teratogenic, particularly in the first trimester. Women of childbearing age should be counseled on its potential effects. Risks of discontinuing lithium therapy must be weighed against effects on the fetus when making decisions regarding lithium therapy during pregnancy.
11. Situations to consider during lithium therapy are listed in Table 11.

Table 11. Situations to Consider During Lithium Therapy

Situation	Factors	Results
Drug interactions	Diuretics	
	Thiazides	↑ Li Cp; avoid use to reduce toxicity
	Furosemide	Little effect
	Amiloride	Little effect
	NSAIDs	↑ Li Cp; avoid use to reduce toxicity
	Theophylline	↓ Li Cp
	ACEIs	↑ Li Cp; avoid use to reduce toxicity
	Neuromuscular blockers	Li prolongs action
	Neuroleptics	Li may potentiate EPS
	Carbamazepine	↑ CNS toxicity
Thyroid	Li ↓ synthesis and release of thyroid hormone	Hypothyroidism
Pregnancy	↑ GFR	↓ Li Cp
Aging	↓ GFR	↓ Li requirements
	↑ Sensitivity to ADRs	Li toxicity
↓ Renal function	↓ GFR, ↑ creatinine and BUN	↑ Li Cp
Dehydration, salt restriction, and extrarenal salt loss	↑ Sodium reabsorption	↑ Li Cp

ACEI = angiotensin-converting enzyme inhibitor; ADR = adverse drug reaction; BUN = blood urea nitrogen; EPS = extrapyramidal symptoms; GFR = glomerular filtration rate; NSAID = nonsteroidal anti-inflammatory drug.

C. Anticonvulsants for Bipolar Disorder: These are also considered mood-stabilizing drugs that reduce manic and depressive episodes. Refer to the Neurology chapter for additional drug-specific details.

1. Divalproex: It is as effective as lithium in acute and prophylactic management. It appears to be good for rapid cyclers but may not be as effective during depressive episodes. It is also beneficial for patients with dysphoric mania, mixed episodes, or a history of substance use disorder. Target serum concentrations are 50–125 mcg/mL. The serum concentration can be checked 3–5 days after initiation or after a change of dose. Hypoalbuminemia increases the risk of increased free concentrations. Nonresponse to treatment is common if the dose is too low; however, the free fraction increases as the serum concentration is increased (above 100–125 mcg/mL). Dose-related adverse effects that occur at serum concentrations greater than 80 mcg/mL include neurotoxicity, sedation, hair loss, and thrombocytopenia. Life-threatening pancreatitis can occur but rarely (less than 5%). It can recur with reinitiation of valproate. The extended-release product has lower bioavailability than the enteric-coated preparation. The dose should be increased by 8%–20% when converting to the extended-release product.

2. Carbamazepine: This drug also appears effective for acute mania and maintenance therapy, particularly in patients with a history of head injury. Equetro is approved by the FDA for acute manic and mixed episodes. Although the same serum concentration range as for seizures (4–12 mcg/mL) should be used, keep in mind that clinicians may push it higher on the basis of tolerability and effect. Carbamazepine can also be added to lithium for patients who have not responded to monotherapy.

3. Lamotrigine: This drug has been approved for maintenance therapy. It appears particularly effective against the depressed phase of bipolar disorder. It is less effective than other mood stabilizers in the manic phase.

    a. A Stevens-Johnson type rash occurs in about 0.3% of adults and 1% of children. Lamotrigine must be discontinued if a rash occurs and should never be rechallenged. Risk increases with rapid dose titrations, high doses, young age, and concurrent use of valproic acid. The rash most commonly occurs within the first 2–8 weeks of therapy.

    b. The dose titration must be halved if lamotrigine is given with valproate and doubled if given with carbamazepine because of increased lamotrigine metabolism. The titration period is lengthy, so the onset of therapeutic effect can be delayed. For this reason, lamotrigine is not helpful in the acute setting.

    c. Lamotrigine has been associated with aseptic meningitis in adult and pediatric patients. Patients who experience headache, fever, chills, nausea, vomiting, stiff neck, rash, abnormal sensitivity to light, drowsiness, or confusion while taking lamotrigine should contact their health care professional right away. In 15 of 40 identified cases of aseptic meningitis, symptoms returned when patients were rechallenged with lamotrigine. Symptoms have occurred 1–42 days after the drug is started, and many of the patients required hospitalization.

4. Topiramate is also being used for bipolar disorder, but comparative data with other anticonvulsants are unavailable. It should be used with caution, however, because it has been linked with depression. Other anticonvulsants, including levetiracetam and oxcarbazepine, are being used for bipolar disorder, but data about efficacy are scarce. Data for gabapentin suggest it is ineffective.

D. Antipsychotics for Bipolar Disorder: Antipsychotics, particularly SGAs, have mood stabilizing properties. They can be used alone or with anticonvulsant mood stabilizers to treat bipolar symptoms. Metabolic adverse effects associated with antipsychotic use should be considered when medications are administered long term (see Schizophrenia section).

1. Acute treatment: Antipsychotics treat acute symptoms of mania, including psychosis, aggression, or irritation. They are often combined with a traditional mood stabilizer for severe symptoms. All atypical antipsychotics have received FDA approval for use in acute mania or mixed episodes except

for brexpiprazole, clozapine, and iloperidone. For acute mania, the Canadian Network for Mood and Anxiety Treatments/International Society for Bipolar Disorders (CANMAT/ISBD) guidelines include olanzapine, risperidone, quetiapine, aripiprazole, ziprasidone, asenapine, and paliperidone extended release among first-line agents.

2. Bipolar depression: Both quetiapine and lurasidone are approved for treatment of bipolar depression. Data for aripiprazole suggest it is suboptimal for the treatment of bipolar depression.

3. Maintenance treatment: Risperdal Consta and Abilify Maintena have been approved for use in bipolar maintenance as monotherapy. The CANMAT/ISBD guidelines additionally recommend olanzapine and quetiapine.

E. Benzodiazepines for Bipolar Disorder: These agents are acutely helpful for agitation but are not as helpful for the core symptoms, nor do they prevent relapses. They are particularly useful for insomnia, hyperactivity, and agitation. Lorazepam or diazepam is often used in the acute setting, but long-term therapy is not recommended.

F. Antidepressants for Bipolar Disorder:
1. Use of these agents in bipolar disorder is controversial. There is a potential for switching to the manic phase, particularly in patients with type I bipolar disorder. The risk appears greater with TCAs and SNRIs than with SSRIs or bupropion. Because individual patients with bipolar disorder might benefit from antidepressants, the ISBD stopped short of recommending against any use of antidepressants. Antidepressants should not be used as monotherapy, and their use should be minimized in general. Antidepressants should not be used in bipolar depression if symptoms of mania are also present. The Systematic Treatment Enhanced Program for Bipolar Disorder trials found no statistically significant increased episodes of depression in patients taking mood stabilizers who discontinued their antidepressants. Patients with bipolar disorder taking mood stabilizers who received either paroxetine or bupropion were no more likely to achieve remission or have a durable recovery than those receiving placebo. They were also no more likely to experience a switch to a manic phase (N Engl J Med 2007;356:1711-22).
2. Fluoxetine in combination with olanzapine is approved to treat depression associated with type I bipolar disorder.

G. Type II Bipolar Disorder: The depressive phase tends to be more debilitating. Patients are usually functional during hypomanic episodes. Lithium is a first-line agent, but it may not achieve remission as monotherapy and takes time to relieve symptoms. Quetiapine is preferred for acute symptom treatment. Lurasidone may also be used. Lamotrigine is a reasonable alternative for longer-term symptom control, but because of its slow titration schedule, it is not useful in the acute setting. Other mood stabilizers can be used but may not be as efficacious as for type I. Antidepressants are used more commonly but should be used with caution, and never as monotherapy. Olanzapine and fluoxetine may thus be an option.

Patient Cases

Questions 12–15 pertain to the following case.

C.P. is a recent Iraq war veteran who has been treated successfully with paroxetine for his major depression for the past 3 weeks. He presents to the clinic experiencing nightmares, "feeling on edge all the time," and having flashbacks of his time in the war. He is evaluated and given a diagnosis of posttraumatic stress disorder (PTSD). He has no history of substance dependence and has no significant medical history.

12. Which recommendation is most appropriate at this time?
    A. Continue paroxetine because it treats both PTSD and major depression.
    B. Discontinue paroxetine and initiate sertraline, which treats both PTSD and major depression.
    C. Continue paroxetine and add lorazepam for the anxiety symptoms.
    D. Discontinue paroxetine and initiate buspirone for the anxiety symptoms.

13. C.P. has been adherent to the medication you recommended earlier, but he still feels very irritable and has been aggressive at times at work toward others. Which adjunctive medication is most appropriate in this patient?
    A. Buspirone.
    B. Clonazepam.
    C. Divalproex.
    D. Lithium.

14. After 8 months of treatment, C.P. is not responding to the medication you recommended. Having heard a lot about buspirone, he wonders whether this medication might be helpful for his conditions. Which is the most accurate statement for this patient?
    A. Buspirone may be helpful for the nightmares.
    B. Buspirone may work as quickly as 3 days.
    C. Buspirone is convenient because of its once-daily dosing.
    D. Buspirone does not have much dependence potential.

15. C.P. returns to the clinic and states that his depressive and anxiety symptoms are much improved. However, he is concerned that his girlfriend, who has OCD, is not doing well on her treatment with lorazepam. If you were also treating the girlfriend, which is the most appropriate medication you would initiate?
    A. Clomipramine.
    B. Amitriptyline.
    C. Imipramine.
    D. Nortriptyline.

IV. ANXIETY AND RELATED DISORDERS (OCD, PTSD)

A. Overview of Anxiety Disorders
   1. Generalized anxiety disorder (GAD) is characterized by 6 months or more of excessive worry or anxiety, generally with an unidentified cause.
   2. Panic disorder is characterized by discrete periods of sudden, intense fear or terror and feelings of impending doom. Usually, the precipitating cause is unknown, but the patient can become conditioned to believe it is attributable to some environmental cause.
   3. Agoraphobia: Intense fear in two or more settings (mostly in the open or in public). These settings include using public transportation, being in open spaces, being in enclosed spaces, standing in line or being in a crowd, and being outside the home alone.
   4. Social anxiety disorder is characterized by marked and persistent fear and anxiety in social or performance situations that are recognized as excessive or unreasonable. These situations are either avoided or endured with intense anxiety.
   5. Specific phobias are characterized by intense fear or anxiety induced by a specific object.
   6. OCD used to be classified as an anxiety disorder, but now, it has its own designation. It is characterized by obsessive or intrusive thoughts that cannot be controlled and that are repetitive. Compulsions are ritualistic behaviors (e.g., washing the hands, combing the hair, cleaning the house).
   7. PTSD also used to be classified as an anxiety disorder. It has been moved to a category titled "Trauma- and Stressor-Related Disorders." PTSD follows a traumatic event. It is characterized by increased arousal and avoidance of stimuli that approximate the original traumatic event.

B. Pharmacotherapeutic Options for Anxiety and Related Disorders
   1. Benzodiazepines: These drugs have anxiolytic properties, and some have preventive efficacy for panic attacks. They are not effective for all anxiety disorders. Depending on the choice of agent, the onset can be very rapid, as outlined below. The high-potency, short half-life agents are the most rapidly acting. They are effective for treating the acute somatic and autonomic symptoms of anxiety, but do not adequately address the underlying cognitive and psychological pathology.
      a. Pharmacologically, they share, to various degrees, five properties: (1) anxiolytic, (2) hypnotic, (3) muscle relaxation, (4) anticonvulsant, and (5) amnesic actions. Tolerance of the anxiolytic action is uncommon. Benzodiazepines are differentiated by their half-life (plus or minus active metabolites) and potency. If they are thought of as short half-life/high-potency versus long half-life/lower-potency drugs, the following distinctions can be made:
         i. Short half-life/high potency: These are usually more rapid-acting agents that provide quicker control of the symptoms. However, tolerance of the hypnotic effect develops rapidly, withdrawal problems are common, and interdose breakthrough symptoms can occur. These are often used for acute management and later replaced with longer half-life agents.
         ii. Long half-life/low potency: These drugs produce longer-lasting effects throughout the day, and although withdrawal symptoms may be less pronounced, they do occur. Interdose breakthrough symptoms are less likely; however, more "hangover" symptoms occur in the morning. These agents can accumulate in older adult patients.
         iii. Table 12 compares the half-lives and potencies of the five main/most commonly prescribed benzodiazepines.

Table 12. Half-lives and Potency of the Most Commonly Prescribed Benzodiazepines

Agent	Half-life (hr)	Dose (mg)
Alprazolam (Xanax)	6–12	0.5
Chlordiazepoxide (Librium)	5–30 (act. met.)	25
Clonazepam	20–50	0.5
Diazepam (Valium)	20–100 (act. met.)	10
Lorazepam (Ativan)	10–18	1

act. met. = active metabolite.

b. The primary issues associated with benzodiazepines are tolerance and dependence. Tolerance of the hypnotic actions occurs within days. Dependence occurs within weeks to months of continued use. Abrupt cessation can lead to withdrawal problems. For this reason, it is generally recommended that treatment periods be restricted to 3–4 months, or about the time of an adequate trial on an antidepressant. After this time, the patient is tapered off the drug to avoid withdrawal and supplementation with other agents. Benzodiazepine tapers can take months to more than 1 year to complete. In practice, many of these patients go on to use these drugs for long periods. Often, these patients are not in remission, despite treatment with maintenance medications. In patients with a history of substance use disorder or risk factors for substance use disorder, the situation is different. In these patients, try to avoid the use of benzodiazepines because patients may begin to show an abusive pattern of use.

2. Antidepressants: SSRIs are also effective for several anxiety disorders. They are the agents of choice for long-term treatment of anxiety disorders. Venlafaxine has been approved for the treatment of generalized anxiety and social anxiety disorders. Duloxetine is also approved for GAD. Some initial symptoms may be improved within days, but the full benefit of treatment may take weeks, as for depression treatment. Tricyclic antidepressants have preventive efficacy for panic disorder and anxiolytic activity. **Important note:** About 25% of these patients experience a hyper-stimulatory response to antidepressants, which can be confused with a worsening of the anxiety symptoms. This response is more common when therapy is first begun. Using low doses at first can help. Antidepressants can also be helpful for anxiety that accompanies depression.

3. Buspirone: This drug has anxiolytic properties, but clinicians' opinions are divided on its real value in treating GAD. It has little efficacy for other anxiety disorders. The main drawback to buspirone is its long onset of action (weeks). In the meantime, the anxiety must be covered with another agent. Some clinicians will use short-term benzodiazepines as a bridge until buspirone takes effect.

4. Miscellaneous agents

   a. β-Blockers are sometimes used to block the peripheral symptoms of panic disorder or performance anxiety.

   b. MAOIs can be effective for the treatment of panic disorder when the patient also has atypical depression. However, these drugs are seldom used because of the potential for serious adverse effects.

   c. Antihistamines with sedating properties (e.g., hydroxyzine) can help reduce physical symptoms of anxiety

   d. Barbiturates are seldom used. They are often less effective and can be lethal if taken in overdose.

   e. Antipsychotics are not considered first-line agents for the treatment of anxiety disorders. Selected SGAs can be useful as add-on therapy for OCD, GAD, and PTSD.

5. CBT should be an integral part of any therapeutic plan for treating anxiety disorders.

C. Recommended Therapy for Specific Anxiety and Related Disorders
 1. Generalized anxiety disorder
    a. Antidepressants: These are considered first-line agents. These include the SSRIs (escitalopram, paroxetine, and sertraline), the SNRIs (duloxetine and venlafaxine), and imipramine
    b. Benzodiazepines: This class of drugs is rapidly effective; if possible, try to discontinue in 3–4 months, or once the patient has remittance of symptoms. Long-term therapy is common but not recommended. Benzodiazepines can be taken in combination with either antidepressants or buspirone as a bridge until these drugs start to take effect. They are more effective against somatic symptoms than against the underlying psychic pathology.
    c. Buspirone: Good when benzodiazepines should be avoided (e.g., in patients with a history of substance use disorder); takes 2–4 weeks to be effective
    d. Pregabalin: Considered a second-line agent behind antidepressants. Limited data suggest comparable efficacy with venlafaxine and benzodiazepines.
    e. CBT or another type of psychotherapy should generally be included with pharmacotherapy.
    f. In treatment-refractory patients, augmentation with quetiapine, olanzapine, or risperidone can be tried. Valproate also shows promise.
 2. Panic disorder
    a. Antidepressants: First-line therapy. These include the SSRIs (escitalopram, fluoxetine, fluvoxamine, paroxetine, sertraline), venlafaxine, and duloxetine.
    b. Benzodiazepines: High-potency agents; effective; rapid onset
    c. Not effective: Buspirone, β-blockers, antihistamines, antipsychotics, bupropion, trazodone
    d. CBT and other psychotherapies are effective.
    e. Patients with panic disorder tend to have a higher sensitivity to physical symptoms. For this reason, these patients should be initiated on low doses of antidepressants—as low 25 mg of sertraline or 5 mg of paroxetine.
 3. Obsessive-compulsive disorder
    a. Serotonergic agents are effective—SSRIs (escitalopram, fluoxetine, fluvoxamine, paroxetine, and sertraline) and clomipramine
    b. CBT may be effective, but it is secondary to pharmacotherapy.
    c. Alone, SSRIs often fail to control OCD completely. Not many other drugs help. Augmentation with haloperidol or an SGA (olanzapine, quetiapine, or risperidone) may help. In general, high doses need to be used.
 4. Posttraumatic stress disorder
    a. SSRIs (fluoxetine, sertraline, and paroxetine) are considered first-line agents.
    b. Augment with other agents to treat specific symptoms (e.g., intermittent explosive behavior with β-blockers or mood stabilizers).
       i. Prazosin is used to treat PTSD-associated nightmares.
       ii. Anticonvulsants for aggression, anger, and depression (valproic acid, carbamazepine, lamotrigine, topiramate)
       iii. Atypical antipsychotics for psychotic symptoms (olanzapine, quetiapine, risperidone)
    c. Benzodiazepines are sometimes used acutely for sleep disturbances, but use should be very limited. Most data analyses indicate a lack of efficacy. Benzodiazepines have dissociative and disinhibiting properties and may worsen non-hyperarousal symptoms. Benzodiazepines may thus interfere with the fear conditioning aspects of psychotherapy.
    d. As with all other anxiety disorders, psychotherapy is integral. Trauma-focused CBT and exposure therapy are preferred.

5. Social anxiety disorder
   a. CBT is the most important modality.
   b. Antidepressants: First-line medication for treatment; SSRIs (escitalopram, fluvoxamine, paroxetine, sertraline) and venlafaxine. Response to antidepressants tends to be slow (up to 12 weeks) and has a flat dose-response curve.
   c. Clonazepam may be used as an adjunct.
   d. Gabapentin and pregabalin are used as second- or third-line agents.
6. Specific phobias
   a. Not treated with medication
   b. Systematic desensitization and other behavioral approaches often effective

---

Patient Cases

Questions 16–18 pertain to the following case.

C.D. is a 38-year-old kindergarten teacher who presents to the clinic today with noticeable dark circles under her eyes. She has difficulty with sleep, mainly with staying asleep. It takes her about 20 minutes to fall asleep, but after about 2 hours, she wakes up and cannot fall asleep again for several hours. This pattern has taken a toll on her job, and she feels tired all the time. She once took diphenhydramine for sleep but had to miss work because of extreme drowsiness in the morning. She wonders whether she can take any other medications. Her other medical problems include hypothyroidism (levothyroxine 125 mcg at bedtime), hypertension (hydrochlorothiazide 25 mg in the morning), chronic back pain (ibuprofen 800 mg three times daily), and MDD (citalopram 20 mg in the morning).

16. Which agent is most likely contributing to C.D.'s insomnia?
    A. Citalopram.
    B. Hydrochlorothiazide.
    C. Ibuprofen.
    D. Levothyroxine.

17. Which medication used for insomnia is most appropriate to recommend for C.D.?
    A. Eszopiclone.
    B. Trazodone.
    C. Temazepam.
    D. Zaleplon.

18. Which is the best example of an adverse effect that should concern C.D. when using zolpidem?
    A. Orthostasis.
    B. Disorientation.
    C. Abnormal behaviors while asleep.
    D. Seizures with high doses of the drug.

V. INSOMNIA

A. Normal Sleep Patterns and Neurochemistry/Physiology of Sleep
   1. We spend about one-third of our lives asleep. The amount of sleep required varies from individual to individual and changes with age.
   2. Sleep difficulties are common, with up to 35% of the population affected. Of interest, 4%–5% of the population may experience hypersomnia.
   3. People with sleep problems usually experience one or more of the following: insomnia, daytime sleepiness, or abnormal sleep behaviors.
   4. The sleep-wake cycle in humans usually lasts 25 hours, which means that with the 24-hour day-night cycle of the earth's rotation, there must be some internal clock resetting. This resetting is accomplished by cues such as clocks and daylight, which tell the time of day.
   5. The neural networks regulating sleep-wake cycles are located in the brainstem, basal forebrain, and hypothalamus, with projections to the cortex and thalamus.
   6. The reticular activating system maintains wakefulness, and when activity here declines, sleep occurs.
   7. Several neurotransmitters are involved in the sleep-wake cycle. Norepinephrine, acetylcholine, histamine, and neuropeptides operate in the hypothalamus during wakefulness. Neuronal systems in the raphe nuclei, solitary tract, ventricular thalamus, anterior hypothalamus, and basal forebrain promote sleep. As the reticular activating system slows down, serotonin neurotransmission in the raphe nuclei reduces sensory input and inhibits motor activity. Norepinephrine is involved in dreaming, whereas serotonin is active during non-dreaming sleep.
   8. A lot of brain activity occurs during sleep; simultaneous electroencephalograms, electro-oculograms, and electromyograms characterize sleep stages. These are used to measure sleep latency (time to sleep onset), number of awakenings, number of stage shifts during the night, and latency to rapid eye movement (REM). These recordings are termed polysomnography. Stages are as shown in Table 13.

Table 13. Sleep Stages

State	Characteristics
Wakefulness	Low-voltage EEG, random eye movements, high muscle tone
Non-REM sleep	Low muscle tone, few eye movements
Stage 1	Transition between wakefulness and sleep, low-voltage desynchronized EEG, lasts 0.5–7.0 minute
Stage 2	Low-voltage EEG with sleep spindles and K-complexes
Stages 3 and 4	High-amplitude, slow-wave EEG, "delta sleep"
REM sleep	Low-voltage, mixed-frequency EEG, low muscle tone, REMs, autonomic fluctuations in heart rate and perspiration, and dreaming reported in 80%–90% of subjects

EEG = electroencephalogram; REM = rapid eye movement.

   9. Sleep architecture is cyclic. Passing from wakefulness to stage 4 non-REM sleep takes about 45 minutes in young adults. Rapid eye movement usually occurs within 90 minutes of falling asleep; at first, REM lasts 5–7 minutes, but it gets progressively longer through the night. The sleep cycle (non-REM stages 1–4 and REM), which lasts about 70–120 minutes, is repeated four to six times a night. The typical young adult spends about 75% of his or her time in non-REM.
   10. Sleep patterns change with age. Older adult patients experience less delta sleep, REM sleep, and total sleep time. They have more nocturnal awakenings and total time awake at night. The incidence of sleep pathology may be as high as 40%.

B. Sleep Disorders
1. The *DSM-5* recognizes several sleep-wake disturbances: insomnia disorder, hypersomnia disorder, narcolepsy, obstructive sleep apnea, hypopnea, central sleep apnea, sleep-related hypoventilation, circadian rhythm sleep-wake disorders, non-REM sleep arousal disorders, nightmare disorder, REM sleep behavior disorder, restless legs syndrome, substance/medication-induced sleep disorder, and several other or unspecified sleep-wake disorders.
2. Insomnia
    a. Insomnia is defined as an inability to initiate or maintain sleep, and it can be associated with problems during the daytime. About one-third of the U.S. population experiences insomnia, with half of those saying it is serious.
    b. More than 40% of those suffering from insomnia self-medicate with over-the-counter medications (discussed below) or with other substances (e.g., alcohol).
    c. Insomnia can be classified according to symptom duration as in Table 14.

Table 14. Types of Insomnia

Type	Duration (wk)	Likely Causes
Transient	< 1	Acute situational or environmental stressors
Short term	< 4	Continued personal stress
Chronic	> 4	Psychiatric illness, substance use disorder
		Behavioral causes (poor sleep hygiene)
		Medical causes, primary sleep disorder (e.g., sleep apnea, restless legs syndrome; these are no longer recognized by the *DSM-5* as insomnia)

    d. Transient insomnia is most often associated with acute stressors. It resolves once the acute stressors are removed. Pharmacotherapy may be used for a few days until the situation resolves.
    e. Short-term insomnia is also most often associated with an acute stressor, but it is ongoing. Here, it is important to initiate good sleep hygiene (as below) and avoid stimulants such as caffeine. Pharmacotherapy may be indicated, especially if on an intermittent basis (e.g., skip it after 2 or 3 good nights of sleep). Therapy for 7–10 days is usually sufficient.
    f. Chronic insomnia should be carefully evaluated for an underlying medical or psychiatric cause. If a cause is not present, a common type of chronic insomnia is chronic psychophysiologic insomnia, which is a behavioral problem. The person has usually developed poor sleep hygiene, and the bedroom is associated with an alerting response. Behavioral therapy is important, but pharmacotherapy can be useful in short courses and intermittently. The development of chronic insomnia is a complex process and can be difficult to treat. Pharmacotherapy can be part of the overall treatment approach, but there is no consensus about how effective it is when used long term. Ramelteon, eszopiclone, and zolpidem controlled release all contain language in the package labels suggesting they can be used chronically.
    g. The evaluation of insomnia should include an assessment of medical and psychiatric status. Medical causes are many and include thyroid disease and therapy with medications that can interfere with sleep. Several psychiatric conditions can interfere with sleep, including affective and anxiety disorders.
    h. For all types of insomnia, patients can be instructed about good sleep hygiene. These principles are listed below:
        i. Maintain regular bedtimes and awakenings.
        ii. Do not go to bed unless you are sleepy.
        iii. Sleep long enough to avoid feeling tired, but no more.

    iv. Optimize the bedroom conditions (e.g., light, temperature, noise).

    v. Develop a bedtime ritual that allows you to unwind.

    vi. If you cannot go to sleep, or if you awaken and cannot go back to sleep, do not stay in bed more than 15–20 minutes; get up and do something else until you are sleepy.

    vii. Do not go to bed hungry, but do not stuff yourself before bed; try a small snack.

    viii. Avoid activities in the bedroom except for sleeping and sex.

    ix. Do not lie there and watch the clock; get one without a luminous dial.

    x. Avoid naps during the day.

    xi. Avoid stimulants such as caffeine and nicotine throughout the day.

    xii. Avoid alcohol because it can lead to "fragmented" sleep.

    xiii. Exercise regularly during the day, but not close to bedtime.

C. Pharmacotherapy of Insomnia

    1. Pharmacotherapy is indicated for all forms of insomnia as long as it is part of an overall plan to deal with the causes and is used for well-defined periods. It should be considered adjunctive therapy only for short-term or chronic insomnia.

    2. Agents that can depress respiration should be avoided in patients with respiratory disorders, a history of substance use disorder, or obstructive sleep apnea. Ramelteon should be avoided in patients with severe sleep apnea.

    3. There are several classes of sedative-hypnotics: barbiturates, which are no longer indicated; nonbarbiturates (e.g., chloral hydrate), which have only limited indications; benzodiazepines; and the non-benzodiazepines zolpidem, zaleplon, and eszopiclone, which are often used in clinical practice. Ramelteon is a melatonin receptor 1 and melatonin receptor 2 agonist. Suvorexant is an orexin receptor antagonist.

    4. Benzodiazepines: In general, they are safe, effective, and well tolerated by most patients, but they are not considered first line. Although all members of this class can be used as sedatives, only five are FDA approved and marketed as such. These five are primarily used as sedative-hypnotics because they are rapidly absorbed and produce central nervous system actions more quickly than most anxiety agents. The sedative-hypnotic benzodiazepines are listed in Table 15. They are primarily differentiated by their onset of action and half-life in the body. According to their half-life, they are classified as short acting (half-life less than 6 hours), intermediate acting (half-life 6–24 hours), and long acting (half-life more than 24 hours). These are important parameters when selecting therapy. For instance, someone with problems initiating sleep would most likely benefit from an agent with a quick onset but short duration of action. Someone with problems maintaining sleep in the middle of the night might respond better to a drug with a longer half-life. Table 15 compares the benzodiazepines available in the United States.

Table 15. Benzodiazepines for Insomnia

Drug (Trade)	Usual Dose (mg)	Half-life (hr)	Duration
Triazolam (Halcion)	0.125–0.25	2–6	Short
Temazepam (Restoril)	15–30	8–20	Intermediate
Estazolam (Prosom)	1–2	8–24	Intermediate
Flurazepam (Dalmane)	15–30	48–120	Long
Quazepam (Doral)	7.5–15	48–120	Long

5. These drugs are usually well tolerated. However, several problems still exist.

   a. Tolerance: Tolerance can develop, particularly when the drugs are used consistently for long periods. These drugs are not indicated for chronic use; however, newer evidence is emerging that they may be effective for longer periods than originally thought. Most are effective for 2–4 weeks and, in some cases, longer. An intermittent pattern of use can reduce the development of tolerance. In addition, most people without a history of substance use disorder do not escalate their doses.

   b. Residual daytime sedation: This is a common complaint of patients using these drugs. It is especially likely with agents having a long half-life. Dose is also an important factor; always use the lowest effective dose.

   c. Rebound insomnia: This can occur when the drug is discontinued abruptly. Insomnia is usually worse than baseline and usually lasts for 1–2 days; tapering the drug may minimize its effect. It is most common after the use of short- and intermediate-acting agents.

   d. Anterograde amnesia: All benzodiazepines appear to impair the acquisition and encoding of new information. They may also impair memory storage and recall. Dosage may be important.

   e. Be careful when using benzodiazepines in older adult patients because benzodiazepines can cause memory problems, increase the risk of falls, and accumulate (agents with a long half-life). Try to avoid use in this population. Idiosyncratic reactions can occur in older adult and pediatric populations with benzodiazepine use.

   f. Withdrawal: Physical dependence will occur if these agents are used long enough. Symptoms of withdrawal include worsening insomnia, anxiety, muscle twitches, photophobia, tinnitus, auditory and visual hypersensitivity, and seizures. Minimize by gradually tapering the drug at discontinuation.

Table 16. Non-benzodiazepines for Insomnia

Drug	$t_{1/2}$ (hr)	Administration (minutes before sleep)	Indications			CDS Scheduling
			Sleep Onset	Sleep Maintenance	Chronic Therapy	
Doxepin (Silenor)	Doxepin: 15.3 Nordoxepin: 31	30		X		Not controlled
Eszopiclone (Lunesta)	6	Immediately	X	X	X	C-IV
Ramelteon (Rozerem)	1-2.6	30	X		X	Not controlled
Suvorexant (Belsomra)	12	30	X	X		C-IV
Zaleplon (Sonata)	1	Immediately	X			C-IV
Zolpidem (Ambien)	1.4–6.5 (see below)	Immediately	X	X (CR only)		C-IV

6. Doxepin (Silenor) is a tricyclic antidepressant indicated for the treatment of impaired sleep maintenance. The doses used are lower than those used to treat depression. Chances for morning effects are high because of the long half-life of both doxepin and its active metabolite, nordoxepin.

7. Eszopiclone (Lunesta): This non-benzodiazepine is a $GABA_A$ agonist. Its half-life is 6 hours, so morning effects could result if it is taken late in the night. This drug can be used for chronic insomnia. On May 1, 2014, the FDA reduced the starting dose to 1 mg to minimize the amount of next-day

impairment. Patients should be counseled to use caution when driving or performing activities that require alertness, particularly with the 2- to 3-mg doses. It should be taken immediately before bed and when the patient will be in bed for at least 7–8 hours. C-IV

8. Ramelteon (Rozerem): Melatonin agonist (no activity at the GABA or benzodiazepine receptor). Duration is 2–5 hours. To date, there is no evidence that this melatonin agonist is associated with dependence or tolerance, and it may be used long term. This drug can be used long term for chronic insomnia. It is primarily metabolized by CYP1A2, but inducers and inhibitors of 2C9 and 3A4 can also affect it.

9. Suvorexant (Belsomra) is a newly approved (August 2014) orexin receptor antagonist. It will be available in 2015. The neuropeptide orexin promotes wakefulness. By blocking the OX1R and OX2R receptors, suvorexant both decreases sleep latency and promotes sleep maintenance. It should be taken within 30 minutes of bedtime, and with at least 7 hours of sleep time. It is metabolized by CYP3A4, and the dose must be decreased in patients taking concomitant 3A4 inhibitors.

10. Zaleplon: This is a non-benzodiazepine with a similar pharmacology to zolpidem (see below) and a very short half-life. For patients with sleep maintenance problems, it might not last as long. However, it has a shorter half-life (about 1 hour) and may cause fewer problems in the morning, especially if given late. It shortens onset to sleep, but does not prolong sleep time or number of awakenings. It is indicated only for short-term treatment of insomnia. It has been used in trials for up to 5 weeks. C-IV

11. Zolpidem: This non-benzodiazepine sedative-hypnotic modulates the GABA$_A$ receptor complex.
    a. Compared with benzodiazepines, zolpidem lacks anticonvulsant action, muscle-relaxant properties, and respiratory depressant effect; it also has a lower risk of tolerance and withdrawal. It should still be avoided in obstructive sleep apnea. It is a good choice for patients in whom benzodiazepines should be avoided.
    b. Zolpidem is available as an immediate release tablet (IR), controlled release tablet (CR), sublingual tablet (Edluar, Intermezzo), and sublingual spray (Zolpimist). The pharmacokinetics and indications vary based upon the dosing form. The sublingual spray has a shorter onset of action, but that of the sublingual tablet is comparable to both the IR and CR tablets.
    c. Indications vary by dosage form. All are indicated to decrease sleep latency. The CR tablets are indicated to improve sleep maintenance and can be used for longer-term therapy. Intermezzo is indicated as a "prn" treatment for patients who have difficulty falling back to sleep as long as 4 hours or more remain.
    d. The FDA has reduced the dosing recommendations to limit next-day impairment. The dosing differs based upon the gender and degree of debility. For women, the nightly dose is 5 mg (IR) or 6.25 mg (CR). For men, it is 5–10 mg (IR) or 6.25–12.5 mg (CR). Debilitated patients should receive 5 mg (IR) or 6.25 mg (CR). Patients should be maintained on the lowest dose needed to benefit.

12. Patients should be warned about the potential risk of engaging in abnormal activities while asleep when taking sedative-hypnotics. Such behaviors may include driving, eating, having sex, or talking on the phone while asleep (with amnesia for the event). Other cautions include anaphylaxis and decreased respiratory drive.

13. Taking any of the agents listed in Table with food can delay onset of effects, thus prolonging the time to onset of sleep and increasing the risk of hangover effects in longer-acting agents. Doxepin should be separated from meals by 3 hours.

14. Over-the-counter medications: These are most often antihistamines (doxylamine or diphenhydramine) that are both sedating and anticholinergic. They are possibly effective, but not as effective as benzodiazepines. Their regular use is not recommended. In fact, some data suggest that they do not maintain efficacy beyond a few days. They are associated with a higher incidence of daytime sedation than short- or intermediate-acting benzodiazepines. Diphenhydramine has been a popular agent when benzodiazepines were contraindicated. However, caution should be used in older adult patients because an

anticholinergic action can worsen dementia or other medical conditions. In addition, it should not be administered with the cholinesterase inhibitors used for Alzheimer disease.

15. Other non-benzodiazepines: In some situations, antidepressants such as trazodone may be used as sedative-hypnotics. These can be effective, and often, the dose required is lower than that used for depression. However, efficacy has not been fully established through clinical trials. Trazodone has been popular for managing insomnia caused by SSRI antidepressants (see discussion in Depression section). It is also popular by itself as a sleep agent because the potential for dependence is low. However, it is associated with considerable adverse effects, and the data for long-term use are scant.

Patient Cases

Questions 19–22 pertain to the following case.
L.M. is a 50-year-old patient with a 25-year history of alcohol dependence who was found unconscious after his last drinking binge. He was first admitted to the medical unit for alcohol withdrawal symptoms before being transferred to the substance dependence unit. His last drink was 6 hours ago, and fluids have been started. He has had three alcohol withdrawal seizures in the past and an episode of delirium tremens. He also has significant hepatitis, and liver function tests show aspartate aminotransferase (AST) of 220 IU/L and alanine aminotransferase (ALT) of 200 IU/L.

19. Which symptom are you most likely to observe in the medical unit?
    A. Alcohol craving.
    B. Delirium tremens.
    C. Increased heart rate.
    D. Seizures.

20. Which agent is best for alcohol withdrawal symptoms in L.M. for intramuscular administration?
    A. Chlordiazepoxide.
    B. Clonazepam.
    C. Diazepam.
    D. Lorazepam.

21. Before administering fluids with glucose, which agent is most important to administer?
    A. Folate.
    B. Multivitamin supplement.
    C. B_{12}.
    D. Thiamine.

22. Which medication is best to use in L.M. for alcohol dependence?
    A. Acamprosate.
    B. Diazepam.
    C. Disulfiram.
    D. Naltrexone.

VI. SUBSTANCE USE DISORDERS

A. Alcohol
   1. Acute withdrawal
      a. Characteristic symptoms occur after alcohol discontinuation. The symptoms that develop, how quickly they develop, and the degree of severity depend on the level of alcohol abuse and a person's characteristics. Not all patients develop delirium tremens, nor do all develop seizures. However, it is difficult to predict, so detoxification should always be supervised. A history of alcohol withdrawal problems suggests that inpatient detoxification is indicated.
      b. Table 17 lists the stages of acute alcohol withdrawal.

Table 17. Stages of Acute Alcohol Withdrawal

Stage	Onset	Symptoms
1	6–12 hr	Mild tremors, irritability, mild agitation, restlessness, tachycardia, nausea, sweating
2	12–24 hr	Marked tremors, hyperactivity, hyper-alertness, increased startle response, pronounced tachycardia, insomnia, nightmares, illusions, hallucinations, alcohol cravings
3	12–48 hr	More severe symptoms than observed during stage 2; seizures may occur
4	3–5 days	Delirium tremens: Confusion, agitation, tremor, insomnia, tachycardia, sweating, hyperpyrexia

      c. Delirium tremens, which can be life threatening, should be considered a potential medical emergency and treated promptly.
      d. The seizures that occur are often difficult to control. Status epilepticus can develop; thus, it is important to ensure that these patients have intravenous access. Benzodiazepines are first line for seizure prevention in alcohol withdrawal compared with other anticonvulsants.
   2. Treatment of acute alcohol withdrawal
      a. The degree of symptoms and the resulting treatment level should be individualized, and an accurate history regarding amount, duration, and past withdrawal symptoms including seizures and delirium tremens should guide treatment. If it is believed that complications may arise, treatment should take place in an inpatient setting.
      b. Because of cross-tolerance, benzodiazepines can be used therapeutically to prevent and/or treat withdrawal symptoms. Several dosing regimens are used (Table 18).
         i. Symptom-driven treatment using the Clinical Institute Withdrawal Assessment for Alcohol scale (CIWA-Ar) is the most common method. The CIWA-Ar consists of seven items and has a range of 0–67. The higher the score, the more severe the symptoms. The patient's CIWA-Ar score is determined every hour. Patients are typically treated if the score is greater than 8–10 (depending on protocol). This protocol has been shown to be efficacious and results in lower total benzodiazepine use.
         ii. Scheduled dosing: For severe alcohol withdrawal, fixed-dose benzodiazepine therapy is used for 2–3 days, regardless of symptoms, with supplementation according to the hourly CIWA-Ar score. The benzodiazepine can then be tapered for 3–4 days until symptoms have abated.
         iii. Loading-dose (front loaded) protocol: A new approach during recent years uses a loading-dose strategy for diazepam. Diazepam is given in a dose of 10–20 mg every 1–2 hours until the symptoms of withdrawal are alleviated. Most patients will need two or three doses, especially those with a history of seizures during withdrawal, in which case three doses should be used. The half-life of diazepam is long, and most patients will not need subsequent doses in this protocol once symptoms are relieved. Of course, patients should be monitored closely.

    iv. Chlordiazepoxide is considered the "classic" benzodiazepine for treating alcohol withdrawal because it was used first. It has no proven advantages over the other agents. Its long half-life may cause unnecessary sedation, particularly in patients with liver dysfunction. Conversely, patients with a high risk of withdrawal seizures or delirium tremens may need a long-acting benzodiazepine.

    v. <u>Lorazepam</u> is preferred in most situations. Its shorter half-life allows for tighter control of dosing with minimal risk of oversedation.

Table 18. Benzodiazepines in the Treatment of Acute Alcohol Withdrawal

Drug	CIWA-Ar Dosing	Fixed-Dose Regimen	Comments
Lorazepam (Ativan)	2–4 mg PO/IV/IM	2 mg every 6 hr x 4; then 1 mg every 6 hr x 8	Preferred medication, particularly for liver disease; no active metabolites
Diazepam (Valium)	10–20 mg PO/IV/IM[a]	10 mg every 5 hr x 4; then 5 mg every 6 hr x 8	Decrease dose for liver disease
Chlordiazepoxide (Librium)	50–100 mg PO/IV	50 mg every 6 hr x 4; then 25 mg every 6 hr x 8	Long acting; decrease dose for liver disease

[a]IM administration of diazepam is unreliable.

IM = intramuscular(ly); IV = intravenous(ly); PO = orally.

    c. Nutritional considerations
        i. Thiamine: This should be given to all patients to prevent Wernicke-Korsakoff syndrome—100 mg intramuscularly on admission and then orally for 3 days; always give the first dose before glucose because it is a cofactor for the metabolism of glucose.
        ii. Magnesium: Assess by serum chemistry; if low, give intravenous supplement.
        iii. Electrolytes: Assess by serum chemistry and add to intravenous solutions as indicated (e.g., potassium).
        iv. Vitamins: These patients are usually undernourished; a good multivitamin may be indicated (folate and vitamin B_{12} should be monitored).
    d. Fluid therapy: The patient may initially be overhydrated, but usually, fluid deficit will follow; replace fluids, usually with intravenous 5% dextrose solution with half-normal saline plus other electrolytes (e.g., potassium, phosphate).
    e. Hallucinations: Benzodiazepine will usually manage hallucinations effectively; if not, give haloperidol; however, be cautious because haloperidol can lower the seizure threshold.
    f. Seizures: Benzodiazepine will usually prevent seizures. Higher doses (and/or increased frequency) of benzodiazepines can be used if the patient has a history of seizures. If a seizure occurs during withdrawal, increasing the benzodiazepine dose and slowing the taper are options. Other antiepileptics may be used to treat status epilepticus, but their efficacy varies.
    g. Other agents
        i. β-Blockers: These agents help with vital signs and blood pressure.
        ii. α-Agonists (e.g., clonidine): These agents may help with some of the withdrawal symptoms.
  3. Chronic therapy
    a. Disulfiram: This drug blocks acetaldehyde dehydrogenase, and if alcohol is used with it, the person will develop symptoms that include nausea/vomiting, flushing, and headache, among others. Adherence is critical, and disulfiram is usually reserved for patients with considerable motivation for adherence. Caution should be exercised in patients with liver disease, particularly if is severe or the patient has cirrhosis. Disulfiram has been associated with hepatotoxicity, although it is not known whether patients with existing liver disease are at an increased risk.

b. Naltrexone: This drug can also be used chronically and has been shown to reduce cravings. If used, it should be combined with CBT. Liver toxicity is associated with this drug. The extended-release injectable suspension (Vivitrol) is available in an intramuscular formulation and is approved for **the treatment of alcohol dependence in patients who are able to abstain from alcohol in an outpatient setting before treatment initiation.**

c. Acamprosate (Campral): This drug is a structural analog of GABA. It, too, reduces cravings. It is not metabolized by the liver; however, it must be taken three times daily.

B. Opioid Dependence

1. In 2013, 1.5 million people used prescription pain relievers for nonmedical reasons. Most (53%) get their drugs free from friends or relatives. The number of people who received treatment for nonmedical use of prescription pain relievers was 746,000, up from 360,000 in 2002. In 2012, 16,007 deaths attributable to overdose with opioid analgesics occurred, accounting for 72% of all deaths caused by overdoses with pharmaceuticals.

2. The potential for abuse led the Drug Enforcement Administration to reclassify products containing hydrocodone and acetaminophen from C-III to C-II, effective October 6, 2014.

3. Opioid withdrawal is not life threatening in absence of concomitant medical conditions. Early symptoms may resemble flu and include agitation, anxiety, muscle aches, yawning, sweating, rhinorrhea, and lacrimation. Later symptoms include abdominal cramping, diarrhea, piloerection, dilated pupils, nausea, and vomiting.

    – Pharmacologic therapies for opioid addiction include maintenance therapy with methadone, an opioid agonist; antagonist therapy with naltrexone; detoxification with medications given in rapid taper (e.g., methadone, buprenorphine, or clonidine) to prepare the patient for antagonist or counseling therapy; and partial agonist therapy with buprenorphine or buprenorphine/naloxone.

4. The use of buprenorphine came about as a result of the Drug Abuse Treatment Act of 2000 (DATA), which allows qualifying physicians to apply for a waiver to treat opioid addiction outside an opioid treatment program using schedule III, IV, and V medications that are FDA approved for this indication.

    a. Only two formulations that qualify under DATA 2000 are FDA approved for opioid dependence: buprenorphine (available as sublingual tablets [Subutex]) and buprenorphine/naloxone (available in 4:1 ratio dosing increments as sublingual tablets [Zubsolv], sublingual film [Suboxone], and buccal film [Bunavail]).

    b. Buprenorphine is a partial agonist at the opioid mu receptor and an antagonist of the kappa receptor. The mu receptor binding affinity is higher than that of full opioid agonists with a lower intrinsic activity. Thus, it will displace morphine, methadone, and other opioid drugs but only gives a fraction of effect that levels out with increasing doses—a ceiling effect. This allows patients enough effect to "feel normal" but minimizes functional impairment. It also makes the drug safer in overdose situations. At high enough doses, the kappa antagonist properties could precipitate withdrawal.

    c. The addition of naloxone reduces abuse potential because naloxone is less potent when given sublingually than by injection. Thus, if the medication is used as intended (sublingually), the likelihood of withdrawal symptoms is low as opposed to dissolving and injecting it.

5. Treatment with buprenorphine involves three phases: induction, stabilization, and maintenance. Buprenorphine/naloxone is the preferred agent for most patients, including those taking short-acting opioids (hydromorphone, oxycodone, heroin). Patients taking long-acting opioids (methadone, long-acting morphine, long-acting oxycodone) should be tapered to methadone 30 mg/day or less or the equivalent, and transitioned to buprenorphine first. It is recommended that these patients be switched to the combination after no more than 2 days on buprenorphine monotherapy.

a. Patients should not be intoxicated or feeling effects from their last dose of opioid (~12–24 hours since the last dose of short-acting opioid). They must also be screened for other substance use disorder and for appropriateness of buprenorphine therapy. Patients may feel like they are going through early stages of withdrawal. In these cases, the opioid receptors are not fully occupied, and the buprenorphine is less likely to induce withdrawal.

b. Patients need to receive concomitant counseling and nonpharmacologic treatment support during treatment. Part of the DATA 2000 waiver requires that physicians be able to refer the patient to appropriate supportive services. Counseling should consider all psychosocial factors.

c. Induction phase: Find the minimum dose of buprenorphine that minimizes cravings for opioids but prevents withdrawal symptoms. The first dose should be given in the office and the patient observed for 2 hours. The patient is given the 4/1 dose of buprenorphine/naloxone. If withdrawal symptoms are not relieved or return before the 2-hour period, a second dose of 4/1 is given, and the daily dose is established at 8/2. The dose established during the induction phase depends on the presence of withdrawal symptoms on subsequent days, to a maximum of 32/8.

d. Stabilization phase: Reached when the patient is without withdrawal symptoms, is not experiencing adverse effects of buprenorphine/naloxone, and no longer has uncontrollable symptoms of craving. Toxicology screens can be used to verify that the patient is not using opioids. Patients should be seen weekly until stable. Doses can be adjusted in 2/0.5 to 4/1 increments. Most patients are maintained on 16/4–24/6.

e. Maintenance: Once the minimum dose needed to maintain abstinence is reached, the buprenorphine/naloxone therapy can be maintained indefinitely. Nonpharmacologic modalities should continue during this time.

f. Discontinuation: This should be considered only if the patient is psychologically and medically stable, is able to maintain a drug-free lifestyle, and no longer feels the drug is necessary to remain abstinent. The medication should be tapered slowly to avoid withdrawal symptoms.

6. Buprenorphine is metabolized by CYP3A4. Use caution with other medications that either induce or inhibit 3A4.

C. Tobacco Dependence
1. Tobacco use is the top cause of preventable morbidity and mortality.
2. It increases the risk of cardiovascular disease (including stroke), chronic obstructive pulmonary disease, and cancer (both lung and non-lung).
3. According to the 2012–2013 National Annual Tobacco Survey, 21.3% of Americans use a tobacco product every day or on most days, and 19.2% used some form of combustible tobacco product. Cigarettes are the most commonly used product. Rates have greatly declined over the past decade. There are more former smokers than there are current smokers.
4. Smoking cessation counseling is not consistently offered and tends to be directed to patients with tobacco-related conditions. Interventions lasting as few as 3 minutes make a difference. Patient counseling can help prime patients who are unwilling to quit to consider quitting and act on it in the future.
5. As of January 2015, the Joint Commission will require inpatient psychiatric services to screen for tobacco use (TOB-1), offer or provide treatment for tobacco dependence (TOB-2), and provide or offer treatment for tobacco dependence at discharge (TOB-3).
6. It takes an average of seven attempts for a patient to quit successfully.
7. Willingness to quit should be assessed via the five A's: *ask* about tobacco use, *advise* to quit, *assess* willingness to attempt to quit, *assist* in quit attempt, and *arrange* for follow-up.
8. Motivational interviewing is a successful technique that can help identify barriers to change and help the patient overcome them.

9. The five R's can be used to increase motivation to quit: *relevance, risks, rewards, roadblocks,* and *repetition.*
10. Quit lines such as 1-800-QUIT-NOW can facilitate attempts.
11. Seven pharmacologic agents (five nicotine and two non-nicotine) are available to help. They should be used with nonpharmacologic modalities to increase the success of quitting.
12. A usual pack contains 20 cigarettes.
13. Nicotine replacement therapy (NRT): All forms are equally efficacious. Patients should be advised to stop smoking completely before initiating. It comes in the following forms:
    a. Patch: For patients who smoke more than 10 cigarettes/day, start with 21 mg/day for 2 weeks, then 14 mg/day for 2 weeks, then 7 mg/day for 2 weeks. Those who smoke 10 cigarettes/day or less, start with 14 mg/day for 6 weeks, then 7 mg/day for 2 weeks. Patches may be used for longer periods if needed to improve success. It is recommended to change the patch upon awakening every day. Rotate sites.
    b. Gum: The gum should be chewed until a "peppery" or flavored taste develops; then "park" the gum between the cheek and gum to facilitate buccal absorption. The gum should be chewed and parked for 30 minutes or until the flavor is gone. The maximum number of pieces of gum is 24 pieces in 24 hours. At least 9 pieces of gum should be used daily to increase the chances of quitting. Patients who smoke 25 cigarettes/day or more should use the 4-mg dose. Those who smoke fewer than 25 cigarettes should use the 2-mg dose. One piece of gum should be used every 1–2 hours for the first 6 weeks of therapy, followed by 1 piece every 2–4 hours for weeks 7–9, then 1 piece every 4–6 hours for weeks 10–12. Acidic beverages (e.g., coffee, juices, and soft drinks) interfere with buccal absorption and should be avoided at least 15 minutes before using the gum. Adverse effects include soreness, dyspepsia, hiccups, and jaw ache. They are usually mild and can be corrected with changes in chewing technique.
    c. Lozenge: Patients who smoke their first cigarette within 30 minutes of waking should use the 4-mg strength. Otherwise, the 2-mg dose is used. The lozenge should be dissolved in the mouth rather than being chewed or swallowed. The frequency of use and tapering are the same as for the gum. Adverse effects are also similar. At least 9 lozenges should be used at the beginning to increase chances of quitting. Only 1 lozenge should be used at one time. No more than 5 lozenges within 6 hours, maximum 20 lozenges/24 hours.
    d. Inhaler: Available by prescription only. Each puff delivers 4 mg. Each cartridge delivers 80 inhalations. The recommended dosing is 6–16 cartridges/day. The best results are obtained if the contents of the cartridges are continuously puffed over about 20 minutes. Recommended treatment length is 3 months, with reduction in frequency during the past 6–12 weeks. As with the gum and lozenges, patients should not drink acidic beverages or eat within 15 minutes of using the inhaler. Delivery decreases at less than 40°F, so the inhaler should be kept in an inner pocket in cold weather. The most common adverse effects are sore throat, coughing, and rhinitis. Inhalers should be avoided in patients with reactive airway diseases.
    e. Nasal spray: Available by prescription only. The dose is 0.5 mg delivered to each nostril. One to two doses should be used hourly, up to five doses. The 24-hour maximum is 40 doses. At least eight doses should be used at the start of therapy. Each bottle contains 100 doses. Recommended length of therapy is 3–6 months, with tapering. Risk of dependency is higher than with other forms of nicotine replacement. Inhaling, sniffing, and swallowing can increase the risk of nasal irritation and should thus be avoided when taking the spray. Nasal irritation can occur in up to 94% of patients. Although it can resolve, a significant number of patients may have it as much as 8 weeks into therapy. It is not recommended for use in patients with reactive airway diseases or nasal conditions.
    f. Nicotine patches can be used with the as-needed dosage forms to increase the chances of quitting.

g. Patients with a history of cardiovascular disease can use nicotine replacement therapies.

h. The treatment of choice in pregnant women is nonpharmacologic. Nicotine has a pregnancy category D rating. NRT has not been shown to be effective in pregnant women.

14. Bupropion sustained release (SR): Bupropion SR should be initiated 7 days before the quit date. Treatment should last for at least 8 weeks but can be continued for up to 6 months to increase chances of quitting. It can also be combined with the nicotine patch if needed.

15. Varenicline: It is a nicotine receptor partial agonist. It blocks the effects of nicotine from smoking. It should be started 1 week before the quit day, although patients can choose to quit smoking up to 35 days after initiating varenicline. It should be continued for a total of 12 weeks. If the patient is successful at smoking cessation, it can be continued for another 12 weeks. Varenicline carries a black box warning for neuropsychiatric symptoms, including depression, suicidal ideation, suicide, psychosis, mood disturbance, and hostility. This can occur in patients with or without preexisting psychiatric conditions. It is associated with an increase in cardiovascular events, particularly in patients with preexisting cardiovascular disease. It must be used with caution in patients with a CrCl less than 30 mL/minute/1.73 m^2. Combining it with NRT increases adverse effects. It can be combined with bupropion.

16. Other agents used include clonidine and nortriptyline.

17. Patients who were unsuccessful in quitting on one form of pharmacologic therapy should be tried on a different method.

REFERENCES

Depression

1. American Psychiatric Association (APA). Practice Guideline for the Treatment of Patients with Major Depressive Disorder, 3rd ed. Washington, DC: APA, 2010. Available at http://psychiatryonline. org/guidelines.aspx. Accessed October 11, 2014. This is the current guideline of the American Psychiatric Association.

2. American Psychiatric Association (APA). Diagnostic and Statistical Manual of Mental Disorders, 5th ed. (DSM-5). Washington, DC: APA, 2013.

3. Teter CJ, Kando JC, Wells BG. Major depressive disorder. In: DiPiro JT, Talbert RL, Hayes PE, et al. Pharmacotherapy: A Pathophysiologic Approach, 9th ed. New York: McGraw-Hill, 2014:chap 51.

Bipolar Disorder

1. American Psychiatric Association (APA). Diagnostic and Statistical Manual of Mental Disorders, 5th ed. (DSM-5). Washington, DC: APA, 2013.

2. Drayton SJ, Pelic CM. Bipolar disorder. In: DiPiro JT, Talbert RL, Hayes PE, et al. Pharmacotherapy: A Pathophysiologic Approach, 9th ed. New York: McGraw-Hill, 2014:chap 52.

3. Pacchiarotti I, Bond DJ, Baldessarini RJ, et al. The International Society for Bipolar Disorders (ISBD) Task Force Report on Antidepressant Use in Bipolar Disorders. 2013;170:1249-62.

4. Yatham LN, Kennedy SH, Parikh SV, et al. Canadian Network for Mood and Anxiety Treatments (CANMAT) and International Society for Bipolar Disorders (ISBD) collaborative update of CANMAT guidelines for the management of patients with bipolar disorder: update 2013. Bipolar Disord 2013;15:1-44.

Schizophrenia

1. Buchanan RW, Kreyenbuhl JM, Kelly DL, et al. The 2009 schizophrenia PORT psychopharmacological treatment. Recommendations and summary statements. Schizophrenia Bull 2010;36:71-93.

2. Crismon ML, Argo TR, Buckley PF. Schizophrenia. In: DiPiro JT, Talbert RL, Hayes PE, et al. Pharmacotherapy: A Pathophysiologic Approach, 9th ed. New York: McGraw-Hill, 2014:chap 50.

Anxiety Disorders

1. Bandelow B, Zohar J, Hollander E, et al. World Federation of Societies of Biological Psychiatry (WFSBP) guidelines for the pharmacological treatment of anxiety, obsessive-compulsive and post-traumatic stress disorders, first revision. World J Biol Psychiatry 2008;9:248-312.

2. Melton ST, Kirkwood CK. Anxiety disorders I: generalized anxiety, panic, and social anxiety disorders. In: DiPiro JT, Talbert RL, Hayes PE, et al. Pharmacotherapy: A Pathophysiologic Approach, 9th ed. New York: McGraw-Hill, 2014:chap 53.

3. Kirkwood CK, Melton ST, Wells BG. Anxiety disorders II: posttraumatic stress disorder and obsessive-compulsive disorder. In: DiPiro JT, Talbert RL, Hayes PE, et al. Pharmacotherapy: A Pathophysiologic Approach, 9th ed. New York: McGraw-Hill, 2014:chap 54.

Insomnia

1. Dopp JM, Philips BG. Sleep disorders. In: DiPiro JT, Talbert RL, Hayes PE, et al. Pharmacotherapy: A Pathophysiologic Approach, 9th ed. New York: McGraw-Hill, 2014:chap 55.

2. Sateia M, Nowell P. Insomnia. Lancet 2004;364:1959-73. This is a good review of the pathophysiology and treatment of insomnia. It also includes a discussion of nondrug interventions.

3. Schutte-Rodin S, Broch L, Buysse D, et al. Clinical guideline for the evaluation and management of chronic insomnia in adults. J Clin Sleep Med 2008;4:487-504.

Substance Use Disorders

1. Doering P, Li RM. Substance-related disorders I: overview, depressants, stimulant and hallucinogens. In: DiPiro JT, Talbert RL, Hayes PE, et al. Pharmacotherapy: A Pathophysiologic Approach, 9th ed. New York: McGraw-Hill, 2014:chap 48.

2. Doering P, Li RM. Substance-related disorders II: alcohol, nicotine, and caffeine. In: DiPiro JT, Talbert RL, Hayes PE, et al. Pharmacotherapy: A Pathophysiologic Approach, 9th ed. New York: McGraw-Hill, 2014:chap 49.

3. Fiore MC, Jaén CR, Baker TB, et al. Treating tobacco use and dependence: 2008 update—a clinical practice guideline. Rockville, MD: U.S. Department of Health and Human Services; 2008 May.

4. Kosten T, O'Connor P. Management of drug and alcohol withdrawal. N Engl J Med 2003;348:1786-95.

5. McNicholas L. Clinical Guidelines for the Use of Buprenorphine in the Treatment of Opioid Addiction TIP 40. Rockville, MD: U.S. Department of Health and Human Services, 2004.

6. Miller NS. Detoxification and Substance Abuse Treatment. TIP 45. Rockville, MD: U.S. Department of Health and Human Services, 2013.

7. Reoux JP, Miller K. Routine hospital alcohol detoxication practice compared to symptom triggered management with an objective withdrawal scale (CIWA-Ar). Am J Addict 2000;9:135-44.

8. Sullivan JT, Sykora K, Schneiderman J, et al. Assessment of alcohol withdrawal: the revised clinical institute withdrawal assessment for alcohol scale (CIWA-Ar). Br J Addict 1989;84:1353-7.

ANSWERS AND EXPLANATIONS TO PATIENT CASES

1. Answer: A
Benztropine or another anticholinergic should be given to reverse the symptoms of EPS (neck stiffness, extreme restlessness) (Answer A is correct). Haloperidol is an FGA and would be expected to worsen the symptoms (Answer B is incorrect). Although the incidence of EPS is low with quetiapine, it will not help resolve this patient's current symptoms (Answer D is incorrect). Propranolol is useful for akathisia but not for other types of EPS (Answer C is incorrect).

2. Answer: B
Risperidone has less risk of EPS than haloperidol/FGAs, but it has the greatest risk among the SGAs (Answer A is incorrect). Risperidone is effective for negative symptoms, like other SGAs, and can be dosed once daily after reaching the target dose. However, for this patient with a significant history of nonadherence, the most likely reason for initiating risperidone is to eventually convert him to the long-acting injection formulation (Risperdal Consta), given twice a month (Answer B is correct; Answers C and D are incorrect).

3. Answer: C
Risperidone is more likely to cause EPS than are other SGAs (Answer C is correct). Risperidone may cause some sedation but not appreciably so (Answer A is incorrect). Anticholinergic effects are minimal with risperidone (Answer B is incorrect). Although all antipsychotics can potentially cause QTc prolongation, they rarely cause problems in patients without risk factors (Answer D is incorrect).

4. Answer: D
Quetiapine is most appropriate, given the patient's history of dystonia and akathisia with haloperidol (Answer D is correct). Quetiapine has a lower risk of causing EPS than FGAs such as fluphenazine (Answer B is incorrect). Clozapine and olanzapine have low risks of EPS as well, but clozapine is reserved for treatment-resistant cases (Answer A is incorrect). Olanzapine is not preferred because of the significant metabolic risks in this young patient (Answer C is incorrect).

5. Answer: C
Paroxetine has the most interaction with this patient's current medications because of its interaction with hydrocodone by inhibition of the CYP2D6 isoenzyme (Answer C is correct). This will result in a lack of analgesic effects from the opiate. Fluvoxamine is a CYP1A2 inhibitor that does not interact with thiazides, metformin, or opiates (Answer B is incorrect). Citalopram has no appreciable effects on any of this patient's medications (Answer A is incorrect). The effect of sertraline, although it may compete with that of hydromorphone (metabolite of hydrocodone) through CYP3A4, is less than that of paroxetine (Answer D is incorrect).

6. Answer: C
Mirtazapine is appropriate because it can improve this patient's insomnia and poor appetite (Answer C is correct). In addition, mirtazapine has no drug-drug interactions with the patient's current medications. Bupropion, fluoxetine, and venlafaxine would worsen her insomnia (Answers A, B, and D are incorrect). At doses greater than 150 mg daily, venlafaxine would worsen hypertension (Answer D is incorrect), and bupropion would worsen decreased appetite (Answer A is incorrect).

7. Answer: B
The citalopram dose should be increased to 40 mg/day because this patient has had some initial response to the drug (improvement in insomnia and appetite) but may not have reached the maximal tolerated dose (Answer B is correct). The patient has been taking citalopram for only 4 weeks, possibly at a subtherapeutic dose (Answer A is incorrect). Bupropion can be added later, after the patient has reached a maximal tolerated dose of citalopram for 6–8 weeks (which is a therapeutic trial) (Answer C is incorrect). Switching SSRIs may also be an option after the maximal tolerated dose of citalopram is reached (Answer D is incorrect).

8. Answer: B
The patient still needs an antidepressant, and discontinuing citalopram without an alternative agent at 6 months is inappropriate (Answer A is incorrect). Bupropion can be added to treat the anorgasmia and may even provide augmentation effects (Answer B is correct). Switching to a different SSRI may also produce the same adverse

effect because the anorgasmia appears to be caused by serotonergic activity (Answer C is incorrect). Switching to mirtazapine is not appropriate because the patient has had a therapeutic response and has been doing well for 6 months (Answer D is incorrect).

9. Answer: C
Lithium should be initiated to treat the current manic phase and prevent future episodes (Answer C is correct). Carbamazepine is effective for maintenance treatment but considered second or third line for acute mania (Answer A is incorrect). Divalproex is also good for maintenance treatment, but given this patient's history of hepatitis C, it is not a good choice (Answer B is incorrect). Lamotrigine is also effective for maintenance but not for treating the patient's current manic phase (Answer D is incorrect).

10. Answer: B
Coarse tremor may indicate lithium toxicity and would require an immediate evaluation of the patient's lithium concentration (Answer B is correct). Lithium can cause hypothyroidism, severe acne, and weight gain, but these can generally be managed with lifestyle modifications or medications (Answers A, C, and D are incorrect).

11. Answer: C
This patient appears to have symptoms of lithium toxicity, and a lithium concentration should be ordered immediately (Answer C is correct). Certainly, medications that may worsen the condition (e.g., lisinopril, zolpidem, ibuprofen) may be discontinued later (Answers A, B, and D are incorrect).

12. Answer: A
Paroxetine should be continued at this time because the patient is being successfully treated for depression, and paroxetine is considered a first-line agent for PTSD (Answer A is correct). Sertraline also treats PTSD, but there is no reason to discontinue paroxetine (Answer B is incorrect). Adding adjunctive agents such as lorazepam and buspirone is not indicated because paroxetine was initiated only 3 weeks ago (Answers C and D are incorrect).

13. Answer: C
Anticonvulsants such as divalproex sodium are often used to treat symptoms of irritability and aggression in

patients with PTSD (Answer C is correct). Buspirone is generally ineffective for these symptoms of PTSD and is used for GAD (Answer A is incorrect). Clonazepam can be used for short periods for anxiety; however, it is generally not used to target these symptoms of aggression (Answer B is incorrect). Lithium may be able to control the mood lability, but it requires close monitoring (Answer D is incorrect).

14. Answer: D
Buspirone is not a benzodiazepine and does not have much dependence potential (Answer D is correct). Buspirone does not work in relieving nightmares (Answer A is incorrect), and it is dosed three times daily (Answer C is incorrect). It also takes about 2 weeks for the onset of effect (Answer B is incorrect).

15. Answer: A
Clomipramine is the most serotonergic drug of the choices provided and is highly effective for OCD (Answer A is correct; Answers B–D are incorrect).

16. Answer: D
The patient is taking levothyroxine at nighttime, which is most likely contributing to the patient's insomnia (Answer D is correct). Hydrochlorothiazide and ibuprofen are not significantly associated with causing insomnia (Answers B and C are incorrect). Citalopram may contribute to insomnia in certain patients, but this patient is taking it in the morning, which decreases the risk (Answer A is incorrect).

17. Answer: A
The patient does not want a drug with significant daytime sedation, but she needs a drug that will help her stay asleep throughout the night. Eszopiclone is the best option (Answer A is correct). Trazodone has a long half-life that will help her stay asleep but has fewer efficacy data for insomnia (Answer B is incorrect). Temazepam causes daytime sedation (Answer C is incorrect). Zaleplon does not cause daytime sedation, but the short half-life of the drug will not help her stay asleep (Answer D is incorrect).

18. Answer: C
Zolpidem and other sedative-hypnotics have been associated with abnormal behaviors such as eating, driving, having sex, and talking on the telephone while asleep

(Answer C is correct). Zolpidem may cause orthostasis and disorientation, but when taken appropriately, it does not cause significant problems (Answers A and B are incorrect). Zolpidem at high doses has been associated with seizures, but this patient has no history of drug abuse or of using high doses of medications (Answer D is incorrect).

19. Answer: C
The initial symptoms of alcohol withdrawal include hemodynamic instability such as elevated heart rate and blood pressure (Answer C is correct). Alcohol craving, delirium tremens, and seizures generally occur after 12 hours of abstinence (Answers A, B, and D, respectively, are incorrect).

20. Answer: D
Lorazepam can be given intramuscularly and is appropriate because of the patient's liver abnormalities (Answer D is correct). Lorazepam undergoes glucuronidation and does not rely on oxidative pathways for metabolism. Chlordiazepoxide and diazepam are not available in intramuscular formulations and should be avoided in patients with liver disease (Answers A and C are incorrect). Clonazepam is generally not used for alcohol withdrawal and is not given intramuscularly (Answer B is incorrect).

21. Answer: D
Thiamine should be administered before fluids containing glucose to prevent Wernicke-Korsakoff syndrome (Answer D is correct). Folate, a multivitamin supplement, and B_{12} are also helpful but can be given after fluids (Answers A–C are incorrect).

22. Answer: A
Given the patient's liver disease, acamprosate is most appropriate because it does not rely on hepatic metabolism (Answer A is correct). Disulfiram and naltrexone are not generally recommended in patients with liver disease (Answers C and D are incorrect). Diazepam is not used for alcohol dependence but is used during alcohol withdrawal (Answer B is incorrect).

ANSWERS AND EXPLANATIONS TO SELF-ASSESSMENT QUESTIONS

1. Answer: B

Fluoxetine's adverse effect profile most closely counteracts the patient's symptoms. She additionally has anxiety, so fluoxetine may concomitantly relieve her symptoms of anxiety and allow her to stop taking benzodiazepine (Answer B is correct). Paroxetine can increase appetite and cause somnolence (Answer D is incorrect), as can mirtazapine (Answer C is incorrect). Although her suicidal ideation is intermittent and passive, desipramine can be fatal in an overdose situation (Answer A is incorrect).

2. Answer: B

Duloxetine is the best choice because it is also indicated for diabetic neuropathy (Answer B is correct). Although nortriptyline is also used to treat neuropathy, it is not a good choice in a patient with cardiovascular disease. It could also cause weight gain (Answer C is incorrect). Although bupropion is either weight neutral or can lead to some weight loss, the data are not strong for use in neuropathy (Answer A is incorrect). Sertraline is safe in this patient and could be used as an alternative to citalopram, but it has no utility in the treatment of neuropathy (Answer D is incorrect).

3. Answer: D

This patient is experiencing serotonin syndrome (myoclonus, agitation, diaphoresis). The symptoms are probably caused by adding dextromethorphan to paroxetine. In addition to the serotonergic activity of both agents, paroxetine inhibits CYP2D6, which is responsible for metabolizing dextromethorphan. This further increases the serotonergic activity (Answer D is correct). None of the other choices represents a combination of serotonergic agents, nor do they interact in a fashion that would cause a rise in serotonergic activity (Answers A–C are incorrect).

4. Answer: C

This patient is experiencing an acute depressive episode despite therapeutic lithium concentrations. He has been taking lithium for 5 years, which is long enough to derive any antidepressant effects. Quetiapine is FDA indicated for depression associated with bipolar disorder (Answer C is correct). Its onset of action is more rapid than that of lamotrigine, which requires a slow titration to reach therapeutic doses (Answer B

is incorrect). Unlike data for unipolar depression, data for aripiprazole suggest it is not effective for bipolar depression (Answer A is incorrect). The efficacy of antidepressants in treating type I bipolar disorder is questionable, and treatment with an SNRI could lead to a switch to mania (Answer D is incorrect).

5. Answer: A

This patient is experiencing hypothyroidism, as indicated by her elevated TSH. This is probably induced by lithium (Answer A is correct). Although olanzapine can cause a metabolic syndrome with glucose intolerance and obesity, it would not cause an elevation in her TSH (Answer C is incorrect). Lithium-induced hypothyroidism is not dose-dependent, and the patient's lithium concentration is on the lower side of the 0.6–1.0 mEq/L maintenance range (Answer B is incorrect). Yasmin (ethinyl estradiol/drospirenone) is not associated with elevations in TSH (Answer D is incorrect).

6. Answer: B

This patient's presentation and laboratory results are consistent with acute pancreatitis. Although the incidence is rare, divalproex can cause pancreatitis. Patients who develop pancreatitis on divalproex that resolves when the patient is off the agent should not be rechallenged (Answer B is correct). Neither aripiprazole nor lamotrigine is associated with pancreatitis (Answers A and C are incorrect). This patient's lamotrigine dose should be lowered to prevent Stevens-Johnson syndrome. Despite lamotrigine's temporal relationship with prednisone, it is not likely contributing to the current clinical picture (Answer D is incorrect).

7. Answer: D

The symptoms most closely resemble akathisia. The treatment of choice in this case is a lipophilic β-blocker such as propranolol (Answer D is correct). Benztropine is an anticholinergic agent that can be used for other movement disorders, such as dystonias or Parkinsonian symptoms, but it is not effective for acathisia (Answer A is incorrect). Benzodiazepines are also used to treat akathisia, but they are not the best choice given this patient's history of alcohol use disorder (Answer C is incorrect). Dantrolene is used for neuroleptic malignant syndrome (Answer B is incorrect).

8. Answer: B
This patient is experiencing severe tardive dyskinesia. The symptoms involve the orofacial muscles and came on slowly after antipsychotics had been initiated. The symptoms improved with antipsychotic dose reduction. The antipsychotic of choice in patients with severe tardive dyskinesia is clozapine because of its low to nonexistent incidence of tardive dyskinesia (Answer B is correct). Chlorpromazine is also an FGA associated with tardive dyskinesia (Answer A is incorrect). Although risperidone is associated with a lesser degree of EPS, it can cause tardive dyskinesia (Answer D is incorrect). Although quetiapine has a low incidence of tardive dyskinesia, it is not the agent of choice in severe tardive dyskinesia, particularly in a patient whose therapy with an FGA (perphenazine) and an SGA (olanzapine) has previously failed (Answer C is incorrect).

9. Answer: D
This patient has diabetes, dyslipidemia, and obesity, all factors that contribute to metabolic syndrome. With her family history of early coronary artery disease, she would best be served by an antipsychotic with a low incidence of metabolic syndrome. Of the antipsychotics listed, ziprasidone is the best choice (Answer D is correct). Olanzapine is associated with a high incidence of metabolic syndrome (Answer A is incorrect). Quetiapine has a lower incidence but can still cause metabolic abnormalities (Answer C is incorrect). Paliperidone is the major metabolite of risperidone and has a similar pharmacologic profile. Like risperidone, it is associated with an elevated incidence of galactorrhea (Answer B is incorrect).

10. Answer: A
This patient has panic disorder. Benzodiazepines more rapidly treat the acute physical symptoms and fear that occur with panic disorder (Answer A is correct). Selective serotonin reuptake inhibitors such as paroxetine are first-line treatment for preventing panic attacks but take time to achieve full efficacy (Answer D is incorrect). Buspirone is not effective for panic attacks (Answer B is incorrect). Hydroxyzine may offer some sedation, but it is ineffective to treat the underlying anxiety disorder (Answer C is incorrect).

11. Answer: D
An antidepressant is the first-line treatment for GAD. Venlafaxine is the agent of choice for several reasons. It has demonstrated efficacy against GAD. In addition, it may offer some relief against this patient's vasomotor symptoms (Answer D is correct). Fluoxetine is an effective choice for GAD but is a strong inhibitor of CYP2D6. This would decrease the efficacy of tamoxifen (Answer B is incorrect). Bupropion is also an inhibitor of CYP2D6 and is not effective against most anxiety disorders (Answer A is incorrect). Pregabalin may be effective for GAD, but it is generally used as a second- or third-line agent (Answer C is incorrect).

12. Answer: B
This patient primarily has difficulty with sleep onset and would benefit from an agent that decreases sleep latency and does not prolong sleep. Ramelteon is the only one of the listed agents that does this. Older adults can have difficulty with circadian rhythm, and a melatonin analog may help regulate this. It is also indicated for treatment of chronic insomnia if needed for a prolonged period (Answer B is correct). Although eszopiclone decreases time to sleep, it is also designed to improve sleep maintenance and may result in hangover effects (Answer A is incorrect). Suvorexant also treats sleep maintenance, but it can cause a hangover effect (Answer C is incorrect). Zolpidem received recent labeling changes for reduced doses and has reduced metabolism in older adults (Answer D is incorrect).

13. Answer: D
To avoid withdrawal symptoms, patients taking long-acting opioids should be tapered to the equivalent of methadone 30 mg/day or less before being switched to a buprenorphine regimen (Answer D is correct). Initiating a patient on buprenorphine at higher doses of methadone may precipitate withdrawal because of the higher binding affinity of buprenorphine for the mu receptor with less activity and the added antagonism at the kappa receptor (Answer B is incorrect). Patients taking long-acting opioids such as methadone should be switched to buprenorphine monotherapy before being advanced to buprenorphine/naloxone (Answer A is incorrect). Naltrexone monotherapy is not appropriate because it can precipitate withdrawal (Answer C is incorrect).

14. Answer: D

This patient has alcoholic hepatitis, as indicated by his AST and ALT values. Presumably, these would improve with abstinence. Liver function is intact, as evidenced by his albumin, PT, and platelet values. Naltrexone can be given to patients with hepatic dysfunction. Hepatic function would need to be monitored (Answer D is correct). Disulfiram should be used with caution in patients with active liver disease. It also requires a strong commitment on the patient's part to abstain from drinking and may be less effective. This patient has a history of several failed attempts (Answer C is incorrect). The acamprosate dose should be reduced to 333 mg orally three times daily for a CrCl of 30–50 mL/minute/1.73 m^2 (Answer A is incorrect). Chlordiazepoxide is used during acute alcohol detoxification but has no role in maintenance therapy (Answer B is incorrect).

15. Answer: A

This patient's previous quit attempt with nicotine gum was probably unsuccessful because the gum strength (2 mg) and frequency of use (less than 9 pieces/day) were too low to support a successful attempt. Thus, his previous use of nicotine gum is not a true treatment failure. Nevertheless, he has concomitant depression, so bupropion is a reasonable choice (Answer A is correct). His MI is not a contraindication to using nicotine products; thus, nicotine gum could be added to bupropion if monotherapy fails (Answers B and C are incorrect). Coronary artery disease is not a contraindication to varenicline therapy, but because bupropion has not been previously used, it should be tried first (Answer D is incorrect).

Endocrine and Metabolic Disorders

Brian K. Irons, Pharm.D., FCCP, BCACP, BC-ADM

Texas Tech University Health Sciences Center
School of Pharmacy
Lubbock, Texas

ENDOCRINE AND METABOLIC DISORDERS

BRIAN K. IRONS, PHARM.D., FCCP, BCACP, BC-ADM

TEXAS TECH UNIVERSITY HEALTH SCIENCES CENTER
SCHOOL OF PHARMACY
LUBBOCK, TEXAS

Learning Objectives

1. Differentiate between the diagnostic and classification criteria for various endocrine and metabolic disorders, including type 1 and type 2 diabetes mellitus, diabetes insipidus, polycystic ovary syndrome, obesity, and disorders of the thyroid, adrenal, and pituitary glands.
2. Review the various therapeutic agents used in treating endocrine and metabolic disorders.
3. Select appropriate treatment and monitoring options for a given patient presenting with one of the above endocrine or metabolic disorders.
4. Recommend appropriate therapeutic management for secondary complications from diabetes or thyroid disorders.

Self-Assessment Questions

Answers and explanations to these questions can be found at the end of this chapter.

1. A 66-year-old Hispanic man with a history of myocardial infarction, dyslipidemia, and hypertension received a diagnosis of type 2 diabetes mellitus (DM). After 1 month of exercise and dietary changes and no diabetes medications, his hemoglobin A1C and fasting glucose concentration today are 11.5% and 362 mg/dL, respectively. He weighs 123.8 kg, with a body mass index (BMI) of 42 kg/m². Which set of drugs is best to initiate?

    A. Metformin and glipizide.
    B. Glipizide and insulin glulisine.
    C. Pioglitazone and acarbose.
    D. Insulin detemir and glulisine.

2. A 21-year-old patient is given a diagnosis of type 1 DM after the discovery of elevated glucose concentrations (average 326 mg/dL) and is showing signs and symptoms of hyperglycemia. Her weight is 80 kg. Which is the most appropriate initial dosage of rapid-acting insulin before breakfast for this patient? Assume a total daily insulin (TDI) regimen of 0.5 unit/kg/day.

    A. 2 units.
    B. 4 units.
    C. 7 units.
    D. 14 units.

3. A patient with type 2 DM has a blood pressure reading of 152/84 mm Hg, a serum creatinine of 1.8 mg/dL, and two recent spot urine albumin/creatinine concentrations of 420 and 395 mg/g. Which class of drugs (barring any contraindications) is best to initiate in this patient?

    A. Thiazide diuretic.
    B. Dihydropyridine calcium channel blocker.
    C. Angiotensin receptor blocker (ARB).
    D. Nondihydropyridine calcium channel blocker.

4. Regarding propylthiouracil (PTU) and methimazole in the treatment of hyperthyroidism, which statement is most appropriate?

    A. PTU is clinically superior to methimazole in efficacy.
    B. PTU may be associated with greater liver toxicity than methimazole.
    C. Both agents are equally efficacious in the treatment of Hashimoto's disease.
    D. Both medications should be administered three times daily.

5. Which medication is the most appropriate choice for a patient with a diagnosis of Cushing's syndrome who did not experience adequate symptom relief after surgical resection for a pituitary adenoma?

    A. Ketoconazole.
    B. Spironolactone.
    C. Hydrocortisone.
    D. Bromocriptine.

6. A physician is asking for a recommendation for initial therapy for a patient with type 2 DM. The physician states that metformin is no longer an option for this patient. An A1C obtained today is 9.4% (personal goal 7%), and the patient's estimated glomerular filtration rate (eGFR) is 29 mL/min. Which of the following agents would be the best recommendation?

    A. Canagliflozin.
    B. Alogliptin.
    C. Glargine.
    D. Exenatide.

7. A 76-year-old woman recently given a diagnosis of Hashimoto's disease presents with mild symptoms of lethargy, weight gain, and intolerance to cold. Her thyroid-stimulating hormone (TSH) level is 12.2 mIU/L, and her free thyroxine (T_4) is below normal limits. Her current weight is 47 kg. She has a history of hypertension and underwent a coronary artery bypass surgery 2 years ago. Which would be the most appropriate initial treatment for this patient?

    A. Levothyroxine 25 mcg once daily.

    B. Levothyroxine 75 mcg once daily.

    C. Liothyronine 25 mcg once daily.

    D. Liothyronine 75 mcg once daily.

8. A woman with type 2 DM has an A1C of 8.6%. She is receiving insulin glargine (60 units once daily at bedtime) and insulin aspart (8 units before breakfast, 7 units before lunch, and 12 units before dinner). She is consistent in her carbohydrate intake at each meal. Her morning fasting plasma glucose (FPG) and premeal blood glucose (BG) readings have consistently averaged 112 mg/dL. Her bedtime readings are averaging between 185 and 200 mg/dL. Which is the best insulin adjustment to improve her overall glycemic control?

    A. Increase her prebreakfast aspart to 10 units.

    B. Increase her predinner aspart to 14 units.

    C. Increase her bedtime glargine to 65 units.

    D. Increase her prelunch aspart to 9 units.

9. A 53-year-old woman with a history of Graves' disease underwent ablative therapy 3 years ago. She experienced significant symptom relief and became euthyroid. Her thyroid laboratory values today include TSH 0.12 mIU/L (normal 0.5–4.5 mIU/L) and a free T_4 concentration of 3.8 g/dL (normal 0.8–1.9 ng/dL). She states that many of her previous symptoms have returned but are mild. Which would be the most appropriate treatment for her condition?

    A. Methimazole.

    B. Thyroidectomy.

    C. Propylthiouracil.

    D. Metoprolol.

10. A 65-year-old man with type 2 DM has been receiving metformin 1000 mg twice daily for the past 2 years. His A1C today is 7.8%. His morning fasting blood glucose (FBG) readings are consistently at goal. His after-meal glucose readings average 190–200 mg/dL. Which option would be most appropriate for this patient?

    A. Increase metformin to 1000 mg three times daily.

    B. Add insulin glargine 10 units once daily.

    C. Switch from metformin to insulin glargine 10 units once daily.

    D. Add saxagliptin 5 mg once daily.

11. A 34-year-old woman has a BMI of 33 kg/m². With dietary changes, she has lost 2 lb in 6 months. She exercises regularly but is unable to do more because she has two jobs and young children. Her medical history is significant for depression, type 2 DM, and substance abuse. Her current medications include metformin 1000 mg twice daily, aspirin 81 mg once daily, and sertraline 100 mg once daily. She is most concerned about weight loss. Which would be the best recommendation to help her lose weight?

    A. Continue her diet and exercise routine; additional intervention is unwarranted.

    B. Initiate lorcaserin 10 mg twice daily.

    C. Initiate phentermine/topiramate 3.75/23 mg once daily.

    D. Initiate orlistat 120 mg three times daily with meals.

12. A 53-year-old Hispanic woman has a BMI of 44 kg/m² and a history of gestational diabetes. Her mother and sister both have type 2 DM. Two weeks ago she had an A1C of 7.4%. Her fasting glucose concentration is 178 mg/dL. She is asymptomatic. Which is the best course of action?

    A. Diagnose type 2 DM and begin treatment.

    B. Diagnose type 1 DM and begin treatment.

    C. Obtain another A1C today.

    D. Obtain another glucose concentration another day.

13. A 42-year-old man has a history of type 2 DM. His current therapy includes metformin 1000 mg twice daily, glyburide 10 mg twice daily, and aspirin 81 mg once daily. Today, his A1C is 6.9%, blood pressure is 126/78 mm Hg, and fasting lipid panel is as follows: total cholesterol 212 mg/dL, low-density lipoprotein cholesterol (LDL-C) 98 mg/dL, high-density lipoprotein cholesterol (HDL-C) 45 mg/dL, and triglycerides (TG) 145 mg/dL. Which would be the most appropriate choice for this patient?

A. Add insulin detemir 10 units once daily.

B. Add lisinopril 10 mg once daily.

C. Add atorvastatin 10 mg once daily.

D. Add fenofibrate 145 mg once daily.

BPS Pharmacotherapy Specialty Examination Content Outline

This chapter covers the following sections of the Pharmacotherapy Specialty Examination Content Outline:

1. Domain 1: Patient-Centered Pharmacotherapy
   a. Task 1 with Knowledge of:
      1) Anatomy, physiology, and pathophysiology
      2) Disease processes, including drug-induced diseases
      3) Pharmacology and toxicology
      5) Evidence-based standards of care and clinical pathways
      7) Allergies and adverse drug reactions
      11) Interpretation of laboratory tests, diagnostics, and procedures
      12) Drug interactions
      14) Nonpharmacologic treatments
      15) Preventive care (e.g. screening, immunizations)
      17) Patient-specific goals of care and prioritization of needs
   b. Task 4 with Knowledge of:
      1) Response to therapy and implications for therapeutic goals
      2) Interpretation of laboratory tests, diagnostics, and procedures
      3) Changes in patient clinical status
      4) Disease progression or resolution
      5) Drug interactions
      6) Adverse drug reactions
   c. Systems and Patient-Care Problems:
      - Thyroid Disorders
      - Diabetes Insipidus
      - Pituitary Gland Disorders
      - Adrenal Gland Disorders
      - Obesity
      - Polycystic Ovary Syndrome
      - Diabetes Mellitus (Type 1 and 2)
      - Treatment of DM Complications
2. Domain 3: System-based Standards and Population-based Pharmacotherapy
   a. Task 1 with Knowledge of
      2) Laws and regulations

Endocrine and Metabolic Disorders

I. THYROID DISORDERS

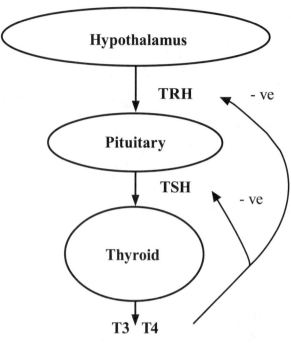

Figure 1. Hypothalamus-pituitary-thyroid axis.[a]

[a]T_4 is converted to T_3 by peripheral tissue. Only unbound (free) thyroid hormone is biologically active.

T_3 = triiodothyronine; T_4 = thyroxine; TRH = thyrotropin-releasing hormone; TSH = thyroid-stimulating hormone; - ve = negative feedback loop.

Patient Case

1. A 43-year-old woman has received a diagnosis of Graves' disease. She is reluctant to try ablative therapy and wants to attempt oral pharmacotherapy first. Her thyroid laboratory values today include TSH 0.22 mIU/L (normal 0.5–4.5 mIU/L) and a free T_4 concentration of 3.2 ng/dL (normal 0.8–1.9 ng/dL). She is anxious and always feels warm when others say it is too cold. Which would be considered the best drug for initial treatment of her condition?

    A. Lugols solution.

    B. Propylthiouracil (PTU).

    C. Atenolol.

    D. Methimazole.

A. Hyperthyroid Disorders (Thyrotoxicosis)
    1. Classification
        a. Toxic diffuse goiter (Graves' disease): Most common hyperthyroid disorder
            i.   Autoimmune disorder
            ii. Thyroid-stimulating antibodies directed at thyrotropin receptors mimic thyroid-stimulating hormone (TSH) and stimulate triiodothyronine/thyroxine (T_3/T_4) production.
        b. Pituitary adenomas: Produce excessive TSH secretion that does not respond to normal T_3 negative feedback
        c. Toxic adenoma: Nodule in thyroid, autonomous of pituitary and TSH

    d. Toxic multinodular goiter (Plummer disease): Several autonomous follicles that, if large enough, cause excessive thyroid hormone secretion

    e. Painful subacute thyroiditis: Self-limiting inflammation of the thyroid gland caused by viral invasion of the parenchyma, resulting in the release of stored hormone

    f. Drug induced (e.g., excessive exogenous thyroid hormone dosages, amiodarone therapy)

2. Diagnosis

    a. Elevated free T_4 serum concentrations

    b. Suppressed TSH concentrations (except in TSH-secreting adenomas)

    c. If examination and history do not provide the exact etiology, radioactive iodine uptake may be used.

        i. Radioactive iodine uptake elevated if thyroid gland is actively and excessively secreting T_4 and/or T_3: Graves' disease, TSH-secreting adenoma, toxic adenoma, multinodular goiter

        ii. Radioactive iodine uptake is suppressed in disorders caused by thyroiditis or hormone ingestion.

    d. Can also assess for the presence of various thyroid-related antibodies (thyroid stimulating, thyrotropin receptor, or thyroperoxidase), thyroglobulin, and thyroid biopsy

3. Clinical presentation

    a. Weight loss or increased appetite

    b. Lid lag

    c. Heat intolerance

    d. Goiter

    e. Fine hair

    f. Heart palpitations or tachycardia

    g. Nervousness, anxiety, insomnia

    h. Menstrual disturbances (lighter or more infrequent menstruation, amenorrhea) caused by hypermetabolism of estrogen

    i. Sweating or warm, moist skin

    j. Exophthalmos, pretibial myxedema in Graves' disease

4. Therapy goals

    a. Minimize or eliminate symptoms, improve quality of life.

    b. Minimize long-term damage to organs (heart disease, arrhythmias, sudden cardiac death, bone demineralization, and fractures).

    c. Normalize free T_4 and TSH concentrations.

5. Therapeutics

    a. Ablative therapy: Treatment of choice for Graves' disease, toxic nodule, multinodular goiter: Radioactive iodine ablative therapy and surgical resection for adenomas according to patient preferences or comorbidities. Ablative therapy often results in hypothyroidism.

    b. Antithyroid pharmacotherapy usually reserved for

        i. Those awaiting ablative therapy or surgical resection

          (a) Depletes stored hormone

          (b) Minimizes risk of posttreatment hyperthyroidism caused by thyroiditis

        ii. Those who are not an ablative or surgical candidates (e.g., serious cardiovascular disease, candidate unlikely to be adherent to radiation safety)

        iii. When ablative therapy or surgical resection fails to normalize thyroid function

        iv. Those with a high probability of remission with oral therapy for Graves' disease

          (a) Mild disease

          (b) Small goiter

          (c) Low or negative antibody titers

     v. Those with limited life expectancy

     vi. Those with moderate to severe active Graves' ophthalmopathy

  c. Thioureas (i.e., propylthiouracil [PTU], methimazole)

     i. Mechanism of action: Inhibits iodination and synthesis of thyroid hormones; PTU may block T_4/T_3 conversion in the periphery as well.

     ii. Dosing

       (a) PTU

          (1) Initial: 100 mg by mouth three times daily

          (2) Maximal: 400 mg three times daily

          (3) Once euthyroid, may reduce to 50 mg two or three times daily

       (b) Methimazole

          (1) Preferred agent for Graves' disease according to the American Association of Clinical Endocrinologists (AACE) for most patients unless in first trimester of pregnancy, then use PTU

             (A) American Thyroid Association recommends PTU in first trimester because of risk of embryopathy.

             (B) Switch to methimazole in second trimester.

          (2) Initial: 10–20 mg by mouth once daily

          (3) Maximal: 40 mg three times daily

          (4) Once euthyroid, may reduce to 5–10 mg/day

       (c) Monthly dosage titrations as needed (based on symptoms and free T_4 concentrations); TSH may remain low months after therapy starts.

     iii. Adverse effects

       (a) Hepatotoxicity risk with PTU (boxed warning): AACE recommends baseline liver function tests. Routine evaluation of liver function while receiving antithyroid agents has not been shown to prevent severe hepatotoxicity.

       (b) Rash

       (c) Arthralgias, lupus-like symptoms

       (d) Fever

       (e) Agranulocytosis early in therapy (usually within 3 months): AACE recommends baseline complete blood cell count (CBC); no routine monitoring recommended. May repeat if patient becomes febrile or develops pharyngitis.

     iv. Efficacy

       (a) Slow onset in reducing symptoms (weeks). Maximal effect may take 4–6 months.

       (b) Neither drug appears superior to the other in efficacy.

       (c) On a milligram-to-milligram basis, methimazole is 10 times more potent than PTU.

       (d) Remission rates low: 20%–30%. Remission is defined as normal TSH and T_4 for 1 year after discontinuing antithyroid therapy.

       (e) Therapy duration in Graves' disease (oral agents unlikely to cause remission in those with nodular thyroid disease)

          (1) Usually 12–18 months; length of trial may not affect remission rate.

          (2) Consider trial off oral therapy if TSH is normal; antibody titers may help guide decision.

          (3) Monitor thyroid concentrations every 1–3 months for up to 12 months for relapse (abnormal TSH or T_4 return).

  d. Nonselective β-blockers (primarily propranolol; sometimes nadolol)

     i. Mechanism of action: Blocks many hyperthyroidism manifestations mediated by β-adrenergic receptors. Also may block (less active) T_4 conversion to (more active) T_3.

      ii. Propranolol dosing
        (a) Initial: 20–40 mg by mouth three or four times daily
        (b) Maximal: 240–480 mg/day
      iii. Adverse effects (see Hypertension section in Cardiology II chapter)
      iv. Efficacy
        (a) Used primarily for symptomatic relief (e.g., palpitations, tachycardia, tremor, anxiety)
        (b) Guidelines recommend use in symptomatic older adults and in others with heart rates greater than 90 beats/minute or existing cardiovascular disease, and consider use in all symptomatic patients. Recommended for use before ablative iodine therapy also in those who are extremely symptomatic or have a free T_4 two to three times the upper limit of normal.
        (c) Poor remission rates: 20%–35%
        (d) Primary role is treatment of thyroiditis, which is usually self-limiting, and for acute management of symptoms during thyroid storm (see below).
        (e) Alternatives to β-blockers: Clonidine, nondihydropyridine calcium channel blocker
  e. Iodines and iodides (e.g., Lugols solution, saturated solution of potassium iodide)
      i. Mechanism of action: Inhibits the release of stored thyroid hormone. Minimal effect on hormone synthesis. Helps decrease vascularity and size of gland before surgery.
      ii. Dosing
        (a) Lugols solution (6.3–8 mg iodide per drop)
        (b) Saturated solution of potassium iodide (38–50 mg iodide per drop)
        (c) Potassium iodide tablets: (130-mg tablets contain 100 mg of iodide)
        (d) Usual daily dosage: 120–400 mg mixed with juice or water, split three times daily
      iii. Adverse effects
        (a) Hypersensitivity
        (b) Metallic taste
        (c) Soreness or burning in mouth or tongue
        (d) Do not use in the days before ablative iodine therapy (may reduce uptake of radioactive iodine).
      iv. Efficacy
        (a) Limited efficacy after 7–14 days of therapy because thyroid hormone release will resume
        (b) Primary use is temporary before surgery (7–10 days) to shrink the gland.
        (c) Can be used after ablative therapy (3–7 days) to inhibit thyroiditis-mediated release of stored hormone
        (d) Used acutely in thyroid storm

B. Subclinical Hyperthyroidism
  1. Definition: Low (below lower limit of reference range) or undetectable TSH with normal T_4
  2. Risk
    a. Associated with elevated risk of atrial fibrillation in patients older than 60 years
    b. Associated with elevated risk of bone fracture in postmenopausal women
    c. Conflicting data about mortality risk
  3. Treatment (based on 2011 guidelines) similar to treating overt hyperthyroidism
    a. Oral antithyroid drug therapy alternative to ablative therapy in young patients with Graves' disease
    b. β-Blockers may be of benefit in controlling cardiovascular morbidity, especially with atrial fibrillation.
  4. If untreated, screen regularly for the development of overt hyperthyroidism (elevated free T_4 concentrations).

C. Thyroid Storm
1. Severe and life-threatening decompensated thyrotoxicosis. Mortality rate may be as high as 20%.
2. Precipitating causes: Trauma, infection, antithyroid agent withdrawal, severe thyroiditis, postablative therapy (especially if inadequate pretreatment)
3. Presentation: Fever, tachycardia, vomiting, dehydration, coma, tachypnea, delirium
4. Pharmacotherapy
   a. PTU
      i. 500- to 1000-mg loading dose, then 250 mg every 4 hours
      ii. Blocks new hormone synthesis
      iii. Can use methimazole 60–80 mg daily
   b. Iodide therapy 1 hour after PTU initiation (dosed as above) to block hormone release
   c. β-Blocker therapy: Propranolol or esmolol commonly used to control symptoms and block conversion of T_4 to T_3
   d. Acetaminophen as antipyretic therapy, if needed (avoid nonsteroidal anti-inflammatory drugs [NSAIDs] because of displacement of protein-bound thyroid hormones)
   e. Corticosteroid therapy: Prednisone 300 mg intravenous loading dose then 100 mg every 8 hours (or equivalent dosages of, e.g., dexamethasone, hydrocortisone). Prophylaxis against relative adrenal insufficiency and may block conversion of T_4 to T_3.

Patient Case

2. A 63-year-old woman has Hashimoto's disease. Her thyroid laboratory values today include the following: TSH 10.6 mIU/L (normal 0.5–4.5 mIU/L) and a free T_4 concentration of 0.5 ng/dL (normal 0.8–1.9 ng/dL). She feels consistently run down and has dry skin that does not respond to the use of hand creams. Which would be considered the best drug for initial treatment of her condition?

A. Levothyroxine.

B. Liothyronine.

C. Desiccated thyroid.

D. Methimazole.

D. Hypothyroid Disorders
1. Classification
   a. Hashimoto's disease: Most common hypothyroid disorder in areas with iodine sufficiency
      i. Autoimmune-induced thyroid injury resulting in decreased thyroid secretion
      ii. Disproportionately affects women
   b. Iatrogenic: Thyroid resection or radioiodine ablative therapy for treatment of hyperthyroidism
   c. Iodine deficiency most common cause worldwide
   d. Secondary causes
      i. Pituitary insufficiency (failure to produce adequate TSH secretion, referred to by some as central or secondary hypothyroidism)
      ii. Drug induced (e.g., amiodarone, lithium)
2. Diagnosis
   a. Low free T_4 serum concentrations
   b. Elevated TSH concentrations, usually above 10 mIU/L (normal or low if central hypothyroidism is the etiology)
   c. Thyroid antibodies such as antithyroid peroxidase and antithyroglobulin autoantibodies
   d. Screen patients older than 60, especially women (there are many different screening recommendations by various professional groups with little consensus).

3. Clinical presentation
   a. Cold intolerance
   b. Dry skin
   c. Fatigue, lethargy, weakness
   d. Weight gain
   e. Bradycardia
   f. Slow reflexes
   g. Coarse skin and hair
   h. Periorbital swelling
   i. Menstrual disturbances (more frequent or longer menstruation, painful menstruation, menorrhagia) caused by hypometabolism of estrogen
   j. Goiter (primary hypothyroidism)
4. Therapy goals
   a. Minimize or eliminate symptoms; improve quality of life.
   b. Minimize long-term damage to organs (myxedema coma, heart disease).
   c. Normalize free T_4 and TSH concentrations.
5. Therapeutics
   a. Levothyroxine (drug of choice)
      i. Mechanism of action: Synthetic T_4
      ii. Dosing
         (a) Initial
            (1) In otherwise healthy adults, 1.6 mcg/kg (use ideal body weight) per day.
            (2) In patients 50–60 years of age, consider 50 mcg/day.
            (3) In those with existing cardiovascular disease, consider 12.5–25 mcg/day.
         (b) Usually dosed in the morning on an empty stomach 30–60 minutes before breakfast or at bedtime 4 hours after last meal; dosed separately from other medications (particularly calcium or iron supplements and antacids)
         (c) Dosage titration based on response (control of symptoms, normalization of TSH and free T_4)
         (d) Can increase or decrease in 12.5- to 25-mcg/day increments
         (e) Daily requirements are higher in pregnancy (separate guidelines available for treating thyroid disorders in pregnancy).
      iii. Monitoring
         (a) 4–8 weeks is appropriate to assess patient response in TSH after initiating or changing therapy (about a 7-day half-life for T_4). May take longer for TSH to achieve steady-state concentrations
         (b) Use free T_4 rather than TSH if central or secondary hypothyroidism; obtain sample before daily dosing of levothyroxine.
      iv. Adverse effects
         (a) Hyperthyroidism
         (b) Cardiac abnormalities (tachyarrhythmias, angina, myocardial infarction)
         (c) Linked to risk of fractures (usually at higher dosages or oversupplementation)
      v. Efficacy: If levothyroxine is properly dosed, most patients will maintain TSH and free T_4 in the normal ranges and experience symptomatic relief.
      vi. Considered drug of choice because of its adverse effect profile, cost, lack of antigenicity, and uniform potency
      vii. Bioequivalency
         (a) AACE recommends brand-name levothyroxine (none of the other thyroid preparations below are supported by AACE).

       (b)   Although legal, guidelines recommend against changing from brand to generic and vice versa. It is recommended to stay with one product throughout therapy.

       (c)   TSH concentrations in bioequivalence testing were never performed; small changes in T_4 between products may result in significant changes in TSH. Pharmacokinetic studies were conducted in normal subjects with normal thyroid function.

    b.   Liothyronine (synthetic T_3), liotrix (synthetic T_4/T_3), desiccated thyroid are not recommended by leading professional organizations or clinical guidelines.

E.   Subclinical Hypothyroidism
1.   Definition: Elevated TSH (above upper limit of reference range) with normal T_4. Often the result of early Hashimoto's disease
2.   Risk
    a.   TSH greater than 7.0 mIU/L in older adults associated with elevated risk of heart failure
    b.   TSH greater than 10 mIU/L associated with elevated risk of coronary heart disease
3.   Treatment of subclinical hypothyroidism is controversial because benefits in identified patients are inconclusive. An association between the use of levothyroxine and a reduction in heart disease in younger patients (40–70 years of age) does appear to exist, but not in older patients (older than 70 years).
4.   Whom to treat
    a.   TSH between 4.5 and 10 mIU/L and
       i.   Symptoms of hypothyroidism
       ii.   Antithyroid peroxidase antibodies present
       iii.   History of cardiovascular disease, heart failure, or risk factors for such
    b.   Initial daily dosages of 25–75 mcg recommended
5.   If untreated, screen regularly for the development of overt hypothyroidism (decreased free T_4 concentrations).

F.   Myxedema Coma
1.   Severe and life-threatening decompensated hypothyroidism. Mortality rate 30%–60%
2.   Precipitating causes: Trauma, infections, heart failure, medications (e.g., sedatives, narcotics, anesthesia, lithium, amiodarone)
3.   Presentation: Coma is not required and is uncommon, despite terminology; altered mental state (very common); diastolic hypertension; hypothermia; hypoventilation
4.   Pharmacotherapy
    a.   Intravenous thyroid hormone replacement
       i. T_4: 100- to 500-mcg loading dose, followed by 75–100 mcg/day, until patient can tolerate oral therapy. Lower the initial dose in frail patients or in patients with established cardiovascular disease.
       ii.   Some advocate the use of T_3 over T_4, given that T_3 is more biologically active and that T_4/T_3 conversion may be suppressed in myxedema coma. Cost and availability limit intravenous T_3 use.
    b.   Antibiotic therapy: Given common infectious causes, some advocate empiric therapy with broad-spectrum antibiotics.
    c.   Corticosteroid therapy
       i.   Hydrocortisone 100 mg every 8 hours (or equivalent steroid)
       ii.   Can be discontinued if random cortisol concentration not depressed

II. PITUITARY GLAND DISORDERS

Table 1. Basic Pituitary Gland (Anterior) Hormone Physiology

Anterior Pituitary Hormone	Primary Functions	Hypothalamic Stimulator	Primary Secretion Inhibitor
Growth hormone (GH)	Promote tissue growth	GH-releasing hormone	Somatostatin Elevated insulin-like growth factor-1
Adrenocorticotropic hormone (ACTH)	Stimulate adrenal cortisol and androgen release	Corticotropin-releasing hormone	Cortisol
Thyroid-stimulating hormone (TSH)	Metabolic stability	Thyrotropin-releasing hormone	Triiodothyronine
Prolactin	Regulate lactation	Thyrotropin-releasing hormone	Dopamine
Follicle-stimulating hormone	Maturation of ovarian follicles Sperm production	Gonadotropin-releasing hormone	Inhibin Estrogens
Luteinizing hormone	Secretion of sex steroids	Gonadotropin-releasing hormone	Estrogens and progestins Testosterone

A. Classification (focus on the common anterior pituitary disorders)
  1. Hypersecretory diseases
     a. Acromegaly and gigantism: Usually caused by growth hormone (GH)-secreting pituitary adenoma
     b. Hyperprolactinemia
        i. Most common cause is prolactinomas (prolactin-secreting pituitary tumor).
        ii. Drug induced (e.g., serotonin reuptake inhibitors and some antipsychotics)
        iii. Central nervous system lesions
  2. Hyposecretory disease
     a. GH deficiency
        i. Congenital abnormality caused by GH gene deletion, GH-releasing hormone deficiency
        ii. Other causes are pituitary aplasia, head trauma, and central nervous system infection.
        iii. Idiopathic
     b. Panhypopituitarism: Result of partial or complete loss of anterior and posterior pituitary function. Can be caused by primary pituitary tumor, ischemic necrosis of the pituitary, trauma from surgery, or irradiation. Results in adrenocorticotropic hormone (ACTH) deficiency, GH deficiency, hypothyroidism, gonadotropin deficiency

B. Acromegaly
  1. Diagnosis and clinical presentation
     a. Failure of an oral glucose tolerance test (OGTT) to suppress GH serum concentrations but with elevated insulin-like growth factor-1 (IGF-1). (GH serum concentrations alone are unreliable, given the pulsatile pattern of release in the body.)
     b. Clinical presentation (Note: Disease has a very slow onset, and many symptoms do not appear for years.)
        i. Excessive sweating
        ii. Osteoarthritis, joint pain, paresthesias, or neuropathies
        iii. Coarsening of facial features

      iv.   Increased hand volume or ring size, increased shoe size

      v.   Hypertension, heart disease, cardiomyopathy

      vi.   Sleep apnea

      vii.   Type 2 diabetes mellitus (DM)

2. Therapy goals

   a.   Reduce GH and IGF-1 concentrations.

   b.   Decrease mortality.

   c.   Improve clinical symptoms.

   d.   Normalize IGF-1 concentrations and suppressed GH concentrations after OGTT.

3. Therapeutics

   a.   Treatment of choice is surgical resection of tumor, if causative.

   b.   Pharmacotherapy usually reserved for

      i.   Control before surgery or irradiation

      ii.   When surgery is not possible (usually requires lifelong pharmacotherapy)

      iii.   Surgical failures or relapses after period of remission after surgery

   c.   Dopamine agonists (e.g., bromocriptine, cabergoline)

      i.   Mechanism of action: Dopamine agonist that, in acromegaly, causes paradoxical decrease in GH production

      ii.   Dosing (bromocriptine, most commonly used agent)

         (a)   Initial: 1.25 mg/day by mouth

         (b)   Maximal: 20–30 mg/day (can titrate once or twice weekly as needed)

      iii.   Adverse effects

         (a)   Fatigue, dizziness, nervousness

         (b)   Diarrhea, abdominal pain

      iv.   Efficacy: Normalization of IGF-1 concentrations in about 10% of patients. More than 50% of patients experience symptomatic relief.

   d.   Somatostatin analog (e.g., octreotide)

      i.   Mechanism of action: Blocks GH secretion; 40 times more potent than endogenous somatostatin

      ii.   Dosing

         (a)   Initial: 50–100 mcg subcutaneously every 8 hours

         (b)   Maximal: Little benefit greater than 600 mcg/day

         (c)   If response to above, can be changed to long-acting octreotide formulation administered once monthly

      iii.   Adverse effects

         (a)   Diarrhea, nausea, cramps, flatulence, fat malabsorption

         (b)   Arrhythmias

         (c)   Hypothyroidism

         (d)   Biliary tract disorders

         (e)   Changes in serum glucose concentrations (usually reduces)

      iv.   Efficacy: 50%–60% of patients experience normalization of IGF-1 concentrations with good symptomatic relief as well. May shrink tumor mass in some patients

   e.   GH receptor antagonist (e.g., pegvisomant)

      i.   Mechanism of action: GH derivative binds to liver GH receptors and inhibits IGF-1.

      ii.   Dosing

         (a)   Initial: 40 mg once-daily subcutaneous injection loading dose and then 10 mg once daily

         (b)   Maximal: 30 mg/day

      iii.   Adverse effects

         (a)   Nausea, vomiting

(b) Flu-like symptoms

(c) Reversible elevations in hepatic transaminase

    iv. Efficacy: More than 95% of patients attain normal IGF-1 concentrations, and most have improved symptoms.

Patient Case

3. A 28-year-old woman presents with acne, facial hair growth, and irregular menses that have lasted for 6–7 months. She has diagnoses of hypertension and depression. Her pituitary and thyroid tests have all come back negative. Her current medications include atenolol and fluoxetine. Her prolactin level today is 112 ng/mL (normal 15–25 ng/mL). Which is the most likely cause of her elevated prolactin level?

    A. Atenolol.

    B. Prolactin-secreting adenoma.

    C. Pregnancy.

    D. Fluoxetine.

C. Hyperprolactinemia

    1. Causes

        a. Direct: Pituitary tumor (lactotroph adenoma)

        b. Indirect: Drug induced (most frequent nontumor cause), renal failure, hypothyroidism, breastfeeding

        c. Potential causative drugs: Typical antipsychotics, opiates, nondihydropyridine calcium channel blocker, antidepressants

    2. Diagnosis and clinical presentation

        a. Elevated serum prolactin concentrations. May be challenging to find specific etiology (unless drug induced)

        b. Clinical presentation

            i. Amenorrhea, anovulation, infertility, hirsutism, and acne in women

            ii. Erectile dysfunction, decreased libido, gynecomastia, and reduced muscle mass in men

            iii. Headache, visual disturbances, bone loss

    3. Therapy goals

        a. Normalize prolactin concentrations

        b. Normalize gonadotropin secretion

        c. Symptomatic relief

    4. Therapeutics

        a. Treatment of choice is surgical resection of tumor, if causative.

        b. Pharmacotherapy usually reserved for

            i. Control before surgery or irradiation

            ii. When surgery is not possible (usually requires lifelong pharmacotherapy)

            iii. Surgical failures or relapses after period of remission after surgery

        c. Discontinue causative agent if drug induced.

            i. Recheck prolactin concentration 3 days after discontinuation.

            ii. Select agent with similar action but no known effect on prolactin concentrations.

            iii. If discontinuation of causative agent not feasible, consider dopamine agonist.

        d. Dopamine agonists

            i. Cabergoline (preferred agent per Endocrine Society guidelines, long-acting oral agent; adverse effect profile similar to that of bromocriptine)

                (a) Initial: 0.5 mg once weekly

     (b) Maximal: 4.5 mg/week
    ii. Bromocriptine (see above)
    iii. Efficacy: May restore fertility in more than 90% of women. Cabergoline may be easier for patients to take, given weekly administration.
    iv. Consider taper or discontinuation after 2 years of therapy if asymptomatic, prolactin concentrations normalized, and no tumor remnant by imagery.

  5. GH deficiency: Diagnosis and clinical presentation
    a. Decreased GH concentrations after provocative pharmacologic challenge (e.g., insulin, clonidine, GH-releasing hormone)
    b. Clinical presentation
     i. Delayed growth velocity or short stature
     ii. Central obesity
     iii. Immaturity of the face or prominence of the forehead

  6. Therapy goals
    a. Increased growth velocity
    b. Increased final adult height when treating children

  7. Therapeutics: Recombinant GH (somatropin)
    a. Dosing
     i. Depends on which of the various products are selected (dosed subcutaneously or intramuscularly once daily)
     ii. When to discontinue therapy on the basis of growth velocity is controversial.
     iii. Once- or twice-monthly long-acting depot formulation is also available.
    b. Adverse effects
     i. Arthralgias, injection site pain
     ii. Rare but serious cases of idiopathic intracranial hypertension have been reported.
    c. Efficacy: All products are considered equally efficacious.

III. ADRENAL GLAND DISORDERS

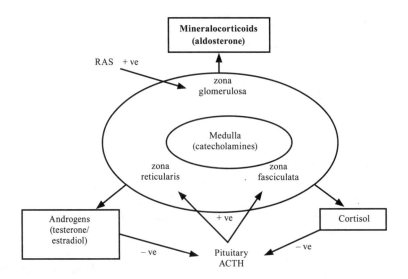

Figure 2. Basic adrenal cortex hormone physiology.

ACTH = adrenocorticotropic hormone; RAS = renin-angiotensin system; + ve = positive stimulation; - ve = negative feedback.

Patient Case

4. A 44-year-old man has consistently high blood pressure (e.g., 172/98 mm Hg today) despite documented adherence to two maximal-dose blood pressure medications. He has frequent headaches, increased thirst, and fatigue. His urine free cortisol is 45 mcg/24 hours (normal range 20–90), and his plasma aldosterone/renin ratio is 125 (normal is less than 25). Which condition is the most likely cause of this patient's uncontrolled hypertension?

   A. Cushing's syndrome.

   B. Addison's disease.

   C. Hyperprolactinemia.

   D. Hyperaldosteronism.

A. Hypersecretory Cortisol Diseases (a.k.a. Cushing's syndrome)
1. Classification
   a. ACTH dependent: Result of excessive ACTH secretion
      i. Pituitary corticotroph adenoma (Cushing's disease)
      ii. Ectopic ACTH syndrome (extrapituitary tumor)
   b. ACTH independent: Result of excessive cortisol secretion or exogenous steroids
      i. Unilateral adrenocortical tumors
      ii. Bilateral adrenal hyperplasia or dysplasia
      iii. Exogenous steroid administration
2. Diagnosis and clinical presentation
   a. Presence of hypercortisolism through 24-hour urinary free cortisol concentration
   b. Differentiate etiology (key to treatment options).
      i. Complex and beyond the scope of this chapter
      ii. Plasma ACTH concentrations (normal or elevated in ACTH dependent)
      iii. Pituitary magnetic resonance imaging (MRI) (Cushing's syndrome vs. ectopic ACTH syndrome)
      iv. Overnight dexamethasone suppression test
      v. 24-hour urinary free cortisol
   c. Clinical presentation
      i. Central obesity and facial rounding quite common
      ii. Peripheral obesity and fat accumulation
      iii. Myopathies
      iv. Osteoporosis, back pain, compression fracture
      v. Abnormal glucose tolerance or diabetes
      vi. Amenorrhea and hirsutism in women
      vii. Lower abdominal pigmented striae (red to purple)
      viii. Hypertension (principal cause of morbidity and mortality)
3. Therapy goals
   a. Reduce morbidity and mortality and eliminate cause.
   b. Reverse clinical features.
   c. Normalize biochemical changes (when possible).
   d. Achieve long-term control without recurrence (remission when possible).
4. Therapeutics
   a. If excessive exogenous corticosteroid use is causative, discontinue or minimize use.
   b. Surgical resection of causative area or tumor is usual treatment of choice. Pharmacotherapy is usually reserved on the basis of the same criteria listed earlier for pituitary adenomas.

   c. Pasireotide

      i. Mechanism of action: Somatostatin analog blocks ACTH secretion from pituitary, leading to decreased circulating cortisol levels (better selectivity to pertinent somatostatin receptors than other analogs such as octreotide). Generally not effective for adrenal causative Cushing's syndrome. Main role is in Cushing's disease, but role per guidelines is yet to be determined.

     ii. Dosing: 0.6–0.9 mg twice-daily subcutaneous injection (dosage adjustments based on urinary free cortisol and symptom improvements)

    iii. Adverse effects: Hyperglycemia, hypocorticalism, diarrhea, nausea, gallstones, headache, bradycardia

    iv. Obtain an electrocardiogram, a fasting plasma glucose (FPG), an A1C, liver function tests, and a gallbladder ultrasound before initiating therapy.

     v. Self-monitor blood glucose (BG) values every week for first 2–3 months, then periodically obtain liver function tests 1–2 weeks after starting therapy, then obtain them monthly for 2–3 months and then every 6 months. Repeat gallbladder ultrasonography at 6- to 12-month intervals.

   d. Ketoconazole

      i. Mechanism of action: In addition to its antifungal activity, it hinders cortisol production by inhibiting 11- and 17-hydroxylase.

     ii. Dosing

        (a) Initial: 200 mg twice daily by mouth

        (b) Maximal: 400 mg three times daily

    iii. Adverse effects

        (a) Gynecomastia

        (b) Abdominal discomfort

        (c) Reversible hepatic transaminase elevations

   e. Mitotane

      i. Mechanism of action: Inhibits 11-hydroxylase but also has some direct adrenolytic activity

     ii. Dosing

        (a) Initial: 500–1000 mg/day by mouth (some use much higher daily dosages, but they are not well tolerated)

        (b) Maximal: 9–12 g/day

    iii. Adverse effects

        (a) Adrenocortical atrophy: Can persist upon discontinuation and, in severe cases, may necessitate androgen and glucocorticoid replacement

        (b) Anorexia

        (c) Ataxia

        (d) Abdominal discomfort

        (e) Lethargy

   f. Etomidate

      i. Mechanism of action: Similar to ketoconazole, inhibits 11-hydroxylase

     ii. Dosing

        (a) Initial: 0.03 mg/kg intravenously, followed by a 0.1-mg/kg/hour infusion

        (b) Maximal: 0.3 mg/kg/hour

    iii. Adverse effects

        (a) Pain at injection site

        (b) Nausea and vomiting

        (c) Myoclonus

        (d) Psychoses

iv. Given route of administration is usually reserved for when rapid control of cortisol levels is needed and oral therapy is problematic.

g. Metyrapone (by compassionate use only)

i. Mechanism of action: Hinders secretion of cortisol by blocking final step in cortisol synthesis by inhibiting 11-hydroxylase activity

ii. Dosing

(a) Initial: 500 mg three times daily by mouth

(b) Average dosage in Cushing's syndrome is 2000 mg/day, but it is about 4000 mg in ectopic ACTH syndrome.

iii. Adverse effects

(a) Hypoadrenalism

(b) Hypertension

(c) Worsening of hirsutism and acne if present before treatment

(d) Headache

(e) Abdominal discomfort

h. Efficacy is measured by control of symptoms and normalization of 24-hour urine free cortisol concentrations.

i. Glucocorticoid replacement may be necessary if circulating cortisol is reduced to lower than physiological concentrations.

j. Mifepristone for hyperglycemia associated with endogenous Cushing's syndrome. Proposed to limit binding of cortisol. May reduce insulin requirements and improve clinical symptoms associated with hyperglycemia

B. Hyperaldosteronism: Primary Aldosteronism

1. Classification

a. Bilateral adrenal hyperplasia (70% of cases)

b. Aldosterone-producing adenoma (30% of cases)

2. Diagnosis and clinical presentation

a. Elevated plasma aldosterone/renin ratio

b. Other features: Hypernatremia, hypokalemia, hypomagnesemia, glucose intolerance

c. Clinical presentation (can be asymptomatic)

i. Hypertension

ii. Muscle weakness or fatigue

iii. Headache

iv. Polydipsia

v. Nocturnal polyuria

3. Therapy goals (same as earlier for Cushing's syndrome)

4. Therapeutics

a. Spironolactone (drug of choice)

i. Mechanism of action: Competitively inhibits aldosterone biosynthesis

ii. Dosing

(a) Initial: 25–50 mg/day by mouth

(b) Maximal: 400 mg/day

iii. Adverse effects

(a) Hyperkalemia

(b) Gynecomastia

(c) Abdominal discomfort

b. Eplerenone and amiloride are alternatives to spironolactone.

C. Hyposecretory Adrenal Disorders
1. Classification
    a. Primary adrenal insufficiency (a.k.a. Addison's disease)
        i. Caused by autoimmune disorder, infection, or infarction
        ii. Results in cortisol, aldosterone, and androgen deficiencies
    b. Secondary adrenal insufficiency
        i. Exogenous steroid use (from chronic suppression); oral, inhaled, intranasal, and topical administration
        ii. Surgery, trauma, infection, infarction
        iii. Results in impaired androgen and cortisol production
2. Diagnosis and clinical presentation (focus on Addison's disease)
    a. Abnormal rapid cosyntropin (synthetic ACTH) stimulation test (blunted increase in cortisol concentrations) suggests adrenal insufficiency.
    b. Clinical presentation
        i. Hyperpigmentation (caused by elevated ACTH concentrations)
        ii. Weight loss
        iii. Dehydration
        iv. Hyponatremia, hyperkalemia, elevated blood urea nitrogen (BUN)
3. Therapy goals (same as above for Cushing's syndrome)
4. Therapeutics
    a. Steroid replacement (replace cortisol loss)
        i. Oral administration is commonly dosed to mimic normal cortisol production circadian rhythm.
        ii. Two-thirds administered in the morning and one-third in the evening
            (a) This may cause periods of transient adrenal insufficiency or variable serum concentrations in some patients.
            (b) Daily cortisol production in average patient: 5–10 mg/m^2
    b. Hydrocortisone: 15 mg/day (may reduce need for fludrocortisone compared with using cortisone or prednisone)
        i. Cortisone acetate: 20 mg/day
        ii. Prednisone: 2.5 mg/day
        iii. Dexamethasone: 0.25–0.75 mg/day
    c. Fludrocortisone (replaces loss of mineralocorticoid): 0.05–0.2 mg/day by mouth
    d. For women with decreased libido or low energy levels because of androgen deficiency, dehydroepiandrosterone (DHEA): 25–50 mg/day
    e. Efficacy can be measured by symptom improvement.
    f. Note that during times of stress or illness, corticosteroid dosages must be increased. Dosage and route of administration depend on level of stress to the body.

Table 2. Comparative Glucocorticoid Dosing

Glucocorticosteroid	Relative Equivalent Dosing (mg)
Cortisone	25
Hydrocortisone	20
Prednisone	5
Prednisolone	5
Triamcinolone	4
Methylprednisolone	4
Dexamethasone	0.75

IV. OBESITY

A. Recent Guidelines

1. American College of Cardiology/American Heart Association (ACC/AHA) and the Obesity Society (TOS) 2013 guidelines. First significant guideline since 1998. Most of the below therapeutic agents were approved for obesity after the guideline was initiated and are not included.

2. Endocrine Society 2015 guidelines. Focused on new obesity agents. No specific recommendations of a particular agent over another but a good review of the therapeutic options.

B. Classification

1. Based on BMI
2. Normal: BMI 18.5–24.9 kg/m^2
3. Overweight: BMI 25.0–29.9 kg/m^2
4. Obesity
   a. Class I: BMI 30.0–34.9 kg/m^2
   b. Class II: BMI 35.0–39.9 kg/m^2
   c. Class III: BMI 40 kg/m^2 or greater

C. Therapy Goals

1. Weight loss: Initial goal 5%–10% decrease from baseline weight over 6 months
2. Maintain lower weight in the long term.
3. Limit weight-induced comorbidities (e.g., type 2 DM, hypertension, cardiovascular disease).

D. Nonpharmacologic Therapy (aimed at providing an energy deficit)

1. Increased physical activity: 200–300 minutes per week
2. Dietary options: Any diet that has proven weight reduction data available is appropriate. No specific recommendations of one diet over another. Individualize according to patient preferences.
   a. Strive for at least a 500-kcal/day deficit.
   b. 1200–1800 kcal/day for women
   c. 1500–1800 kcal/day for men
3. Behavioral intervention: Per ACC/AHA/TOS guidelines: Preferably in-person, high-intensity (at least 14 sessions in 6 months) comprehensive weight loss intervention through group or individual sessions with a professional (e.g., dietitian, exercise specialist, health counselor)
4. Surgery: Usually reserved for severely obese (BMI greater than 40) or lower BMIs with existing comorbidities
   a. Gastric bypass
   b. Gastric banding

Patient Case

5. A patient is taking the maximal daily dose of phentermine/topiramate for treatment of obesity. The patient's baseline BMI is 36 kg/m^2 and weight is 255 lb. What would be the minimum weight loss to occur to consider continuing treatment with this agent?

   A. 7 lb.
   B. 13 lb.
   C. 17 lb.
   D. 26 lb.

E. Pharmacotherapy
   1. Always in conjunction with diet, physical activity, and behavioral therapy
   2. Medications should be reserved for those not achieving or sustaining weight reduction with adequate lifestyle modifications or in those who are obese or have BMI at least 27 kg/m^2 with significant weight-related comorbidities (e.g., diabetes, hypertension).
   3. Medication selected according to risk-benefit profile should be Food and Drug Administration (FDA) approved. Approved agents should provide after 1 year at least a statistically significant 5% weight loss difference from placebo, and at least 35% of treated subjects should achieve at least a 5% weight loss from baseline and twice that of placebo-treated subjects.
   4. Orlistat
      a. Mechanism of action: Reduced absorption of fat by inhibition of gastric and pancreatic lipases
      b. Dosing
         i.   Prescription: 120 mg three times daily during or up to 1 hour after meals
         ii. Over the counter: 60 mg three times daily during or up to 1 hour after meals
      c. Adverse effects
         i.   Gastrointestinal (GI) tract: Flatulence, oily stools, loose stools, fecal urgency or incontinence (very dependent on fat content of meal)
         ii. Reduced absorption of fat-soluble vitamins (A, D, E, and K): Use vitamin supplement before or well after use.
         iii. Hepatotoxicity, kidney stones
      d. Efficacy: 35%–54% of patients taking a prescription-strength product attained at least a 5% weight loss after 1 year of therapy, and 16%–25% attained at least a 10% weight loss.
   5. Lorcaserin (Schedule IV)
      a. Mechanism of action: Reduced hunger by stimulating serotonin 2C receptors in the brain. Previous serotonin agonists used for obesity (e.g., fenfluramine) were nonselective and caused cardiac and pulmonary problems.
      b. Dosing: 10 mg twice daily
      c. Adverse effects: Headache, dizziness, nausea, dry mouth, constipation, memory or attention disturbances, hypoglycemia in patients with diabetes
      d. Efficacy: 4.5%–6% weight loss from baseline; 47% attained at least a 5% loss, and 23% attained at least a 10% weight loss. In overweight patients with diabetes, up to a 1% reduction in A1C
      e. Discontinue use if at least a 5% weight loss is not achieved after 12 weeks of use.
      f. Avoid concurrent use with serotonergic drugs, including selective serotonin reuptake inhibitors.
   6. Phentermine/extended-release topiramate (Schedule IV)
      a. Mechanism of action: Phentermine promotes appetite suppression and decreased food intake secondary to its sympathomimetic activity. Mechanism of topiramate is unknown but may cause appetite suppression and satiety through increased γ-aminobutyrate activity.
      b. Dosing (phentermine/topiramate): Should be taken in the morning to avoid insomnia
         i.   Initial: 3.75/23 mg daily for 2 weeks; then increase to 7.5/46 mg daily
         ii. If at least a 3% weight loss not achieved after 12 weeks, can discontinue or increase to 11.25/69 mg daily for 2 weeks; then increase to 15/92 mg daily if tolerated
         iii. If at least a 5% weight loss not achieved with 15/92 mg daily, discontinue use. Taper when discontinuing to avoid seizures.
         iv. Dosing in moderate hepatic or renal impairment: Do not exceed 7.5/46 mg daily.
      c. Adverse effects: Dry mouth, paresthesia, constipation, dysgeusia, insomnia, attention and memory disturbances, increased heart rate
      d. In women of childbearing age, obtain a negative pregnancy test before initiating and monthly thereafter because of fetal toxicity. Stress the importance of adequate contraception during use.

    e.   Efficacy: 9%–10% weight loss from baseline; 60%–70% attained at least a 5% weight loss after 1 year of treatment, and 37%–48% attained at least a 10% weight loss.

7. Bupropion/naltrexone

    a.   Mechanism of action: Reuptake inhibitor of dopamine and norepinephrine (bupropion) and opioid antagonist (naltrexone)

    b.   Dosing (8 mg naltrexone/90 mg bupropion tablets)

        i.   Dosage escalation at weekly intervals by 1 tablet daily

        ii.   Initially 1 tablet once daily

        iii.   Target dosage 2 tablets twice daily

    c.   Adverse effects: Nausea, constipation, headache, vomiting, dizziness, insomnia, dry mouth

    d.   Precautions and contraindications: Uncontrolled hypertension, seizure disorders, anorexia nervosa or bulimia, drug or alcohol withdrawal. Avoid with chronic use of opioids.

    e.   Efficacy: 5%–6% weight loss from baseline; 40%–55% attained at least a 5% weight loss after 56 weeks of therapy, 20%–25% attained at least a 10% weight loss.

    f.   Discontinue use if at least a 5% weight loss is not achieved after 12 weeks of use.

8. Liraglutide

    a.   Mechanism of action: Glucagon-like peptide-1 (GLP-1) agonist (part of incretin system). Thought to cause satiety and delay gastric emptying. Used in treatment of type 2 DM (see below).

    b.   Dosing (administered subcutaneously via pen device)

        i.   Target dosage higher in obesity than in treatment of diabetes. Brand name product for obesity is not approved for diabetes and vice versa.

        ii.   Initially 0.6 mg once daily, increase by 0.6 mg at weekly intervals.

        ii.   Target dosage for obesity is 3 mg daily.

    c.   Adverse effects: Nausea, vomiting, diarrhea, constipation, dyspepsia

    d.   Precautions and contraindications

        i.   See below in Diabetes Mellitus section.

        ii.   Obesity formulation should be avoided in patients receiving insulin (increased risk for hypoglycemia).

        iii.   Do not use with other GLP-1 agonists used in the treatment of DM.

    e.   Efficacy

        i.   Patients without diabetes: 8%–9% weight loss from baseline; 60%–65% attained at least a 5% weight loss after 56 weeks of treatment, and about 33% attained at least a 10% weight loss.

        ii.   Patients with diabetes: 6% weight loss from baseline; 54% attained at least a 5% weight loss after 56 weeks of treatment, and 25% attained at least a 10% weight loss. Only minimally more effective at A1C reduction than standard diabetes dosage (see below for diabetes dosing).

    f.   Discontinue use if at least a 4% weight loss is not experienced after 16 weeks of therapy or if patient cannot tolerate the target 3-mg daily dosage.

9. Diethylpropion or phentermine monotherapy (Schedule IV)

    a.   Should be used only for a limited time, up to 3 months, and avoid in those with abuse potential.

    b.   Adverse effects: Increased blood pressure, constipation, increased heart rate, dysrhythmias, abuse potential (avoid in patients with hypertension or history of cardiovascular disease)

10. Other issues

    a.   Concurrent use of obesity medications has not been studied.

    b.   Comparative studies between agents are lacking (although liraglutide has been shown to reduce weight better than orlistat).

    c.   Long-term safety of all agents is unknown.

    d.   Consider chronic medication. Weight loss after continuation of agent is not sustained.

11. Off-label medications used but not well studied specifically for obesity: selective serotonin reuptake inhibitors, zonisamide, metformin, pramlintide

V. POLYCYSTIC OVARY SYNDROME

A. Background and Classification
   1. May be a cause of infertility in up to 20% of infertile couples
   2. Mainly considered to be caused by androgen excess or hyperandrogenism
   3. Underlying cause appears to be insulin resistance (in obese and nonobese patients), with subsequent compensatory insulin hypersecretion or increased insulin action. This increased action stimulates androgen secretion by the ovaries or adrenal cells, leading to increased luteinizing hormone (LH) secretion but normal or low follicle-stimulating hormone (FSH) levels, with a subsequent decrease in follicular maturation and anovulation.
   4. Has several potential comorbidities with endocrine and cardiovascular implications (e.g., type 2 DM, obesity)
   5. May affect 6%–10% of women, making it one of the most prevalent endocrine disorders in young women
   6. No clear consensus on classifying polycystic ovary syndrome (PCOS), although some rate it from mild to severe
   7. Endocrine Society has the only recent guideline on PCOS diagnosis and treatment.

B. Diagnosis
   1. Still somewhat under debate; no clear consensus
   2. 1990 National Institutes of Health (NIH) criteria
      a. Hyperandrogenism or hyperandrogenemia
      b. Oligoovulation (infrequent or irregular ovulation)
      c. Exclusion of other secondary causes, particularly adrenal hyperplasia, Cushing syndrome, hyperprolactinemia
   3. 2003 Rotterdam criteria: Presence of at least two of the following and ruling out secondary causes
      a. Menstrual irregularity (oligoovulation or anovulation)
      b. Hyperandrogenism (clinical or biochemical signs)
      c. Polycystic ovaries (by transvaginal ultrasonography)
      d. Recommended by the Endocrine Society's guideline
   4. 2006 Androgen Excess Society: Follow 1990 NIH criteria but recognize concerns brought about from the Rotterdam criteria.

C. Clinical Presentation
   1. Clinical signs of hyperandrogenism: Hirsutism, acne, pattern alopecia (can vary by ethnicity)
   2. Biochemical signs of hyperandrogenism (should not be used as sole criteria because 20%–40% of patients with PCOS may be in the normal range)
      a. Elevated free or total serum testosterone
      b. LH/FSH ratio greater than 2
   3. Infrequent, irregular (e.g., late), or no ovulation, leading to irregular menses
   4. Infertility despite unprotected and frequent intercourse during the past year
   5. In obese patients, prediabetes (impaired glucose tolerance [IGT]) or type 2 DM may be present.

D. Therapy Goals
   1. Normalize ovulation and menses.
   2. Improve fertility in those who want to become pregnant.
   3. Limit clinical signs.
   4. Reduce progression to type 2 DM (perhaps cardiovascular disease).

E. Nonpharmacologic Therapy: Weight loss (5%–10%) important in overweight or obese patients.

F. Pharmacotherapy
   1. Fertility improvement
      a. Clomiphene citrate
         i. Mechanism of action: Induces ovulation as a selective estrogen receptor modulator that improves LH-FSH secretion
         ii. Dosing
            (a) 50 mg/day for 5 days starting on the third or fifth day of the menstrual cycle
            (b) Increase to 100 mg if ovulation does not occur after first cycle of treatment.
            (c) Maximal daily dosage 150–200 mg/day
         iii. Adverse effects: Flushing, GI discomfort, vision disturbances, vaginal dryness, multiple pregnancies
         iv. Drug of choice for infertility per Endocrine Society's guideline
      b. Gonadotropin (e.g., recombinant FSH) or recombinant gonadotropin-releasing hormone therapy with or without clomiphene
         i. Mechanism of action: Normalize LH/FSH ratio to stimulate ovulation.
         ii. Dosing: Many dosing strategies used
         iii. Adverse effects: Multiple pregnancies, ovarian hypertrophy, miscarriage, mood swings, breast discomfort
   2. Symptomatic improvement
      a. Hormonal contraceptives: Endocrine Society first-line therapy for menstrual abnormalities, hirsutism, or acne
      b. Metformin
         i. Effective for metabolic and glycemic abnormalities if present
         ii. Alternative to hormonal contraception for irregular menses when hormonal contraceptives are contraindicated
         iii. Little data to support use for increased fertility (may improve pregnancy rate but not shown to improve rates of live births)
      c. Spironolactone
      d. Pioglitazone: Questionable if benefits outweigh risks in PCOS. Not recommended in Endocrine Society's guidelines

VI. DIABETES MELLITUS

A. Consensus Recommendations
   1. American Diabetes Association (ADA). Updated yearly in the January supplement of Diabetes Care (www.diabetes.org)
   2. American College of Endocrinology/American Association of Clinical Endocrinologists (ACE/AACE)
   3. Canadian Diabetes Association
   4. Various European groups
   5. For the remainder of this section, unless otherwise noted, the ADA recommendations will be followed.

B. Classification
   1. Type 1 DM
      a. Attributable to cellular-mediated β cell destruction leading to insulin deficiency (insulin needed for survival)

    b. Accounts for 5%–10% of DM

    c. Formerly known as insulin-dependent diabetes, juvenile-onset diabetes

    d. Prevalence in the United States: 0.12% (about 340,000)

    e. Usually presents in childhood or early adulthood but can present in any stage of life

    f. Usually symptomatic with a rapid onset in childhood, but a slower onset can occur in older adults

2. Type 2 DM

    a. Results primarily from insulin resistance in muscle and liver, with subsequent defect in pancreatic insulin secretion, although GI, brain, liver, and kidneys are all involved in the pathophysiology

    b. Accounts for 90%–95% of DM

    c. Formerly known as non–insulin-dependent diabetes, adult-onset diabetes

    d. Prevalence in the United States: 7.8% (about 23.6 million and growing)

    e. Often asymptomatic, with a slow onset over 5–10 years. Rationale for early, frequent screening of those at risk (below) and initial assessment for complications at diagnosis

    f. Disturbing increased trends in type 2 DM in children and adolescents attributed to rise in obesity

3. Maturity-onset diabetes of the young

    a. Result of genetic disorder leading to impaired secretion of insulin with little or no impairment in insulin action

    b. Onset usually before age 25 and may mimic type 1 or 2 DM

4. Gestational diabetes

    a. Glucose intolerance occurring during pregnancy

    b. Prevalence: 1%–14% of pregnancies (complicates about 4% of pregnancies)

    c. Newer diagnostic criteria (see below) will probably improve the diagnosis and change the prevalence.

    d. Most common in third trimester

5. Prediabetes

    a. IGT

    b. Impaired fasting glucose (IFG)

6. Other DM types

    a. Genetic defects in β cell function or insulin action

    b. Diseases of the pancreas (e.g., pancreatitis, neoplasia, cystic fibrosis)

    c. Drug or chemical induced (e.g., glucocorticoids, nicotinic acid, protease inhibitors, atypical antipsychotics)

Patient Case

6. A 64-year-old African American woman has had a 12-kg (27-lb) weight increase during the past year, primarily because of inactivity and a poor diet. Her BMI is 44 kg/m². Her mother and sister both have type 2 DM. Her fasting glucose concentration today is 212 mg/dL. Which is the best course of action?

    A. Diagnose type 2 DM and begin treatment.

    B. Diagnose type 1 DM and begin treatment.

    C. Obtain another glucose concentration today.

    D. Obtain another glucose concentration another day.

C. Screening for DM

    1. Type 1 DM

        a. Symptomatic patients

        b. Asymptomatic patients at higher risk

           i. Relatives with type 1 DM

        ii.   Measure islet autoantibodies to assess risk of type 1 DM

        iii. If screen is positive for antibodies, counsel on symptoms of hyperglycemia and risk of DM. Consider enrollment in observational study.

  2. Type 2 DM

     a. Age 45 or older, repeat every 3 years if normal

     b. Screen regardless of age if BMI is 25 kg/m^2 or greater (23 kg/m^2 or greater in Asian Americans) and at least one of the following risk factors:

        i.   History of cardiovascular disease

        ii.   A1C is 5.7% or greater, IGT, or IFG in previous testing

        iii. History of PCOS

        iv. High-density lipoprotein cholesterol (HDL-C) less than 35 mg/dL or triglycerides (TG) greater than 250 mg/dL

        v.   Hypertension

        vi. Women with a diagnosis of gestational diabetes or women who delivered a baby weighing more than 4.1 kg (9 lb)

        vii. High-risk ethnicity: African American, Latino, Native American, Asian American, Pacific Islander

        viii. First-degree relative with type 2 DM

        ix. Physical inactivity

  3. Gestational DM

     a. Screen at first prenatal visit for undiagnosed type 2 DM in all patients with type 2 DM risk factors present.

     b. Screen at 24–28 weeks' gestation using a 75-g OGTT.

     c. If a diagnosis of gestational DM is made, screen for diabetes 6–12 weeks after delivery.

     d. Continue to screen patients who have had gestational DM every 3 years for type 2 DM for life.

D. DM Diagnosis

  1. Type 1 and type 2 DM diagnosis

     a. Glycemic values in nonpregnant patients

        i.   FPG

           (a) Easy and preferred method

           (b) 126 mg/dL or greater

        ii.   Random plasma glucose

           (a) 200 mg/dL or greater with symptoms of hyperglycemia

           (b) Common hyperglycemia symptoms include polyuria, polydipsia, and unexplained weight loss.

           (c) Prudent to verify with A1C concentration

        iii. OGTT

           (a) Plasma glucose concentration obtained 2 hours after a 75-g oral glucose ingestion

           (b) 200 mg/dL or greater

           (c) More sensitive and specific than FPG but more cumbersome to perform

        iv. With an abnormal test result, the patient should be retested (preferably with the same test, but it can be any of the above on a subsequent day or by obtaining an A1C unless unequivocal hyperglycemia is noted).

        v.   A1C (glycated hemoglobin)

           (a) 6.5% or greater

           (b) Confirmed by repeating (unless unequivocal hyperglycemia is noted), although interval for repeating test is not provided

        (c) May be less sensitive than FPG in identifying mild diabetes but does not require fasting and has less variability from day to day

        (d) A1C values may be inaccurate in patients with anemia, chronic malaria, sickle cell anemia, pregnancy, or significant blood loss or recent blood transfusion.

    b. Other useful diagnostic tests if type of DM is in question

      i. C-peptide (measure of endogenous insulin secretion, usually negligible in type 1 DM and normal or elevated early in type 2 DM)

      ii. Presence of islet cell autoantibodies, autoantibodies to insulin, glutamic acid decarboxylase, or tyrosine phosphatase (all suggest autoimmune activity)

2. Gestational diabetes diagnosis: Glycemic values in pregnancy

    a. Updated and simplified diagnostic criteria

    b. "One-step" approach: 75-g OGTT at 24–28 weeks' gestation

      i. Fasting: 92 mg/dL or greater

      ii. 1 hour after OGTT: 180 mg/dL or greater

      iii. 2 hours after OGTT: 153 mg/dL or greater

    c. "Two-step" approach: 50-g OGTT (nonfasting) at 24–28 weeks' gestation

      i. If 1 hour after 50-g OGTT is less than 140 mg/dL, no further workup.

      ii. If greater than or equal to 140 mg/dL, then perform additional fasting OGTT using 100 g (see ADA guidelines for diagnostic glucose criteria).

3. Prediabetes diagnosis (high-risk population)

    a. IFG: FPG between 100 and 125 mg/dL

    b. IGT: 2-hour plasma glucose after OGTT (75 g) between 140 and 199 mg/dL

    c. A1C between 5.7% and 6.4%

Patient Case

7. A 56-year-old man with type 2 DM is receiving metformin 1000 mg twice daily. He has no other chronic diseases or history of cardiovascular disease. His current vital signs and laboratory results are as follows: blood pressure 148/78 mm Hg, pulse 74 bpm, A1C 6.9%. Which agent if added to the current regimen has the potential to reduce both microvascular and macrovascular complications in this patient?

    A. Insulin glargine.

    B. Lisinopril.

    C. Glyburide.

    D. Niacin.

E. Goals of Diabetes Management in Nonpregnant Adults

    1. Primary goal is to prevent the onset of acute or chronic complications.

    2. Acute complications: Hypoglycemia, diabetic ketoacidosis (DKA), hyperglycemic hyperosmolar nonketotic syndrome

    3. Chronic complications

      a. Microvascular: Retinopathy, nephropathy, and neuropathy

      b. Macrovascular: Cardiovascular, cerebrovascular, and peripheral vascular diseases

    4. Glycemic therapy goals

      a. A1C less than 7.0% (Note: The ACE/AACE guidelines recommend 6.5% or less.)

        i. Obtain every 6 months in patients at goal A1C and every 3 months in those over goal.

    ii.   Less stringent A1C targets may be appropriate in those with a short life expectancy (e.g., terminal cancer), advanced diabetic complications, long-standing diabetes that is difficult to control (e.g., frail older adults with a history of hypoglycemia at risk of falls), or extensive other comorbidities. (In such situations, a higher A1C [e.g., less than 8%] may be sufficient to limit the risk of acute complications of hyperglycemia such as dehydration and electrolyte deficiencies.)

  b. FPG or premeal 80–130 mg/dL. Frequency of monitoring depends on regimen, type of DM, and current glycemic control.

  c. Peak postprandial glucose (1–2 hours after a meal) less than 180 mg/dL

5. Nonglycemic therapy goals

  a. Blood pressure less than 140/90 mm Hg (updated in 2015 ADA guidelines to be more consistent with Eighth Joint National Committee recommendations)

    i.   Lower blood pressure goals may be appropriate in younger patients, if albuminuria is present, and/or those with hypertension with additional cardiovascular risk factors

    ii.   Suggested lower blood pressure goal is less than 130/80 mm Hg.

  b. Lipids

    i.   ADA: No specific LDL-C goal is currently recommended (updated by ADA in 2015 to be consistent with ACC/AHA recommendations)

    ii.   ACC/AHA 2013 guidelines suggest lowering LDL-C by 30%–49% in patients with diabetes 40–75 years of age and by at least 50% if 10-year risk of cardiovascular event is at least 7.5%.

    iii. No specific TG or HDL-C goals are currently recommended.

F. Goals for Gestational Diabetes

1. Primary goal is to prevent complications to mother and child.

2. Glycemic therapy goals (more stringent)

  a. FPG of 95 mg/dL or less

  b. 1-hour postprandial glucose 140 mg/dL or less

  c. 2-hour postprandial glucose 120 mg/dL or less

3. Potential complications of hyperglycemia during pregnancy

  a. Mother: Hypertension, preeclampsia, type 2 DM after pregnancy

  b. Fetus/child: Macrosomia, hypoglycemia, jaundice, respiratory distress syndrome

G. Benefits of Optimizing Diabetes Management in Nonpregnant Adults

1. Glycemic control

  a. Reduce the risk of developing retinopathy, nephropathy, and neuropathy in type 1 and type 2 DM.

  b. Prospective studies, specifically designed to assess optimizing glycemic control and effect on cardiovascular events, have not shown little or no reduction in cardiovascular outcomes.

  c. However, the "legacy" effect seen in the Diabetes Control and Complications Trial in type 1 DM and the UK Prospective Diabetes Study in type 2 DM suggests early control has future cardiovascular benefit.

  d. No profound benefit of very aggressive glycemic control in type 2 DM (A1C less than 6.5%)

2. Blood pressure control: Reduction in both macrovascular and microvascular complications

3. Lipid control: Reduction in LDL-C with moderate-intensity statin therapy reduces cardiovascular complications.

Patient Case

8. A patient weighing 110 lb has been given a diagnosis of type 1 DM. The physician wants to start at a total daily insulin (TDI) of 0.4 unit/kg/day with a combination of long- and rapid-acting insulin. The patient is unwilling to estimate his or her carbohydrate intake at this time. Which would be the most appropriate initial basal insulin regimen?

   A. 30 units of insulin glargine once daily.

   B. 20 units of insulin detemir once daily.

   C. 10 units of insulin aspart once daily.

   D. 10 units of insulin glargine once daily.

H. Therapeutic Management of Type 1 DM
   1. Insulin agents
      a. Categorized on the basis of duration after injection
         i. Short acting: Regular human insulin
         ii. Rapid acting: Insulin aspart, lispro, glulisine, and inhaled insulin
         iii. Intermediate acting: Neutral protamine Hagedorn (NPH)
         iv. Long acting: Insulin glargine and detemir; cannot be mixed with other insulins
      b. Combination insulins (intermediate or long-acting, regular or rapid acting): 70/30, 75/25
      c. Higher insulin concentration products
         i. More frequently used in type 2 DM patients needing significant daily insulin dosages
         ii. U-300 glargine (300 units/mL), U-200 degludec (200 units/mL), U-200 lispro (200 units/mL), U-500 regular insulin (500 units/mL)

Table 3. Characteristics of U-100 (100 units/mL) Insulins[a]

Category	Drug Name	Clarity	Onset	Injection Time Before Meal (minutes)	Peak (hours)	Duration (hours)
Short acting	Regular	Clear	30–60 minutes	30	2–3	4–6
Rapid acting	Aspart Lispro Glulisine Inhaled insulin	Clear	15–30 minutes	15 (inhaled insulin at beginning of meal)	1–3	2–5
Intermediate acting	Neutral protamine hagedorn	Cloudy	1–2 hours	N/A	4–8	10–20
Long acting	Detemir Glargine Degludec	Clear	2–4 hours 1–2 hours 1–2 hours	N/A	6–8 "Peakless" "Peakless"	6–24 ~24 24–42

[a]Note: The above times are dependent on the source of data and intersubject variability.

N/A = not applicable.

      d. Glycemic target
         i. Regular- and short-acting insulins target postprandial glucose concentrations.
         ii. Intermediate- and long-acting insulins target fasting glucose concentrations.

    e. Inhaled insulin may cause bronchospasm and is contraindicated in patients with asthma, chronic obstructive pulmonary disease, or lung cancer. Requires spirometry testing at baseline, at 6 months of therapy, and annually thereafter.

2. Management of insulin therapy
   a. First step is to estimate total daily insulin (TDI) requirements.
   b. Weight-based estimate if insulin naive
      i. 0.3–0.6 unit/kg/day
     ii. Requirements higher if treating DKA near initial diagnosis of DM
    iii. Honeymoon phase shortly after treatment initiation often requires lower daily insulin needs.
   c. One common approach is to use older insulin formulations (NPH and regular insulin).
      i. Two-thirds of TDI given before morning meal. Two-thirds of this is given as NPH and one-third as regular insulin.
     ii. One-third of TDI given before the evening meal (or regular given before a meal and NPH at bedtime). Again, two-thirds of this is given as NPH and one-third as regular insulin.
    iii. Advantages: Daily insulin injection frequency two or three times daily and inexpensive
    iv. Disadvantages: Does not mimic natural insulin secretion pattern; prone to hypoglycemic events
   d. Another approach is basal/bolus insulin therapy (a.k.a. physiologic insulin therapy).
      i. Use of newer insulin analogs to better mimic natural insulin secretion patterns
     ii. Provides day-long basal insulin to prevent ketosis and control FPG
    iii. Provides bolus insulin to control postprandial hyperglycemia
    iv. Basal insulins: Insulin glargine once daily or insulin detemir once or twice daily
     v. Bolus insulins: Rapid-acting insulin
    vi. Basal requirements are 50% of estimated TDI.
    vii. Bolus requirements are 50% of estimated TDI split three ways before meals.
      (a) Provides initial estimate of prandial insulin needs
      (b) Typically, patients begin to estimate bolus requirements given the amount of carbohydrates to be ingested.
    viii. Advantages over NPH plus regular approach: More physiologic, less hypoglycemia, more flexible to patient mealtimes
    ix. Disadvantages: Cost and increased frequency and number of daily injections (rapid-acting and basal insulin must be injected separately). Note: The same process of basal/bolus insulin therapy can apply to a patient with type 2 DM who is receiving intensive insulin therapy with or without oral DM medications.
   e. Correctional insulin needs
      i. Always a need to correct for hyperglycemic excursions, despite optimal basal/bolus therapy
     ii. "1800 rule": 1800/TDI = # mg/dL of glucose lowering per 1 unit of rapid-acting insulin.
      (a) For example, if TDI is 60 units, 1800/60 = 30, suggesting 1 unit of rapid-acting insulin will reduce BG concentrations by 30 mg/dL.
      (b) Also referred to as insulin sensitivity
      (c) Some advocate the "1500 rule" when using regular human insulin (i.e., 1500/TDI).
    iii. More patient-specific than traditional sliding-scale insulin
   f. Continuous subcutaneous insulin infusion (insulin pump)
      i. Device allows very patient-specific hourly basal dosing and bolus insulin dosing.
     ii. Uses rapid-acting insulins
    iii. Requires patient education and carbohydrate counting
   g. Assessing therapy and dosage adjustment
      i. Know the goals for fasting and postprandial glucose concentrations.

      ii.   Identify when patient is at goal and not at goal (hypoglycemia or hyperglycemia). Look for consistent trends rather than isolated events.

      iii.   Identify which insulin affects problematic glucose concentrations.

      iv.   Adjust insulin dosage or patient behavior accordingly.

      v.   Same process for treating type 2 DM applies (see below).

3.   Amylin analog

   a.   Mechanism of action: Amylin is cosecreted with insulin and has effects similar to those of GLP-1 described below.

   b.   Pramlintide is currently the only agent in this class available in the United States. Can be used in either type 1 or type 2 DM as adjunctive therapy in patients receiving insulin

   c.   Dosing

      i.   Type 1 DM

         (a) Initial: 15 mcg subcutaneously immediately before main meals

         (b) Must reduce dosage of preprandial rapid-acting, short-acting, or combination insulin products by 50%

         (c) Maximal daily dosage: 60 mcg with each meal

         (d) Dosage should be titrated in 15-mcg increments, as tolerated, but no more rapidly than every 3 days.

      ii.   Type 2 DM

         (a) Initial: 60 mcg subcutaneously immediately before main meals

         (b) As above, must reduce preprandial insulins by 50%

         (c) Maximal daily dosage: 120 mcg with each meal

         (d) Dosage should be titrated in 60-mcg increments, as tolerated, but no more rapidly than every 3–7 days.

      iii.   Use of prefilled pens is strongly recommended, when possible, rather than using a syringe and vial, to reduce the risk of dosing errors (dosing instructions with U-100 syringes and vial in package insert).

      iv.   Cannot be mixed with insulin products; requires increased frequency of daily injections

   d.   Adverse effects

      i.   Black box warning for severe hypoglycemia, especially in patients with type 1 DM

      ii.   Nausea, vomiting, anorexia, headache

   e.   Contraindications and precautions

      i.   Substantial gastroparesis

      ii.   History of poor adherence or monitoring of BG

      iii.   A1C greater than 9%

      iv.   Hypoglycemia unawareness or frequent bouts of hypoglycemia

   f.   Efficacy

      i.   A 0.5%–1% reduction in A1C

      ii.   Very effective at controlling postprandial glucose excursions

Patient Cases

9. A 55-year-old man with type 2 DM for 6 months has been receiving metformin 1000 mg twice daily since being diagnosed. His A1C today is 8.2%. His morning fasting blood glucose (FBG) readings are consistently at goal. His after-meal glucose readings average 210–230 mg/dL. The patient states is worried about his weight and does not want to add a medication that may increase it. Which option would be most appropriate for this patient?

   A. Glyburide.

   B. Liraglutide.

   C. Pioglitazone.

   D. Insulin glargine.

10. A 66-year-old man has had type 2 DM for 4 years. His A1C today is 7.7%. He has altered his diet, and he states that he has been exercising regularly for months. He is taking metformin 1000 mg twice daily. Which would be the best choice to help optimize his glycemic control?

   A. Continue current medications and counsel to improve his diet and exercise.

   B. Discontinue metformin and initiate exenatide 5 mcg twice daily.

   C. Add bromocriptine 0.8 mg at bedtime.

   D. Add sitagliptin 100 mg once daily to his metformin therapy.

I. Therapeutic Management of Type 2 DM
   1. Given the progressive nature of type 2 DM, a stepwise approach is usually needed.
   2. 2012 ADA treatment recommendations and recent 2015 updates to the 2012 recommendations for hyperglycemia emphasize a patient-centered approach to care, considering patient preferences, needs, and values.
   3. Metformin remains the initial drug of choice, unless it is contraindicated or adverse effects preclude its use, if improvements in exercise and diet early after diagnosis fail to control hyperglycemia.
   4. If metformin monotherapy fails to allow the patient to attain or maintain glycemic control, adding other agents is based on several criteria and weighs the advantages and disadvantages of the various oral and injectable agents.
      a. Efficacy in lowering A1C (also focus on ability to lower fasting or postprandial glucose concentrations or both)
      b. Risk of hypoglycemia
      c. Effects on weight
      d. Adverse effect profile
      e. Cost
   5. Sulfonylureas, thiazolidinediones (TZDs), dipeptidyl peptidase-4 (DPP-4) inhibitors, sodium glucose cotransporter-2 (SGLT-2) inhibitors, GLP-1 agonists, and basal insulin are preferred over less efficacious or agents with a higher adverse risk profile.
   6. Initial insulin therapy: Use insulin early with any of the following baseline characteristics:
      a. A1C greater than 10%
      b. Glucose greater than 300–350 mg/dL
      c. Hyperglycemic symptoms
      d. Presence of urine ketones

7. Adding insulin to existing oral DM agents
   a. Common to add a basal insulin regimen to existing oral agents when hyperglycemia still not controlled but do not want to switch to all-insulin regimen
   b. Weight-based dosing: For example, 0.1–0.2 unit/kg/day (higher dosages if significant hyperglycemia exists)
   c. Can increase basal insulin based on fasting glucose concentrations
   d. Can add bolus insulin to one or more meals if postprandial glucose is of concern
   e. Insulin secretagogues should be lowered in dosage or discontinued altogether when bolus insulin added to reduce risk of hypoglycemia.
   f. TZDs should be lowered or discontinued when basal or bolus insulin is added to regimen because of increased risk of edema.

8. Changing from oral DM medications to insulin-only management (e.g., because of adverse effects, contraindications, lack of efficacy of oral medications)
   a. Can follow NPH/regular insulin or basal/bolus approach similar to that in type 1 DM described earlier
   b. The TDI requirements in type 2 DM are usually much higher than in type 1 DM because of insulin resistance.

9. Changing from NPH to long-acting insulin (either insulin glargine or detemir)
   a. If adequate glycemic control is already attained, initiate insulin glargine at 80% of total daily NPH dose.
   b. Detemir may be initiated by a unit-to-unit conversion and may require higher daily insulin dosages after conversion, but this is determined by glycemic response.

J. Therapeutic Agents in Type 2 DM
   1. Metformin (biguanide)
      a. Mechanism of action: Reduces hepatic gluconeogenesis. Also favorably affects insulin sensitivity and, to a lesser extent, intestinal absorption of glucose
      b. Dosing
         i. Initial: 500 mg once or twice daily (once daily with extended-release formulation)
         ii. Maximal daily dose: 2550 mg (more commonly, 2000 mg/day)
         iii. Can increase at weekly intervals as necessary
         iv. Small initial dosage and slow titration secondary to GI disturbances
      c. Adverse effects
         i. Common: Nausea, vomiting, diarrhea, epigastric pain
         ii. Less common: Decrease in vitamin B_{12} levels, lactic acidosis (rare)
         iii. Signs or symptoms of lactic acidosis include acidosis, nausea, vomiting, increased respiratory rate, abdominal pain, shock, and tachycardia.
      d. Contraindications and precautions (because of risk of lactic acidosis)
         i. Renal impairment (contraindicated because of increased risk of lactic acidosis)
            (a) U.S. package insert: Serum creatinine 1.5 mg/dL or greater in men and 1.4 mg/dL or greater in women or reduced creatinine clearance (CrCl)
            (b) CrCl and estimated glomerular filtration rate (eGFR) cutoffs are not well established; differ depending on guideline or package insert. Would discontinue or not initiate if CrCl is less than 30 mL/minute.
         ii. Age 80 years or older (use caution and carefully assess renal function)
         iii. High risk of cardiovascular event or hypoxic state
         iv. Hepatic impairment
         v. Congestive heart failure (especially if prone to exacerbations)

        vi. Interrupt therapy if undergoing procedures using iodinated contrast dye because of risk of nephrotoxicity. Reinitiate after 48 hours and after normal serum creatinine concentrations are achieved.

    e. Efficacy
- i. 1%–2% A1C reduction
- ii. Some benefit in TG reduction and weight loss
- iii. Considered first-line therapy unless contraindicated on the basis of adverse effect profile, reduction in A1C, cost, and limited data that it reduces cardiovascular events in overweight patients

2. Sulfonylureas
   - a. Mechanism of action: Bind to receptors on pancreatic β cells, leading to membrane depolarization, with subsequent stimulation of insulin secretion (insulin secretagogue)
   - b. First-generation agents seldom used today (e.g., chlorpropamide, tolbutamide)
   - c. Second-generation agents (e.g., glyburide, glipizide, glimepiride). Dosage titration: Can increase at weekly intervals as necessary
   - d. Adverse effects
     - i. Common: Hypoglycemia, weight gain
     - ii. Less common: Rash, headache, nausea, vomiting, photosensitivity
   - e. Contraindications and precautions
     - i. Hypersensitivity to sulfonamides
     - ii. Patients with hypoglycemic unawareness
     - iii. Poor renal function (glipizide may be a better option than glyburide or glimepiride in older adults or in those with renal impairment because drug or active metabolites are not renally eliminated)
   - f. Efficacy
     - i. 1%–2% A1C reduction
     - ii. Note: For this and all medications used to treat hyperglycemia, the absolute decrease in A1C is larger for higher baseline A1C values and smaller for lower A1C values.

Table 4. Second-Generation Sulfonylurea Dosing Strategies

Drug	Initial Dosage	Maximal Daily Dosage (mg)
Glyburide (nonmicronized)	2.5–5.0 mg once or twice daily	20
Glyburide (micronized)	1.5–3 mg once or twice daily	12
Glipizide	5 mg once or twice daily (once daily with extended release)	40 (little improved efficacy above 20 mg/day)
Glimepiride	1–2 mg once daily	8

3. Meglitinides
   - a. Mechanism of action: Very similar to that of sulfonylureas in increasing insulin secretion from the pancreas but with a more rapid onset and shorter duration of activity
   - b. Glucose-dependent activity
   - c. Two currently available: Repaglinide and nateglinide
   - d. Dosing
     - i. Repaglinide
       - (a) Initial: 0.5–1 mg 15 minutes before meals
       - (b) Maximal daily dosage: 16 mg

    ii. Nateglinide
        (a) 120 mg before meals
        (b) 60 mg if A1C near goal
    iii. Repaglinide can be increased in weekly intervals if needed.

e. Adverse effects: Hypoglycemia (though less than with sulfonylureas), weight gain, upper respiratory infection

f. Contraindications and precautions
    i. Hypersensitivity
    ii. Caution in concomitant use of repaglinide and gemfibrozil: Can lead to greatly increased repaglinide levels

g. Efficacy
    i. 0.5%–1.5% A1C reduction (repaglinide reduces A1C more than nateglinide)
    ii. Most effective on postprandial glucose excursions

4. TZDs (often called glitazones)
  a. Mechanism of action
    i. Peroxisome proliferator–activated receptor γ-agonist
    ii. Increases expression of genes responsible for glucose metabolism, resulting in improved insulin sensitivity

  b. Two agents available: Pioglitazone and rosiglitazone
    i. In September 2010, the FDA initiated restricted access to rosiglitazone because of continued concerns about its cardiovascular safety. Rosiglitazone was restricted to patients unable to attain glycemic control with other agents and when pioglitazone is not used for medical reasons.
    ii. In November 2013, the FDA removed some prescribing and dispensing restrictions for rosiglitazone after evaluating clinical trial data. The impact of this change and the availability of the agent remain unknown.

  c. Dosing
    i. Pioglitazone
        (a) Initial: 15 mg once daily
        (b) Maximal daily dosage: 45 mg
    ii. Dosage titration is slow, and the maximal effect of a dosage change may not be observed for 8–12 weeks.

  d. Adverse effects
    i. Weight gain
    ii. Fluid retention (particularly peripheral edema), worse with insulin use and dose dependent. Edema less responsive to diuretic therapy. May cause macular edema
    iii. Risk of proximal bone fractures; use caution in patients with existing osteopenia or osteoporosis (discontinuation reduces risk)
    iv. Possible risk of bladder cancer with pioglitazone (dosage and duration of use dependent). Data are contradictory.
    v. Increased risk of heart failure
        (a) Boxed warning.
        (b) More than 2-fold higher relative risk, although absolute risk is quite small
    vi. Both agents have been withdrawn from some countries in Europe.

  e. Contraindications and precautions
    i. Hepatic impairment
    ii. Class III/IV heart failure (symptomatic heart failure)
    iii. Existing fluid retention

  f. Efficacy

    i. 0.5%–1.4% A1C reduction

    ii. Both drugs increase HDL-C, but pioglitazone has a more favorable effect in reducing LDL-C and TG compared with rosiglitazone.

5. DPP-4 inhibitors

  a. Mechanism of action: Inhibits the breakdown of GLP-1 secreted during meals, which in turn increases pancreatic insulin secretion, limits glucagon secretion, slows gastric emptying, and promotes satiety

  b. Dosing

    i. Sitagliptin: 100 mg once daily

      (a) Reduce dosage with CrCl between 30 and 50 mL/minute to 50 mg once daily.

      (b) Reduce dosage with CrCl less than 30 mL/minute to 25 mg once daily.

    ii. Saxagliptin: 5 mg once daily.

      (a) Reduce dosage with CrCl of 50 mL/minute or less to 2.5 mg once daily.

      (b) Reduce dosage when coadministered with strong CYP3A4/5 inhibitor (e.g., ketoconazole) to 2.5 mg once daily.

    iii. Linagliptin: 5 mg once daily (no dosage adjustment for renal impairment)

    iv. Alogliptin: 25 mg once daily

      (a) Reduce dosage with CrCl between 30 and 60 mL/minute to 12.5 mg once daily.

      (b) Reduce dosage with CrCl less than 30 mL/minute to 6.25 mg once daily.

  c. Adverse effects

    i. Upper respiratory and urinary tract infections, headache, severe joint pain

    ii. Hypoglycemia with monotherapy is minimal, but frequency is increased with concurrent sulfonylurea therapy (can lower dosage of sulfonylurea when initiating)

    iii. Sitagliptin has had some postmarketing reports of acute pancreatitis, angioedema, Stevens–Johnson syndrome, and anaphylaxis.

    iv. Saxagliptin (but not alogliptin or sitagliptin) shown to have an increased risk for heart failure hospitalization (studies still pending on linagliptin)

  d. Contraindications and precautions

    i. Previous hypersensitivity to the agents

    ii. History of pancreatitis

  e. Efficacy: 0.5%–0.8% reduction in A1C, considered weight neutral

6. SGLT-2 inhibitor

  a. Mechanism of action: Increases urinary glucose excretion by blocking normal reabsorption in the proximal convoluted tubule. Has some effect on delaying GI glucose absorption

  b. Dosing

    i. Canagliflozin

      (a) 100 mg once daily before the first meal of the day

      (b) Maximal daily dosage: 300 mg

      (c) Reduce dosage with CrCl between 45 and 59 mL/minute to 100 mg daily.

      (d) Discontinue or do not initiate if eGFR is less than 45 mL/min/1.73 m^2.

    ii. Dapagliflozin

      (a) 5 mg once daily in the morning (with or without food)

      (b) Maximal daily dosage: 10 mg

      (c) Discontinue or do not initiate if eGFR is less than 60 mL/min/1.73 m^2.

    iii. Empagliflozin

      (a) 10 mg once daily in the morning (with or without food)

      (b) Maximal daily dosage: 25 mg

      (c) Discontinue or do not initiate if eGFR is less than 45 mL/min/1.73 m^2.

    c. Adverse effects
        i. Increased urination
        ii. Urinary tract infections
        iii. Genital mycotic infections
        iv. Hypotension
        v. Increased hypoglycemia risk with concomitant insulin or insulin secretagogue
        vi. Class is linked with rare cases of euglycemic diabetic ketoacidosis
        vii. Possible increased bone fracture risk/decreased bone mineral density with canagliflozin
    d. Contraindications and precautions
        i. Significant renal impairment (varies as above by agent)
        ii. Suggested to ensure euvolemia before initiating agent, given its diuretic effect especially in older adults, patients with existing renal impairment or already low blood pressure, or patients receiving diuretics
    e. Efficacy
        i. 0.3%–1.0% reduction in A1C
        ii. Effect on both fasting and postprandial glucose concentrations
        iii. Mild weight loss

Patient Case

11. A 66-year-old man is given a diagnosis today of type 2 DM. Two weeks ago, his A1C was 7.5%, and his serum creatinine was 1.8 mg/dL (estimated CrCl 25 mL/minute). He has a history of hypertension, dyslipidemia, and systolic heart failure (New York Heart Association class III, ejection fraction 33%). He has 2+ pitting edema bilaterally. In addition to improvements in diet and exercise, which is the best drug to initiate?

    A. Linagliptin.
    B. Pioglitazone.
    C. Exenatide.
    D. Metformin.

---

    7. GLP-1 analogs
        a. Mechanism of action: Synthetic analog of human GLP-1 that binds to GLP-1 receptors, resulting in glucose-dependent insulin secretion, reduction in glucagon secretion, and reduced gastric empty-ing; promotes satiety
        b. Approved agents: Exenatide, liraglutide, dulaglutide, and albiglutide
        c. Dosing
            i. Exenatide
               (a) Twice-daily formulation (pen)
                   (1) Initial: 5 mcg subcutaneously twice daily, administered no more than 60 minutes before morning and evening meals
                   (2) Maximal dosage: 10 mcg twice daily
                   (3) Dosage titration from 5 to 10 mcg twice daily after 1 month if tolerated
               (b) Once-weekly formulation (single-dose tray or pen, each containing lyophilized powder and diluent)
                   (1) 2 mg subcutaneously once weekly
                   (2) Powder must be reconstituted by patient immediately before injection.

    ii. Liraglutide (pen)
      (a) 0.6 mg subcutaneously once daily for 1 week (regardless of mealtime)
      (b) Dosage titration from 0.6 to 1.2 mg/day if tolerated
      (c) Maximal daily dosage: 1.8 mg/day
    iii. Albiglutide (pen containing lyophilized powder and diluent)
      (a) 30 mg subcutaneously once weekly
      (b) Dosage titration to 50 mg once weekly if tolerated and requires improved glycemic control
      (c) Patient must reconstitute powder via diluent in pen delivery device. Must be injected within 8 hours of reconstituting.
    iv. Dulaglutide (pen and single-dose syringe)
      (a) 0.75 mg subcutaneously once weekly
      (b) Dosage titration to 1.5 mg once weekly for additional glycemic control
    v. For each of the once-weekly formulations: Can administer a missed dose if within 3 days of the missed dose; if longer time period, wait until the next regularly scheduled weekly dose.
  d. Adverse effects
    i. Nausea, vomiting, diarrhea very common but can subside or cease over time
    ii. Hypoglycemia common with concurrent sulfonylurea (consider reduction in sulfonylurea dose)
    iii. Postmarketing reports of pancreatitis and acute renal failure or impairment
  e. Contraindications and precautions
    i. Impaired renal function: CrCl less than 30 mL/minute for either exenatide formulation; less than 15 mL/minute for albiglutide, less specific for liraglutide
    ii. History of severe GI tract disorder, particularly gastroparesis
    iii. History of pancreatitis
    iv. For liraglutide, albiglutide, once-weekly exenatide, dulaglutide: Contraindicated in patients with a personal or family history of medullary thyroid carcinoma (adverse effect found in rodent studies but not in humans)
  f. Efficacy
    i. A 0.5%–1.5% reduction in A1C
    ii. Effects on postprandial hyperglycemia better than on fasting glucose concentrations with once- or twice-daily formulations
    iii. Improved A1C, fasting glucose reduction, and nausea or vomiting with once-weekly compared with twice-daily exenatide formulation
    iv. Modest weight loss
8. α-Glucosidase inhibitors
  a. Mechanism of action: Slows the absorption of glucose from the intestine to the bloodstream by slowing the breakdown of large carbohydrates into smaller absorbable sugars
  b. Two agents available: Acarbose and miglitol
  c. Dosing (both agents dosed similarly)
    i. Initial: 25 mg three times daily at each meal
    ii. Maximal daily dosage: 300 mg
    iii. Slow titration, increasing as tolerated every 4–8 weeks to minimize GI adverse effects
  d. Adverse effects
    i. Flatulence, diarrhea, abdominal pain
    ii. Increased liver enzymes observed with high dosages of acarbose
  e. Contraindications and precautions: Inflammatory bowel disease, colonic ulcerations, intestinal obstruction

    f. Efficacy
- i. 0.5%–0.8% reduction in A1C, also shown to decrease body weight
- ii. Targets postprandial glucose excursions
- iii. May not be as effective in patients using low-carbohydrate diets

9. Bile acid sequestrant: Colesevelam is the only studied and approved drug in this class.
   a. Mechanism of action
      - i. Bile acid sequestrant used primarily for cholesterol management. Its mechanism to reduce serum glucose concentrations is not clearly understood. Thought to be an antagonist to the farnesoid X receptor, which subsequently reduces hepatic gluconeogenesis. By reducing bile acid absorption, colesevelam reduces farnesoid X receptor activity.
      - ii. Used in conjunction with insulin or oral DM medications
   b. Colesevelam is the only studied and approved drug in this class.
   c. Dosing: Six 625-mg tablets once daily or 3 625-mg tablets twice daily
   d. Adverse effects: Constipation, dyspepsia, nausea, myalgia
   e. Contraindications and precautions
      - i. Contraindicated in patients with a history of bowel obstruction, serum TG concentration greater than 500 mg/dL
      - ii. Caution in patients with swallowing disorders (large pill), dysphasia, gastric mobility disorders, and serum TG concentrations greater than 300 mg/dL
   f. Efficacy: A 0.3%–0.5% reduction in A1C

10. Bromocriptine
    a. Mechanism of action: Not clearly understood. Agonist for dopamine receptor D_2 is thought to reset circadian rhythm, which may reduce caloric intake and storage. Other effects may be through α_1 antagonism, α_2-agonistic properties, and modulation of serotonin and prolactin.
    b. Dosing
       - i. Initial: 0.8 mg once daily on waking; take with food (increases bioavailability)
       - ii. Maximal daily dosage: 4.8 mg
       - iii. Titrate weekly by 0.8 mg/day as tolerated and according to response.
       - iv. Tablet strength is different from that of generic formulations currently on the market.
    c. Adverse effects: Nausea, somnolence, fatigue, dizziness, vomiting, headache, orthostatic hypotension, syncope
    d. Contraindications and precautions
       - i. Can limit the effectiveness of agents used to treat psychosis or exacerbate psychotic disorders
       - ii. Should not be used in nursing mothers or patients with syncopal migraines
       - iii. Concomitant use with dopamine antagonists (e.g., neuroleptic agents) may limit the efficacy of both agents.
    e. Efficacy
       - i. 0.1%–0.6% reduction in A1C
       - ii. Possible cardiovascular benefit

Table 5. Comparison of Therapies for Type 2 DM Hyperglycemia Added to Metformin

Agent or Class	Primary Glycemic Effect	Benefits	Limitations and Precautions
Sulfonylurea	Fasting and prandial	Efficacy Cost	Weight gain Hypoglycemia risk Hastens β cell dysfunction
Meglitinide	Prandial	Prandial focus Use in kidney impairment	Hypoglycemia risk Weight gain Mealtime dosing
Pioglitazone	Fasting and prandial	Improves insulin sensitivity and pancreatic function Low risk of hypoglycemia Possible cardiovascular benefit Cost	Weight gain and edema Risk of heart failure Risk of osteoporosis Possible bladder cancer risk?
α-Glucosidase inhibitor	Prandial	No systemic absorption Prandial focus Weight loss	GI adverse effect profile Mealtime dosing Modest A1C effect
DPP-4 inhibitor	Prandial	Well tolerated Weight neutral	Possible pancreatitis risk? Modest A1C effect Possible increased heart failure risk with saxagliptin Cost
GLP-1 agonist	Once- or twice-daily formulations have prandial focus Once-weekly formulations affect both fasting and prandial	Greater effect on prandial glucose Weight loss Efficacy Improves pancreatic function	Nausea and vomiting Injection site effects Questionable pancreatitis or thyroid cancer risk? Cost
Colesevelam	Prandial	Lipid benefits No systemic absorption	Large pill size and burden GI adverse effect profile Small decrease in A1C Avoid with high triglycerides
Bromocriptine	Fasting and prandial	Low risk of hypoglycemia Possible cardiovascular benefit	Small decrease in A1C CNS adverse effects
SGLT-2 inhibitors	Fasting and prandial	Low risk of hypoglycemia Efficacy Weight loss Possible cardiovascular benefit	Urinary tract and genital infections Diuresis Euglycemic DKA
Amylin agonist	Prandial	Modest weight loss Efficacy on postprandial glucose	High risk of hypoglycemia Must be taken with insulin Frequent injections Injection site effects GI adverse effects
Insulin	Basal: fasting Bolus: prandial	Significant A1C reduction Flexibility in dosing strategies and titration	Hypoglycemia Weight gain Injection site effects

CNS = central nervous system; DPP-4 = dipeptidyl peptidase type-4; GI = gastrointestinal; GLP = glucagon-like peptide; SGLT = sodium glucose cotransporter, DKA = diabetic ketoacidosis.

Information adapted from Inzucchi S, Bergenstal R, Buse J. Management of hyperglycemia in type 2 diabetes: a patient-centered approach. Diabetes Care 2012;35:1364-79; and Garber A, Agrahamson M, Barzilay J, et al. American Association of Clinical Endocrinologists' comprehensive diabetes management algorithm 2013 consensus statement. Endocr Pract 2013;19(suppl 2):1-48.

K. Treatment of inpatient DM (non–critically ill)
  1. Joint guidelines from the ADA and AACE. The Endocrine Society also has guidelines (2016 ADA recommendations added new subsection dedicated to the issue).
  2. Strong association between admission hyperglycemia and worse inpatient outcomes and length of stay. Outcomes worse in those who have stress-related hyperglycemia or not known to previously have diabetes.
  3. Glycemic goals
     a. Less than 140 mg/dL fasting or premeal
     b. Less than 180 mg/dL random glucose
  4. Treatment
     a. Assess glucose concentrations before meals and at bedtime if eating (every 4–6 hours if taking nothing by mouth [NPO]).
     b. Threshold for initiating therapy is 180 mg/dL or greater.
     c. Subcutaneous insulin administration per guidelines is the most practical way to improve hyperglycemia.
     d. Oral diabetes agents are generally not recommended unless patient is clinically stable and eating regularly, and no significant precautions or contraindications for use exist.
     e. Use of sliding scale insulin alone is not recommended.
     f. Basal/bolus insulin therapy as described above in the treatment of type 1 DM is recommended unless patient is NPO. If NPO, use basal insulin alone.

VII. TREATMENT OF DM COMPLICATIONS

Patient Case

12. A patient with newly diagnosed type 2 DM is screened for diabetic nephropathy. The following laboratory values are obtained today: blood pressure 129/78 mm Hg, heart rate 78 beats/minute, urine albumin/creatinine 27 mg/g, and estimated CrCl 94 mL/minute. Which would be the most appropriate treatment strategy?

A. No change in therapy is warranted.

B. Add an angiotensin-converting enzyme (ACE) inhibitor.

C. Add an ARB.

D. Reduce daily protein intake.

A. Hypoglycemia
  1. Degree of intervention depends on glucose concentrations and presence of symptoms.
  2. Symptoms are very patient-specific but may include anxiousness, sweating, nausea, tachycardia, hunger, clammy skin, and many others.
  3. Consequences of significant hypoglycemia are most worrisome in the very young, older adults, and those with established heart disease.
  4. Definition
     a. Plasma glucose less than 70 mg/dL with or without symptoms
     b. Hypoglycemic unawareness: Low glucose without symptoms
  5. Mild to moderate hypoglycemia
     a. Oral ingestion of 15–20 g of glucose or equivalent
     b. Repeat glucose concentration in 15 minutes and, if still less than 70 mg/dL, repeat ingestion of glucose.
     c. Once glucose is normalized, ingest snack or meal.

6. Severe hypoglycemia (altered consciousness, needs assistance from others)
   a. Glucagon 1 mg intramuscularly
   b. Intravenous dextrose if patient does not respond to glucagon
   c. Raise glucose targets for several weeks.

B. Diabetic Ketoacidosis
   1. More common in type 1 DM but can occur in type 2 DM
   2. Usually occurs because of a precipitating factor that stresses the body, resulting in increased counter-regulatory hormones
      a. Inappropriate (including nonadherence) or inadequate insulin therapy and infection are the two most common causes.
      b. Other causes: Myocardial infarction, pancreatitis, stroke, drugs (e.g., corticosteroids)
   3. Results in significant hyperglycemia, dehydration, and ketoacidosis
   4. Common signs and symptoms: Polyuria, polydipsia, vomiting, dehydration, weakness, altered mental status, coma, abdominal pain, Kussmaul respirations, tachycardia, hyponatremia, hyperkalemia
   5. Treatment
      a. Treat underlying cause if known.
      b. Fluid replacement
         i. 0.45%–0.9% sodium chloride, depending on baseline serum sodium concentrations
         ii. Change to 5% dextrose with 0.45% sodium chloride when serum glucose is less than 200 mg/dL.
      c. Insulin
         i. Goal is to stop ketosis, not to normalize glucose concentrations.
         ii. Intravenous bolus: 0.1 unit/kg
         iii. Intravenous infusion
            (a) 0.1 unit/kg/hour (increase if not a 50- to 75-mg/dL drop in serum glucose in the first hour)
            (b) Alternatively, 0.14 unit/kg/hour if no insulin bolus is given
            (c) If not at least a 10% decrease in serum glucose attained in first hour, give 0.14 unit/kg intravenous bolus.
            (d) Reduce infusion rate to 0.02–0.05 unit/kg/hour when serum glucose reaches 200 mg/dL and keep glucose between 150 and 200 mg/dL until DKA resolves.
         iv. Interrupt insulin treatment if baseline serum potassium is less than 3.3 mEq/L and until corrected.
      d. Potassium
         i. Potassium 20–30 mEq/L of intravenous fluid if baseline serum potassium greater than 3.3 but less than 5.3 mEq/L
         ii. Hold if 5.3 mEq/L or greater initially. Monitor and replace as needed.
         iii. Potassium 20–30 mEq/hour if baseline less than 3.3 mEq/L (while holding insulin)
      e. Intravenous bicarbonate if serum pH less than 6.9
      f. DKA considered resolved and can be converted to subcutaneous insulin when serum glucose is less than 200 mg/dL and at least two of the following:
         i. Venous pH greater than 7.3
         ii. Serum bicarbonate of 15 mEq/L or greater
         iii. Calculated anion gap of 12 mEq/L or less

C. Nephropathy
   1. Screen annually with random spot collection of urine albumin/creatinine ratio, starting at diagnosis in type 2 DM and after 5 or more years in type 1 DM.
      a. Normal: Less than 30 mg/g (or micrograms per milligram)
      b. Increased urinary albumin excretion (albuminuria) 30 mg/g or greater

  c. Two of three specimens greater than 30 mg/g obtained over a 3- to 6-month period is consistent with diagnosis of albuminuria.

  d. ADA in 2013 no longer uses terms *microalbuminuria* and *macroalbuminuria*.

 2. Estimated CrCl yearly as well

 3. Use of angiotensin-converting enzyme (ACE) inhibitors or ARBs considered initial treatment of choice if urine albumin/creatinine levels are greater than 30 mg/g.

 4. Dietary protein restriction as renal function declines

D. Retinopathy

 1. Screen annually with dilated and comprehensive eye examinations, starting at diagnosis in type 2 DM and after 5 or more years in type 1 DM.

 2. Frequency can be reduced to every 2–3 years after one or more normal examinations.

 3. No specific pharmacotherapy is recommended except to adequately control glucose concentrations and blood pressure.

E. DM Neuropathies

 1. Can have nerve damage in any area of the body but commonly affects the lower extremities.

 2. Screen for distal polyneuropathy using monofilament once yearly.

  a. Screen after 5 years of type 1 DM and at diagnosis with type 2 DM.

  b. Diminished sensitivity is a significant risk factor for diabetes-related foot ulcer and increases the need for frequent visual inspection by patients if it exists.

 3. Treatment of neuropathies is for symptomatic improvement and does not prevent progression.

 4. Symptoms are patient specific but may include numbness, burning, tingling sensation, or pain.

 5. Neuropathic pain

  a. Tricyclic antidepressants (amitriptyline, desipramine)

   i. Effective but limited because of anticholinergic effects; some recommend using secondary amine tricyclic antidepressants (e.g., desipramine, nortriptyline) because they may have less anticholinergic effect than tertiary amines (e.g., amitriptyline, imipramine).

   ii. Daily dosage is less than dosages used for depression.

  b. Anticonvulsants (gabapentin, lamotrigine, pregabalin)

   i. Comparative data on gabapentin and pregabalin against tricyclic antidepressants show similar efficacy with fewer adverse effects. Adverse effect profile is still significant (e.g., fatigue, dizziness).

   ii. Pregabalin is the only anticonvulsant approved for use in DM neuropathic pain and is recommended by the American Academy of Neurology in its 2011 guideline.

  c. Selective serotonin reuptake inhibitor/selective serotonin and norepinephrine reuptake inhibitor (duloxetine, paroxetine, citalopram)

   i. Duloxetine is the only approved agent in this category.

   ii. Duloxetine data compared with amitriptyline data show similar efficacy and expected higher anticholinergic adverse effects with amitriptyline.

   iii. Duloxetine may provide better pain reduction, with tolerability similar to that of pregabalin.

  d. Tramadol/acetaminophen: As effective as gabapentin; different adverse effect profile

  e. Opioids: Tapentadol extended release is the only approved agent in this class; no head-to-head efficacy studies

 6. Gastroparesis

  a. Autonomic neuropathy causes nausea and vomiting after meals because of delayed gastric emptying.

  b. Nonpharmacologic strategies

   i. More frequent but smaller meals

   ii. Homogenize food.

    c. Pharmacologic treatment
      i. Metoclopramide: 10 mg before meals. Risk of tardive dyskinesia or extrapyramidal reactions
      ii. Erythromycin: 40–250 mg before meals

F. Cardiovascular Disease
  1. Most common cause of morbidity and mortality as well as health care expenditures in DM complications
  2. Proper DM management should always focus on cardiovascular disease risk reduction (review cardiovascular chapters).
  3. Stress and continually assess the blood pressure and lipid goals described earlier.
  4. Blood pressure management
    a. Often requires more antihypertensive medications
    b. Hypertensive regimen should include an ACE inhibitor or an ARB.
    c. Administration of at least one antihypertensive in the evening may improve blood pressure and reduce cardiovascular outcomes.
  5. Lipid management
    a. Assess fasting lipid profile annually or as needed to monitor adherence.
    b. Statin therapy recommendations are based on age and cardiovascular risk.
      i. Moderate-dose statin therapy is recommended for all patients age 40 or older without cardiovascular risk factors (e.g., LDL-C greater than or equal to 100 mg/dL, high blood pressure, smoker, overweight, or obese).
      ii. High-dose statin therapy is recommended for those age 40–75 with existing cardiovascular risk factors (moderate- or high-dose statin if greater than 75 years of age).
      iii. High-dose statin therapy is recommended for all patients with existing cardiovascular disease (e.g., previous cardiovascular event or acute coronary syndrome).
      iv. For patients with acute coronary syndrome and LDL-C greater than 50 mg/dL who cannot tolerate high-dose statin, consider moderate-dose statin plus ezetimibe.
      v. Statin doses are consistent with ACC/AHA lipid guidelines
  6. Antiplatelet therapy
    a. Low-dose aspirin (75–162 mg/day)
      i. With existing cardiovascular disease
      ii. For primary prevention if 10-year risk is greater than 10% (includes most patients regardless of gender 50 years of age or older who have at least one cardiovascular risk factor)
    b. Clopidogrel for those intolerant of aspirin therapy

G. Preventive Immunizations
  1. Annual influenza vaccine
  2. Pneumococcal polysaccharide vaccine
  3. Hepatitis B vaccine

VIII. OTHER DIABETES MEDICATION ISSUES

A. Former FDA Risk Evaluation and Mitigation Strategy for Rosiglitazone (removed November 2013)
  1. The strategy limited use and distribution of rosiglitazone because of concerns of increased myocardial events.
  2. Subsequent review of clinical trial data suggests no increased risk for myocardial infarction, resulting in strategy being removed.
  3. Despite removal of the strategy, rosiglitazone remains unavailable.

B. In the wake of the rosiglitazone safety issue, the FDA now requires all newly approved diabetes medications to prove cardiovascular safety.
   1. At least 2 years of safety data that includes cardiovascular events as an end point and independent adjudication of events
   2. Necessary to study in older adults and in those with some degree of renal impairment and those with more advanced diabetes.
   3. Cardiovascular safety data for many of the newer DPP-4 inhibitors, GLP-1 agonists, insulins, and SGLT-2 inhibitors are still pending.

IX. DIABETES INSIPIDUS

A. Diabetes insipidus (DI) is usually a result of decreased production of antidiuretic hormone, also known as vasopressin, in the case of central DI or a lack of ADH effect in the kidneys (nephrogenic DI).
B. Classification
   1. Central or neurogenic
      a. Idiopathic
      b. Trauma (brain injury)
      c. Neoplasm
      d. Hypodipsia
      e. Genetic abnormality
   2. Nephrogenic
      a. Genetic abnormality
      b. Acquired (more common)
         i. Drug-induced (e.g., lithium, amphotericin B, foscarnet, cidofovir)
         ii. Kidney disease (e.g., polycystic kidney disease, obstruction)
         iii. Electrolyte disorder (hypercalcemia, hypokalemia)
C. Diagnosis
   1. Elevated urine volume (greater than 3 L/day)
   2. Decreased urine osmolarity (less than 200 mOsm/kg)
   3. Response to water deprivation (may help differentiate between nephrogenic and central etiology in non–critically ill patient)
D. Signs and symptoms
   1. Polydipsia
   2. Polyuria or nocturia
   3. Weakness or lethargy
   4. Confusion or delirium (if severe)
E. Treatment
   1. Treat underlying cause if known
   2. Central DI
      a. Desmopressin: 5–20 mcg intranasally once to twice daily
      b. Adjunctive therapies: Chlorpropamide, carbamazepine
   3. Nephrogenic DI
      a. Thiazide diuretic
      b. Dietary sodium restriction
      c. Indomethacin

REFERENCES

Thyroid

1. Garber J, Cobin R, Gharib H, et al. Clinical practice guidelines for hypothyroidism in adults: co-sponsored by the American Association of Clinical Endocrinologists and the American Thyroid Association. Thyroid 2012;22:1200-35.

2. Jonklaas J, Talbert RL. Thyroid disorders. In: Talbert RL, DiPiro JT, Matzke GR, et al., eds. Pharmacotherapy: A Pathophysiologic Approach, 8th ed. New York: McGraw-Hill, 2011:chap 84. Available at www.accesspharmacy.com/content. aspx?aID=7991868. Accessed October 11, 2012.

3. Pearce E, Farwell A, Braverman L. Thyroiditis. N Engl J Med 2005;348:2646-55.

4. Rahn R, Burch H, Cooper D, et al. Hyperthyroidism and other causes of thyrotoxicosis: management guidelines of the American Thyroid Association and American Association of Clinical Endocrinologists. Endocr Pract 2011;17:e1-65.

5. Razvi S, Weaver J, Butler T, et al. Levothyroxine treatment of subclinical hypothyroidism, fatal and nonfatal cardiovascular events, and mortality. Arch Intern Med 2012;172:811-7.

6. Rodondi N, Newman A, Vittinghoff E, et al. Subclinical hypothyroidism and the risk of heart failure, other cardiovascular events, and death. Arch Intern Med 2005;165:2460-6.

7. Surks M, Ortiz E, Daniels G, et al. Subclinical thyroid disease: scientific review and guidelines for diagnosis and management. JAMA 2004;291:228-38.

8. Wall C. Myxedema coma: diagnosis and treatment. Am Fam Physician 2000;62:2485-90.

9. Walsh J, Bremner A, Bulsara M, et al. Subclinical thyroid dysfunction as a risk factor for cardiovascular disease. Arch Intern Med 2005;165:2467-72.

10. Stagnaro-Green A, Abalovich M, Alexander E, et al. Guidelines of the American Thyroid Association for the diagnosis and management of thyroid disease during pregnancy and postpartum. Thyroid 2011;21:1081-125.

Pituitary

1. Melmed S, Casanueva F, Hoffman A, et al. Diagnosis and treatment of hyperprolactinemia: an Endocrine Society clinical practice guideline. J Clin Endocrinol Metab 2011;96:273-88.

2. Thorogood N, Baldeweg S. Pituitary disorders: an overview for the general physician. Br J Hosp Med 2008;69:198-204.

3. Jordan JK, Sheehan A, Yanovski JA, et al. Pituitary gland disorders. In: DiPiro JT, Talbert RL, Yee GC, et al., eds. Pharmacotherapy: A Pathophysiologic Approach, 9th ed. New York, NY: McGraw-Hill, 2014:chap 60. Available at http://accesspharmacy. mhmedical.com/content.aspx?bookid=689&Sectionid=45310512. Accessed October 7, 2015.

Adrenal

1. Biller B, Grossman A, Stewart P, et al. Treatment of adrenocorticotropin-dependent Cushing's syndrome: a consensus statement. J Clin Endocrinol Metab 2008;93:2454-62.

2. Shalet S, Mukherjee A. Pharmacological treatment of hypercortisolism. Curr Opin Endocrinol Diabetes Obes 2008;15:234-8.

3. Dietrich E, Smith SM, Gums JG, et al. Adrenal gland disorders. In: DiPiro JT, Talbert RL, Yee GC, et al., eds. Pharmacotherapy: A Pathophysiologic Approach, 9th ed. New York, NY: McGraw-Hill, 2014:chap 59. Available at http://accesspharmacy. mhmedical.com/content.aspx?bookid=689&Sectionid=45310511. Accessed October 7, 2015.

4. Treatment of Cushing's syndrome: an Endocrine Society clinical practice guideline. J Clin Endocrinol Metab 2015;100:2807-31.

Obesity

1. Fidler M, Sanchez M, Raether B, et al. A one-year randomized trial of lorcaserin for weight loss in obese and overweight adults: the BLOSSOM trial. J Clin Endocrinol Metab 2011;96:3067-77.

2. Foster G, Wyatt H, Hill J, et al. Weight and metabolic outcomes after 2 years on a low-carbohydrate versus low-fat diet. Ann Intern Med 2010;153:147-57.

3. Jensen M, Ryan D, Apovian C, et al. 2013 AHA/ACC/TOS guideline for the management of overweight and obesity in adults: a report of the American College of Cardiology/American Heart Association Task Force on Practice Guidelines and the Obesity Society. J Am Coll Cardiol 2014;63:2985-3023.

4. Apovian C, Aronne L, Bessesen D, et al. Pharmacological management of obesity: an Endocrine Society clinical practice guideline. J Clin Endocrinol Metab 2015;100:342-62.

Polycystic Ovary

1. Legro R, Arslanian, S, Ehrmann D, et al. Diagnosis and treatment of polycystic ovary syndrome: an Endocrine Society clinical practice guideline. J Clin Endocrinol Metab 2013;98:4565-92.

2. Nestler J. Metformin for the treatment of the polycystic ovary syndrome. N Engl J Med 2008;358:47-54.

3. Norman R, Dwailly D, Legro R, et al. Polycystic ovary syndrome. Lancet 2007;370:685-97.

4. Radosh L. Drug treatment for polycystic ovary syndrome. Am Fam Physician 2009;79:671-6.

Diabetes Mellitus and Insipidus

1. American Diabetes Association (ADA). Standards of medical care in diabetes—2016: classification and diagnosis of diabetes. Diabetes Care 2016;39(suppl 1):S13-22.

2. American Diabetes Association (ADA). Standards of medical care in diabetes—2016: glycemic targets. Diabetes Care 2016;39(suppl 1):S39-46.

3. American Diabetes Association (ADA). Standards of medical care in diabetes—2016: approaches to glycemic treatment. Diabetes Care 2016;39(suppl 1):S52-9.

4. American Diabetes Association (ADA). Standards of medical care in diabetes—2016: cardiovascular disease and risk management. Diabetes Care 2016;39(suppl 1):S60-71.

5. American Diabetes Association (ADA). Standards of medical care in diabetes—2016: microvascular complications and foot care. Diabetes Care 2016;39(suppl 1):S72-80.

6. Inzucchi S, Buse J, Ferrannini E, et al. Management of hyperglycemia in type 2 diabetes, 2015: a patient-centered approach. Diabetes Care 2015;38:140-9.

7. Bril V, England J, Franklin G, et al. Evidence-based guideline: treatment of painful diabetic neuropathy: report of the American Academy of Neurology, the American Association of Neuromuscular and Electrodiagnostic Medicine, and the American Academy of Physical Medicine and Rehabilitation. Neurology 2011;76:1-8.

8. Camilleri M. Diabetic gastroparesis. N Engl J Med 2007;356:820-9.

9. The Diabetes Control and Complications Trial/Epidemiology of Diabetes Interventions and Complications (DCCT/EDIC) Study Research Group. Intensive diabetes treatment and cardiovascular disease in patients with type 1 diabetes. N Engl J Med 2005;353:2643-53.

10. Handelsman Y, Bloomgarden Z, Grunberger G, et al. American Association of Clinical Endocrinologists and American College of Endocrinology: clinical practice guidelines for developing a diabetes mellitus comprehensive care plan 2015. Endocr Pract 2015;21:1-87.

11. Kitabchi A, Umpierrez G, Miles J, et al. Hyperglycemic crises in adult patients with diabetes. Diabetes Care 2009;32:1335-43.

12. Seaquist E, Anderson J, Childs B, et al. Hypoglycemia and diabetes: a report of a workgroup of the American Diabetes Association and the Endocrine Society. Diabetes Care 2013;36:1384-95.

13. Skyler J, Bergenstal R, Bonow R, et al. Intensive glycemic control and the prevention of cardiovascular events: implications of the ACCORD, ADVANCE, and VA diabetes trials. Diabetes Care 2009;32:187-92.

14. American Association of Clinical Endocrinologists and American Diabetes Association. Consensus statement on inpatient glycemic control. Endocr Pract 2009;15:1-17.

15. American Diabetes Association (ADA). Standards of medical care in diabetes—2016: diabetes care in the hospital. Diabetes Care 2016;39(suppl 1):S99-104.

16. Blevins L, Wand G. Diabetes insipidus. Crit Care Med 1992;20:69-79.

17. Chessman KH, Matzke GR. Disorders of sodium and water homeostasis. In: DiPiro JT, Talbert RL, Yee GC, et al., eds. *Pharmacotherapy: A Pathophysiologic Approach, 9th ed.* New York, NY: McGraw-Hill, 2014:chap 34. Available at http://accesspharmacy.mhmedical.com.ezproxy.ttuhsc.edu/content.aspx?bookid=689&Sectionid=48811473. Accessed October 9, 2015.

ANSWERS AND EXPLANATIONS TO PATIENT CASES

1. Answer: D

Given this patient's reluctance to undergo ablative therapy, usually the most common treatment, oral therapy is warranted. Methimazole is recommended over PTU (Answer B) because it is associated with a lower risk of hepatotoxicity, although it may not be more efficacious. Answer A is incorrect because iodine therapy is indicated in this type of case only before surgery or during an acute case of thyroid storm. Answer C is incorrect because although β-blockers might provide some symptomatic relief, they would do little to stabilize this patient's thyroid levels.

2. Answer: A

This patient has hypothyroidism on the basis of her elevated TSH and low free T_4, caused by Hashimoto's disease. Levothyroxine is the drug of choice for this condition, given its adverse effect profile, cost, antigenicity profile, and uniform potency. Although liothyronine can be used for hypothyroidism, its potential for increasing the risk of cardiovascular complications makes it second line (Answer B). Answer C is also incorrect, given its increased antigenicity compared with levothyroxine. Answer D is incorrect because it is an agent used to treat hyperthyroidism.

3. Answer: D

Fluoxetine, a selective serotonin reuptake inhibitor, may cause drug-induced hyperprolactinemia. Answer A is incorrect because β-blockers are not associated with an elevated risk of the condition. Given the patient's normal pituitary and thyroid tests, it is unlikely that Answer B, prolactin-secreting adenoma, is correct. Answer C is incorrect because pregnancy is not associated with an elevated risk of the condition.

4. Answer: D

Because the aldosterone/renin ratio and blood pressure are high, hyperaldosteronism is the most likely disease listed. Cushing's syndrome and hyperaldosteronism can be secondary causes of hypertension. In this case, the patient's free 24-hour urine cortisol is normal, but it would be elevated if he had Cushing's syndrome; therefore, Answer A is incorrect. Answer B is incorrect because Addison's disease is a result of cortisol deficiency and is not associated with hypertension. Answer C, hyperprolactinemia, is unlikely, given the patient's presentation and his abnormal aldosterone/renin ratio.

5. Answer: B

The minimal weight loss after 12 weeks of therapy with phentermine/topiramate should be 5%; otherwise, the medication should be discontinued. Given this patient's baseline weight, a minimum of 13 lb is necessary to continue therapy. The other answers provided are too low (Answer A), or they exceed the 5% minimal expectation (Answer C and Answer D).

6. Answer: D

Unless the patient has significant symptoms of hyperglycemia (none noted in this case), a subsequent evaluation for hyperglycemia by a fasting glucose concentration, a random glucose concentration, an OGTT, or an A1C is warranted; therefore, Answer A and Answer B are incorrect. Answer C is incorrect because a subsequent test for hyperglycemia should not be performed on the same day according to ADA guidelines.

7. Answer: B

Improved blood pressure control has been associated with both a decrease in microvascular complications (e.g., nephropathy) and macrovascular (e.g., myocardial infarction) complications. Answers A and C address only hyperglycemia, which may improve microvascular complications but not macrovascular complications. Answer D, niacin, has not been shown to reduce either complication in patients with diabetes.

8. Answer: D

This patient weighs 50 kg (110 lb). 0.4 unit/kg/day × 50 kg = 20 units of TDI. When using insulin analogs, 50% of the TDI dose should be used as an initial estimate of the patient's basal insulin needs; therefore, 10 units is needed. Glargine is a once-daily, long-acting basal insulin. Although they include basal insulin, Answer A and Answer B are incorrect because of the higher-than-estimated dosage. Answer C is incorrect because insulin aspart is used for bolus insulin dosing, not for basal therapy, unless the patient is using an insulin pump.

9. Answer: B

GLP-1 agonists have shown to mildly reduce weight when used to treat hyperglycemia in patients with type 2 DM. Each of the other options, a sulfonylurea (Answer A), a thiazolidinedione (Answer C), or insulin (Answer D), are all associated with weight gain.

10. Answer: D

The usual next step in therapy for a patient no longer able to maintain adequate glycemic control with monotherapy is to add agents. Answer A is incorrect because the patient is already exercising and still has uncontrolled hyperglycemia. Answer B is incorrect because one agent, particularly metformin, would not normally be changed to another unless a patient was experiencing adverse effects of the original agent. Answer C, bromocriptine, is not likely to provide sufficient glycemic control given this patient's current A1C.

11. Answer: A

In this case, the initiation of medications to treat a patient with newly diagnosed hyperglycemia is complicated by the patient's many comorbidities. Normally, metformin, Answer D, would be the initial treatment of choice, but the patient's renal function is poor, and metformin should not be used. Answer C, exenatide, is also incorrect because it, too, should not be used in patients with significant renal impairment. Given the patient's existing edema and history of heart failure, pioglitazone (Answer B) is contraindicated because it can aggravate the conditions. Answer A, linagliptin, is the most appropriate choice because the A1C is not markedly elevated, and renal function does not need to be considered.

12. Answer: A

Current recommendations call for the use of an ACE inhibitor or ARB if a patient has elevated urinary albumin excretion. This patient's blood pressure is at goal (less than 140/90 mm Hg) and urine albumin/creatinine is normal (less than 30 mg/g). No additional therapy in necessary. Answer B and Answer C are incorrect because the patient's blood pressure is well controlled, and the urine albumin/creatinine is normal. Answer D is incorrect because protein restriction is used only after a significant decrease in CrCl, and this patient has normal renal function.

ANSWERS AND EXPLANATIONS TO SELF-ASSESSMENT QUESTIONS

1. Answer: D
According to the ADA guidelines, patients with this degree of hyperglycemia should be initiated on insulin therapy, and Answer D provides an appropriate basal and bolus insulin combination. This patient's A1C is greater than 10%, and his fasting glucose is greater than 300–350 mg/dL. Answer A and Answer C are not optimal because dual therapy with oral agents is unlikely to bring this patient to his glycemic goal. Answer B is also not optimal because the combination of a sulfonylurea and rapid-acting insulin would increase the risk of hypoglycemia and would be unlikely to bring about a sufficient reduction in A1C.

2. Answer: C
This patient's TDI requirement is 40 units (80 kg × 0.5 unit/kg/day). Half of this is initially used for basal insulin requirements and half for bolus insulin requirements before meals. The 20 units for bolus requirements should initially be divided equally between three meals (i.e., 6–7 units). The other three answers would provide either too much or too little estimated insulin at each meal.

3. Answer: C
This patient has an elevated blood pressure, poor renal function, and two urine albumin/creatinine concentrations above 30 mg/g. According to the ADA and the clinical literature, the best classes of medications for patients with this condition are ARBs and ACE inhibitors. Answer A (thiazide diuretic) is not appropriate because this class of medications is not more beneficial than agents that block the renin-angiotensin system. Answer B, a dihydropyridine calcium channel blocker, is not best because this class has not been shown to be beneficial in type 1 and type 2 DM and proteinuria. Answer D, a nondihydropyridine calcium channel blocker, is an alternative to agents that block the renin-angiotensin system, but it should not be used instead of these agents unless a patient has contraindications to them.

4. Answer: B
Unlike methimazole, PTU has a boxed warning about the risk of hepatotoxicity. Answer A is incorrect because neither agent is considered more efficacious than the other. Answer C is incorrect because Hashimoto's disease is a result of hypothyroidism, not hyperthyroidism. Methimazole is dosed once daily, whereas PTU is usually dosed up to three times daily, making Answer D incorrect.

5. Answer: A
Ketoconazole is used in patients with Cushing's syndrome because it reduces cortisol synthesis. Answer B, spironolactone, is used in patients with hyperaldosteronism. Answer C is inappropriate because Cushing's syndrome results in cortisol concentrations that are too high, and adding a corticosteroid to treat its symptoms could make the problem worse. Bromocriptine, Answer D, is used to treat acromegaly, not Cushing's syndrome.

6. Answer: C
This patient has both significant renal impairment and a markedly elevated A1C. Answers A and D are incorrect because they are both contraindicated in patients with significant renal impairment. Answer B is also incorrect. Although alogliptin can be used in patients with renal impairment at a reduced dosage, it is not likely to provide a sufficient reduction in A1C. Initiating insulin is the best option in this case because it can be used in patients with renal impairment and can be titrated to attain significant reductions in A1C.

7. Answer: A
An older woman with heart disease should be initiated on a lower initial dose of levothyroxine. Answer B is the normal starting dose (i.e., 1.6 mcg/kg), but it is probably too high an initial dose for an older adult with established heart disease. Answer C and Answer D are incorrect because the drug of choice is levothyroxine, and liothyronine is no longer recommended for this condition.

8. Answer: B
For insulin adjustments, determine which BG readings are at goal and which ones are not. For those consistently not at goal, determine which insulin is most affecting the BG readings. In this case, the patient's BG readings are consistently elevated at bedtime, which is probably caused by insufficient predinner prandial (a.k.a. bolus) insulin. Changing the rapid-acting insulin

at other times of the day would not help; therefore, Answer A and Answer D are incorrect. Changing her basal insulin (glargine in this case) would probably not help her bedtime BG, and because her FBG readings have been well controlled, it could lead to hypoglycemia (Answer C).

9. Answer: A

This patient has mild symptoms, and her ablative therapy worked initially but now no longer controls her thyroid levels. Methimazole (Answer A) would be the preferred oral agent, given its dosing frequency and lower risk of hepatotoxicity compared with PTU (Answer C). Thyroidectomy is an option, but it is probably too aggressive for mild Graves' disease; therefore, Answer B is incorrect. Answer D is not optimal; β-blockers, which may provide symptomatic relief, will not significantly affect her thyroid levels.

10. Answer: D

This patient has good control of his fasting glucose but is experiencing postprandial hyperglycemia. An agent that targets postprandial glucose (e.g., a DPP-4 inhibitor) would be most appropriate. Answer A is incorrect because this would exceed the maximal daily dose for metformin. Answer B is incorrect because insulin glargine is a basal insulin that has an effect on FPG but little effect on postprandial glucose. Answer C is incorrect, again because it is a basal insulin and also because it is more appropriate to add medications than to switch to another agent unless the patient is experiencing adverse effects with the first agent.

11. Answer: D

This patient has tried dieting and some exercise, but these are failing to control her weight; thus, her current routine alone is not appropriate, making Answer A incorrect. Answer B, lorcaserin, is approved for the treatment of obesity but should be avoided in patients taking serotonergic agents, in this case sertraline. Answer C is a federally scheduled medication because of its abuse potential with phentermine, and given this patient's history of abuse, it is not the most favorable selection. Orlistat, Answer D, is the only agent listed to which this patient does not have a specific precaution or contraindication with its use.

12. Answer: A

This patient has now had two laboratory glycemic indicators (A1C and FBG) consistent with the diagnosis of diabetes. Answer B is probably incorrect because this patient has several risk factors for developing type 2 DM, including obesity, ethnicity, age, a history of gestational diabetes, and a strong family history of the disease. Answer C is incorrect because there is no need to obtain another A1C reading this soon after the reading just 2 weeks ago, and the A1C can be used in the diagnosis of diabetes. Obtaining another glucose reading on another day (Answer D) is also incorrect, again because there are already two abnormal glycemic indicators; therefore, another is not necessary to confirm the diagnosis.

13. Answer: C

According to the ADA, moderate-dose statin therapy is recommended for patients older than 40 years with diabetes but without other cardiovascular risk factors. The updated 2015 ADA guidelines are similar to newer guidelines from the ACC/AHA, who also advocate moderate-intensity statin therapy. In this case, the patient's glycemic and blood pressure readings are at goal (less than 7.0% and less than 140/90 mm Hg, respectively). Adding insulin (Answer A) and adding a blood pressure medication (Answer B) are not necessary. Answer D is incorrect because there is no need for fibrate therapy in this patient; the HDL-C and TG are under control.

Nephrology

John M. Burke, Pharm.D., FCCP, BCPS

St. Louis College of Pharmacy
St. Louis, Missouri

NEPHROLOGY

JOHN M. BURKE, PHARM.D., FCCP, BCPS

ST. LOUIS COLLEGE OF PHARMACY
ST. LOUIS, MISSOURI

Learning Objectives

1. Categorize acute kidney injury (AKI) as prerenal, intrinsic, or postrenal, based on patient history, physical examination, and laboratory values.
2. Identify risk factors for AKI.
3. Formulate preventive strategies to decrease the risk of developing AKI in specific patient populations.
4. Formulate a therapeutic plan to manage AKI.
5. Identify medications and medication classes associated with acute and chronic kidney damage.
6. Describe characteristics that determine the efficiency of removal of drugs by dialysis.
7. Classify the stage or category of chronic kidney disease (CKD) based on patient history, physical examination, and laboratory values.
8. Identify risk factors for the progression of CKD.
9. Formulate strategies to slow the progression of CKD.
10. Assess for the presence of common complications of CKD.
11. Develop a care plan to manage the common complications observed in patients with CKD (e.g., anemia, secondary hyperthyroidism).

Self-Assessment Questions

Answers and explanations to these questions can be found at the end of this chapter.

1. A 75-year-old man (weight 92.5 kg, height 73 inches) presents to your institution with abdominal pain and dizziness. He has a brief history of gastroenteritis and has had nothing to eat or drink for 24 hours. His blood pressure (BP) reading while sitting is 120/80 mm Hg, which drops to 90/60 mm Hg when standing. His heart rate is 90 beats/minute. His basic metabolic panel shows sodium (Na) 135 mEq/L, chloride (Cl) 108 mEq/L, potassium (K) 4.7 mEq/L, CO_2 26 mEq/L, blood urea nitrogen (BUN) 40 mg/dL, serum creatinine (SCr) 1.5 mg/dL, and glucose 188 mg/dL. He has no known drug allergies. Which is the best approach to treat this patient?

    A. Administer furosemide 40 mg intravenously × 1.
    B. Insert Foley catheter to check for residual urine.
    C. Administer fluid bolus (500 mL of normal saline solution).
    D. Administer insulin lispro 3 units subcutaneously.

2. A 44-year-old man is admitted with gram-negative bacteremia. He receives 4 days of parenteral aminoglycoside therapy and develops acute tubular necrosis (ATN). Antibiotic therapy is adjusted on the basis of culture and sensitivity results. Which set of laboratory data is most consistent with this presentation?

    A. BUN/SCr ratio greater than 20:1, urine sodium less than 10 mOsm/L, fractional excretion of sodium (FENa) less than 1%, specific gravity more than 1.018, and hyaline casts.
    B. BUN/SCr ratio greater than 20:1, urine sodium more than 20 mOsm/L, FENa more than 3%, specific gravity 1.010, no casts visible.
    C. BUN/SCr ratio of 10–15:1, urine sodium more than 40 mOsm/L, FENa more than 1%, specific gravity less than 1.015, muddy casts.
    D. BUN/SCr ratio of 10–15:1, urine sodium less than 10 mOsm/L, FENa less than 1%, specific gravity more than 1.018, muddy casts.

3. A patient with chronic kidney disease (CKD) category G4 (estimated creatinine clearance [eCrCl] of 25 mL/minute) has received a diagnosis of gram-positive bacteremia, which is susceptible only to drug X. There are no published reports on how to adjust the dose of drug X in patients with impaired kidney function. Review of the drug X package insert shows that it has significant renal elimination, with 40% excreted unchanged in the urine. The usual dose for drug X is 600 mg/day intravenously and is provided as 100 mg/mL in a 6-mL vial. Which is the best dose (in milliliters of drug X) to give this patient?

    A. 3.6.
    B. 4.1.
    C. 4.5.
    D. 5.5.

4. A 45-year-old man (weight 59 kg, height 70 inches) has a long history of cancer and malnutrition. His SCr is 0.5 mg/dL. He is to be given carboplatin,

for which an accurate estimate of kidney function is critical. Which is the best method for assessing kidney function in this patient?

   A. Cockcroft-Gault equation.

   B. Modification of Diet in Renal Disease (MDRD) study equation.

   C. 24-hour urine collection.

   D. Iothalamate study.

5. A 59-year-old patient who has had category G5 CKD for 10 years is maintained on chronic hemodialysis. He has a history of hypertension, coronary artery disease (CAD), mild congestive heart failure (CHF), and type 2 diabetes mellitus. Medications are as follows: epoetin 10,000 units intravenously three times/week at dialysis, renal multivitamin once daily, atorvastatin 20 mg/day, insulin, and calcium acetate 1334 mg three times/day with meals. Laboratory values are as follows: hemoglobin 9.2 g/dL, intact parathyroid hormone (PTH) 300 pg/mL, Na 140 mEq/L, K 4.9 mEq/L, SCr 7.0 mg/dL, calcium 9 mg/dL, albumin 3.5 g/dL, and phosphorus 4.8 mg/dL. He has a serum ferritin concentration of 80 ng/mL and a transferrin saturation (TSAT) of 14%. Mean corpuscular volume, mean corpuscular hemoglobin concentration, and white blood cell count (WBC) are all normal. He is afebrile. Which is the best approach to managing anemia in this patient?

   A. Increase epoetin.

   B. Add oral iron.

   C. Add intravenous iron.

   D. Maintain current regimen; patient is at goal.

6. A 60-year-old (72-kg) patient with a history of diabetes and hypertension is in the intensive care unit after having a myocardial infarction about 1 week ago with secondary heart failure. He now has pneumonia. He has been hypotensive for the past 5 days. Before his admission 1 week ago, he had an SCr of 1.0 mg/dL. His urine output has been steadily declining for the past 3 days, despite adequate hydration, with 700 mL of urine output in the past 24 hours. His medications since surgery include intravenous dobutamine, nitroglycerin, and cefazolin. Yesterday, his BUN and SCr were 32 and 3.1 mg/dL, respectively; today, they are

41 and 3.9 mg/dL. His urine osmolality is 290 mOsm/kg. His urine sodium is 40 mEq/L, and there are tubular cellular casts in his urine. Which is the most likely renal diagnosis?

   A. Prerenal azotemia.

   B. ATN.

   C. Acute interstitial nephritis (AIN).

   D. Hemodynamic/functional-mediated acute kidney injury (AKI).

7. You are evaluating a study comparing epoetin and darbepoetin in terms of their efficacy on mean hemoglobin concentrations. Both drugs are initiated at the recommended dose, and the hemoglobin concentration is checked at 4 weeks. Fifty patients are in each group. The mean hemoglobin in the epoetin group is 12.1 g/dL, and in the darbepoetin group, it is 12.2 g/dL. Which statistical test is best for this comparison?

   A. A paired t-test.

   B. An independent (unpaired) t-test.

   C. An analysis of variance.

   D. A chi-square test.

8. A pharmacoeconomic study is performed to compare the use of erythropoiesis-stimulating agents with various hemoglobin concentrations. The primary outcome of this study was cost per quality-adjusted life-year gained. Which is the best description of this economic evaluation?

   A. Cost minimization.

   B. Cost-effectiveness.

   C. Cost-benefit.

   D. Cost-utility.

9. A 58 year-old woman is being evaluated for AKI. Laboratory data reveal a serum sodium 134 mEq/L, BUN 35 mg/dL, SCr 1.8 mg/dL, urine sodium 24 mEq/L, and urine Cr 14.3 mg/dL. Which is the best estimate of this patient's fractional excretion of sodium (FENa)?

   A. 0.8%.

   B. 1.25%.

   C. 2.3%.

   D. 4.4%.

10. A 55-year-old man has a history of hypertension. His estimated glomerular filtration rate (eGFR) is 48 mL/min/1.73 m². Urine albumin:Cr ratio (ACR) is 28 mg/g. According to the Kidney Disease: Improving Global Outcomes (KDIGO) guidelines, which of the following is this patient's goal blood pressure?

    A. Less than 130/80 mm Hg.

    B. Less than 140/90 mm Hg.

    C. Less than 140/80 mm Hg.

    D. Less than 130/90 mm Hg.

11. A 66 year-old man has an eGFR of 55 mL/min/1.73 m². His albumin:Cr ratio is 100 mg/g. His hemoglobin is currently 13.2 g/dL, with normal red blood cell indices without treatment. What is the recommended frequency of monitoring of hemoglobin in this patient?

    A. At least every month.

    B. At least every 3 months.

    C. At least every 6 months.

    D. At least every 12 months.

12. A 68-year-old patient has diabetes, hypertension, and an eGFR of 40 mL/min/1.73 m². Medications include a renal multivitamin once daily, simvastatin, lisinopril, and hydrochlorothiazide. Laboratory values are as follows: hemoglobin 11.2 g/dL, immunoassay for PTH 200 pg/mL, Na 138 mEq/L, K 4.9 mEq/L, calcium 8.6 mg/dL, albumin 3.5 g/dL, phosphorus 5.8 mg/dL, and 25-hydroxyvitamin D 45 ng/mL. Which of the following is best to prevent CKD–mineral bone disorder (MBD) in this patient?

    A. Ergocalciferol.

    B. Calcium acetate.

    C. Calcitriol.

    D. Cinacalcet.

BPS Pharmacotherapy Specialty Examination Content Outline
This chapter covers the following sections of the Pharmacotherapy Specialty Examination Content Outline:
1. Domain 1: Patient-Specific Pharmacotherapy
    a. Tasks 1.1–1.4, 1.7, 1.9–1.11, 1.14, 1.15, 1.17, 4.1–4.6
    b. Systems and Patient Care Problems
        i. Acute Kidney Failure (AKI) or Acute Renal Failure (ARF)
        ii. Drug-Induced Kidney Damage
        iii. Chronic Kidney Disease
        iv. Renal Replacement Therapy (RRT)
        v. Complications of Chronic Kidney Disease
        vi. Dosage Adjustments in Kidney Disease
2. Domain 2: Drug Information and Evidence-Based Medicine, Task 2.2

Abbreviations

ACEI	angiotensin-converting enzyme inhibitor
ACR	albumin/creatinine ratio
ADA	American Diabetes Association
AIN	acute interstitial nephritis
AKI	acute kidney injury
AKIN	Acute Kidney Injury Network
APD	automated peritoneal dialysis
ARB	angiotensin II receptor blocker
ATN	acute tubular necrosis
BPH	benign prostatic hypertrophy
BUN	blood urea nitrogen
CAPD	continuous ambulatory peritoneal dialysis
CCPD	continuous cycling peritoneal dialysis
CHF	congestive heart failure
CKD	chronic kidney disease
CKD-MBD	chronic kidney disease–mineral bone disorder
CrCl	creatinine clearance
CVVH	continuous venovenous hemofiltration
CVVHD	continuous venovenous hemodialysis
CVVHDF	continuous venovenous hemodiafiltration
ESAs	erythropoiesis-stimulating agents
ESKD	end-stage kidney disease
FDA	U.S. Food and Drug Administration
FENa	fractional excretion of sodium
GFR	glomerular filtration rate
HD	hemodialysis
HTN	hypertension
IV	intravenous(ly)
IVP IV	push
IVPB	IV piggyback
JNC	Joint National Committee
KDIGO	Kidney Disease: Improving Global Outcomes
KDOQI	Kidney Disease Outcomes Quality Initiative
NS	normal saline solution
NSAID	nonsteroidal anti-inflammatory drug
PTH	parathyroid hormone
RBC	red blood cell count
RIFLE	risk, injury, failure, loss, and end-stage kidney disease
RRT	renal replacement therapy
SC	sieving coefficient
SCr	serum creatinine
TIBC	total iron-binding capacity
TSAT	transferrin saturation
URR	urea reduction ratio
WBC	white blood cell count

Patient Cases

1   A 48-year-old African American man is admitted to the intensive care unit after an acute myocardial infarction. He has a history of type 2 diabetes mellitus, hypertension, and tobacco use. Current medications include metformin 500 mg orally twice daily, lisinopril 20 mg/day, nicotine patch 14 mg/day applied each morning, and aspirin 81 mg/daily. Before admission, his kidney function was normal (serum creatinine [SCr] 1.0 mg/dL); however, during the past 24 hours, his kidney function has declined (blood urea nitrogen [BUN] 20 mg/dL, SCr 2.1 mg/dL). His urine shows muddy casts. He has been anuric for 6 hours. His current blood pressure (BP) is 110/70 mm Hg. He has edema and pulmonary congestion. Which is the best assessment of this patient's kidney function?

A.   26.2 mL/minute (creatinine clearance [CrCl] using the Cockcroft-Gault equation).

B.   44 mL/minute/1.73 m^2 (glomerular filtration rate [GFR] using the abbreviated Modification of Diet in Renal Disease [MDRD] study equation).

C.   23.1 mL/minute/70 kg (CrCl using the Brater equation).

D.   Assumed CrCl of less than 10 mL/minute.

2.   Which is the most likely cause of impaired kidney function in this patient?

A.   Prerenal azotemia.

B.   Intrinsic renal disease.

C.   Postrenal obstruction.

D.   Functional acute kidney injury (AKI).

3.   Which medication is best to discontinue at this time because of its potential adverse effect on kidney function?

A.   Lisinopril.

B.   Nicotine patch.

C.   Metformin.

D.   Aspirin.

4.   Which intervention is most appropriate to add at this time?

A.   Intravenous 0.9% sodium chloride (NaCl).

B.   Hydrochlorothiazide.

C.   Furosemide.

D.   Fluid restriction.

I. ACUTE KIDNEY INJURY OR ACUTE RENAL FAILURE

A. Definitions and Background
1. Acute kidney injury (AKI) is defined as an acute decrease in kidney function or glomerular filtration rate (GFR) over hours, days, or even weeks and is associated with an accumulation of waste products and (usually) volume.
   a. Common definitions
      i. An increase in SCr of 0.5 mg/dL or greater
      ii. A decrease of 25% or greater in estimated GFR (eGFR)
      iii. An increase of 1 mg/dL or more in SCr in patients with chronic kidney disease (CKD)
      iv. Urine output less than 0.5 mL/kg/hour for at least 6 hours
   b. The Acute Kidney Injury Network (AKIN): Diagnostic criteria require one of the following within a 48-hour period:
      i. An absolute increase in SCr of more than 0.3 mg/dL
      ii. An increase in baseline SCr by 50% or more
      iii. Urine output of less than 0.5 mL/kg/hour for more than 6 hours
   c. Can further classify into stages 1–3 on the basis of degree of SCr rise and urine output
   d. Stratifying AKI using risk, injury, failure, loss, and end-stage kidney disease (RIFLE) criteria. Developed by the Acute Dialysis Quality Initiative (ADQI) Group. Uses change in baseline SCr/GFR or urine output (Table 1)

Table 1. Stratification of AKI

RIFLE Classification		Common Criteria	AKIN Criteria	
Classification	**SCr or GFR Criteria**	**Urine Output**	**Stage**	**SCr or GFR Criteria**
R Risk of renal dysfunction	SCr increase to 1.5 times baseline *or* GFR decrease by >25%	Less than 0.5 mL/kg/hour for >6 hours	1	SCr increase to >0.3 mg/dL or 1.5–1.9 times baseline
I Injury to kidney	SCr increase to 2 times baseline *or* GFR decrease by >50%	Less than 0.5 mL/kg/hour for > 12 hours	2	SCr increase to 2–2.9 × baseline
F Failure of kidney function	SCr increase to 3 × baseline *or* GFR decrease by >75% *or* SCr >4 mg/dL with acute rise of >0.5 mg/dL	Less than 0.3 mL/kg/hour for >24 hours *or* Anuria for 12 hours	3	SCr increase to ≥3 times baseline or SCr >4 mg/dL with an acute increase of >0.5 mg/dL; or on RRT
L Loss of kidney function	Complete loss of kidney function for >4 weeks			
E End-stage kidney disease	Complete loss of kidney function for >3 months			

AKIN = Acute Kidney Injury Network; GFR = glomerular filtration rate; RRT = renal replacement therapy; SCr = serum creatinine.

   e. Common complications include fluid overload and acid-base and electrolyte abnormalities.
   f. Urine output classification
      i. Anuric: Less than 50 mL/24 hours; associated with worse outcomes
      ii. Oliguric: 50–500 mL/24 hours
      iii. Nonoliguric: More than 500 mL/24 hours; associated with better patient outcomes and easier to manage because of fewer problems with volume overload

2. Community-acquired AKI
   a. Low incidence (0.02%) in otherwise healthy patients
   b. As high as 13% incidence among patients with CKD
   c. Usually has a very high survival rate (70%–95%)
   d. Single insult to the kidney, often drug induced
   e. SCr may return to baseline but may lead to development or progression of CKD
3. Hospital-acquired AKI
   a. Has a moderate incidence (2%–5%) and moderate survival rate (30%–50%)
   b. Single or multifocal insults to the kidney
   c. Can still be reversible
4. Intensive care unit–acquired AKI: 5%–6% of patients in intensive care develop AKI during unit stay, and patients who develop this condition have a low survival rate (10%–30%).
5. Estimating kidney function in AKI
   a. Difficult because commonly used SCr-based equations (Cockcroft-Gault, Modification of Diet in Renal Disease [MDRD], and Chronic Kidney Disease Epidemiology Collaboration [CKD-EPI]) are not appropriate (assume stable SCr)
   b. Equations by Brater and Jeliffe are probably more accurate than the Cockcroft-Gault equation but have not been rigorously tested.
   c. Can do a urine collection in nonoliguria by obtaining a SCr before and after the collection and averaging these values for the calculation

B. Risk Factors Associated with AKI
   1. Preexisting CKD (eGFR less than 60 mL/minute/1.73 m^2)
   2. Volume depletion: Vomiting, diarrhea, poor fluid intake, fever, diuretic use, intravascular or effective volume depletion (e.g., congestive heart failure [CHF], liver disease with ascites)
   3. Use of nephrotoxic agents or medications
      a. Intravenous radiographic contrast
      b. Aminoglycosides and amphotericin
      c. Nonsteroidal anti-inflammatory drugs (NSAIDs) and cyclooxygenase-2 (COX-2) inhibitors
      d. Angiotensin-converting enzyme inhibitors (ACEIs) and angiotensin II receptor blockers (ARBs)
      e. Cyclosporine and tacrolimus
   4. Obstruction of the urinary tract

C. Classifications of AKI (Table 2)
   1. Prerenal AKI
      a. Initially, the kidney is undamaged.
      b. Characterized by hypoperfusion to the kidney
         i. Systemic hypoperfusion: Hemorrhage, volume depletion, drugs, CHF
         ii. Isolated kidney hypoperfusion: Renal artery stenosis, emboli
      c. Physical examination: Hypotension, signs of volume depletion
      d. Urinalysis will initially be normal (no sediment) but concentrated
   2. Functional AKI
      a. Kidney is undamaged; often classified as prerenal azotemia
      b. Caused by reduced glomerular hydrostatic pressure; often without hypotension
      c. In general, medication-related (cyclosporine, ACEIs and ARBs, and NSAIDs) or seen in patients with low effective blood flow (patients with CHF, patients with liver disease, and older adults) who cannot compensate for alterations in afferent and efferent tone
      d. Concentrated urine

3. Intrinsic AKI
   a. Kidney is damaged, and damage can be linked to the structure involved: Small blood vessels, glomeruli, renal tubules, and interstitium.
   b. Most common cause is acute tubular necrosis (ATN); other causes include acute interstitial nephritis (AIN), vasculitis, and acute glomerulonephritis.
   c. History: Identifiable insult, drug use, infections
   d. Physical examination: Normotensive, euvolemic, or hypervolemic depending on the cause; check for signs of allergic reactions or embolic phenomenon.
   e. Urinalysis will reflect damage; urine generally is not concentrated.
4. Postrenal AKI
   a. Kidney is initially undamaged. Bladder outlet obstruction is the most common cause of postrenal AKI. Lower urinary tract obstruction may be caused by calculi. Ureteric obstructions may be caused by clots or intraluminal obstructions. Extrarenal compression can also cause postrenal disease. Elevated intraluminal pressure upstream of the obstruction will result in damage if the obstruction is not relieved.
   b. History: Trauma, benign prostatic hyperplasia, cancers
   c. Physical examination: Distended bladder, enlarged prostate
   d. Urinalysis may be nonspecific.

Table 2. Classifications of Acute Kidney Injury

	Prerenal and Functional	**Intrinsic (ATN and AIN)**	**Postrenal**
History and clinical presentation	Volume depletion Renal artery stenosis CHF Hypercalcemia NSAID, ACEI, and ARB use Cyclosporine	Long-standing renal hypoperfusion Nephrotoxins (e.g., contrast or antibiotics) Vasculitis Glomerulonephritis	Kidney stones BPH Cancers
Physical examination	Hypotension Dehydration Petechia if thrombotic Ascites	Rash, fever (with AIN)	Distended bladder Enlarged prostate
Serum BUN/SCr ratio	Greater than 20:1	15:1	15:1
Urine sodium	Less than 20 mEq/L	Greater than 40 mEq/L	Greater than 40 mEq/L
FENa	Less than 1%	Greater than 2%	Greater than 2%
Urine osmolality	High urine osmolarity	Low urine osmolarity	Low urine osmolarity
Urine sediment	Normal	Muddy brown granular casts; tubular epithelial casts	Variable; may be normal
Urinary WBC	Negative	2–4+	Variable
Urinary RBC	Negative	2–4+	1+
Proteinuria	Negative	Positive	Negative

ACEI = angiotensin-converting enzyme inhibitor; AIN = ARB = angiotensin II receptor blocker; ATN = acute tubular necrosis; BPH = benign prostatic hypertrophy; BUN = blood urea nitrogen; CHF = congestive heart failure; FENa = NSAID = nonsteroidal anti-inflammatory drug; RBC = red blood cell count; SCr = WBC = white blood cell count.

e. Calculation of fractional excretion of sodium (FENa – percentage of Na filtered at the glomerulus that is excreted in the urine).

$$FENa\ (\%) = \frac{(Urine\ Na)/Serum\ Na)}{(Urine\ Cr)/(SCr)} \times 100$$

D. Prevention of AKI
   1. Avoid nephrotoxic drugs when possible.
   2. Ensure adequate hydration.
   3. Educate patient.
   4. Use drug therapies to decrease the incidence of contrast-induced nephropathy (see "II. Drug-Induced Kidney Damage").

E. Treatment and Management of Established AKI
   1. Prerenal azotemia: Correct primary hemodynamics.
      a. Normal saline if volume depleted
      b. Pressure management if needed
      c. Blood products if needed
   2. Intrinsic: No specific therapy universally effective
      a. Eliminate the causative hemodynamic abnormality or toxin.
      b. Avoid additional insults.
      c. Manage fluid and electrolytes to prevent volume depletion or overload and electrolyte imbalances.
      d. Nutrition support is important, but no specific recommendations are widely accepted.
      e. Medical therapy
         i. Loop diuretics: Recommend not using to prevent AKI (Kidney Disease: Improving Global Outcomes [KDIGO], Grade 1B) and suggest not using to treat AKI, except to manage hypervolemia (KDIGO, Grade 2C)
         ii. Fenoldopam: Suggest not using to prevent or treat AKI (KDIGO, Grade 2C)
         iii. Dopamine: Recommend not using low-dose dopamine to prevent or treat AKI (KDIGO, Grade 1A)
         iv. Atrial natriuretic peptide: Suggest not using to prevent (KDIGO, Grade 2C) or treat (KDIGO, Grade 2B) AKI
         v. Recombinant human insulin-like growth factor-1: Recommend not using to prevent or treat AKI (KDIGO, Grade 1B)
   3. Postrenal AKI: Relieve obstruction. Early identification is important. Consult urology or radiology.
   4. Indications for renal replacement therapy (RRT) in AKI
      a. Blood urea nitrogen (BUN) greater than 100 mg/dL
      b. Volume overload unresponsive to diuretics
      c. Uremia or encephalopathy
      d. Life-threatening electrolyte imbalance: Hyperkalemia, hypermagnesemia
      e. Refractory metabolic acidosis

Patient Cases

5. A 67-year-old man is referred for intermittent chest pain. His medical history is significant for KDIGO Category G3a CKD, type 2 diabetes mellitus, and hypertension. Medications include enalapril, hydrochlorothiazide, and pioglitazone. Laboratory values include SCr 1.8 mg/dL, glucose 189 mg/dL, hemoglobin 12 g/dL, and hematocrit 36%. His physical examination is normal. The plan is to undergo elective cardiac catheterization. Which approach is the best choice for hydration?

    A. 0.45% NaCl.

    B. 0.9% NaCl.

    C. 5% dextrose/0.45% NaCl.

    D. Oral hydration with water.

6. After the administration of radiocontrast, which is the optimal time to reevaluate renal function to assess for possible contrast-associated nephropathy?

    A. 6 hours.

    B. 24 hours.

    C. 4 days.

    D. 7 days.

II. DRUG-INDUCED KIDNEY DAMAGE

A. Introduction: Drugs can cause kidney damage through many mechanisms. Evaluate potential drug-induced nephropathy on the basis of the period of ingestion, patient risk factors, and the propensity of the suspected agent to cause kidney damage.

    1. Risk factors
        a. History of CKD
        b. Advanced age
    2. Epidemiology
        a. 7% of all drug toxicities
        b. 18%–27% of AKI in hospitals
        c. 1%–5% of NSAID users in community
        d. Most implicated medications: Aminoglycosides, NSAIDs, ACEIs, intravenous contrast dye, amphotericin
    3. The kidneys are at elevated risk of toxic injury because:
        a. High exposure to toxin: Kidney receives 20%–25% cardiac output.
        b. Autoregulation and specialized blood flow through glomerulus
        c. High intrarenal drug metabolism
        d. Tubular transport processes
        e. Concentration of solutes (i.e., toxins) in tubules
        f. High energy requirements of tubule epithelial cells
        g. Urine acidification
    4. Pseudonephrotoxicity
        a. Drugs that inhibit the tubular secretion of Cr: Trimethoprim, cimetidine
        b. Drugs that increase BUN: Corticosteroids, tetracycline
        c. Drugs that interfere with Cr assay: Cefoxitin and other cephalosporins

B. Acute Tubular Necrosis
   1. Most common drug-induced kidney disease in the inpatient setting
   2. Aminoglycoside nephrotoxicity
      a. Incidence: 1.7%–58% of patients
      b. Pathogenesis
         i. Caused by proximal tubular damage leading to obstruction of the lumen
         ii. Cationic charge of drug leads to binding to tubular epithelial cells and uptake into those cells.
         iii. Accumulation of phospholipids and toxicity
      c. Presentation
         i. Gradual rise in SCr concentrations and decrease in GFR after 6–10 days of therapy
         ii. Patients usually have nonoliguric kidney failure.
         iii. Wasting of electrolytes (i.e., hypokalemia and hypomagnesemia) may occur.
      d. Risk factors
         i. Related to dosing: Large total cumulative dose, prolonged therapy, trough concentration exceeding 2 mg/L, recent previous aminoglycoside therapy
         ii. Concurrent use of other nephrotoxins (cyclosporine, amphotericin B, diuretics, vancomycin)
         iii. Patient related: Preexisting kidney disease or damage, advanced age, poor nutrition, shock, gram-negative bacteremia, liver disease, hypoalbuminemia, obstructive jaundice, dehydration, and K and Mg deficiencies
      e. Prevention
         i. Avoid use in high-risk patients.
         ii. Maintain adequate hydration.
         iii. Limit the total cumulative aminoglycoside dose.
         iv. Avoid use of other nephrotoxins.
         v. Use extended-interval (once-daily) dosing; monitor these and other high-risk patients closely.
   3. Radiographic contrast media nephrotoxicity related to intravenous contrast use
      a. Incidence
         i. Third leading cause of inpatient AKI
         ii. Less than 2% and up to 50% of patients, depending on risk
         iii. Associated with a high (34%) in-hospital mortality rate
      b. Pathogenesis
         i. Renal ischemia caused by alteration in intrarenal hemodynamics
            (a) Osmotic diuresis and dehydration. Contrast media based on osmolality: High-osmolar contrast media about 2000 mOsm/kg, low-osmolar contrast media 600–800 mOsm/kg, iso-osmolar contrast media 290 mOsm/kg
            (b) Some contrast agents also cause systemic hypotension on injection and renal vasoconstriction caused by the release of adenosine, endothelin, and other vasoconstrictors.
         ii. Direct tubular toxicity caused by reactive oxygen species; directly influenced by tubular flow rates and duration of exposure of tubules
      c. Presentation
         i. Initial transient osmotic diuresis, followed by tubular proteinuria
         ii. SCr rises within 24 hours and peaks 2–5 days after the procedure.
         iii. 50% of patients develop oliguria, and some will need dialysis.
      d. Risk factors for toxicity
         i. Preexisting kidney disease (SCr more than 1.5 mg/dL or CrCl less than 60 mL/minute)
         ii. Diabetes mellitus
         iii. Volume depletion
         iv. Age 75 years and older

       v. Anemia

      vi. Conditions with decreased blood flow to the kidney (e.g., CHF)

     vii. Hypotension

   viii. Other nephrotoxins

      ix. Large doses of contrast (more than 140 mL) or hyperosmolar contrast agents

e. Prevention

       i. Volume expansion with either intravenous isotonic saline or sodium bicarbonate (KDIGO recommendation, Grade 1A) beginning 6–12 hours before procedure; maintain urine output greater than 150 mL/hour.

      ii. Use an alternative imaging study, if possible.

     iii. Discontinue nephrotoxic agents and avoid diuretics.

     iv. Use low-osmolar or iso-osmolar contrast agents in patients at risk (KDIGO recommendation, Grade 1B).

      v. Medications used to prevent contrast-induced nephropathy

         (a) *N*-Acetylcysteine (NAC): Antioxidant and vasodilatory mechanism. Accumulation of glutathione takes time, so it may not be as effective in emergency cases. Various dosing recommendations. Widely used. Conflicting evidence. Considered safe. May use oral NAC in combination with intravenous hydration (KDIGO suggestion, Grade 2D)

         (b) Ascorbic acid: Antioxidant. One large study showed benefit when used immediately before. Not confirmed. Give oral ascorbic acid 3 g before procedure and 2 g twice daily for two doses after procedure. May have role in emergency cases

         (c) Theophylline: Do not use (KDIGO suggestion, Grade 2C).

         (d) Fenoldopam: Do not use (KDIGO recommendation, Grade 1B).

         (e) Prophylactic hemodialysis (HD) and hemofiltration: Do not use (KDIGO suggestion, Grade 2C).

f. The Joint National Committee (JNC) standards on medication management regarding radiologic contrast media

       i. Treated as a drug

      ii. Subject to all the standards for medication management in a health system

g. Nephrogenic systemic fibrosis (also known as nephrogenic fibrosing dermopathy)

       i. Rare but associated with gadolinium-based agents used in high doses for magnetic resonance angiogram

      ii. Occurs in patients with moderate CKD to end-stage kidney disease (ESKD) given intravenous contrast, and systemic acidosis seems to be a risk factor (Magnevist, Omniscan, and OptiMARK considered inappropriate for use in patients with AKI or CKD).

     iii. Onset 2–18 days after exposure

     iv. Presents as burning; itching; swelling, hardening, or tightening of skin; skin patches; spots on eyes; joint stiffness; and muscle weakness

      v. Can cause organ damage, and deaths have occurred

      vi. In 2010, the U.S. Food and Drug Administration (FDA) required the addition of a warning to prescribing information.

4. Cisplatin and carboplatin nephrotoxicity

a. Incidence: 6%–13% with appropriate dosing and administration

b. Pathogenesis: Complex; direct tubular toxins

c. Presentation

       i. SCr peaks 10–12 days after therapy starts but may continue to rise with subsequent cycles of therapy.

        ii. Renal Mg wasting is common (may be severe with central nervous system symptoms) and may be accompanied by hypokalemia and hypocalcemia.

        iii. May result in irreversible kidney damage

    d. Risk factors for toxicity: Many courses of cisplatin, advanced patient age, dehydration, concurrent nephrotoxins, kidney irradiation, alcohol abuse

    e. Prevention

        i. Avoid concurrent use of nephrotoxins.

        ii. Use smallest dose possible and decrease frequency of administration.

        iii. Aggressive intravenous hydration: 1–4 L within 24 hours of high-dose cisplatin or carboplatin

        iv. Amifostine: Cisplatin-chelating agent that should be considered in patients at risk of nephrotoxicity

  5. Amphotericin B nephrotoxicity

    a. Incidence

        i. Increases as cumulative dose increases

        ii. Approaches 80% with cumulative doses of 4 g or more

    b. Pathogenesis

        i. Direct proximal and distal tubular toxicity

        ii. Arterial vasoconstriction

    c. Presentation

        i. Manifests after administration of 2–3 g

        ii. Loss of tubular function leads to electrolyte wasting (especially K^+, Na^+, and Mg^{2+}) and distal tubular acidosis.

        iii. Patients may need substantial K^+ and Mg^{2+} replacement.

        iv. SCr increases and GFR decreases because of a decrease in kidney blood flow from vasoconstriction caused by amphotericin.

    d. Risk factors for toxicity: Existing kidney dysfunction, high average daily doses, diuretic use, volume depletion, concomitant nephrotoxins, rapid infusion

    e. Prevention

        i. Avoid other nephrotoxins (especially cyclosporine) and limit the total cumulative dose.

        ii. Intravenous hydration with 0.9% NaCl at least 1 L/day before each dose

        iii. Use a liposomal product in high-risk patients.

C. Functional (Hemodynamically Mediated) AKI

  1. Caused by a decrease in intraglomerular pressure through the vasoconstriction of afferent arterioles or the vasodilation of efferent arterioles

  2. ACEIs and ARBs

    a. Pathogenesis

        i. Vasodilation of the efferent arteriole

        ii. Leads to a decrease in glomerular hydrostatic pressure and a resultant decrease in GFR

    b. Presentation

        i. Exerts a predictable dose-related reduction in GFR

        ii. SCr is usually expected to rise by up to 30%.

           (a) Usually occurs within 2–5 days

           (b) Usually stabilizes in 2–3 weeks

           (c) Increases greater than 30% may be detrimental.

           (d) Usually reversible on drug discontinuation

    c.   Risk factors for toxicity: Patients with bilateral (or unilateral with a solitary kidney) renal artery stenosis, decreased effective kidney blood flow (CHF, cirrhosis), preexisting kidney disease, and volume depletion

    d.   Prevention

        i.   Initiate therapy with low doses and gradually titrate upward.

        ii.   Switch to long-acting agents once tolerance is established.

        iii.   Initially, monitor kidney function and SCr concentrations daily for inpatients, weekly for outpatients.

        iv.   Avoid use of concomitant diuretics, if possible, during therapy initiation.

        v.   Avoid use of concomitant NSAIDs.

3.   Nonsteroidal anti-inflammatory drugs (NSAIDs)

    a.   Incidence: Estimates indicate that 500,000–2.5 million people develop NSAID-induced nephrotoxicity annually in the United States.

    b.   Pathogenesis

        i.   Vasodilatory prostaglandins help maintain glomerular hydrostatic pressure by afferent arteriolar dilation, especially in times of decreased kidney blood flow.

        ii.   Administration of an NSAID in the setting of decreased kidney perfusion reduces this compensatory mechanism by decreasing the production of prostaglandins, resulting in afferent vasoconstriction and reduced glomerular blood flow.

    c.   Presentation

        i.   Can occur within days of starting therapy

        ii.   Patients generally have low urine volume and Na; may also observe an increase in BUN, SCr, K^+, edema, and weight

    d.   Risk factors for toxicity: Preexisting kidney disease, systemic lupus erythematosus, high plasma renin activity (e.g., CHF, hepatic disease), diuretic therapy, atherosclerotic disease, and advanced age

    e.   Prevention

        i.   Use therapies other than NSAIDs when appropriate (e.g., acetaminophen for osteoarthritis).

        ii.   COX-2–specific inhibitors have not been shown to cause less kidney dysfunction, and they increase cardiovascular complications.

    f.   Treatment

        i.   If NSAID-induced AKI is suspected, discontinue drug and give supportive care.

        ii.   Avoid use of concomitant medications affecting the renin-angiotensin-aldosterone system.

        iii.   Recovery is usually rapid.

4.   Cyclosporine and tacrolimus

    a.   Incidence

        i.   The 5-year risk of developing CKD after transplantation of a nonrenal organ ranges from 7% to 21%.

        ii.   The occurrence of kidney failure in the transplant recipient population increases the risk of death fourfold.

    b.   Pathogenesis

        i.   Caused by a dose-related hemodynamic mechanism; calcineurin inhibitors may also cause chronic interstitial nephritis through a separate mechanism that is not dose related.

        ii.   Causes vasoconstriction of afferent arterioles through possible increased activity of various vasoconstrictors (thromboxane A_2, endothelin, sympathetic nervous system) or decreased activity of vasodilators (nitric oxide, prostacyclin)

        iii.   Increased vasoconstriction from angiotensin II may also contribute.

        iv.   Effects usually resolve with a dose reduction.

c. Presentation
   i. Can occur within days of starting therapy
   ii. SCr rises and eGFR decreases.
   iii. Patients often have hypertension, hyperkalemia, and hypomagnesemia.
   iv. A biopsy is often needed for kidney transplant recipients to distinguish drug-induced injury from acute allograft rejection.
d. Risk factors for toxicity include advanced age, high initial cyclosporine dose, kidney graft rejection, hypotension, infection, and concomitant nephrotoxins.
e. Prevention
   i. Monitor serum cyclosporine and tacrolimus concentrations closely.
   ii. Use lower doses in combination with other nonnephrotoxic immunosuppressants (e.g., steroids, mycophenolate mofetil).
   iii. Calcium channel blockers *may* help antagonize the vasoconstrictor effects of cyclosporine by dilating afferent arterioles.

D. Tubulointerstitial Disease
   1. Involves the renal tubules and the surrounding interstitium
   2. Onset can be acute or chronic.
      a. Acute onset generally involves interstitial inflammatory cell infiltrates, rapid loss of kidney function, and systemic symptoms (i.e., fever and rash).
      b. Chronic onset shows interstitial fibrosis, slow decline in kidney function, and no systemic symptoms.
   3. Acute allergic interstitial nephritis
      a. Cause of up to 3% of all AKI cases; caused by an allergic hypersensitivity reaction that affects the interstitium of the kidney
      b. Many medications and medication classes can cause this type of kidney failure, including β-lactams and the NSAIDs (although the presentations are different).
         i. Penicillins: Classic presentation of acute allergic interstitial nephritis. Signs and symptoms occur about 1–2 weeks after therapy initiation and include fever, maculopapular rash, eosinophilia, pyuria, hematuria, and proteinuria. Eosinophiluria may also be present.
         ii. NSAIDs: Onset much more delayed; typically begins about 6 months into therapy. Usually occurs in older adults on chronic NSAID therapy. Patients usually do not have systemic symptoms.
      c. Kidney biopsy may be needed to confirm diagnosis.
      d. Treatment includes discontinuing the offending agent and possibly initiating steroid therapy.
   4. Chronic interstitial nephritis
      a. Often progressive and irreversible
      b. Lithium
         i. Toxicity results from a duration-related decrease in response to antidiuretic hormone after long-term use (more than 10 years of therapy).
         ii. Clinical presentation
            (a) Often asymptomatic, with slow progression over years
            (b) May be recognized by slow increases in blood pressure (BP) or BUN and SCr
         iii. Risks include long duration of use, elevated serum concentrations, and repeated episodes of AKI from lithium toxicity.
         iv. Prevention is accomplished by maintaining the lowest serum lithium concentrations possible, avoiding dehydration, and monitoring kidney function closely.
      c. Cyclosporine and tacrolimus: Presents later in therapy (about 6–12 months) than hemodynamically mediated toxicity

5. Papillary necrosis
   a. Form of chronic interstitial nephritis affecting the papillae, causing necrosis of the collecting ducts
   b. Results from the long-term use of analgesics
      i. "Classic" example was with products that contained phenacetin.
      ii. Occurs more often with combination products
      iii. Products containing caffeine may also increase risk.
   c. Evolves slowly as time progresses
   d. Affects women more often than men
   e. Difficult to diagnose, and much controversy remains about risk, prevention, and cause

E. Postrenal (Obstructive) Nephropathy
   1. Results from obstruction of the flow of urine after glomerular filtration
   2. Renal tubular obstruction
      a. Caused by intratubular precipitation of tissue degradation products or precipitation of drugs or their metabolites
         i. Tissue degradation products
            (a) Uric acid intratubular precipitation after tumor lysis after chemotherapy
            (b) Drug-induced rhabdomyolysis leading to intratubular precipitation of myoglobin
            (c) Results in rapid decline in kidney function, with resultant oliguric or anuric kidney failure
         ii. Drug precipitation: Sulfonamides, methotrexate, acyclovir, ascorbic acid; needlelike crystals observed in leukocytes found on urinalysis can prompt diagnosis.
      b. Prevention includes pretreatment hydration, maintenance of high urinary volume, and alkalinization of the urine.
   3. Extrarenal urinary tract obstruction
      a. BPH can be worsened by anticholinergics.
      b. Bladder outlet or ureteral obstruction from fibrosis after cyclophosphamide for hemorrhagic cystitis
   4. Nephrolithiasis
      a. Usually does not affect GFR, so does not have the classic signs and symptoms of nephrotoxicity
      b. Some medications contribute to the formation of kidney stones: Triamterene, sulfadiazine, indinavir, and ephedrine derivatives.

F. Glomerular Disease
   1. Proteinuria is the hallmark of glomerular disease and may occur with or without a decrease in GFR.
   2. A few distinct drugs can cause glomerular disease.
      a. NSAIDs: Associated with acute allergic interstitial nephritis
      b. Heroin: Can be caused by direct toxicity or toxicity from additives or infection from injection, and ESKD develops in most cases.
      c. Parenteral gold: Results from immune complex formation along glomerular capillary loops

III. CHRONIC KIDNEY DISEASE

A. Background
   1. Prevalence: According to the 2015 U.S. Renal Data System Annual Report, 14% of adults (20 years or older) in the National Health and Nutrition Examination Survey population (2007–2012) have CKD. There were 468,386 patients on dialysis in 2013 and 193,262 transplant recipients. Incidence rate is flat, so growth in the number of patients with ESKD results mainly from the longer life span of these patients.
   2. Definition of CKD
      a. According to the National Kidney Foundation Kidney Disease Outcome Quality Initiative (KDOQI), CKD is kidney damage for more than 3 months, as defined by structural or functional abnormality of the kidney, with or without decreased GFR. Manifested by either pathologic abnormalities or markers of kidney damage—including abnormalities in the composition of blood or urine or abnormalities in imaging tests—*or* GFR less than 60 mL/minute/1.73 m² for 3 months, with or without kidney damage (Table 3).

Table 3. KDOQI Stages in CKD

Stage of Renal Disease	Damage	GFR (mL/minute/1.73 m²)
Increased risk of developing kidney disease	Risk factors for CKD (diabetes, HTN, family history)	≥90
Stage 1	Kidney damage with normal GFR	≥90
Stage 2	Kidney damage with mild decrease in GFR	60–89
Stage 3	Moderate decrease in GFR	30–59
Stage 4	Severe decrease in GFR	15–29
Stage 5	Kidney failure	<15

CKD = chronic kidney disease; GFR = glomerular filtration rate; HTN = hypertension; KDOQI = Kidney Disease Outcome Quality Initiative

      b. According to the KDIGO clinical practice guideline for the evaluation and management of CKD, CKD is defined as abnormalities of kidney structure or function for more than 3 months. These abnormalities may be seen as persistent markers of kidney damage or GFR less than 60 mL/minute/1.73 m² (Table 4).

Table 4. KDIGO Categories in CKD

GFR Category	Terms	GFR (mL/minute/1.73 m²)
G1	Kidney damage with normal or high GFR	≥90
G2	Kidney damage with mildly decreased GFR	60–89
G3a	Mildly to moderately decreased GFR	45–59
G3b	Moderately to severely decreased GFR	30–44
G4	Severely decreased GFR	15–29
G5	Kidney failure	<15

GFR = glomerular filtration rate; KDIGO = Kidney Disease: Improving Global Outcomes.

B. Etiology
   1. Diabetes (40% of new cases of ESKD in the United States)
   2. Hypertension (25% of new cases)
   3. Glomerulonephritis (10%)
   4. Others: Urinary tract disease, polycystic kidney disease, lupus, analgesic nephropathy, unknown

C. Risk Factors
1. Susceptibility (associated with an increased risk but not proved to cause CKD): Advanced age, reduced kidney mass, low birth weight, racial or ethnic minority, family history, low income or education, systemic inflammation, and dyslipidemia; mostly not modifiable
2. Initiation (directly cause CKD): Diabetes, hypertension, autoimmune disease, polycystic kidney diseases, and drug toxicity; may be modifiable by drug therapy
3. Progression (result in faster decline in kidney function): Hyperglycemia, elevated BP, proteinuria, and smoking

---

Patient Cases

7. A 55-year-old man has a history of hypertension and newly diagnosed type 2 diabetes mellitus. He denies alcohol use but does smoke cigarettes (1 pack/day). His medications include atenolol 50 mg/day and a multivitamin. At your pharmacy, his BP is 149/92 mm Hg. His albumin/creatinine ratio (ACR) is 400 mg/g. A recent SCr is 1.9 mg/dL, which is consistent with a value measured 3 months earlier. His eGFR is 50 mL/minute/1.73 m^2. Which is the best assessment of his kidney disease based on KDIGO criteria?

   A. Category G2.
   B. Category G3a.
   C. Category G3b.
   D. Category G4.

8. Assuming that nonpharmacologic approaches have been optimized, which action is best to limit the progression of his kidney disease?

   A. Add nifedipine.
   B. Add diltiazem.
   C. Add enalapril.
   D. Increase atenolol.

9. Enalapril was added to this patient's regimen. Two weeks later, he presents back to his physician. His BP is 139/89 mm Hg. A repeat SCr is 2.3 mg/dL, and serum potassium is 5.2 mEq/L. Which is the best recommendation for this patient?

   A. Change enalapril to diltiazem ER. Monitor BP, SCr, and K in 2 weeks.
   B. Add chlorthalidone 50 mg/day. Monitor BP, SCr, and K in 2 weeks.
   C. Change enalapril to valsartan.
   D. Increase atenolol.

10. A study compared the use of an angiotensin receptor blocker alone or in combination with an ACEI in patients with CKD. AKI occurred in 80 of 724 (11%) patients receiving monotherapy and in 130 of 724 patients (18%) receiving combination therapy. Based on this information, what is the number of patients needed to harm?

   A. 7.
   B. 15.
   C. 50.
   D. 105.

$$\frac{i}{.18-.11} \qquad \frac{1}{.07} \qquad \frac{1}{18-11} \qquad \frac{1}{7}$$

D. Albuminuria or Proteinuria
   1. Marker of kidney damage, progression factor, and cardiovascular risk factor. Can be classified as in Table 5

Table 5. KDIGO Categories of Albuminuria

Category	Classification	ACR (mg/g)	Daily Excretion (mg/24 hours)
A1	Normal to mildly increased	<30	<30
A2	Moderately increased	30–300	30–300
A3	Severely increased albuminuria	>300	>300
	Nephrotic-range proteinuria		>3000

Note: Classified as "normal" or "increased urinary albumin excretion" in American Diabetes Association. Diabetes Care 2015;38(suppl 1): S58-S66.

ACR = albumin/creatinine ratio; KDIGO = Kidney Disease: Improving Global Outcomes.

   2. Assessment for proteinuria: Usually assessed by measuring urinary ACR. Spot urine: Untimed sample is adequate for adults and children (screening test).

E. Assessment of Kidney Function
   1. Serum creatinine (SCr)
      a. Avoid use as the sole assessment of kidney function.
      b. Depends on age, sex, weight, and muscle mass
      c. All laboratories now use "standardized" SCr traceable to isotope dilution mass spectrometry, which decreases variability in results between laboratories.
   2. Measurement of GFR: Inulin, iothalamate, and others are very rarely used in clinical practice.
   3. Measurement of CrCl through urine collection
      a. Reserve for vegetarians, patients needing dietary assessment, or those with abnormal muscle mass (e.g., patients with low muscle mass, patients with amputations) or when documenting need to start or continue dialysis.
      b. Urine collection yields a better estimate in patients with very low muscle mass.
      c. In most cases, equations overestimate kidney function because SCr concentrations are low in patients with very low muscle mass.
   4. Estimated CrCl using Cockcroft-Gault equation (mL/minute): Overestimates GFR

   $$CrCl = \frac{[(140 - age) \times body\ weight]}{[SCr \times 72]} \times (0.85\ if\ female)$$

   Although controversial, ideal body weight is often used in place of actual body weight for obese patients.

   5. eGFR with MDRD study data equation
      a. eGFR (mL/minute/1.73 m^2) in patients with known CKD (GFR less than 90 mL/minute/1.73 m^2)
      b. Isotope dilution mass spectrometry–traceable four-variable MDRD formula correlates well with the original MDRD formula; simpler to use:

      $$eGFR\ (mL/minute/1.73\ m^2) = 175 \times SCr^{-1.154} \times age^{-0.203} \times (0.742\ if\ female) \times (1.212\ if\ African\ American)$$

      c. This equation is available at http://nkdep.nih.gov/lab-evaluation/gfr-calculators.shtml (accessed October 29, 2015) or www.kidney.org.

6. CKD-EPI equation: Alternative equation based on race, sex, SCr range, and age. More accurate at GFRs greater than 60 mL/minute/1.73 m^2. Available at www.kidney.org/professionals/KDOQI/gfr_calculator (accessed October 29, 2015)

7. For children, use the modified Schwartz "Bedside" formula.

F. Diabetic Nephropathy
   1. Pathogenesis
      a. Hypertension (systemic and intraglomerular)
      b. Glycosylation of glomerular proteins
      c. Genetic links
   2. Diagnosis
      a. Long history of diabetes
      b. Proteinuria
      c. Retinopathy (suggests microvascular disease)
   3. Monitoring
      a. Type 1 diabetes mellitus: Begin annual monitoring for albuminuria 5 years after diagnosis.
      b. Type 2 diabetes mellitus: Begin annual monitoring for albuminuria immediately (do not know how long patient has had diabetes mellitus).
   4. Management and slowing progression
      a. Aggressive BP management
         i. Goal BP readings in patients with diabetes

Group	Severity of Albuminuria	Goal Blood Pressure (maximum)	Level of Evidence
ADA 2015	Any	140/90 mm Hg[a]	B
KDIGO	Normal to mild albuminuria	140/90 mm Hg	1B
KDIGO	Moderate to severe albuminuria	130/80 mm Hg	2D
JNC 8	Any	140/90 mm Hg	E

[a]Systolic BP less than 130 mm Hg and diastolic BP less than 80 mm Hg may be appropriate in some patients.

ADA = American Diabetes Association; JNC = Joint National Committee; KDIGO = Kidney Disease: Improving Global Outcomes.

         ii. ACEIs or ARBs are preferred and should be used with any degree of proteinuria, even if the patient is not hypertensive.
            (a) Use moderate to high doses with proteinuria.
            (b) Hold ACEI or ARB if serum potassium is greater than 5.6 mEq/L or if there is a rise in SCr greater than 30% after initiation.
            (c) Increased risk of hyperkalemia if combined with direct renin inhibitor
         iii. Most patients will need diuretic in combination (thiazide with stages 1–3 and loop diuretics in stages 4 and 5). If BP is greater than 160/100 mm Hg, start with a two-drug regimen.
         iv. Calcium channel blockers (nondihydropyridine) are second line to ACEIs and ARBs. Data are emerging for combined therapy.
         v. Dietary Na consumption should be less than 2.4 g/day. Modify Dietary Approaches to Stop Hypertension (DASH) diet to limit K intake as well.
      b. Intensive blood glucose control. Glycosylated hemoglobin (A1C) less than 7%. Less aggressive with more advanced CKD
      c. Protein restriction: Data are insufficient in diabetes, but 0.8 g/kg/day might slightly reduce progression and decrease the risk of ESKD. Patients should avoid high-protein diets.

G. Nondiabetic Nephropathy
1. Management of hypertension
   a. BP goals
      i. KDIGO guidelines

Target Group	Severity of Albuminuria	Goal Blood Pressure (maximum)	Level of Evidence
Nondiabetic CKD	Normal to mild albuminuria	140/90 mm Hg	1B
Nondiabetic CKD	Moderate to severe albuminuria	130/80 mm Hg	2D moderate 2C severe

CKD = chronic kidney disease.

      ii. JNC 8 guidelines: Patients 18 years and older with CKD: Goal BP less than 140/90 mm Hg (Grade E, Expert Opinion)
   b. If proteinuric and hypertensive, use ACEI *or* ARB. Often need to add (or start with) combination. Diuretic is usual second drug. Monitor serum potassium.
2. Minimize protein in diet. Controversial. May slow progression according to MDRD study but may also impair nutrition. Very low-protein diet may increase mortality.

H. Other Guidelines to Slow Progression
1. Hyperlipidemia
   a. Assessment
      i. Newly identified CKD: Recommend evaluation of lipid profile (KDIGO, Grade 1C).
      ii. Follow-up measurement of lipid levels not necessary for most patients (not graded)
   b. Treatment recommendations (KDIGO)

Target Group	Treatment Recommendation	Grade
Adults ≥50 years of age, GFR category G1–G2	Statin	1B
Adults ≥50 years of age, GFR category G3a–G5	Statin or statin/ezetimibe	1A
Adults 18–49 years of age with CKD before dialysis or transplant with CAD, diabetes, stroke, or estimated risk of coronary death or MI >10%	Statin	2A
Adults on therapy when dialysis initiated	Continue statin or statin/ezetimibe	2C
Adults with dialysis-dependent CKD	Do *not* start therapy	2A
Adult kidney transplant recipients	Statin	2A

CAD = coronary artery disease; CKD = chronic kidney disease; GFR = glomerular filtration rate.

KDIGO guideline for lipid management in CKD. Kidney Int 2014;85:1303-9.

2. Smoking cessation.

Patient Cases

11. A 70-year-old man is being assessed for HD access. He has a history of diabetes mellitus and hypertension but is otherwise healthy. Which dialysis access has the lowest rate of complications and the longest life span and is thus the best access to use?

    A. Subclavian catheter.

    B. Tenckhoff catheter.

    C. Arteriovenous graft.

    D. Arteriovenous fistula.

12. A patient undergoing long-term HD experiences intradialytic hypotension. After nonpharmacologic approaches have been optimized, which medication is best to manage his low BP?

    A. Levocarnitine.

    B. NaCl tablets.

    C. Fludrocortisone.

    D. Midodrine.

13. A patient with CKD on peritoneal dialysis presents with fever and abdominal pain. She also notes that her peritoneal dialysate has become cloudy. Laboratory evaluation of dialysate reveals many white blood cells, primarily neutrophils. Gram stain and culture of the fluid are ordered. According to the 2010 recommendations for peritoneal dialysis–related peritonitis, which is the best empiric therapy for this patient?

    A. Intravenous metronidazole plus gentamicin.

    B. Cefazolin plus ceftazidime instilled intraperitoneally.

    C. Intravenous clindamycin plus vancomycin.

    D. Vancomycin instilled intraperitoneally.

IV. RENAL REPLACEMENT THERAPY

   A. Indications for RRT
      1. A: Acidosis (not responsive to bicarbonate)
      2. E: Electrolyte abnormality (hyperkalemia, hyperphosphatemia)
      3. I: Intoxication (boric acid, ethylene glycol, lithium, methanol, phenobarbital, salicylate, theophylline)
      4. O: Fluid overload (symptomatic [pulmonary edema])
      5. U: Uremia (pericarditis and weight loss)

   B. Two Primary Modes of Dialysis
      1. Hemodialysis: Most common modality in United States
      2. Peritoneal dialysis

C. Hemodialysis (intermittent for ESKD)
1. Access
    a. Arteriovenous fistula: Preferred access
        i.   Natural, formed by anastomosis of artery and vein
        ii. Lowest incidence of infection and thrombosis, lowest cost, longest survival
        iii. Takes weeks or months to "mature"
    b. Arteriovenous graft
        i.   Usually synthetic (polytetrafluoroethylene)
        ii. Often used in patients with vascular disease
    c. Catheters
        i.   Commonly used if permanent access unavailable
        ii. Problems include high infection and thrombosis rates. Low blood flow leads to inadequate dialysis.
2. Dialysis membranes
    a. Conventional: Not often used anymore. Small pores, smaller surface area.
    b. High flux (large pores) and high efficiency (large surface area). Can remove drugs that were impermeable to standard membranes (vancomycin). Large amounts of fluid removal (ultrafiltrate)
3. Adequacy
    a. Kt/V: Unitless parameter. K = clearance, t = time on dialysis, and V = volume of distribution of urea. KDOQI set a minimum of 1.2 (target Kt/V of 1.4).
    b. URR: Urea reduction ratio. URR = [(preBUN – postBUN)/preBUN] * 100%. Goal URR is greater than 65% (target URR of 70%).
4. Common complications of HD
    a. Intradialytic
        i.   Hypotension: Related primarily to fluid removal. Common in older adults and in people with diabetes mellitus
             (a) Acute treatment: Trendelenburg position, decrease ultrafiltration rate; administer saline boluses.
             (b) Prevention: Accurately set "dry weight"; limit fluid gains between sessions; midodrine 2.5–10 mg orally before dialysis.
             (c) Less well-studied agents include fludrocortisone, selective serotonin reuptake inhibitors.
        ii. Cramps: Vitamin E 400 international units at bedtime
        iii. Nausea and vomiting
        iv. Headache, chest pain, or back pain
    b. Vascular access complications: Most common with catheters
        i.   Infection: *Staphylococcus aureus* is the most common organism. Need to treat aggressively. May need to remove catheter
        ii. Thrombosis: Suspected with low blood flow. Oral antiplatelet agents for prevention not used because of lack of efficacy. Can treat with alteplase 2 mg or reteplase 0.4 unit per lumen; try to aspirate after 30 minutes; may repeat dose after 120 minutes
5. Factors that affect the efficiency of HD
    a. Type of dialyzer used (changes in membrane surface area and pore size)
    b. Length of therapy
    c. Dialysis flow rate
    d. Blood flow rate

D. Continuous RRT for AKI
   1. Continuous venovenous hemofiltration (CVVH): Removes fluid and solutes by convection rather than by diffusion
      a. Drug removal depends on ultrafiltrate production rate and protein binding of drug. Predict drug removal by the sieving coefficient (SC):

$$SC = \frac{\text{Concentration of drug in ultrafiltrate}}{\text{Concentration of drug in blood}}$$

      b. Requires replacement fluid because of high ultrafiltration rate
   2. Continuous venovenous hemodialysis (CVVHD): Dialysate flows countercurrent to blood flow, and solute is removed by diffusion.
   3. Continuous venovenous hemodiafiltration (CVVHDF): Ultrafiltration and dialysis; solute is removed by both convection and diffusion. Requires both replacement fluid and dialysate.

E. Peritoneal Dialysis
   1. Peritoneal dialysis membrane is 1–2 m² (approximates the body surface area) and consists of the vascular wall, the interstitium, the mesothelium, and the adjacent fluid films. From 1.5 to 3 L of peritoneal dialysate fluid may be instilled in the peritoneum (fill), allowed to dwell for a specified time, and then drained.
   2. Solutes and fluid diffuse across the peritoneal membrane.
   3. Peritoneal dialysis is usually *not* used to treat AKI in adults.
   4. Peritonitis
      a. Infection of the peritoneal cavity. Patient technique and population variables influence the infection rate. Older adults or those with diabetes have a higher infection rate. Peritonitis is a main cause of failure of peritoneal dialysis. Diagnosed based on the cell count and differential of the peritoneal dialysate (more than 100 WBC/mm³ and more than 50% neutrophils).
      b. Treatment based on ISPD guidelines
         i. Most common gram-positive organisms include *Staphylococcus epidermis, S. aureus,* and streptococci. Most common gram-negative organisms include *Escherichia coli* and *Pseudomonas aeruginosa.*
         ii. Empiric treatment should cover gram-positive and gram-negative bacteria.
            (a) Intraperitoneal administration of vancomycin or first-generation cephalosporin *and* intraperitoneal third-generation cephalosporin or aminoglycoside
            (b) Adjust as needed based on culture and sensitivity.
   5. Types of peritoneal dialysis
      a. Continuous ambulatory peritoneal dialysis (CAPD): Classic. Requires mechanical process, which requires many manual exchanges throughout the day. Can disrupt daytime routine
      b. Automated peritoneal dialysis (APD): Many variants exist, but continuous cycling peritoneal dialysis (CCPD) is the most common. Patient undergoes many exchanges during sleep by a cycling machine. May have one or two dwells during day. Minimizes potential contamination. Lowest incidence of peritonitis

Patient Cases

14. A 60-year-old patient on HD has had end-stage kidney disease for 10 years. His HD access is a left arteriovenous fistula. He has a history of hypertension, coronary artery disease (CAD), mild CHF, type 2 diabetes mellitus, and a seizure disorder. Medications are as follows: epoetin alfa 14,000 units intravenously three times/week at dialysis, a renal multivitamin once daily, atorvastatin 20 mg/day, insulin, calcium acetate 2 tablets three times/day with meals, phenytoin 300 mg/day, and intravenous iron 100 mg/month. Laboratory values are as follows: hemoglobin 10.2 g/dL, immunoassay for PTH 800 pg/mL, Na 140 mEq/L, K 4.9 mEq/L, Cr 7.0 mg/dL, calcium 9.5 mg/dL, albumin 2.5 g/dL, and phosphorus 7.8 mg/dL. Serum ferritin is 550 ng/mL, and transferrin saturation (TSAT) is 32%. The red blood cell count (RBC) indices are normal. His white blood cell count (WBC) is normal, and he is afebrile. Which is most likely to be contributing to relative epoetin resistance in this patient?

    A. Iron deficiency.
    B. Hyperparathyroidism.
    C. Phenytoin therapy.
    D. Infection.

15. In addition to diet modification and emphasizing adherence, which is the best approach to managing this patient's hyperparathyroidism?

    A. Increase calcium acetate.
    B. Change calcium acetate to sevelamer and add cinacalcet.
    C. Hold calcium acetate and add intravenous vitamin D analog.
    D. Add intravenous vitamin D analog.

V. MANAGING THE COMPLICATIONS OF CHRONIC KIDNEY DISEASE

A. Anemia
   1. Several factors are responsible for anemia in CKD: Decreased erythropoietin production (most important), shorter life span of red blood cells, blood loss during dialysis, iron deficiency, anemia of chronic disease, and renal osteodystrophy.
   2. Prevalence: 26% of patients with a GFR greater than 60 mL/minute have anemia, compared with 75% of patients with a GFR less than 15 mL/minute.
   3. Signs and symptoms: Similar to those of anemia associated with other causes
   4. Treatment: Treatment of anemia in CKD can decrease morbidity and mortality, reduce left ventricular hypertrophy, increase exercise tolerance, and increase quality of life.
   5. Recent studies suggest that treatment with erythropoiesis-stimulating agents (ESAs) to high hemoglobin concentrations (greater than 13 g/dL) increases cardiovascular events. Most recently, the Trial to Reduce Cardiovascular Events with Aranesp Therapy failed to show a benefit in outcomes, but treatment with ESAs was associated with increased stroke (N Engl J Med 2009;361:2019-32).
      a. Anemia workup: Initiate evaluation when CrCl is less than 60 mL/minute *or* when hemoglobin is less than 13 g/dL (men) or less than 12 g/dL (women)
         i. Hemoglobin and hematocrit monitoring recommendations
            (a) Stage 3 CKD: At least annually
            (b) Stage 4 and 5 (nondialysis): At least twice per year
            (c) Stage 5 (dialysis): At least every 3 months
         ii. Mean corpuscular volume

      iii. Reticulocyte count

      iv. Iron studies

         (a) TSAT (serum iron/TIBC × 100): Assesses available iron

         (b) Ferritin: Measures stored iron

      v. Serum vitamin B_{12} and folate levels

      vi. Stool guaiac

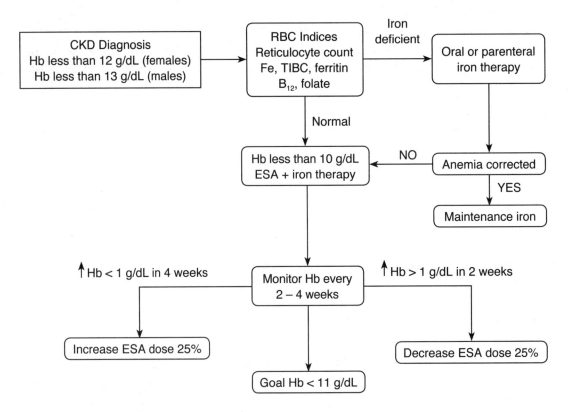

Figure 1. Management of anemia of CKD based on KDIGO and KDOQI guidelines.

TIBC = total iron-binding capacity.

    b. Erythropoiesis-stimulating agents (ESAs) (*Note:* ESAs are under the FDA's Risk Evaluation and Mitigation Strategies program.)

      i. Initiation of ESAs

         (a) Patients with CKD (nondialysis): Not to be initiated if hemoglobin is greater than 10 g/dL. If hemoglobin is less than 10 g/dL, consider the rate of decline in hemoglobin and the need to reduce the likelihood of transfusion (particularly in patients who may receive a renal transplant).

         (b) Patients with CKD (dialysis): Initiate therapy for hemoglobin less than 10 g/dL (KDIGO guidelines recommend avoiding until hemoglobin is less than 9 g/dL).

         (c) Use with caution, if at all, in patients with a history of stroke or cancer (evidence is stronger in nondialysis patients than in dialysis patients with CKD).

      ii. Maintenance of ESAs: Individualize dosing and use the lowest dose of ESA sufficient to reduce the need for red blood cell transfusions; adjust dosing as appropriate.

        iii. Epoetin alfa

            (a) Same molecular structure as human erythropoietin (recombinant DNA technology)

            (b) Binds to and activates erythropoietin receptor

            (c) Administered subcutaneously or intravenously

            (d) Subcutaneous dosage requirement is typically 30% less than intravenous dosage requirement.

        iv. Darbepoetin alfa

            (a) Molecular structure of human erythropoietin has been modified from 3 N-linked carbohydrate chains to 5 N-linked carbohydrate chains; increased duration of activity

            (b) The advantage is less-frequent dosing (e.g., once weekly, once every 2–3 weeks).

            (c) Binds to and activates erythropoietin receptor

            (d) May be administered subcutaneously or intravenously

  c. Therapy goals

      i. Use the lowest possible dose of ESA to prevent blood transfusion.

      ii. In nondialysis patients with CKD, hold or reduce dose when hemoglobin is greater than 10 g/dL.

      iii. In dialysis patients, hold or reduce dose when hemoglobin is greater than 11 g/dL (KDIGO suggests an upper limit of 11.5 g/dL).

      iv. Do not exceed a hemoglobin greater than 13 g/dL

  d. ESA dose adjustment is based on hemoglobin response.

      i. Adjustment parameters are similar for epoetin alfa and darbepoetin alfa.

      ii. Maximal increase in hemoglobin is about 1 g/dL every 2–4 weeks.

      iii. Dosage adjustments upward should not be made more often than every 4 weeks.

      iv. In general, dose adjustments are made in 25% increments (i.e., dosages adjusted upward or downward by 25% according to current dose).

  e. ESA monitoring

      i. Hemoglobin every 2–4 weeks during initiation phase. In maintenance phase of therapy, monitor hemoglobin at least monthly in dialysis patients and at least every 3 months in nondialysis patients with CKD.

      ii. Monitor BP because it may rise (treat as necessary).

      iii. Iron stores (KDIGO, Kidney Int Suppl 2012;2:279)

          (a) Ferritin: Goal is greater than 500 ng/mL.

          (b) TSAT target is greater than 30%.

  f. Common causes of inadequate response to ESA therapy

      i. Iron deficiency is the most common cause of erythropoietin resistance; however, increased use of intravenous iron products has reduced this problem.

      ii. Infection and inflammation

      iii. Other causes include chronic blood loss, hyperparathyroidism, aluminum toxicity, folate or vitamin B_{12} deficiency, malignancies, malnutrition, hemolysis, and vitamin C deficiency.

  g. Iron therapy

      i. Most patients with CKD who are receiving ESAs need parenteral iron therapy (increased requirements, decreased oral absorption).

      ii. For adult patients who undergo dialysis, an empiric cumulative or total dose of 1000 mg is usually given, and equations are rarely used.

      iii. Monitor TSAT and ferritin as noted during erythropoietic therapy.

      iv. Adverse effects

          (a) Anaphylactic-type reactions with iron dextran necessitate test dose. Hypersensitivity reaction may occur with all parenteral iron products.

(b) Hypotension with administration of sodium ferric gluconate, iron sucrose, and ferumoxytol. Monitor during and up to 30 minutes after administration.

(c) Hypertension. Transient increases in BP occur with ferric carboxymaltose.

v. Seven commercial iron preparations are approved in the United States (Table 6).

vi. Oral iron is not recommended in patients with CKD on dialysis.

Table 6. Iron Therapy

Iron Product	Replacement Therapy (TSAT <30% and ferritin <500 ng/mL)	Maintenance Therapy (iron stores in goal)	Initial Test Dose
Iron dextran (high-molecular-weight iron dextran: Dexferrum) (low-molecular-weight iron dextran: INFeD)	IVP: 100 mg IV 3 times/week during HD for 10 doses (1 g) IVPB: 500–1000 mg in 250 mL of NS infused for ≥1 hour (option for non-HD patients)	25–100 mg/week IV × 10 weeks	Yes; 25 mg 1-time test dose
Sodium ferric gluconate complex (Ferrlecit and generic)	125 mg IV 3 times/week during HD for 8 doses (1 g)	31.25–125 mg/week IV × 10 weeks	None needed
Iron sucrose (Venofer)	100 mg IV 3 times/week during HD for 10 doses (1 g) For non-HD CKD, 200 mg IV × 5 doses	25–100 mg/week IV × 10 weeks	None needed
Ferumoxytol (Feraheme)	510 mg at up to 30 mg/second, followed by a second 510-mg IV dose 3–8 days later (all CKD)	N/A	None needed
Ferric carboxymaltose (Injectafer)	15 mg/kg IV up to 750 mg; may repeat after at least 7 days (maximum 1500 mg elemental iron per 2-dose course)	N/A	None needed

CKD = chronic kidney disease; HD = hemodialysis; IV = intravenous; IVP = IV push; IVPB = IV piggyback; N/A = not applicable; NS = normal saline solution; TSAT = transferrin saturation.

B. CKD–Mineral Bone Disorder (CKD-MBD)

1. Pathophysiology: Calcium and phosphorus homeostasis is complex, involving the interplay of hormones affecting the bone, gastrointestinal (GI) tract, kidneys, and parathyroid gland. The process may begin as GFR falls to less than 60 mL/minute. The consequence of CKD-MBD include renal osteodystrophy and vascular calcification. Factors contributing to CKD-MBD include the following:

   a. Hyperphosphatemia

   b. Decreased production of 1,25-dihydroxyvitamin D_3

   c. Reduced absorption of calcium in the gut

   d. Decreased ionized (free) calcium concentrations

   e. Direct stimulation of parathyroid hormone (PTH) secretion

   f. Elevated PTH concentrations cause decreased reabsorption of phosphorus and increased reabsorption of calcium in the proximal tubule. This adaptive mechanism is lost as GFR falls below 30 mL/minute. Important: Calcium is not well absorbed through the gut at this point, and calcium concentrations are maintained by increased bone resorption through elevated PTH. Unabated calcium loss from the bone results in renal osteodystrophy.

2. Prevalence
    a. Main cause of morbidity and mortality in patients undergoing dialysis
    b. Very common
3. Signs and symptoms
    a. Insidious onset: Patients may experience fatigue and musculoskeletal and GI pain; calcification may be visible on radiography; bone pain and fractures can occur if progression is left untreated.
    b. Laboratory abnormalities (Table 7)
        i. Phosphorus
        ii. Corrected calcium (measured Ca + 0.8[4 − serum albumin])
        iii. Intact PTH
        iv. Alkaline phosphatase
        v. 25-hydroxyvitamin D

Table 7. KDIGO Guidelines for Frequency of Laboratory Monitoring in CKD Stages 3–5

	Stage 3 CKD	**Stage 4 CKD**	**Stage 5 CKD**
Calcium	Every 6–12 months	Every 3–6 months	Every 1–3 months
Phosphorus	Every 6–12 months	Every 3–6 months	Every 1–3 months
Intact PTH	Baseline	Every 6–12 months	Every 3–6 months
Alkaline phosphatase	Baseline	Every 12 months	Every 12 months
25-hydroxyvitamin D	Baseline	Baseline	Baseline

CKD = chronic kidney disease; KDIGO = Kidney Disease: Improving Global Outcomes.

4. Treatment
    a. Therapy goals (Table 8)

Table 8. KDIGO Guidelines for Calcium, Phosphorus, and Intact PTH in CKD Stages 3–5

	CKD Stage 3	**CKD Stage 4**	**CKD Stage 5**	**CKD Stage 5 on Dialysis**
Corrected calcium	Normal	Normal	Normal	Normal
Phosphorus	Normal	Normal	Normal	Near normal
Intact PTH	Normal	Normal	Normal	2–9 times upper normal

CKD = chronic kidney disease; KDIGO = Kidney Disease: Improving Global Outcomes; PTH = parathyroid hormone.

    b. Nondrug therapy
        i. Dietary phosphorus restriction 800–1000 mg/day in stage 3 CKD or higher
        ii. Dialysis removes various amounts of phosphorus, depending on treatment modalities; however, by itself it is insufficient to maintain phosphorus balances in most patients.
        iii. Parathyroidectomy: Reserved for patients with unresponsive hyperparathyroidism
    c. Drug therapy
        i. Phosphate binders (Table 9): Take with meals to bind phosphorus in the gut; products from different groups may be used together for additive effect.

Table 9. Phosphate Binders

Product	Dosage Form	Typical Dose
Calcium carbonate	500, 1000, 1250 mg (40% elemental Ca)	1250 mg
Calcium acetate (PhosLo, Phoslyra)	667-mg capsule, tablet 667-mg/5 mL solution (25% elemental Ca)	2001 mg
Sevelamer hydrochloride (Renagel)	400-, 800-mg tablet	800–2400 mg
Sevelamer carbonate (Renvela)	800-mg tablet 0.8-g, 2.4-g packet	800–2400 mg
Lanthanum carbonate (Fosrenol)	500-, 750-, 1000-mg chewable tablet	250–500 mg
Sucroferric oxyhydroxide (Velphoro)	500-mg chewable tablet	500 mg
Aluminum hydroxide	320-mg/5 mL suspension	300–600 mg
Ferric citrate (Auryxia)	210 mg tablet	420 mg

Typical dose is administered 3 times daily with meals.

(a) Aluminum-containing phosphate binders (aluminum hydroxide, aluminum carbonate, and sucralfate) effectively lower phosphorus concentrations. In general, avoid. Not used as often because of aluminum toxicity (adynamic bone disease, encephalopathy, and erythropoietin resistance). Use should be limited to a single short-term (4-week) course.

(b) Calcium-containing phosphate binders (calcium carbonate and calcium acetate)

    (1) Widely used phosphate binder. Calcium binders are often the initial binder of choice for stage 3 and 4 CKD. Calcium or nonionic binders are considered initial binder of choice in stage 5 CKD. Carbonate salt is inexpensive.

    (2) Carbonate is also used to treat hypocalcemia, which sometimes occurs in patients with CKD, and can decrease metabolic acidosis.

    (3) Calcium acetate is a better binder than carbonate and contains less elemental calcium. Less calcium absorption

    (4) Use may be limited by development of hypercalcemia; reduce dose or discontinue.

    (5) Total elemental calcium is 2000 mg/day (1500-mg binder; 500-mg diet).

(c) Sevelamer: A nonabsorbable phosphate binder

    (1) Effectively binds dietary phosphorus

    (2) As with calcium, considered primary therapy in stage 5 CKD. In particular, consider whether the patient has hypercalcemia or whether calcium intake exceeds the recommended dose with calcium-containing binders.

    (3) Decreases low-density lipoprotein cholesterol and increases high-density lipoprotein cholesterol

    (4) Metabolic acidosis may worsen with sevelamer hydrogen chloride (HCl).

(d) Lanthanum carbonate

    (1) As effective as aluminum in phosphate-binding capability. Not widely used, but indications similar to sevelamer

    (2) Flavorless, chewable tablet

    (3) Consider using if patient has hypercalcemia

(e) There are no data indicating that any phosphate binder is superior to another in clinical outcomes (mortality or hospitalization). However, sevelamer and lanthanum do cause less hypercalcemia and reduce calcium burden.

ii. Vitamin D and vitamin D analogs: Suppress PTH synthesis and reduce PTH concentrations; therapy is limited by resultant hypercalcemia.

(a) Ergocalciferol (vitamin D_2): Inactive form of vitamin D. May be used in stage 3–5 CKD for patients with low serum 25-hydroxyvitamin D concentrations; repeat vitamin D levels after 6 months of therapy. Usually doses weekly or monthly (Table 10).

(b) Cholecalciferol (vitamin D_3): Inactive vitamin D. May be used as alternative to ergocalciferol. Usually dosed daily.

Table 10. Ergocalciferol Repletion

Serum 25-hydroxy Vitamin D (ng/mL)	Assessment	Dosing Regimen
Less than 5	Severe deficiency	Weekly oral doses × 12 weeks, then monthly *or* Single intramuscular dose
5–15	Mild deficiency	Weekly oral doses × 4 weeks, then monthly
16–30	Insufficiency	Monthly oral doses

(c) Calcitriol (Calcijex, Rocaltrol): The pharmacologically active form of 1,25-dihydroxy-vitamin D_3 is FDA label approved for the management of hypocalcemia and the prevention and treatment of secondary hyperparathyroidism.
  (1) Oral and parenteral formulations
  (2) Does not require hepatic or renal activation
  (3) Low-dose daily oral therapy reduces hypocalcemia but does not reduce PTH concentrations significantly.
  (4) High incidence of hypercalcemia, limiting PTH suppression
  (5) Dose adjustment at 4-week intervals

(d) Paricalcitol (Zemplar): Vitamin D analog; FDA label approved for the treatment and prevention of secondary hyperparathyroidism
  (1) Parenteral and oral formulations
  (2) Does not require hepatic or renal activation
  (3) Lower incidence of hypercalcemia compared with calcitriol (decreased mobilization of calcium from the bone and decreased absorption of calcium from the gut)

(e) Doxercalciferol (Hectorol): Vitamin D analog; FDA label approved for the treatment and prevention of secondary hyperparathyroidism
  (1) Parenteral and oral formulations
  (2) Prodrug; requires hepatic activation; may have more physiologic levels
  (3) Lower incidence of hypercalcemia compared with calcitriol (decreased mobilization of calcium from the bone and decreased absorption of calcium from the gut)

iii. Cinacalcet HCl (Sensipar): A calcimimetic that attaches to the calcium receptor on the parathyroid gland and increases the sensitivity of receptors to serum calcium concentrations, thus reducing PTH. Especially useful in patients with high calcium and phosphate concentrations and high PTH concentrations when vitamin D analogs cannot be used or cannot be increased

(a) The initial dose is 30 mg, irrespective of PTH concentration.
(b) Monitor serum calcium every 1–2 weeks (risk of hypocalcemia is about 5%); do not initiate therapy if corrected serum calcium is less than 8.4 mg/dL.
(c) Can be used in patients irrespective of phosphate binder or vitamin D analog use

    (d) Caution in patients with seizure disorder (hypocalcemia may exacerbate)

    (e) Adverse effects are nausea (30%) and diarrhea (20%).

    (f) Cinacalcet inhibits cytochrome P450 (CYP) 2D6 metabolism, thereby inhibiting the metabolism of CYP2D6 substrates such that dose reductions in drugs with narrow therapeutic indices may be required (e.g., flecainide, tricyclic antidepressants, thioridazine).

    (g) Cinacalcet is metabolized primarily by CYP3A, so drugs that are potent inhibitors of CYP3A (ketoconazole) may increase cinacalcet concentrations up to twofold.

Patient Case

16. A 40-year-old patient on dialysis with a history of grand mal seizures takes phenytoin 300 mg/day. His albumin concentration is 3.0 g/dL. His total phenytoin concentration is 5.0 mcg/mL. Which is the best interpretation of the phenytoin concentrations?

    A. The concentration is subtherapeutic, and a dose increase is needed.

    B. The concentration is therapeutic, and no dosage adjustment is needed.

    C. The concentration is toxic, and a dose reduction is needed.

    D. The level is not interpretable.

$$\frac{5}{(.1 \cdot 3) + .1}$$

$$\frac{5}{.4} = 12$$

VI. DOSAGE ADJUSTMENTS IN KIDNEY DISEASE

A. Dosages of Many Drugs Will Require Adjustment to Prevent Toxicity in Patients with CKD. Adjustment strategies vary depending on whether the patient is receiving RRT and, if so, the type of RRT. The National Kidney Disease Education Program of the National Institutes of Health/National Institute of Diabetes and Digestive and Kidney Diseases suggests that either eGFR or eCrCl be used for drug dosing. If eGFR is used in very large or small patients, the eGFR should be multiplied by the actual body surface area to obtain eGFR in milliliters per minute.

B. Pharmacokinetic Principles Guiding Therapy Adjustments

    1. Absorption: Oral absorption can be decreased.

        a. Nausea and vomiting

        b. Increased gastric pH (uremia)

        c. Edema

        d. Physical binding of drugs to phosphate binders

    2. Distribution

        a. Changes in concentrations in highly water-soluble drugs occur as extracellular fluid status changes.

        b. Acidic and neutral protein-bound drugs are displaced by toxin buildup. Other mechanisms include conformational changes of the plasma protein–binding site. Phenytoin is a classic example. The "normal" free fraction of phenytoin is 10%. Free fraction can be as high as 30% in patients with ESKD and hypoalbuminemia.

        i. Hypoalbuminemia correction:

          Concentration adjusted = Concentration measured/[(0.2 × measured albumin) + 0.1]

        ii. Renal failure adjustment:

          Concentration adjusted = Concentration measured/[(0.1 × measured albumin) + 0.1]

        iii. Patients have lower total concentrations despite having adequate free concentrations (increased free fraction).

        iv. Dosage adjustment of phenytoin not needed, just a different approach to evaluating concentrations.

    3. Metabolism: Variable changes can occur with uremia; metabolites can accumulate.

    4. Excretion: Decreased

C. Pharmacodynamic Changes Can Also Occur (e.g., patients with CKD can be more sensitive to benzodiazepines).

D. General Recommendations

    1. Patient history and clinical data

    2. Estimate CrCl (Jeliffe or Brater equation in AKI; Cockcroft-Gault or MDRD study equations in stable kidney function).

    3. Identify medications that require modification (Table 11).

Table 11. Dose Adjustments and Precautions in Decreased Kidney Function

Drug Class	Agents Requiring Dose Adjustment
Antibiotics	Almost all antibiotics require dosage adjustment (exceptions: ceftriaxone, clindamycin, linezolid, metronidazole, macrolides, nafcillin)
Anticoagulants	Enoxaparin, fondaparinux, apixaban, rivaroxaban, edoxaban, dabigatran
Cardiac medications	Atenolol, ACEIs, digoxin, nadolol, sotalol; avoid potassium-sparing diuretics if CrCl < 30 mL/minute
Lipid-lowering therapy	Clofibrate, fenofibrate, statins (particularly rosuvastatin)
Narcotics	Codeine, avoid meperidine; other agents may also accumulate
Antipsychotic and antiepileptic agents	Chloral hydrate, gabapentin, lithium, paroxetine, primidone, topiramate, trazodone, vigabatrin, levetiracetam
Hypoglycemic agents	Acarbose, alogliptin, canagliflozin, chlorpropamide, dapagliflozin, exenatide, glyburide, glipizide, insulins, liraglutide, metformin, saxagliptin, sitagliptin
Antiretrovirals	Individualize therapy: Monitor $CD4^+$ counts, viral load, and adverse effects (agents requiring dose adjustment: lamivudine, adefovir, emtricitabine, didanosine, stavudine, tenofovir, and zidovudine)
Miscellaneous	Allopurinol, colchicine, H_2-receptor antagonists, diclofenac, ketorolac, acyclovir, valacyclovir, valganciclovir and terbutaline

ACEI = angiotensin-converting enzyme inhibitor; CrCl = creatinine clearance; H_2 = histamine-2.

    4. Calculate drug doses individualized for the patient.

      a. Published data

      b. Rowland-Tozer estimate

        i. $Q = 1 - [Fe(1 - KF)]$

        ii. Q = kinetic parameter or drug dose adjustment factor

        iii. Fe = fraction of drug excreted unchanged in the urine

        iv. KF = ratio of patient's CrCl to normal (120 mL/minute)

    5. Monitor patient (e.g., kidney function, clinical parameters) and drug concentration (if applicable).

    6. Revise regimen as appropriate.

E. Drug Dosing in HD
1. Dosing changes in patients with HD may be necessary because of accumulation caused by kidney failure *or* because the procedure may remove the drug from the circulation *or* because of pharmacodynamic effects (e.g., BP medication reduction because of intradialytic hypotension).
2. Drug-related factors affecting drug removal during dialysis
   a. Molecular weight: With high-flux membranes, larger molecules (e.g., vancomycin) can be removed compared with conventional filters.
   b. Water soluble: Nonsoluble drugs are not likely to be removed.
   c. Protein binding: Because albumin cannot pass through membranes, protein-bound drugs cannot either.
   d. Volume of distribution: Drugs with a small volume of distribution (less than 1 L/kg) available in central circulation for removal. Large volumes of distribution cannot be removed (digoxin and tricyclic antidepressants), even if the protein binding is very low.
3. Procedure-related factors affecting drug removal
   a. Type of dialyzer: High flux, widely used now
   b. Blood flow rate: Elevated rates increase delivery and maintain gradient across membrane.
   c. Duration of dialysis session
   d. Dialysate flow rate. High rates of flow increase removal by maintaining the gradient across membranes.

REFERENCES

Kidney Disease

1. National Kidney Foundation's Kidney Disease Outcome Quality Initiative (NKF KDOQI). Available at www.kidney.org/professionals/kdoqi/index.cfm.

2. National Kidney Disease Education Program (NKDEP). Available at www.nkdep.nih.gov/.

3. Kidney Disease: Improving Global Outcomes (KDIGO). Available at http://kdigo.org/home/guidelines/.

Acute Kidney Injury

1. Bellomo R, Ronco C, Kellum JA, et al.; the ADQI Workgroup. Acute renal failure—definition, outcome measures, animal models, and information technology needs: the Second International Consensus Conference of the Acute Dialysis Quality Initiative (ADQI) Group. Crit Care 2004;8:R204-R212.

2. Dager W, Halilovic J. Acute kidney injury. In: DiPiro JT, Talbert RL, Yee GC, et al., eds. Pharmacotherapy: A Pathophysiologic Approach, 9th ed. New York: McGraw-Hill, 2014:611-32.

3. Kellum JA. Acute kidney injury. Crit Care Med 2008;36:S141-5.

4. Kidney Disease: Improving Global Outcomes (KDIGO) Acute Kidney Injury Work Group. KDIGO practice guideline for acute kidney injury. Kidney Int Suppl 2012;2:1-138.

5. Mehta RL, Kellum JA, Shah SV, et al. Acute Kidney Injury Network: report of an initiative to improve outcomes in acute kidney injury. Crit Care 2007;11:R31.

6. Palevsky PM, Liu KD, Brophy PD, et al. KDOQI U.S. commentary on the 2012 KDIGO clinical practice guidelines for acute kidney injury. Am J Kidney Dis 2013;61:649-72.

7. Stamatakis MK. Acute kidney injury. In: Chisholm-Burns MA, Wells BG, Schwinghammer TL, et al., eds. Pharmacotherapy: Principles and Practice, 2nd ed. New York: McGraw-Hill, 2010:431-44.

8. Ympa YP, Sakr Y, Reinhart K, et al. Has mortality from acute kidney injury decreased? A systematic review of the literature. Am J Med 2005;118:827-32.

Glomerulonephritis

1. Beck L, Bomback AS, Choi MJ, et al. KDOQI U.S. commentary on the 2012 clinical practice guideline for glomerulonephritis. Am J Kidney Dis 2013;62:403-41.

2. Kidney Disease: Improving Global Outcomes (KDIGO). Glomerulonephritis Work Group. KDIGO clinical practice guideline for glomerulonephritis. Kidney Int Suppl 2012;2:139-274.

3. Lau AH. Glomerulonephritis. In: DiPiro JT, Talbert RL, Yee GC, et al., eds. Pharmacotherapy: A Pathophysiologic Approach, 9th ed. New York: McGraw-Hill, 2014:705-28.

Drug-Induced Kidney Damage

1. Nolin TD, Himmelfarb J. Drug-induced kidney disease. In: DiPiro JT, Talbert RL, Yee GC, et al., eds. Pharmacotherapy: A Pathophysiologic Approach, 9th ed. New York: McGraw-Hill, 2014:687-704.

2. Schweiger MJ, Chambers CE, Davidson CJ, et al. Prevention of contrast induced nephropathy: recommendations for the high risk patient undergoing cardiovascular procedures. Catheter Cardiovasc Interv 2007;69:135-40.

Chronic Kidney Disease and Complications

1. Inker LA, Astor BC, Fox CH, et al. KDOQI commentary on the 2012 Clinical Practice Guideline for the evaluation and management of CKD. Am J Kidney Dis 2014;63:713-35.

2. American Diabetes Association. Standards of medical care in diabetes: 2015: summary of revisions. Diabetes Care 2015;38(suppl 1):S4.

3. American Diabetes Association. Microvascular complications and foot care. Diabetes Care 2015;38(suppl 1):S58-S66.

4. Hudson JQ, Wazny LD. Chronic kidney disease: management of complications. In: DiPiro JT, Talbert RL, Yee GC, et al., eds. Pharmacotherapy: A Pathophysiologic Approach, 9th ed. New York: McGraw-Hill, 2014:633-63.

5. Kidney Disease: Improving Global Outcomes (KDIGO) CKD Work Group. KDIGO 2012 clinical practice guideline for the evaluation and management of chronic kidney disease. Kidney Int Suppl 2013;3:1-150.

6. Levey AS, Coresh J. Chronic kidney disease. Lancet 2012;379:165-80.

7. National Kidney Foundation. KDOQI. Clinical practice guidelines and clinical practice recommendations for diabetes and chronic kidney disease. Am J Kidney Dis 2007;49(suppl 2):S1-180.

8. National Kidney Foundation. K/DOQI clinical practice guidelines for chronic kidney disease: evaluation, classification and stratification. Am J Kidney Dis 2002;39(suppl 1):S1-266.

9. National Kidney Foundation. KDOQI clinical practice guideline for diabetes and CKD: 2012 update. Am J Kidney Dis 2012;60:850-86.

10. National Kidney Foundation. KDOQI clinical practice guidelines on hypertension and antihypertensive agents in chronic kidney disease. Am J Kidney Dis 2004;43(suppl 5):S1.

11. Schonder KS. Chronic and end-stage renal disease. In: Chisholm-Burns MA, Wells BG, Schwinghammer TL, et al., eds. Pharmacotherapy: Principles and Practice, 2nd ed. New York: McGraw-Hill, 2010:445-78.

12. Taler SJ, Agarwal R, Bakris GL, et al. KDOQI U.S. commentary on the 2012 KDIGO clinical practice guideline for management of blood pressure in CKD. Am J Kidney Dis 2013;62:201-13.

13. Wanner C, Tonelli M; KDIGO Lipid Guideline Development Work Group Members. KDIGO clinical practice guideline for lipid management in CKD: summary of recommendation statements and clinical approach to the patient. Kidney Int 2014;85:1303-9.

Anemia of Chronic Kidney Disease

1. Kidney Disease: Improving Global Outcomes (KDIGO) Anemia Work Group. KDIGO clinical practice guideline for anemia in chronic kidney disease. Kidney Int Suppl 2012;2:279-335.

2. Kliger AS, Foley RN, Goldfarb DS, et al. KDOQI U.S. commentary on the 2012 KDIGO clinical practice guideline for anemia in CKD. Am J Kidney Dis 2013;62:849-59. Available at http://www.kidney.org/sites/default/files/docs/kdoqi_commentary_on_kdigo_anemia.pdf. Accessed October 29, 2015.

3. National Kidney Foundation. KDOQI clinical practice guidelines and recommendations for anemia of chronic kidney disease. Am J Kidney Dis 2006;47(suppl 3):S1-146. Available at www2.kidney.org/professionals/KDOQI/guidelines_anemia/. Accessed October 29, 2015.

Mineral and Bone Disorder

1. Kidney Disease: Improving Global Outcomes (KDIGO) CKD-MBD Work Group. KDIGO clinical practice guideline for the diagnosis, evaluation, prevention, and treatment of chronic kidney disease–mineral and bone disorder (CKD-MBD). Kidney Int 2009;76(suppl 113):S1-130.

2. Uhlig K, Berns JS, Kestenbaum B, et al. KDOQI U.S. commentary on the 2009 KDIGO clinical practice guideline for the diagnosis, evaluation, and treatment of CKD–mineral and bone disorder (CKD-MBD). Am J Kidney Dis 2010;55:773-99.

Renal Replacement Therapy

1. Li PK, Szeto CC, Piraino B, et al. Peritoneal dialysis–related infections recommendations: 2010 update. Perit Dial Int 2010;30:393-423.

2. Ballinger AE, Palmer SC, Wiggins KJ, et al. Treatment for peritoneal dialysis-associated peritonitis. Cochrane Database of Systematic Reviews 2014;4:CD005284. doi:10.1002/14651858.CD005284.pub3.

3. Sowinski KM, Churchwell MD, Decker BS. Hemodialysis and peritoneal dialysis. In: DiPiro JT, Talbert RL, Yee GC, et al., eds. Pharmacotherapy: A Pathophysiologic Approach, 9th ed. New York: McGraw-Hill, 2014:665-85.

4. O'Mara NB. Management of patients on dialysis. In: Murphy JE, Lee MW, eds. Pharmacotherapy Self-Assessment Program, 2014 Book 2. Chronic Illnesses. Lenexa, KS: American College of Clinical Pharmacy, 2014:203-207.

Drug Therapy Adjustment in CKD

1. National Kidney Disease Education Program. Chronic kidney disease and drug dosing: information for providers. Revised April 2015. Available at http://nkdep.nih.gov/resources/ckd-drug-dosing-508.pdf. Accessed October 29, 2015.

2. Kappel J, Calissi P. Nephrology: 3. Safe drug prescribing for patients with renal insufficiency. Can Med Assoc J 2002;166:473-7.

3. Mohammad RS, Matzke GR. Drug therapy individualization for patients with chronic kidney disease. In: DiPiro JT, Talbert RL, Yee GC, et al., eds. Pharmacotherapy: A Pathophysiologic Approach, 9th ed. New York: McGraw-Hill, 2014:729-43.

ANSWERS AND EXPLANATIONS TO PATIENT CASES

1. Answer: D

Estimating CrCl in a patient with unstable kidney function is difficult. The Jeliffe or Brater equation has been recommended as preferable to other equations. In this case, the patient is anuric; therefore, a CrCl (GFR) of less than 10 mL/minute (Answer D) should be assumed. Answer A (Cockcroft-Gault) is inappropriate because Cockcroft-Gault should be used only with stable kidney function. The use of MDRD (Answer B) in unstable kidney function is also inappropriate. Although Answer C, the Brater equation, may be used, it would still overestimate kidney function in this patient because the patient is anuric.

2. Answer: B

This patient probably has ATN, which is a type of intrinsic renal failure (Answer B). The rapid rise in SCr, the BUN/SCr ratio of about 10, and the muddy casts all point to ATN. There is no evidence of prerenal causes (hypotension, volume depletion) (Answer A). Naproxen is associated with functional AKI (Answer D), but the urine in these patients is bland without casts. Answer C is incorrect because there is no evidence of obstruction in this patient.

3. Answer: A

One of the strategies in managing AKI is to remove potentially nephrotoxic drugs, either direct toxins or medications that alter intrarenal hemodynamics. It is common to see the following orders for patients in AKI: no ACEIs, ARBs, NSAIDs, or intravenous contrast. However, low-dose aspirin can be continued without adversely affecting kidney function. It is also important to remove (or reduce the dose of) agents that are cleared renally. Metformin, which accumulates in decreased kidney function, should be temporarily discontinued at this time because of an increased risk of lactic acidosis, not because of an adverse effect on kidney function. In this case, lisinopril is most likely to affect kidney function, so it should be discontinued.

4. Answer: C

This patient presents with ATN, anuria, and volume overload. Although loop diuretics have not been shown to improve clinical outcomes in patients with AKI, they may increase urine output, which will help with fluid and electrolyte balance. In addition, this patient is hypervolemic, so a trial of intravenous loop diuretics would be appropriate (Answer C). Adding 0.9% NaCl (Answer A) would worsen fluid overload. Hydrochlorothiazide (Answer B) would not be appropriate because thiazide diuretics are unlikely to be effective with such poor kidney function. Fluid restriction (Answer D) may be necessary if furosemide fails to increase urine output, but it would not be the first-line approach.

5. Answer: B

Intravenous 0.9% NaCl is considered the most effective hydration for the prevention of contrast-induced nephropathy (Answer B). The other solutions, particularly oral, would not be appropriate. Although not listed as a choice, intravenous sodium bicarbonate solutions have also been used in this setting.

6. Answer: B

Contrast-associated nephropathy is associated with an acute rise in BUN and SCr within 24–48 hours, with a peak at 3–5 days. Monitoring of SCr at 24 hours will help identify the development of contrast-associated nephropathy. In contrast, 6 hours is too early to detect a significant change, and waiting more than 48 hours would delay the detection of renal damage.

7. Answer: B

The patient is currently at category 3a CKD (GFR 45–59 mL/minute/1.73 m²), which can be calculated by the MDRD formula or Cockcroft-Gault. The five categories range from mild kidney damage (G1) to kidney failure (G5).

8. Answer: C

Given the diagnosis of diabetes mellitus and the presence of overt proteinuria, this patient probably has diabetic nephropathy. Progression will be accelerated by smoking, poor diabetes control, and poor BP control. In patients with diabetes, a target A1C of less than 7% is associated with a decrease in the rate of disease progression. Blood pressure control of less than 130/80 mm Hg in patients also decreases the progression of kidney disease. The standard of care in patients with diabetic nephropathy is ACEIs (evidence for a reduction in mortality and reduced progression of CKD) or ARBs (evidence for a reduction in progression but no mortality data), so enalapril (Answer C) is the best choice. A nondihydropyridine (Answer B) might be initiated in patients who cannot tolerate ACEI or ARB therapy but would not be a choice yet. Dihydropyridine therapy (Answer A) is not recommended in diabetic nephropathy because of conflicting literature on its efficacy. An increase in atenolol (Answer D) might control BP, but inhibition of the renin-angiotensin system is still the best answer. In addition, a recent meta-analysis evaluating atenolol in hypertensive patients with diabetes mellitus found either no difference or worse outcomes.

9. Answer: B

The BP is not at goal (should be less than 130/80 mm Hg). To improve BP control and increase the effect of the ACEI, chlorthalidone should be added to the regimen (Answer B). Monitoring of SCr and serum potassium is appropriate in this patient. There is less than a 30% increase in SCr, so enalapril should be continued, making Answer A and Answer C inappropriate. Adding chlorthalidone will also counter the tendency for hyperkalemia. Answer D would probably lower BP but would not be the preferred route because renal protection probably would not be improved.

10. Answer: B

Calculation of the number needed to harm (NNH) is similar to the calculation of the number needed to treat but is focused on a negative outcome. In this study, the risk of acute kidney injury was 11% in the monotherapy group and 18% in the combination therapy group, a difference of 7%. The NNH is calculated as 1/(absolute risk increase) = 1/(0.07) = 14.3. So the best estimate is that 1 additional patient would develop AKI for about every 15 patients treated with combination therapy compared with angiotensin receptor blocker therapy alone.

11. Answer: D

A native arteriovenous fistula is the preferred access for chronic HD. If an arteriovenous fistula cannot be constructed, a synthetic arteriovenous graft (Answer C) is considered second line. A subclavian catheter (Answer A) is a poor choice because of the greater risk of infection and thrombosis and because of the poor blood flow obtained through a catheter. A Tenckhoff catheter (Answer B) is incorrect because this is a catheter for peritoneal dialysis.

12. Answer: D

The best-studied agent is midodrine, an α_1-agonist. Levocarnitine (Answer A) has been tried, but data are limited on its benefit. Fludrocortisone (Answer C) is a synthetic mineralocorticoid that is used for hypotension in other situations; however, the primary mechanism is caused by Na and water restriction in the kidney; therefore, this drug is less likely to work. Sodium chloride tablets (Answer B) would not work acutely, and they should generally be avoided.

13. Answer: B

Empiric coverage for the treatment of peritoneal dialysis–related peritonitis should include activity against both gram-positive and gram-negative organisms. Intraperitoneal administration is preferred to intravenous administration. The use of cefazolin will provide activity against *Staphylococcus* unless an area has a high rate of methicillin-resistant organisms. The choice of antibiotic for gram-negative coverage can include a third-generation cephalosporin with activity against *Pseudomonas* (e.g., ceftazidime, cefepime, or an aminoglycoside). Short-term use of an aminoglycoside should not adversely affect residual renal function. For patients with dialysis-related peritonitis, empiric anaerobic coverage is not necessary.

14. Answer: B

Hyperparathyroidism is associated with epoetin resistance in patients on HD (Answer B). Although iron deficiency is the most common cause of epoetin deficiency, the laboratory results in this patient do not indicate iron deficiency (Answer A). Phenytoin therapy (Answer C) has been associated with anemia in other patient populations but not in patients on HD. Infection (Answer D) and inflammation are very common causes of epoetin deficiency in patients on HD, but nothing in this patient's presentation suggests an infectious or inflammatory process.

15. Answer: B

This patient needs treatment for his elevated intact PTH (800 pg/mL), which puts him at high risk of renal osteodystrophy and vascular calcification. He has high serum phosphorus, and although the measured serum calcium concentration is normal, his corrected calcium concentration is elevated according to the presence of hypoalbuminemia (corrected calcium is 10.7 mg/dL).

Current phosphate binder therapy is contributing to calcium exposure; therefore, calcium acetate should be discontinued and sevelamer initiated. Cinacalcet will lower intact PTH and potentially serum calcium. Answer A is incorrect because increasing the calcium acetate may worsen the hypercalcemia. Answer C is incorrect for two reasons. First, the patient needs some type of phosphate binder; second, intravenous vitamin D analogs can worsen hypercalcemia and are not very effective at reducing elevated intact PTH in the presence of hyperphosphatemia. Answer D is incorrect because intravenous vitamin D analogs can worsen hypercalcemia and are not very effective in reducing elevated intact PTH in the presence of hyperphosphatemia. Because this patient also has a seizure disorder, close monitoring of serum calcium concentrations is recommended with the introduction of cinacalcet and discontinuation of calcium acetate. Significant reductions in serum calcium can lower the seizure threshold and potentially worsen seizures.

16. Answer: B
The presence of kidney failure and low albumin results in an increased free fraction of phenytoin. Using the correction equation gives a corrected level of 12.5, which is therapeutic. A free phenytoin concentration can also be drawn.

ANSWERS AND EXPLANATIONS TO SELF-ASSESSMENT QUESTIONS

1. Answer: C
Initial treatment of AKI requires the identification and reversal (if possible) of the insult to the kidney. This patient's symptoms and presentation are consistent with prerenal azotemia because of volume depletion, so fluid administration is the best choice in this case. There is no suggestion of obstruction (e.g., distended abdomen, history of benign prostatic hypertrophy). Diuretic administration would be inappropriate because it would worsen his volume depletion and probably further impair his kidney function. Fluid management is critical to managing AKI, necessitating a careful assessment of the patient. Although his glucose concentration is elevated, insulin is not necessary at this time.

2. Answer: C
The patient has intrinsic azotemia, resulting in damage to the kidneys. Aminoglycosides can cause direct damage to the tubules. The BUN/SCr ratio is normal (an elevated BUN/SCr ratio reflecting hypovolemia is common in prerenal azotemia). Urinary sodium of less than 20 mOsm/L is also a marker of hypovolemia. Fractional excretion of sodium additionally distinguishes prerenal and intrinsic renal damage. A low FENa (less than 1%) in an oliguric patient suggests that tubular function is still intact. A FENa greater than 2% is commonly seen in intrinsic renal failure. The specific gravity is normal in intrinsic renal failure. Elevated specific gravity greater than 1.018 is seen in prerenal failure, reflecting concentrated urine caused by hypovolemia. Cellular debris is often present in intrinsic renal failure because of renal tubular cell death or damage.

3. Answer: B
Application of the Rowland-Tozer equation yields the following calculation:
$Q = 1 - [Fe(1 - KF)]$
$Q = 1 - [0.4(1 - 25/120)]$
$Q = 1 - [0.4(0.79)]$
$Q = 1 - 0.32$
$Q = 0.68$ or 68% of usual dose
Drug X usual dose = 600 mg
Formulation = 100 mg/mL in a 6-mL vial
Adjusted dose = (usual dose) × (Q)
  = (600 mg)(0.68) = 410 mg
Volume drug = (dose)/(concentration) = (410 mg)/(100 mg/mL) = 4.1 mL

4. Answer: C
In most cases, either the Cockcroft-Gault or the MDRD equation is appropriate (and best) to assess kidney function. However, this patient is significantly below his ideal body weight and has malnutrition, so equations will overestimate. An iothalamate study will measure GFR, but it is not used clinically.

5. Answer: C
This patient's hemoglobin is not at goal. Iron studies show the patient is iron deficient, with TSAT less than 30% and ferritin less than 500 ng/mL. Although a trial of oral iron might be indicated in non–dialysis patients with CKD, patients on HD should be given intravenous iron as first line.

6. Answer: B
The BUN/SCr ratio, urine osmolality, and presence of urinary casts all point to ATN. Prerenal and functional AKI look similar in urinalysis. Classically, AIN has eosinophils in the urine.

7. Answer: B
Hemoglobin represents continuous data. Because each treatment is administered to a separate group of patients, the data are not paired (i.e., they are unpaired). Assuming the data are normally distributed, continuous unpaired data should be evaluated using a t-test. Analysis of variance can be used for continuous data, but only when three groups of data are compared. However, a chi-square test is used for nominal data.

8. Answer: D
A cost-utility analysis is an extension of the cost-effectiveness analysis in which outcomes measured are lives saved, adjusted for changes in quality of life, measured as quality-adjusted life-years. A cost minimization study compares the costs and consequences of two or more interventions that have equivalent outcomes, so the primary focus is on cost. A cost-effectiveness analysis compares costs and consequences to determine which treatment can achieve the best outcomes at the lowest cost. A cost-benefit analysis measures costs and consequences in monetary terms. It may be useful to compare costs with unrelated outcomes.

9. Answer: C

Fractional excretion of sodium (FENa) is useful in the assessment of AKI to help differentiate prerenal from acute tubular necrosis. FENa = [(Urine Na)/(Serum Na)]/[(Urine Cr)/(Serum Cr)] × 100 = [(24 mEq/L)/(134 mEq/L)]/[(14.3 mg/dL)/(1.8 mg/dL)] × 100 = 2.3%. This fractional excretion of sodium greater than 2% would be most consistent with ATN.

10. Answer: B

KDIGO provides recommendations for blood pressure goals for patients with CKD based on the severity of proteinuria. This patient is considered to have normal to mildly elevated albuminuria, with an albumin:creatinine ratio less than 30 mg/g. Patients with albuminuria in this category (A1) should have a goal blood pressure of less than 140/90 mm Hg.

11. Answer: D

This patient with an eGFR of 55 mL/min/1.73 m^2 is classified as having stage 3 CKD because his eGFR is less than 60 mL/min/1.73 m^2. He does not currently have anemia based on a hemoglobin concentration greater than 13 g/dL. Therefore, hemoglobin should be monitored based on his CKD stage. For stage 3 CKD, monitoring is recommended at least every 12 months. For patients with stage 4 CKD and stage 5 CKD who are not yet receiving dialysis, monitoring should occur at least every 6 months. Monitoring should occur at least every 3 months once patients in stage 5 CKD are receiving dialysis.

12. Answer: B

Numerous factors can contribute to the development of CKD-MBD, including hyperphosphatemia, hypocalcemia, decreased vitamin D and decreased production of active 1,25-dihydroxyvitamin D, and hyperparathyroidism. Although this patient's PTH level is elevated, it may be related to hyperphosphatemia. Therefore, the first approach would be to administer a phosphate binder, such as calcium acetate, to decrease his serum phosphate concentrations. A calcium-containing phosphate binder, such as calcium acetate, is acceptable with a corrected serum calcium concentration is the low-normal range. Ergocalciferol is not necessary in this patient because the 25-hydroxyvitamin D level is greater than 30 ng/mL, indicating adequate intake. An active vitamin D, such as calcitriol, could be added if the PTH level remains elevated despite normalization of serum phosphate. Cinacalcet is reserved for patients with hyperparathyroidism despite normalization of phosphate in patients with hypercalcemia.

Fluids, Electrolytes, and Nutrition

Leslie A. Hamilton, Pharm.D., BCPS, BCCCP

University of Tennessee
Health Science Center College of Pharmacy
Knoxville, Tennessee

FLUIDS, ELECTROLYTES, AND NUTRITION

LESLIE A. HAMILTON, PHARM.D., BCPS, BCCCP

UNIVERSITY OF TENNESSEE
HEALTH SCIENCE CENTER COLLEGE OF PHARMACY
KNOXVILLE, TENNESSEE

Learning Objectives

1. Calculate the osmolarity of intravenous fluids and compare with normal plasma osmolarity.
2. Recommend an appropriate intravenous fluid regimen and monitoring parameters given a patient clinical scenario.
3. Discuss the appropriate role and risks of hypertonic and hypotonic saline, recommend treatment regimens, and discuss appropriate monitoring parameters to ensure safe and effective use of these intravenous fluids.
4. Assess electrolyte abnormalities and recommend an appropriate pharmacologic treatment plan based on individual patient signs and symptoms.
5. Discuss appropriate indications for the use of enteral nutrition (EN) and parenteral nutrition (PN).
6. Recommend a patient-specific EN formula, infusion rate, and monitoring parameters based on nutritional needs, comorbidities, and clinical condition.
7. Recommend a patient-specific PN formula and monitoring plan based on the type of intravenous access, nutritional needs, comorbidities, and clinical condition.
8. Discuss strategies for preventing complications associated with EN and PN.

Self-Assessment Questions

Answers and explanations to these questions can be found at the end of this chapter.

1. A 74-year-old woman (weight 72 kg) presents to the emergency department with a 3-day history of cough, temperature to 102°F, and lethargy. She has the following vital signs and laboratory values: blood pressure 72/40 mm Hg, heart rate 115 beats/minute, urine output 10 mL/hour, white blood cell count (WBC) 18×10^3 cells/mm³, hemoglobin 12.5 g/dL, and blood urea nitrogen/creatinine ratio (BUN/Cr) 28/1.7 mg/dL (baseline Cr 1.2 mg/dL), blood glucose 82 mg/dL. After a 500-mL fluid bolus of 0.9% sodium chloride, her blood pressure and heart rate are 80/46 mm Hg and 113 beats/minute. Her chest radiograph is consistent with pneumonia. Her medical history includes coronary artery disease and arthritis. Which is the most appropriate treatment at this time?

   A. Furosemide 40 mg intravenously.
   B. 5% albumin 500 mL infused over 4 hours plus norepinephrine titrated to maintain a systolic blood pressure of 90 mm Hg or higher.
   C. 1000-mL fluid bolus with 5% dextrose (D_5W) and 0.9% sodium chloride.
   D. 1000-mL fluid bolus with 0.9% sodium chloride.

2. An order has been received for 3% sodium chloride. Using 0.9% sodium chloride and 23.4% sodium chloride, first determine how much of each is necessary to prepare 1 L of 3% sodium chloride. Second, calculate the osmolarity of 3% sodium chloride. Finally, determine whether the resultant solution should be administered through a central or peripheral intravenous infusion (molecular weight [MW] of sodium chloride is 58.5, osmotic coefficient is 0.93).

   A. Mix 907 mL of 0.9% sodium chloride plus 93 mL of 23.4% sodium chloride; osmolarity = 954 mOsm/L; central intravenous infusion.
   B. Mix 907 mL of 0.9% sodium chloride plus 93 mL of 23.4% sodium chloride; osmolarity = 477 mOsm/L; peripheral intravenous infusion.
   C. Mix 850 mL of 0.9% sodium chloride plus 150 mL of 23.4% sodium chloride; osmolarity = 954 mOsm/L; central intravenous infusion.
   D. Mix 850 mL of 0.9% sodium chloride plus 150 mL of 23.4% sodium chloride; osmolarity = 513 mOsm/L; peripheral intravenous infusion.

3. A 68-year-old man is admitted to the hospital for worsening shortness of breath during the past 2 weeks caused by heart failure. His serum sodium concentration on admission was 123 mEq/L. Other abnormal laboratory values include brain natriuretic peptide 850 pg/mL and Cr 1.7 mg/dL. Chest radiograph is consistent with pulmonary edema. The patient weighs 85 kg on admission, which is up 3 kg from his baseline weight. The patient is not experiencing nausea, headache, or mental status changes. The physician orders 3% sodium chloride to treat the hyponatremia. Which recommendation is best?

A. 3% sodium chloride is an appropriate choice because the hyponatremia is probably acute.

B. A 250-mL bolus of 3% sodium chloride is appropriate if used in combination with furosemide to prevent volume overload.

C. 3% sodium chloride is appropriate as long as the serum sodium does not increase more than 10 mEq/L in 24 hours.

D. The risks of 3% sodium chloride outweigh the potential benefit for this patient.

4. A 55-year-old man with diabetes and kidney disease presents with hyperkalemia. His laboratory values include potassium (K^+) 7.2 mEq/L, calcium (Ca^{2+}) 9 mg/dL, albumin 3.5 g/dL, and blood glucose 302 mg/dL. His electrocardiogram (ECG) is abnormal, with peaked T waves. Which is the best recommendation for initial treatment of his hyperkalemia?

A. Regular insulin 10 units intravenously plus 50 g of glucose intravenously.

B. 10% calcium gluconate 10 mL intravenously over 5 minutes.

C. Kayexalate 15 g mixed with 100 mL of 20% sorbitol every 4 hours as needed.

D. Sodium bicarbonate 50 mEq intravenously over 5 minutes.

5. A 68-year-old woman (weight 60 kg) is admitted to the hospital after a cardioembolic stroke. Her medical history is significant for atrial fibrillation, acute myocardial infarction, and diabetes. She has been unconscious for 48 hours. The medical team decides to start feeding the patient. All of her laboratory values including glucose concentrations are normal. Although she currently has no enteral access, she does have a peripheral intravenous catheter. Which nutritional regimen is best for this patient?

A. Insert a central intravenous catheter and initiate parenteral nutrition (PN) containing 60 g of amino acids (AAs), 500 mL of 10% lipid emulsion, 300 g of dextrose, standard electrolytes, multivitamins, and trace elements in a volume of 2000 mL administered over 24 hours.

B. Insert a central intravenous catheter and initiate PN containing 40 g of AAs, 500 mL of 10% lipid emulsion, 200 g of dextrose, standard electrolytes, multivitamins, and trace elements in a total volume of 2000 mL administered over 24 hours.

C. Insert a nasogastric (NG) or nasoduodenal feeding tube and infuse Isocal (1 kcal/mL) starting at 25 mL/hour and advance to a goal rate of 65 mL/hour.

D. Insert a percutaneous endoscopic gastrostomy feeding tube and infuse Isocal (1 kcal/mL) starting at 25 mL/hour and advance to a goal rate of 100 mL/hour.

6. A 70-year-old man is admitted to the hospital with peritonitis caused by severe inflammatory bowel disease. The patient has received adequate fluid resuscitation, and he is prescribed appropriate antibiotics. The physician wants the patient to have several days of bowel rest, and he or she has consulted the pharmacist to recommend a PN formula to be administered through a central line. The patient is hemodynamically stable, with normal electrolyte concentrations. Weight is 55 kg, prealbumin is 20 mg/dL, BUN/Cr is 20/1.1 mg/dL, and WBC is 17×10^3 cells/mm^3. Assuming that appropriate electrolytes, multivitamins, and trace elements are included, which PN formula, when administered over 24 hours, will best provide this patient adequate calories, AAs, and lipids?

A. AAs 10% 700 mL, dextrose 30% 325 mL, lipid 20% 500 mL.

B. AAs 10% 450 mL, dextrose 70% 400 mL, lipid 10% 500 mL.

C. AAs 10% 800 mL, dextrose 70% 350 mL, lipid 10% 500 mL.

D. AAs 15% 900 mL, dextrose 50% 500 mL, lipid 10% 500 mL.

7. A 59-year-old man has been admitted to the hospital after several days of vomiting and diarrhea. In the emergency department, he had several runs of nonsustained ventricular tachycardia. His plasma potassium on admission was 2.8 mEq/L. After 200 mEq of potassium chloride is infused over 24 hours, his repeat K^+ is 3.2 mEq/L, and he continues to have runs of ventricular tachycardia. Other laboratory values include Na^+ 143 mEq/L, magnesium 1.4 mg/dL, phosphorus 3 mg/dL, Ca^{2+} 9 mg/dL, and ionized Ca^{2+} 1.1 mmol/L. Which suggestion is best to address this patient's continued hypokalemia?

A. Administer potassium chloride 20 mEq intravenously over 1 hour each × 4 doses and recheck K^+.

B. Administer magnesium sulfate as a 2-g slow intravenous infusion over 2 hours.

C. Administer potassium phosphate 15 mmol intravenously over 4 hours.

D. Administer calcium gluconate 2 g intravenously over 5 minutes.

8. Which nutritional strategy can best prevent gut mucosal atrophy and subsequent bacterial translocation?

A. PN enriched with glutamine.

B. PN enriched with branched-chain AAs.

C. Enteral nutrition (EN).

D. Zinc supplementation.

9. A female patient (weight 80 kg) in the intensive care unit has developed acute kidney injury caused by sepsis and requires intermittent hemodialysis on a daily basis to maintain her BUN/Cr at 49/2.5 mg/dL. Currently, she is receiving appropriate antibiotics and is hemodynamically stable. She has also been receiving PN providing 72 g of AAs per day. From the information provided, which is the best recommendation for this patient's protein intake?

A. Reduce AAs to 40 g/day.

B. Reduce AAs to 64 g/day.

C. Increase AAs to 96 g/day.

D. Increase AAs to 160 g/day.

BPS Pharmacotherapy Specialty Examination Content Outline.
This chapter covers the following sections of the Pharmacotherapy Specialty Examination Content Outline

1. Domain 1: Patient-Centered Pharmacotherapy
   a. Task 1, Knowledge statements 1-8, 10-12, 17
   b. Task 3, Knowledge statements 1-3
   c. Task 4, Knowledge statements 1-6
   d. Task 5, Knowledge statement 4

I. FLUID MANAGEMENT

A. Distribution of Total Body Fluid (TBF)

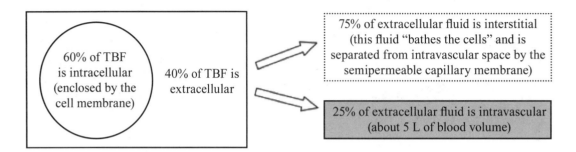

Figure 1. Distribution of total body fluid.
TBF = total body fluid.

1. Estimated as 60% of lean body weight (LBW) in men and 50% in women; a normal adult has about 42 L of fluid
2. Total body water is further divided into intracellular (IC) space and extracellular (EC) space.
   a. About 60% of TBF is IC, and 40% is EC; the IC and EC fluid compartments are separated by cell membranes, which are highly permeable to water.
   b. The EC compartment is also divided into the interstitial (IS) space and the intravascular space; the IS and intravascular fluid compartments are separated by the capillary membrane, which is permeable to almost all solutes except proteins.
      i. 75% of the EC fluid is in the IS space.
      ii. 25% of the EC fluid is in the intravascular space; the EC fluid in the intravascular space is known as plasma and consists of about 3 L; if you also consider about 2 L of fluid found in red blood cells (thus, IC fluid), the total blood volume is about 5 L.
3. The approximate distribution of TBF into the IC and EC compartments with further distribution of the EC fluid into the IS and intravascular compartments is important to remember for determining the distribution of intravenous fluid.

B. Distribution of Intravenous Fluid
   1. Crystalloids are intravenous fluids that can contain water, Na$^+$, chloride (Cl$^-$), and other electrolytes. Lactated Ringer solution is a crystalloid that contains mostly Na$^+$ and Cl$^-$ but also lactate, K$^+$, and Ca^{2+}. Normosol-R and Plasma-Lyte are crystalloids that contain mostly Na$^+$ and Cl$^-$ but also acetate, K$^+$, and Mg^{2+}.
      a. Na and Cl$^-$ do not freely cross into cells, but they will distribute evenly in the EC space.
      b. For 0.9% sodium chloride or lactated Ringer solution, only 25% remains in the intravascular space, and 75% distributes in the IS space; therefore, when 1 L of 0.9% sodium chloride or lactated Ringer solution is administered, about 250 mL of fluid remains in the intravascular compartment.
   2. "Free" water is equivalent to 5% dextrose (D$_5$W).
      a. D$_5$W is metabolized to water and carbon dioxide.
      b. Water can cross any membrane in the body; therefore, it is evenly distributed in TBF ("free" because it is free to cross any membrane).
         i. Many experts avoid administering D$_5$W whenever possible in patients with neurologic injury and elevated intracranial pressure (ICP) because it can cross into cerebral cells, causing a further elevation in ICP.

ii. Some practitioners avoid the use of D$_5$W because of the risk of hyperglycemia, even though D$_5$W contains only 5 g of dextrose/100 mL, which is equivalent to 17 kcal/100 mL.

c. For D$_5$W, 60% distributes to the IC space and 40% to the EC space. Of the 40% distributed to the EC space, 25% remains in the intravascular space, and 75% distributes to the IS space. Therefore, when 1 L of D$_5$W is administered intravenously, about 100 mL of fluid remains in the intravascular compartment.

3. Colloids include packed red blood cells, pooled human plasma (5% albumin, 25% albumin, and 5% plasma protein fraction), semisynthetic glucose polymers (dextran), and semisynthetic hydroxyethyl starch (hetastarch).

a. Colloids are too large to cross the capillary membrane; therefore, they remain primarily in the intravascular space (although a small portion "leaks" into the IS space).

b. Except for 25% albumin, administering 500 mL of colloid results in a 500-mL intravascular volume expansion.

c. Because 25% albumin has an oncotic pressure about 5 times that of normal plasma, it causes a fluid shift from the IS space into the intravascular space. For this reason, 100 mL of 25% albumin results in about 500 mL of intravascular volume expansion. This hyperoncotic solution should generally be avoided in patients requiring fluid resuscitation, because although the intravascular space expands, fluid shifts out of the IS space, potentially causing dehydration. It may be useful in patients who do not require fluid resuscitation but who could benefit from a redistribution of fluid (e.g., ascites, pleural effusions).

d. Hydroxyethyl starch and dextran products have been associated with coagulopathy and kidney impairment. In addition to acute kidney injury, hydroxyethyl starch is associated with increased mortality in critically ill patients (JAMA 2013;309:678-88; N Engl J Med 2012;367:124-34; U.S. Food and Drug Administration [FDA] boxed warning is available at www.fda.gov/biologicsblood-vaccines/safetyavailability/ucm358271.htm. Accessed October 22, 2015).

Table 1. Distribution of IV Fluid

IV Fluid	Infused Volume (mL)	Equivalent Intravascular Volume Expansion (mL)
NS	1000	250
LR	1000	250
Normosol-R	1000	250
D$_5$W	1000	100
Albumin 5%	500	500
Albumin 25%	100	500
Hydroxyethyl starch 6%	500	500

D$_5$W = 5% dextrose; IV = intravenous; LR = lactated Ringer solution; NS = normal saline.

C. Fluid Resuscitation

1. Intravascular fluid depletion can occur as a result of shock (hypovolemic or septic shock) and is associated with reduced cardiac function and organ hypoperfusion.

2. Signs or symptoms (Box 1) usually occur when about 15% (750 mL) of blood volume is lost (e.g., hemorrhage) or shifts out of the intravascular space (e.g., severe sepsis).

3. Fluid resuscitation is indicated for patients with signs or symptoms of intravascular volume depletion.

Box 1. Signs and Symptoms of Intravascular Volume Depletion

Tachycardia (HR > 100 beats/min)
Hypotension (SBP < 80 mm Hg)
Orthostatic changes in HR or BP
Increased BUN/SCr ratio > 20:1
Dry mucous membranes
Decreased skin turgor
Reduced urine output
Dizziness
Improvement in HR and BP after a 500- to 1000-mL fluid bolus

BP = blood pressure; BUN = blood urea nitrogen; Cr = creatinine; HR = heart rate; SBP = systolic blood pressure.

4. The goal of fluid resuscitation is to restore intravascular volume and prevent organ hypoperfusion.

5. Because intravascular volume depletion can cause organ dysfunction and death, prompt resuscitation is necessary.
   a. Intravenous fluids are infused rapidly, preferably through a central venous catheter.
   b. Intravenous fluids are administered as a 500- to 1000-mL bolus, after which the patient is reevaluated; this process is continued as long as signs and symptoms of intravascular volume depletion are improving.

6. Crystalloids (0.9% sodium chloride or lactated Ringer solution) are recommended for fluid resuscitation.
   a. Lactated Ringer solution is historically preferred in surgery and trauma patients, but no evidence suggests superiority over normal saline for fluid resuscitation.
   b. The lactate in lactated Ringer solution is metabolized to bicarbonate and can theoretically be useful for metabolic acidosis; however, lactate metabolism is impaired during shock. Thus, it may be an ineffective source of bicarbonate.
   c. Lactated Ringer solution has been considered a more physiologic amount of Cl (109 mmol/L) than 0.9% sodium chloride (154 mmol/L). Recently (JAMA 2012;308:1566), a Cl-restrictive regimen (e.g., lactated Ringer solution, Plasma-Lyte 148) was associated with a reduction in the incidence of acute kidney injury compared with a standard regimen (e.g., 0.9% sodium chloride, colloids containing Cl 120–130 mmol/L). Although thought provoking, this benefit cannot be attributed solely to differences in Cl content between different intravenous fluids, and causality was not shown in a randomized controlled trial.

7. There is no difference between crystalloids and colloids in the time to achieve fluid resuscitation or in patient outcomes. Colloids have not been shown to be superior to crystalloids and are associated with higher cost and some adverse effects. The following are examples of other, although controversial, uses of colloids:
   a. Colloids may be considered after fluid resuscitation with crystalloid (usually 4–6 L) has failed to achieve hemodynamic goals or after clinically significant edema limits the further administration of crystalloid.
   b. Albumin may be considered in patients with an albumin concentration less than 2.5 g/dL who have required a large volume of resuscitation fluids.
   c. Albumin (theoretically, 25% is preferred) may be considered in conjunction with diuretics for patients with clinically significant edema (e.g., pulmonary edema causing respiratory failure) and an albumin concentration less than 2.5 g/dL, when appropriately dosed diuretics are ineffective.

D. Maintenance Intravenous Fluids
1. Maintenance intravenous fluids are indicated in patients who are unable to tolerate oral fluids.
2. The goal of maintenance intravenous fluids is to prevent dehydration and maintain a normal fluid and electrolyte balance.
3. Maintenance intravenous fluids are typically administered as a continuous infusion through a peripheral or central intravenous catheter.
4. Common methods of estimating the daily volume in children and adults
   a. Administer 100 mL/kg for first 10 kg, followed by 50 mL/kg for the next 10–20 kg (i.e., 1500 mL for the first 20 kg) plus 20 mL/kg for every kilogram greater than 20 kg *or*
   b. Administer 20–40 mL/kg/day (for adults only).
   c. Adjust fluids according to the individual patient's input, output, and estimated insensible loss.
5. A typical maintenance intravenous fluid is D_5W with 0.45% sodium chloride plus 20–40 mEq of potassium chloride per liter. The potassium chloride content can be adjusted for the individual patient.

Patient Cases

Questions 1 and 2 pertain to the following case.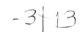

A 65-year-old man (weight 80 kg) with a 3-day history of temperature to 102°F, lethargy, and productive cough is hospitalized for community-acquired pneumonia. His medical history includes hypertension and coronary artery disease. His vital signs include heart rate 104 beats/minute, blood pressure 112/68 mm Hg, and temperature 101.4°F. His urine output is 10 mL/hour, blood urea nitrogen (BUN) 16 mg/dL, Cr 1.7 mg/dL, and white blood cell count (WBC) 10.4×10^3 cells/mm³. Other laboratory values are normal.

1. Which is most appropriate at this time?
   A. Furosemide 40 mg intravenously.
   B. Albumin 25% 100 mL intravenously over 60 minutes.
   C. Lactated Ringer solution 1000 mL intravenously over 60 minutes.
   D. D_5W/0.45% sodium chloride plus potassium chloride 20 mEq/L to infuse at 110 mL/hour.

2. After 2 days of appropriate antibiotic treatment, the patient has a WBC of 9×10^3 cells/mm³, and he is afebrile. His blood pressure is 135/85 mm Hg, and his urine output is now 45 mL/hour. His albumin is 3.2 g/dL, BUN is 14 mg/dL, and Cr is 1.4 mg/dL. All other laboratory values are normal. His appetite is still poor, and he is not taking adequate fluids. He has peripheral intravenous access. Which is most appropriate to initiate?
   A. Peripheral PN to infuse at 110 mL/hour.
   B. Albumin 5% 500 mL intravenously over 60 minutes.
   C. D_5W/0.45% sodium chloride plus potassium chloride 20 mEq/L to infuse at 110 mL/hour.
   D. Lactated Ringer solution to infuse at 110 mL/hour.

II. OSMOLALITY

A. Plasma osmolality is normally 275–290 mOsm/kg.
1. Terminology
   a. Osmolality is a measure of the osmoles of solute per kilogram of solvent (Osm/kg), whereas osmolarity is a measure of osmoles of solute per liter of solution (Osm/L).
   b. Plasma osmolarity (mOsm/L) can be calculated as osmolality × 0.995, showing that there is no clinically significant difference between them (i.e., plasma osmolarity is about 1% lower than plasma osmolality).
2. Plasma osmolality is maintained within a normal range by thirst and secretion of arginine vasopressin (i.e., antidiuretic hormone [ADH]) from the posterior pituitary.
3. Sodium salts are the primary determinant of plasma osmolality and therefore regulate fluid shifts between the IC and EC fluid compartments.
4. Plasma osmolality (in milliosmoles per kilogram) can be estimated: $(2 \times Na^+) + (glucose/18) + BUN/2.8$. Note: Glucose and BUN are in milligrams per deciliter.
5. Increases in plasma osmolality cause an osmotic shift of fluid into the plasma, resulting in cellular dehydration and shrinkage.
6. Decreases in plasma osmolality cause an osmotic shift of fluid into cells, resulting in cellular overhydration and swelling.

B. Intravenous fluids can be classified by their osmolarity relative to plasma.
1. Isotonic fluid does not result in a fluid shift between fluid compartments because the osmolarity is similar to plasma.
2. Hypertonic fluid can cause fluid to shift from the IC to the EC compartment, with subsequent cellular dehydration and shrinkage.
3. Hypotonic fluid with an osmolarity less than 150 mOsm/L can cause fluid to shift from the EC to the IC compartment, with subsequent cellular overhydration and swelling.
   a. Red blood cell swelling can cause cell rupture (i.e., hemolysis).
   b. Brain cells can swell, causing cerebral edema and herniation; this is most likely to occur with acute hyponatremia (occurring in less than 2 days).

C. Definitions
1. Equivalent weight = molecular weight (MW) divided by valence.
   a. A milliequivalent (mEq) = 1/1000 of an equivalent.
   b. Examples of equivalent weight (Table 2)

Table 2. Electrolyte MW, Valence, and Equivalent Weight

Electrolyte	MW	Valence	Equivalent Weight (g)
Sodium	23	1	23
Potassium	39	1	39
Chloride	35.5	1	35.5
Magnesium	24	2	12

MW = molecular weight.

(handwritten: $\frac{}{100\,mL} \times \frac{1}{58.5g} \times \frac{}{1\,equiv}$)

2. Osmoles = number of particles in solution (assuming complete dissociation).
   a. A milliosmole = 1/1000 of an osmole.
   b. Examples of osmoles (Table 3)

Table 3. Osmoles

Salt	Osmoles
NaCl	2
KCl	2
CaCl$_2$	3

CaCl$_2$ = calcium chloride; KCl = potassium chloride; NaCl = sodium chloride.

(handwritten: $\frac{23.4g}{100\,mL} \times \frac{58.5\,equiv}{58.5g} \quad \frac{1000}{1\,equ.}$)

3. Converting MW to milliequivalents

Box 2. Converting MW to Milliequivalents

Convert 23.4% NaCl (concentrated NaCl) to mEq/mL
MW of NaCl = 23 + 35.5 = 58.5 (add MW of Na + Cl)
$\dfrac{23.4\ g}{100\ mL} \times \dfrac{1\ equiv}{58.5\ g} \times \dfrac{1000\ mEq}{1\ equiv} = 4\ mEq/mL$

MW = molecular weight; NaCl = sodium chloride.

D. Calculating the Osmolarity of Intravenous Fluids in Milliosmoles per Liter
   1. The osmotic coefficient can be used to calculate the osmolarity of intravenous fluids because salt forms do not completely dissociate in solution.
      a. With sodium chloride, for example, there is some ionic attraction between Na$^+$ and Cl, so they do not completely dissociate; rather, they are about 93% dissociated in solution (thus, the osmotic coefficient is 0.93).
      b. In clinical practice, most do not consider the osmotic coefficient when calculating the osmolarity of sodium chloride or other electrolytes, and in reality, the osmotic coefficient is probably not clinically relevant (but is used in the following examples for completeness).
   2. Normal saline (0.9% sodium chloride)

Table 4. Calculation for Normal Saline

MW	Osmoles	Osmotic Coefficient
58.5 g/mol	2	0.93
$\dfrac{0.9\ g}{100\ mL} \times \dfrac{1\ mol}{58.5\ g} \times \dfrac{2\ Osm}{1\ mol} \times \dfrac{1000\ mOsm}{1\ Osm} \times \dfrac{1000\ mL}{1\ L} \times 0.93 = 287\ mOsm/L$		

3. D$_5$W (MW 180 g/mol)

(handwritten: $\frac{5g}{100mL} \times \frac{1\,mol}{180g} \times \frac{1\,Osm}{1\,mol} \quad \frac{1000\,mOsm}{1\,mol}$)

Box 3. Calculation for D$_5$W

$\dfrac{5\ g \times}{100\ mL} \times \dfrac{1\ mol}{180\ g} \times \dfrac{1000\ mOsm}{1\ mol} \times \dfrac{1000\ mL}{1\ L} = 278\ mOsm/L$

4. Osmolarity of D$_5$W/normal saline = 287 mOsm/L + 278 mOsm/L = 565 mOsm/L.
5. Osmolarity of normal saline + potassium chloride 20 mEq/L (Box 4)

Box 4. Calculation for NS plus KCl

Step 1: Convert mEq to weight (g)

$$20 \text{ mEq} \times \frac{1 \text{ equiv}}{1000 \text{ mEq}} \times \frac{74.5 \text{ g}}{1 \text{ equiv}} = 1.49 \text{ g of KCl}$$

Step 2: Calculate mOsm/L

$$\frac{1.49 \text{ g}}{L} \times \frac{1 \text{ mol}}{74.5 \text{ g}} \times \frac{2 \text{ Osm}}{1 \text{ mol}} \times \frac{1000 \text{ mOsm}}{1 \text{ Osm}} = 40 \text{ mOsm/L}$$

Step 3: Add osmolarity of NS + KCl = 287 mOsm/L + 40 mOsm/L = 327 mOsm/L

NS = normal saline; KCl = potassium chloride.

III. HYPERTONIC SALINE

A. Concentration: Typically prepared as 3% (954 mOsm/L), 7.5% (2393 mOsm/L), or 23.4% (7462 mOsm/L)

B. Common Uses of Hypertonic Saline
   1. Hypertonic saline is used in traumatic brain injury to reduce an elevated ICP and thereby increase cerebral perfusion pressure.
      a. Typically used if ICP is greater than 20 mm Hg as measured by an ICP monitor
      b. If the serum sodium concentration is close to the upper limit of normal (i.e., 145 mEq/L), it may be preferable to use a lower concentration of hypertonic saline (i.e., 3%).
   2. Hypertonic saline is used for symptomatic hyponatremia (symptoms described in Hyponatremia section below).
      a. Symptoms generally do not occur unless serum sodium is 120 mEq/L or less and increase in severity as Na^+ decreases.
      b. Symptoms of severe hyponatremia include coma and seizures.
      c. In an effort to prevent severe symptoms from occurring, some practitioners treat asymptomatic or moderately symptomatic (e.g., lethargy, confusion) hyponatremia before serum sodium concentrations reach 120 mEq/L or less because of the increased risk of severe symptoms below this concentration.

C. Inappropriate Use of Hypertonic Saline
   1. Chronic asymptomatic hyponatremia
      a. Asymptomatic syndrome of inappropriate secretion of antidiuretic hormone (SIADH) is usually treated with fluid restriction of less than 800 mL of fluid per day.
      b. Hyponatremia is generally a water problem (i.e., an excess of free water) rather than a deficiency of Na; thus, hypertonic saline makes little sense in the absence of symptoms (see Hyponatremia section below).
   2. Hyponatremia associated with severe hyperglycemia (pseudohyponatremia) (i.e., diabetic ketoacidosis)
      a. Typically, serum sodium decreases in a nonlinear fashion in response to hyperglycemia (i.e., Na^+ decreases by about 1.6 mEq/L for every 100-mg/dL elevation in glucose of 100–400 mg/dL, but Na^+ decreases by about 2.4 mEq/L for every 100-mg/dL elevation in glucose above 400 mg/dL).
      b. As hyperglycemia is corrected with insulin, the serum sodium will normalize.
   3. Hyponatremia associated with hypervolemia (i.e., heart failure leads to tissue hypoperfusion, which triggers ADH secretion, causing reabsorption of water from the kidneys and leading to hyponatremia)
      a. In general, this situation is treated with fluid restriction or diuresis.
      b. Symptomatic hyponatremia is uncommon in patients with heart failure.

    c.   Hypertonic saline could be considered in symptomatic patients; however, they may need diuresis to prevent worsening volume overload.

D.   Preparation of Hypertonic Saline

Steps	Example
Choose base solutions	For this example, use concentrated NaCl available as 23.4% vials and sterile water to make 1000 mL of 7.5% HS
Set up alligation	23.4% ⟶ ⟶ ⟶7.5%⟵ 0 ⟶ ⟶

Add and subtract	23.4% ⟶ ⟶ 7.5 parts (from 23.4% NaCl)
	    ⟶7.5%⟵
	0 ⟶ ⟶ 15.9 parts (from sterile water)
	                 23.4 parts total

Divide	7.5 parts/23.4 parts = x/1000 mL; x = 320.5 mL of 23.4% NaCl 15.9 parts/23.4 parts = x/1000 mL; x = 679.5 mL of sterile water

Figure 2. Calculations to prepare hypertonic saline.
HS = hypertonic saline; NaCl = sodium chloride.

E.   Hypertonic Saline Dose
    1.   Dose options for traumatic brain injury
        a.   3% hypertonic saline 250 mL or 2–4 mL/kg intravenously over 1–15 minutes administered for elevated ICP
        b.   23.4% hypertonic saline 30 mL over 20–30 minutes administered for elevated ICP
            i.   Standing orders such as 30 mL every 4–6 hours are *not* recommended.
            ii.   If hypertonic saline is needed for prolonged reduction in ICP, a 3% hypertonic saline concentration is generally recommended.
    2.   Dose options for patients with symptomatic hyponatremia
        a.   Treatment of patients with symptomatic hyponatremia involves a small but quick increase in serum sodium by 0.75–1 mEq/L/hour to a concentration of 120 mEq/L. Then, the infusion can be reduced so that Na^+ increases by 0.5 mEq/L/hour. For severe symptoms, it is reasonable to increase serum sodium by up to 2 mEq/L/hour for a short time, as long as the maximum change of 10–12 mEq in 24 hours is not exceeded. If hypertonic saline is used for mild symptoms, a slower change in serum sodium of 0.5 mEq/L/hour would be appropriate, although some would avoid hypertonic saline altogether.
        b.   Estimate an infusion rate of 3% hypertonic saline by multiplying ideal body weight (IBW) by desired rate of serum sodium increase per hour. (Note: IBW is used to avoid overdosing patients with obesity.)
            i.   For example, 70 kg × 1 mEq/L/hour = 70 mL/hour to increase serum sodium by 1 mEq/L in 1 hour. The infusion can be adjusted to achieve goal changes in serum sodium.
            ii.   Infusion rate of 3% hypertonic saline is generally 1–2 mL/kg/hour.
           iii.   In general, 3% hypertonic saline is not recommended in asymptomatic patients; if used in an asymptomatic patient, the administration rate should generally not exceed 0.5–1 mL/kg/hour.
        c.   Alternatively, some practitioners recommend a 250-mL bolus of 2%–3% hypertonic saline over 30 minutes or 50 mL of 3% hypertonic saline administered as a bolus every 30 minutes for two doses.

F. Administration of Hypertonic Saline
    1. Use central intravenous access because the osmolarity is greater than 900 mOsm/L.
    2. If no central line is available, use 2% hypertonic saline.
    3. Some practitioners use 3% hypertonic saline through a peripheral intravenous access site in an emergency because the osmolarity is close to the cutoff range for peripheral administration. If a peripheral site is used, use a large vein, monitor for phlebitis, and obtain central access as soon as possible.

G. Clinical Goals and Monitoring for Administering Hypertonic Saline in Patients with Symptomatic Hyponatremia
    1. Goals
        a. Stop symptoms (described below).
        b. Safe serum sodium achieved usually in the range of 120–125 mmol/L to avoid adverse neurologic outcomes. Note that the immediate goal for patients with symptomatic hyponatremia is not necessarily a normal serum sodium.
        c. Reached maximum safe amount of change in serum sodium
            i.   Maximum safe amount of change is generally regarded as 10–12 mmol/L (or 10–12 mEq/L) in 24 hours.
            ii. Some practitioners suggest a maximum change of 8 mmol/L in 24 hours.
    2. Monitor serum sodium every 1–4 hours depending on severity of symptoms.

H. Complications of Hypertonic Saline
    1. Osmotic demyelination syndrome (includes central pontine and extrapontine myelinolysis) can occur with rapid correction of hyponatremia.
        a. Characterized initially by lethargy and affective changes, followed by permanent neurologic damage, including paraparesis, quadriparesis, dysarthria, dysphagia, and coma
        b. More likely to occur with rapid correction of chronic hyponatremia than with acute hyponatremia. This partly explains why it is advisable not to administer hypertonic saline in patients with chronic asymptomatic hyponatremia.
        c. Prevent by avoiding changes in serum sodium of more than 10–12 mmol/L in 24 hours or more than 18 mmol/L in 48 hours.
    2. Hypokalemia can occur with large volumes of hypertonic saline.
    3. Hyperchloremic acidosis can result from the administration of chloride salts (i.e., sodium chloride). Can prevent by administering hypertonic saline in a 1:1 or 2:1 ratio of sodium chloride and sodium acetate or using fluid with less chloride content
    4. Hypernatremia
    5. Phlebitis if administered in a peripheral vein
    6. Heart failure
        a. Fluid overload can result from initial volume expansion.
        b. Over time, hypertonic saline can have a diuretic effect, leading to intravascular volume depletion.
    7. Coagulopathy caused by platelet dysfunction
    8. Hypotension if hypertonic saline is administered rapidly

I. Other Considerations When Using Hypertonic Saline
    1. Because hypokalemia can cause hyponatremia, remember to correct K^+ depletion if present. As K^+ is replaced, serum sodium will increase.
    2. If 150 mEq of sodium bicarbonate is added to 850 mL of 0.9% sodium chloride, the resultant solution is equivalent to about 1.6% sodium chloride. When an infusion of 150 mEq of sodium bicarbonate per liter is indicated, it is recommended to add sodium bicarbonate to D_5W or sterile water for injection instead of 0.9% sodium chloride.

IV. HYPOTONIC INTRAVENOUS FLUIDS

A. Hypotonic fluids administered intravenously can cause cell hemolysis and patient death.
   1. Albumin 25% diluted with sterile water to make albumin 5% has an osmolarity of about 60 mOsm/L and can cause hemolysis.
   2. "Quarter normal saline," or 0.225% sodium chloride, has an osmolarity of 77 mOsm/L and can cause hemolysis.

B. Avoid using intravenous fluid with an osmolarity less than 150 mOsm/L.
   1. Sterile water alone should *never* be administered intravenously.
   2. Some prescribers use hypotonic saline for a patient with hypernatremia.
      a. In reality, a patient with hypernatremia generally needs water, not Na^+.
      b. Therefore, for patients with hypernatremia, enteral administration of water is preferable.
      c. If the enteral route is unavailable, recommend D_5W administered intravenously.

C. Prevent a potentially fatal error by recommending one of the following alternatives to 0.225% sodium chloride:
   1. Recommend changing 0.225% sodium chloride to D_5W alone or a combination of D_5W and 0.225% sodium chloride.
   2. Alternatively, if there are concerns related to hyperglycemia with using D_5W (50 g of dextrose or 170 kcal/L), recommend using 2.5% dextrose and 0.225% sodium chloride.
   3. Alternatively, potassium chloride can be added to increase osmolarity.
   4. Recommend administering water enterally (by mouth or feeding tube).
   5. If 0.225% sodium chloride is used, recommend use by central venous line given risk of hemolysis.

V. HYPONATREMIA AND HYPO-OSMOLAL STATES

A. Sodium salts are the primary determinants of plasma osmolality (and subsequent fluid shifts between the IC and EC compartments).
   1. A reduction in serum sodium of less than 136 mEq/L usually correlates with a reduction in plasma osmolality.
   2. Hyponatremia with subsequent hypo-osmolality causes fluid to shift into cells (cellular overhydration). Hypotonic hyponatremia can be divided into three types according to volume status (Table 5).

Table 5. Classification of Hyponatremia

	Hypervolemic Hyponatremia	Euvolemic Hyponatremia	Hypovolemic Hyponatremia
Description	Caused by excess Na^+ and fluid, but fluid excess predominates	Normal total body Na^+ with excess fluid volume (i.e., dilutional)	Deficit of both Na^+ and fluid, but total Na^+ is decreased more than total body water
Example	Heart failure, cirrhosis, nephrotic syndrome	SIADH, medications	Fluid loss (e.g., emesis, diarrhea, fever), third spacing, renal loss (diuretics)
Diagnosis	Urine $Na^+ < 25$ mEq/L indicates edematous disorders (i.e., heart failure, cirrhosis, nephrotic syndrome); urine $Na^+ > 25$ mEq/L indicates acute or chronic renal failure	Urine osmolality > 100 mOsm/kg (indicates impaired water excretion in presence of plasma osmolality < 275 mOsm/kg); urine Na > 40 mEq/L	Urine $Na^+ < 25$ mEq/L indicates nonrenal loss of Na^+ (e.g., emesis, diarrhea); urine $Na^+ > 40$ mEq/L indicates renal loss of Na^+
Treatment	Sodium and water restriction; treat underlying cause; vasopressin receptor antagonists (e.g., conivaptan, tolvaptan), diuretics	If drug-induced SIADH, remove offending agent; fluid restriction; demeclocycline; vasopressin receptor antagonists (e.g., conivaptan, tolvaptan)	Fluid resuscitation (see above)

NA^+ = sodium; SIADH = syndrome of inappropriate secretion of antidiuretic hormone.

3. In select cases, hyponatremia is associated with either a normal or an elevated plasma osmolality.
   a. This is known as pseudohyponatremia because Na^+ content in the body is not actually reduced. Instead, Na^+ shifts from the EC compartment into the cells in an attempt to maintain plasma osmolality in a normal range. Another adaptation to increased plasma osmolality is the shift of water from inside cells to the EC compartment, which further dilutes the Na^+ concentration.
      i. Severe hyperlipidemia can be associated with a normal or elevated plasma osmolality.
      ii. Severe hyperglycemia (i.e., during diabetic ketoacidosis) is associated with an elevated plasma osmolality.
   b. Once the underlying condition is corrected, Na^+ will shift out of the cells, and hyponatremia will resolve.

B. Causes of Hyponatremia
   1. Replacement of lost solute with water
      a. Loss of solute (e.g., vomiting, diarrhea) usually involves the loss of isotonic fluid; therefore, alone, it will not cause hyponatremia.
      b. After the loss of isotonic fluid, hyponatremia can develop when the lost fluid is replaced with water.
      c. A common cause of hyponatremia in hospitals is the postoperative administration of hypotonic fluid.
   2. Volume depletion and organ hypoperfusion stimulate ADH secretion to increase water reabsorption in the collecting tubules, potentially causing hyponatremia.
   3. SIADH and cortisol deficiency are both related to the excessive release of ADH.
   4. Medications, including thiazide diuretics, antiepileptic drugs (e.g., carbamazepine, oxcarbazepine), and antidepressants (especially selective serotonin reuptake inhibitors but also tricyclic antidepressants), can cause hyponatremia. Drug-induced hyponatremia is more likely to occur in older adults and in those who drink large volumes of water.
   5. Renal failure impairs the ability to excrete dilute urine, predisposing to hyponatremia.

C. Symptoms of Hyponatremia (Table 6)

Table 6. Symptoms of Hyponatremia

Serum Sodium (mEq/L)	Clinical Manifestations
120–125	Nausea, malaise
115–120	Headache, lethargy, obtundation, unsteadiness, confusion
< 115	Delirium, seizure, coma, respiratory arrest, death

1. Symptoms are generally attributable to hypo-osmolality, with subsequent water movement into brain cells causing cerebral overhydration.
2. If hyponatremia occurs chronically, cerebral cell swelling is prevented by osmotic adaptation.
    a. Solutes move out of brain cells to prevent the osmotic shift of water into brain cells.
    b. For this reason, patients with chronic hyponatremia may show less severe or no symptoms.
3. Neurologic symptoms are related to the rate of change in the serum sodium and to the degree of change in serum sodium.
4. Acute hyponatremia occurs over 1–3 days.

D. Treatment of Hyponatremia
1. Treat underlying cause.
2. Raise serum sodium at a safe rate, defined as a change no greater than 10–12 mEq/L in 24 hours.
3. Treatment depends on volume status, the presence and severity of symptoms, and the onset of hyponatremia (the latter two have been discussed previously).
    a. If the patient is euvolemic or edematous, there are two treatment options:
        i.   Fluid restriction (to less than 800 mL/day) is the typical first-line recommendation for asymptomatic patients. Note that Na administration is not recommended for asymptomatic patients and can worsen edema.
        ii. Vasopressin antagonists (e.g., intravenous conivaptan, oral tolvaptan) can be used in euvolemic (i.e., SIADH) or hypervolemic (i.e., heart failure) patients to promote aquaresis, increase serum sodium, alleviate symptoms, and reduce weight; however, this approach is costly and has not been shown to improve clinical outcomes (i.e., fall prevention, hospitalization, hospital length of stay, quality of life, mortality) in prospective randomized controlled trials. Vasopressin antagonists are substrates and inhibitors of cytochrome P450 3A4 isoenzymes; monitor for drug interactions with other 3A4 inhibitors that could increase effect and lead to a rapid increase in serum sodium. Fluid restriction in combination with a vasopressin antagonist during the first 24 hours can also increase the risk of overly rapid correction of serum sodium. If needed, fluid restriction can be used after 24 hours. Tolvaptan should not be administered for more than 30 days to minimize risk of liver injury. Monitor for recurrence of hyponatremia once treatment is discontinued.
    b. If patient has intravascular volume depletion, volume must be replaced first with intravenous crystalloids (e.g., 0.9% sodium chloride).
        i.   Until intravascular volume is restored, patient will continue to secrete ADH, causing water reabsorption and subsequent hyponatremia.
        ii. Once intravascular volume is restored, ADH secretion will decrease, causing water to be excreted. This can lead to a rapid correction of serum sodium; careful monitoring is necessary to prevent overly rapid correction.
        iii. Volume status can be assessed by skin turgor, jugular venous pressure, and urine sodium.

    c.   Once intravascular volume is restored, patients who experienced volume depletion, diuretic-induced hyponatremia, or adrenal insufficiency may still need Na^+.

        i.   The amount of Na^+ (in milliequivalents) needed to raise the serum sodium to a safe concentration of about 120 mEq/L is estimated using LBW as follows: $0.5(LBW) \times (120 - Na^+)$ for women (multiply LBW by 0.6 for men). LBW has been estimated using weight in kilograms and height in centimeters for men as $LBW = [(0.3)(kg) + (0.3)(cm) - 29]$ or for women as $LWB = [(0.3)(kg) + (0.4)(cm) - 43]$; formula published in 1966 (J Clin Pathol 1966;19:389).

        ii.   Alternatively, this equation can be modified to estimate the Na^+ deficit in the following manner: $0.5(LBW) \times (140 - Na^+)$ for women (multiply LBW by 0.6 for men). If calculating the Na^+ deficit, it is recommended to administer 25%–50% of the deficit during the first 24 hours to prevent the overly rapid correction of serum sodium.

        iii.   Regardless of the method used to estimate Na^+ replacement, the amount of Na^+ administered should be guided by serial serum sodium concentrations.

    d.   Patients with symptomatic hyponatremia should be treated with hypertonic saline (see Hypertonic Saline section).

    4.   Correct hypokalemia, if present, with hyponatremia.

        a.   Hypokalemia will cause a reduction in serum sodium because Na^+ enters cells to account for the reduction in IC K^+ to maintain cellular electroneutrality.

        b.   Administration of K^+ will correct hyponatremia.

        c.   Use caution when giving K^+ to prevent overly rapid correction of serum sodium.

Patient Cases

Questions 3–5 pertain to the following case.

A 72-year-old woman (weight 60 kg) with a history of hypertension has developed hyponatremia after starting hydrochlorothiazide 3 weeks earlier. She experiences dizziness, fatigue, and nausea. Her serum sodium is 116 mEq/L. Her blood pressure is 86/50 mm Hg and heart rate is 122 beats/minute.

3.   In addition to discontinuing hydrochlorothiazide, which initial treatment regimen is most recommended?

    A.   0.9% sodium chloride infused at 100 mL/hour.

    B.   0.9% sodium chloride 500-mL bolus.

    C.   3% sodium chloride infused at 60 mL/hour.

    D.   23.4% sodium chloride 30-mL bolus as needed.

4.   Which is the best treatment goal for the first 24 hours in correcting the patient's serum sodium from her initial value of 116 mEq/L?

    A.   Increase Na^+ concentration to 140 mEq/L.

    B.   Increase Na^+ concentration to 132 mEq/L.

    C.   Increase Na^+ concentration to 126 mEq/L.

    D.   Maintain serum sodium of 116–120 mEq/L.

5.   One day later, the patient has improved somewhat. Her blood pressure and heart rate are now 122/80 mm Hg and 80 beats/minute. Her serum sodium is 120 mEq/L, and K^+ is 3.2 mEq/L; she still feels tired. She is eating a regular diet. Her ECG is normal. Which is the best recommendation?

    A. D_5W/0.9% sodium chloride plus potassium chloride 40 mEq/L to infuse at 100 mL/hour.

    B.   0.9% sodium chloride infused at 100 mL/hour.

    C.   3% sodium chloride infused at 60 mL/hour.

    D.   Potassium chloride 20 mEq by mouth every 6 hours × 4 doses.

VI. HYPERNATREMIA AND HYPEROSMOLAL STATES

A. Serum sodium greater than 145 mEq/L generally causes hyperosmolality.
   1. The osmotic gradient associated with hypernatremia causes water movement out of cells and into the EC space.
   2. Symptoms are related primarily to the dehydration of brain cells.

B. Causes of Hypernatremia
   1. Loss of water because of fever, burns, infection, renal loss (e.g., diabetes insipidus), gastrointestinal (GI) loss
   2. Retention of Na^+ because of the administration of hypertonic saline or any form of Na^+

C. Prevention of Hypernatremia through Osmoregulation
   1. Plasma osmolality is maintained at 275–290 mOsm/kg, despite changes in water and Na^+ intake.
   2. Hypernatremia is prevented first by the release of ADH, causing water reabsorption.
   3. Hypernatremia is also prevented by thirst.
      a. Hypernatremia occurs primarily in adults with altered mental status who have an impaired thirst response or do not have access to or the ability to ask for water.
      b. Hypernatremia can also occur in infants.

D. Cerebral Osmotic Adaptation
   1. Similar to patients with hyponatremia, patients with chronic hypernatremia can have cerebral osmotic adaptation.
      a. Brain cells take up solutes, Na^+, and K^+, thus limiting the osmotic gradient between the IC and EC fluid compartments.
      b. This prevents cellular dehydration, and it will increase the brain volume toward a normal value, despite hypernatremia.
   2. Because of osmotic adaptation, patients with chronic hypernatremia may be asymptomatic.

E. Symptoms of hypernatremia are primarily neurologic.
   1. Similar to hyponatremia, the symptoms of hypernatremia are related to the rate of increase in plasma osmolality and the degree of increase in plasma osmolality.
   2. Earlier symptoms include lethargy, weakness, and irritability.
   3. Symptoms can progress to twitching, seizures, coma, and death if serum sodium is greater than 158 mEq/L.
   4. Cerebral dehydration can cause cerebral vein rupture with subsequent intracerebral or subarachnoid hemorrhage.

F. Treatment of Hypernatremia
   1. Rapid correction of chronic hypernatremia can result in cerebral edema, seizure, permanent neurologic damage, and death.
      a. With osmotic adaptation, the brain volume is raised toward normal despite an elevated serum osmolarity.
      b. Osmotic adaptation combined with a rapid reduction in plasma osmolality can cause an osmotic gradient, causing water to move into brain cells with subsequent cerebral edema.
   2. In patients with symptomatic hypernatremia, serum sodium should be reduced slowly by no more than 0.5 mEq/L/hour or 12 mEq/L/day.

3. Treat hypernatremia by replacing water deficit slowly over several days to prevent overly rapid correction of serum sodium.
    a. Using LBW, the estimated water deficit (in liters) is $(0.4 \times LBW) \times [(serum\ sodium/140) - 1]$ in women (multiply LBW by 0.5 in men).
    b. Note that in women and men, total body water is typically about 50% and 60%, respectively, of LBW. Thus, some sources recommend a variation on the earlier equation as follows: water deficit = $(0.5 \times LBW) \times [(serum\ sodium/140) - 1]$ in women (multiply LBW by 0.6 in men). However, hypernatremic patients are generally water depleted; thus, the equation using the lower values above (i.e., 40% or 0.4 and 50% or 0.5) is reasonable.
4. Administer free water orally or intravenously as D_5W.
5. If concurrent Na^+ and water depletion occur (e.g., vomiting, diarrhea, diuretic-induced depletion), use a combination of D_5W and 0.225% sodium chloride.
6. If patient is hypotensive because of volume depletion, first restore intravascular volume with 0.9% sodium chloride to restore tissue perfusion. Normal saline is the preferred crystalloid for fluid resuscitation, and in the hypernatremic patient, it is still relatively hypotonic.
7. Patients with severe central diabetes insipidus may require desmopressin (a synthetic analog of ADH) to replace insufficient or absent endogenous ADH.

Patient Case

6. A 74-year-old woman (weight 50 kg) has been receiving Jevity tube feedings at 60 mL/hour for the past 8 days through her gastrostomy feeding tube. She recently had an ischemic stroke; she is responsive but does not communicate. Her serum sodium was 142 mg/dL on the day the Jevity was initiated, and it has risen steadily to 149, 156, and 159 mg/dL on days 3, 4, and 8, respectively, after the start of the tube feedings. Which is the best treatment for her hypernatremia?

    A. Administer sterile water intravenously at 80 mL/hour.

    B. Administer D_5W intravenously at 80 mL/hour.

    C. Administer D_5W/0.2% sodium chloride intravenously at 80 mL/hour.

    D. Administer water by enteral feeding tube 200 mL every 6 hours.

VII. DISORDERS OF K⁺

A. Normal plasma potassium concentrations are 3.5–5 mEq/L.

B. K^+ is the primary IC cation (maintains electroneutrality with Na, the primary EC cation).

C. K^+ balance is maintained between the IC and EC compartments by several factors, including the following:
    1. β_2-Adrenergic stimulation (caused by epinephrine) promotes cellular uptake of K^+.
    2. Insulin promotes cellular uptake of K^+.
    3. Plasma potassium concentration directly correlates with movement of K^+ in and out of cells because of passive shifts based on the concentration gradient across the cell membrane. (A normal response to diarrhea-induced hypokalemia is for K^+ to shift out of the cells passively, minimizing the reduction in plasma potassium concentration.)

D. Normal plasma concentrations of K^+ are maintained by renal excretion.

E. Hypokalemia (K⁺ concentration less than 3.5 mEq/L)
    1. Causes of hypokalemia
        a. Reduced intake seldom causes hypokalemia because renal excretion is minimized because of increased renal tubular absorption.
        b. Increased shift of K⁺ into cells can occur with the following:
            i.   Alkalosis
            ii. Insulin or a carbohydrate load
            iii. β_2-receptor stimulation caused by stress-induced epinephrine release or administration of a β-agonist (e.g., albuterol, dobutamine)
            iv. Hypothermia
        c. Increased GI losses of K⁺ can occur with vomiting, diarrhea, intestinal fistula or enteral tube drainage, and chronic laxative abuse.
        d. Increased urinary losses can occur with mineralocorticoid excess (e.g., aldosterone) and diuretic use (e.g., loop and thiazides).
        e. Hypomagnesemia is commonly associated with hypokalemia caused by increased renal loss of K⁺; correction of plasma potassium requires simultaneous correction of serum magnesium.
    2. Symptoms of hypokalemia generally occur when plasma potassium is below 3 mEq/L and can include the following:
        a. Muscle weakness occurs most commonly in the lower extremities but can progress to the trunk, upper extremities, and respiratory muscles. Muscle weakness in the GI tract can manifest as paralytic ileus, abdominal distention, nausea, vomiting, and constipation.
        b. ECG changes (flattened T waves or elevated U wave)
        c. Cardiac arrhythmias (bradycardia, heart block, ventricular tachycardia, ventricular fibrillation)
        d. Digoxin toxicity can occur despite normal serum digoxin concentrations in the presence of hypokalemia.
        e. Rhabdomyolysis can occur because hypokalemia can cause reduced blood flow to skeletal muscle.
    3. Treatment of hypokalemia
        a. K⁺ deficit can be estimated as 200–400 mEq of K⁺ for every 1-mEq/L reduction in plasma potassium (assuming a normal distribution of K⁺ between EC and IC compartments).
        b. Although the K⁺ deficit can be estimated, K⁺ replacement is guided by K⁺ concentrations; recheck every 2–4 hours if K⁺ is less than 3 mEq/L.
        c. Potassium chloride is the preferred salt in patients with concurrent metabolic alkalosis because these patients typically lose Cl⁻ through diuretics or GI loss. This is the most common presentation of hypokalemia.
        d. Potassium acetate can be administered intravenously, or potassium bicarbonate can be administered orally for patients with a metabolic acidosis that requires frequent K⁺ supplementation.
        e. Guidelines for administering K⁺
            i.   Patients without ECG changes or symptoms of hypokalemia can be treated with oral supplementation.
            ii. Avoid mixing K⁺ in dextrose, which can cause insulin release with a subsequent IC shift of K⁺.
            iii. To avoid irritation, no more than about 60–80 mEq/L should be administered through a peripheral vein.
            iv. Recommended infusion rate is 10–20 mEq/hour to a maximum of 40 mEq/hour.
            v.   Patients who receive K⁺ at rates faster than 10–20 mEq/hour should be monitored using a continuous ECG.

Table 7. K⁺ Replacement

Plasma K⁺ (mEq/L)	Treatment[a]	Comments
3–3.5	Oral KCl 60–80 mEq/day if no signs or symptoms (doses > 60 mEq should be divided to avoid GI adverse effects)	Recheck K⁺ daily
2.5–3	Oral KCl 120 mEq/day (in divided doses) or IV 60–80 mEq administered at 10–20 mEq/hr if signs or symptoms	Monitor K⁺ closely (i.e., 2 hr after infusion)
2–2.5	IV KCl 10–20 mEq/hr	Consider continuous ECG monitoring
< 2	IV KCl 20–40 mEq/hr	Requires continuous ECG monitoring

[a]Treatment doses are for patients with normal kidney function and should be reduced for patients with kidney dysfunction or older adults.
ECG = electrocardiogram; GI = gastrointestinal; KCl = potassium chloride; K⁺ = potassium.

F. Hyperkalemia
  1. Causes of hyperkalemia
     a. Increased intake
     b. Shift of K⁺ from the IC to the EC compartment causes hyperkalemia and can occur with the following:
        i. Acidosis
        ii. Insulin deficiency
        iii. β-Adrenergic blockade
        iv. Digoxin overdose
        v. Rewarming after hypothermia (e.g., after cardiac surgery)
        vi. Succinylcholine
     c. Reduced urinary excretion can occur with:
        i. Kidney dysfunction
        ii. Intravascular volume depletion
        iii. Hypoaldosteronism
        iv. K⁺-sparing diuretics
        v. Angiotensin-converting enzyme inhibitors and angiotensin receptor blockers
  2. Symptoms of hyperkalemia
     a. Muscle weakness or paralysis is caused by changes in neuromuscular conduction; typically occurs when plasma potassium exceeds 8 mEq/L.
     b. Abnormal cardiac conduction can first manifest as peaked, narrowed T waves (typically, when plasma potassium exceeds 6 mEq/L) and widening of the QRS, and it can progress to ventricular fibrillation and asystole.
     c. Not all patients will experience ECG changes, and the initial manifestation of hyperkalemia can be ventricular fibrillation; thus, consider emergency treatment even in patients with no ECG changes if plasma potassium exceeds 6.5 mEq/L.
     d. Conduction disturbances are increased by hypocalcemia, hyponatremia, acidosis, and rapid elevation in the plasma potassium concentration.
  3. Pseudohyperkalemia should be suspected if there is no apparent cause or symptoms of hyperkalemia.
     a. Can occur if K⁺ is released from cells while or after obtaining the blood specimen, usually because of trauma during venipuncture
     b. Can result from measurement of the serum rather than the plasma potassium concentration; caused by K⁺ release during coagulation

4. Treatment of hyperkalemia
   a. Patients with an asymptomatic elevation in the plasma potassium who do not have signs or symptoms can be treated with a cation exchange resin (e.g., sodium polystyrene sulfonate) alone.
   b. Urgent and immediate treatment is required for patients with the following signs or symptoms:
      i. Plasma potassium above 6.5 mEq/L
      ii. Severe muscle weakness
      iii. ECG changes
   c. Calcium should be administered intravenously to patients with symptomatic hyperkalemia to prevent hyperkalemia-induced arrhythmias, even if patients are normocalcemic.
      i. Calcium gluconate can be administered peripherally and is preferred to calcium chloride (CaCl) because of a reduced risk of tissue necrosis; dose is 10 mL (equivalent to 1 g, 90 mg elemental, or 4.65 mEq) of 10% calcium gluconate administered over 2–10 minutes; may repeat in 5 minutes if no improvement in ECG. Calcium chloride can be used if central intravenous access is available; however, the dose should be adjusted because 10 mL (1 g, 270 mg elemental, or 13.6 mEq) provides 3 times the amount of elemental Ca as calcium gluconate.
      ii. Onset is within minutes, but duration is short (30–60 minutes).
      iii. Does not reduce plasma potassium but antagonizes the effect of K^+ in cardiac conduction cells
      iv. Use in urgent circumstances while waiting for other measures (e.g., insulin and glucose) to lower plasma potassium.
      v. Avoid use in patients receiving digoxin because hypercalcemia can precipitate digoxin toxicity, and there are reports of sudden death.
   d. The following treatment options are transient, causing a temporary shift of K^+ from the EC fluid into the cells, and should be used for symptomatic hyperkalemia.
      i. Insulin and glucose
         (a) Dose is regular insulin 10 units intravenously plus 25–50 g of glucose administered as a 50% dextrose intravenous push to prevent hypoglycemia.
         (b) Typically lowers plasma potassium by 0.5–1.5 mEq/L within 1 hour and may last for several hours
         (c) If patients have hyperglycemia, insulin alone can be administered.
         (d) More predictable in patients with kidney failure than sodium bicarbonate or β_2-adrenergic agonists
         (e) Caution with increased risk of insulin errors when used in emergencies (e.g., incorrectly preparing insulin infusions). Errors involving calculations (100 units/mL) and use of 4- or 10-mL syringes instead of an insulin syringe are possible.
      ii. Sodium bicarbonate
         (a) Dose is 50 mEq of intravenous sodium bicarbonate infused slowly over 5 minutes; may repeat in 30 minutes if needed
         (b) May lower plasma potassium within 30–60 minutes and persist for several hours
         (c) The efficacy of bicarbonate is disputed, and it seems least effective in patients with advanced kidney disease; may be effective in patients with underlying metabolic acidosis
      iii. β_2-Adrenergic agonists (e.g., albuterol)
         (a) Dose is albuterol 10–20 mg nebulized over 10 minutes or 0.5 mg intravenously (not available in the United States).
         (b) Will lower plasma potassium by 0.5–1.5 mEq/L
         (c) Onset is within 90 minutes with inhalation.
         (d) Avoid use in patients with coronary ischemia because of risk of tachycardia.
         (e) Up to 40% of patients do not respond to inhaled albuterol; therefore, it is not recommended as a single agent for urgent treatment of hyperkalemia; consider use in combination with insulin.

e. The previous treatment options should be followed by one of the following agents to remove excess K$^+$ from the body.

   i. Diuretics

      (a) Loop or thiazide-type diuretics increase K$^+$ renal excretion.

      (b) Ineffective in patients with advanced kidney disease

   ii. Cation exchange resin

      (a) Exchanges Na$^+$ for K$^+$, resulting in GI excretion of K$^+$. Caution in patients with kidney disease or heart failure caused by Na$^+$ (and subsequent fluid) retention

      (b) Because of its slow onset (2 hours) and unpredictable efficacy, sodium polystyrene sulfonate (Kayexalate) is not indicated for emergency treatment of hyperkalemia.

      (c) Approved by the FDA in 1958, before demonstrated efficacy was required. No controlled trials show efficacy.

      (d) Oral dose of sodium polystyrene sulfonate is 15 g repeated every 6 hours as needed. This can be mixed in 20–100 mL of water or syrup, but it is no longer recommended to mix in 70% sorbitol because of the risk of intestinal necrosis (there are also reports with the premixed 33% sorbitol suspension, but 70% sorbitol appears to have a stronger correlation with intestinal necrosis). Bowel injury is linked to the deposition of drug crystals in the GI tract. Oral sorbitol can prevent constipation associated with the resin; however, the highest risk of intestinal necrosis occurs when administered to patients within 1 week of surgery (occurs in about 1.8% of patients).

      (e) Although the oral route is more effective, 30–50 g can also be given as a retention enema mixed in 100–200 mL of an aqueous vehicle (e.g., water, 10% dextrose) that has been warmed to body temperature and kept in the colon for 30–60 minutes, or up to 3 hours. Irrigate colon after enema. Sorbitol is not recommended as a vehicle for rectal use because of the risk of intestinal necrosis and other serious GI adverse events.

      (f) A recent systematic review found that GI injury is also associated with sodium polystyrene preparations without sorbitol (Am J Med 2013;126:264).

      (g) A new potassium binder was recently approved for use in hyperkalemia. As opposed to sodium polystyrene sulfonate, patiromer (Veltassa) exchanges Ca^{2+} for K$^+$, resulting in GI excretion of K$^+$. As with other binders, caution should be used if patiromer is administered with other medications because it may reduce their absorption. Like sodium polystyrene sulfonate, patiromer should not be used for life-threatening hyperkalemia because it has a slower onset of action.

   iii. Dialysis

      (a) Used when other measures are ineffective or when severe hyperkalemia is present

      (b) Plasma potassium falls by more than 1 mmol/L in the first hour of dialysis and by about 2 mmol/L after 3 hours of dialysis.

      (c) Hemodialysis removes K$^+$ faster than peritoneal dialysis.

      (d) Monitor for rebound increase in K$^+$ after dialysis.

      (e) Used in patients with advanced kidney disease

Patient Case

7. A 61-year-old man is brought to the emergency department with shortness of breath and bilateral lower leg edema. Pertinent vital signs and laboratory values include heart rate 30 beats/minute, blood pressure 102/57 mm Hg, K^+ 7.9 mEq/L, Na^+ 139 mEq/L, glucose 228 mg/dL, Ca^{2+} 8.8 mg/dL, digoxin 2.0 ng/mL, BUN 49 mg/dL, and Cr 2.4 mg/dL. His ECG shows wide QRS and peaked T waves. His medical history includes heart failure, atrial fibrillation, coronary artery disease, peripheral arterial disease, and diabetes. The patient has peripheral intravenous access and an external pacemaker. Which is most appropriate?

    A. Calcium gluconate 10 mL intravenously over 2 minutes.

    B. Insulin 10 units intravenously.

    C. Sodium bicarbonate 50 mEq intravenously over 10 minutes.

    D. Albuterol 10 mg nebulized over 10 minutes.

VIII. DISORDERS OF MAGNESIUM HOMEOSTASIS

A. Normal serum magnesium concentration is 1.7–2.3 mg/dL (1.4–1.8 mEq/L or 0.85–1.15 mmol/L).

B. Hypomagnesemia (serum magnesium concentration less than 1.7 mg/dL)
    1. Usually associated with impaired intestinal absorption (e.g., ulcerative colitis, diarrhea, pancreatitis, chronic laxative abuse), inadequate intake, hypokalemia, or increased renal excretion (e.g., diuretic use)
        a. Common in hospitalized patients
        b. Usually associated with alcoholism and delirium tremens
    2. Often occurs concurrently with hypokalemia and hypocalcemia
    3. Signs and symptoms
        a. Neuromuscular symptoms include tetany, twitching, and seizures.
        b. Cardiovascular symptoms include arrhythmias, sudden cardiac death, and hypertension.
    4. Treatment
        a. Oral supplements (e.g., magnesium oxide, magnesium-containing antacids or laxatives) can be used for asymptomatic patients; however, treatment is limited by the high frequency of diarrhea.
        b. Symptomatic patients should initially be treated with 1–4 g (8–32 mEq) of magnesium sulfate by slow intravenous infusion (about 1 g/hour to avoid hypotension or increased renal excretion because of rapid administration). Initial boluses can be followed by about 0.5 mEq/kg/day added to intravenous fluid and administered as a continuous infusion. For emergency treatment (e.g., torsades), magnesium can be administered by intravenous push. Asymptomatic patients with mild to moderate hypomagnesemia should also be treated with 1–4 g of magnesium sulfate by slow intravenous infusion.
        c. Reduce dose by half in patients with kidney insufficiency.
        d. About half of administered magnesium is excreted in the urine; therefore, magnesium replacement should occur over 3–5 days.

C. Hypermagnesemia (serum magnesium greater than 2.3 mg/dL)
    1. Rarely occurs and is generally associated with chronic kidney disease
    2. Signs and symptoms include nausea, vomiting, bradycardia, hypotension, heart block, asystole, respiratory failure, and death; signs and symptoms rarely occur unless magnesium concentration is greater than 4–5 mg/dL.

3. Treatment
    a. Discontinue all magnesium-containing medications.
    b. Asymptomatic patients with normal kidney function can be treated with 0.9% sodium chloride and loop diuretics.
    c. Symptomatic patients should be treated with 100–200 mg of elemental Ca^{2+} administered intravenously over 5–10 minutes for cardiac stability.
    d. Hemodialysis may be needed for patients with kidney disease.

IX. DISORDERS OF PHOSPHORUS HOMEOSTASIS

A. Normal serum phosphorus concentration is 2.5–4.5 mg/dL.

B. Hypophosphatemia (serum phosphorus concentration less than 3–3.5 mg/dL)
    1. Causes of hypophosphatemia
        a. Increased renal elimination (e.g., diuretics, glucocorticoids, sodium bicarbonate)
        b. Rapidly refeeding patients with chronic malnutrition (see refeeding syndrome in Parenteral Nutrition section)
        c. Respiratory alkalosis
        d. Treatment of diabetic ketoacidosis; phosphorus shifts into the IC compartment as diabetic ketoacidosis is corrected.
    2. Signs and symptoms
        a. Tissue hypoxia can occur because of a decrease in oxygen release to peripheral tissues.
        b. Neurologic manifestations include confusion, delirium, seizures, and coma.
        c. Pulmonary and cardiac symptoms can include respiratory failure, difficulty weaning from mechanical ventilation, heart failure, and arrhythmias.
        d. Other organ systems affected include muscle, hematologic, bone, and kidney.
    3. Prevention and treatment
        a. Prevent hypophosphatemia by supplementing intravenous fluid with 10–30 mmol/L intravenous phosphorus in patients at risk of hypophosphatemia (e.g., malnourished, alcoholism, diabetic ketoacidosis).
        b. Oral phosphorus products (e.g., K-Phos Neutral; also contain K^+ and Na) can be used for asymptomatic patients, but they are poorly absorbed.
        c. Symptomatic patients typically receive 15–30 mmol and sometimes up to 60 mmol (or 0.5–0.75 mmol/kg of IBW) of phosphorus (sodium phosphate or potassium phosphate) administered intravenously over 3–6 hours (maximum rate is 7.5 mmol/hour). Note Na^+ content (4 mEq per 3 mmol of phosphate) and K^+ content (4.4 mEq per 3 mmol of phosphate).
    4. Phosphate shortages
        a. Reserve phosphate products for patients who need them most (e.g., children, neonates, diabetic ketoacidosis, refeeding syndrome, and critically ill patients).
        b. Intravenous fat emulsions contain 15 mmol/L as egg phospholipids. This may be sufficient phosphate for some patients.

C. Hyperphosphatemia
    1. Typically occurs in patients with chronic kidney disease or hypoparathyroidism
    2. In general, patients are asymptomatic, but they can have signs and symptoms including hypocalcemia, ECG changes, paresthesias, and vascular calcifications.
    3. Treatment (see treatment of hyperphosphatemia in the Nephrology chapter)

X. DISORDERS OF CALCIUM HOMEOSTASIS

A. Normal serum calcium concentration is 8.5–10.5 mg/dL (total Ca^{2+} includes bound and unbound Ca^{2+}), and normal ionized calcium is 1.1–1.3 mmol/L (or 4.4–5.3 mg/dL).

B. Distribution of Ca^{2+}
   1. EC fluid contains less than 1% of the total body stores of Ca^{2+}; 99% of total body stores of Ca^{2+} are in skeletal bone.
      a. About half of Ca^{2+} in the EC compartment is bound to plasma proteins (primarily albumin).
      b. The active form of Ca^{2+} is the unbound or ionized Ca^{2+}.
   2. Ionized Ca^{2+} is regulated by parathyroid hormone, phosphorus, vitamin D, and calcitonin.

C. Hypocalcemia
   1. Occurs in patients with chronic kidney disease, hypoparathyroidism, vitamin D deficiency, alcoholism, and hyperphosphatemia, and in patients receiving large amounts of blood products or patients undergoing continuous renal replacement therapy (CRRT [i.e., Ca^{2+} chelates with citrate in blood products or CRRT])
   2. Factors that cause an increase in EC Ca^{2+} binding to albumin (e.g., metabolic alkalosis) can cause a reduction in plasma ionized Ca^{2+} concentration, leading to symptomatic hypocalcemia.
   3. A low serum albumin will cause a falsely low total serum calcium reading, so an adjustment is necessary. Subtract a patient's serum albumin from a normal serum albumin of 4 g/dL, multiply by 0.8 mg/dL, and then add to the total serum calcium concentration to correct the value.
   4. Signs and symptoms include tetany, muscle spasms, hypoactive reflexes, anxiety, hallucinations, lethargy, hypotension, and seizures.
   5. Treatment
      a. Asymptomatic hypocalcemia associated with hypoalbuminemia is typically associated with normal ionized Ca^{2+} concentrations and therefore does not require treatment.
      b. Asymptomatic hypocalcemia can be treated with oral Ca^{2+} supplements at a dose of 2–4 g/day of elemental Ca^{2+} in divided doses; patients may also require vitamin D supplementation.
      c. Symptomatic hypocalcemia is treated with 200–300 mg of elemental Ca^{2+} administered intravenously over 5–10 minutes. This is sometimes followed by a continuous infusion.
         i. Equivalent to 1 g of $CaCl_2$ (273 mg of elemental Ca^{2+}) administered through a central intravenous catheter; peripheral administration of $CaCl_2$ can result in severe limb ischemia
         ii. Equivalent to 2–3 g of calcium gluconate (180–270 mg of elemental Ca^{2+}); preferred for peripheral intravenous administration
         iii. Do not infuse Ca^{2+} at a rate faster than 60 mg of elemental Ca^{2+} per minute; rapid administration, which is not recommended, is associated with hypotension, bradycardia, or asystole.
         iv. The duration of a bolus dose of Ca^{2+} is ideally 1–2 hours. If a continuous infusion is used, the rate should be 0.5–2 mg/kg/hour of elemental Ca^{2+}.
   6. Calcium shortages
      a. If there is a shortage of calcium gluconate, do not add CaCl to PN. Use multielectrolyte products in PN, if possible.
      b. The safety of diluted CaCl administered peripherally is unknown.

D. Hypercalcemia (serum calcium concentration greater than 10.5 mg/dL) is usually related to malignancy or hyperparathyroidism; see Oncology Supportive Care chapter.

XI. ENTERAL NUTRITION

A. Indication and Timing: Enteral nutrition is used in patients at risk of malnutrition in whom it is anticipated that oral feedings will be inadequate for 5–7 days. Malnutrition is associated with poor wound healing and increased risk of infection. According to the American Society for Parenteral and Enteral Nutrition (ASPEN) guidelines, well-nourished adults without excessive metabolic stress can usually tolerate little to no nutrition for up to 7 days. The 2009 ASPEN and Society of Critical Care Medicine (SCCM) guidelines for critically ill patients recommend starting enteral feeding within the first 24–48 hours after ICU admission.

B. EN Contraindications
   1. Complete intestinal obstruction
   2. GI fistula (if a feeding tube cannot be placed distal to the fistula or if high-output fistula, which is defined as greater than 500 mL of output per day)
   3. Extreme short bowel
   4. Severe diarrhea or vomiting
   5. Hemodynamic instability or intestinal ischemia
   6. Paralytic ileus (however, many patients can be fed through the small bowel, despite an ileus)
   7. Note: The absence of bowel sounds is *not* a contraindication for the provision of EN (i.e., positive bowel sounds are not required for EN initiation). EN promotes gut motility.

C. EN Administration Routes
   1. Orogastric tubes are preferred in patients with nasal or facial trauma or sinusitis, but they are uncomfortable for alert patients.
   2. Nasogastric (NG) tubes are the most common tubes for short-term enteral access, and they can be used for stomach decompression in addition to feeding.
      a. Prolonged use can cause sinusitis or nasal mucosal ulceration.
      b. Patients with a gastric ileus will not tolerate NG feedings and will have an increased risk of aspiration.
   3. Nasoduodenal tubes are smaller and more flexible than NG tubes.
      a. Ideally, the tip is placed past the pyloric sphincter to improve tube feeding tolerance and prevent aspiration.
      b. These tubes, which are smaller than NG tubes, will clog if not flushed appropriately.
      c. Patients with a gastric ileus may tolerate this type of feeding tube.
   4. Nasojejunal tubes are advanced into the fourth portion of the duodenum or past the ligament of Treitz.
   5. Gastrostomy tubes (also known as percutaneous endoscopic gastrostomy tubes) are placed through the abdominal wall into the stomach for patients requiring long-term feeding.
   6. Jejunostomy tubes are placed through the abdominal wall into the jejunum, usually to facilitate immediate postoperative or postinjury feeding.

D. EN Delivery
   1. Gravity control refers to delivery with tubing that is fitted with a roller clamp to allow infusion into the stomach as desired.
   2. Continuous infusion by an enteral feeding pump is usually used in hospitals because of the lower risk of aspiration compared with bolus feedings; must be used for duodenal or jejunal feedings
   3. Cyclic feedings are administered continuously for 10–12 hours (overnight) to facilitate patient mobility during the daytime.
   4. Intermittent bolus feedings of 100–300 mL for 30–60 minutes every 4–6 hours can be used only for feeding tubes ending in the stomach in stable patients.

E. Benefit of EN

1. EN is preferred in patients with a functional GI tract because it is associated with a lower risk of infection than PN. Early administration of EN is associated with lower rates of infection and shorter lengths of stay.

2. GI mucosal atrophy occurs with an absence of EN or oral nutrition. This can increase the risk of bacterial translocation because of gut bacteria crossing the weakened intestinal barrier.

F. EN Formulations

1. Typically contain carbohydrate, fat, protein, electrolytes, water, vitamins, and trace elements in varying amounts

2. Intact or polymeric formulas are used in patients with normal digestive processes, and they typically contain 1–1.2 kcal/mL. Examples include Osmolite and Isocal.

   a. These are generally inexpensive and an appropriate first choice for many patients.

   b. Some polymeric formulas are concentrated for patients requiring fluid restriction and contain 2 kcal/mL. Examples include Novasource 2.0, TwoCal HN, and Deliver 2.0.

   c. Some polymeric formulas are designed for oral administration and are used to supplement the patient's diet. Examples include Boost and Ensure.

3. Elemental formulas are easily digested by patients with impaired digestive capacity or malabsorption (e.g., short bowel, pancreatic insufficiency); they are typically more expensive than polymeric EN. Examples include Peptamen, Vital HN, and Vivonex TEN.

4. Some EN contains fiber for patients with constipation. Examples include Ultracal and Jevity.

5. Disease-specific EN

   a. EN formulations for patients with renal failure are typically concentrated (i.e., 2 kcal/mL to adhere to fluid restrictions) and can contain differing amounts of protein and electrolytes. Examples include Novasource Renal and Nepro.

   b. Some EN products designed for patients with respiratory failure have more calories from fat (40%–55% of total calories) and fewer from carbohydrates to reduce the production of CO_2 and facilitate ventilator weaning. However, excessive CO_2 production is caused primarily by overfeeding with total calories rather than the total amount of dextrose; therefore, these more expensive formulations may be unnecessary as long as the patient is not being overfed; examples include Pulmocare, Respalor, and NutriVent.

   c. EN formulations for patients with diabetes have more calories from fat, fewer calories from carbohydrates, and added fiber to improve glycemic control. Examples include Diabetisource AC and Glucerna.

   d. EN formulations for patients with hepatic failure and hepatic encephalopathy contain more branched-chain AAs and less aromatic AAs, which may improve encephalopathy (controversial). NutriHep is an example.

   e. EN for highly stressed patients (e.g., trauma, burn injury, acute respiratory distress syndrome, sepsis) is enhanced with protein, arginine, glutamine, omega-3 fatty acids, nucleotides, or beta-carotene. These enteral formulations are designed to improve immune function and clinical outcomes. Examples (although not interchangeable) include Impact, Impact Glutamine, and Oxepa.

G. EN Complications

1. Improper tube placement or displacement

2. Clogged feeding tubes

   a. Prevent by flushing feeding tube before, between, and after the administration of each drug.

   b. Unclog feeding tubes with warm water, pancreatic enzymes, or sodium bicarbonate.

3. Aspiration
   a. Prevent by keeping the head of bed elevated at 30–45 degrees.
   b. Prevent by monitoring gastric residuals and holding infusion if gastric residual volume is greater than 250–500 mL.
      i. Prevent delays in gastric emptying using an EN formula with less fat.
      ii. Gastric motility can be increased with metoclopramide (5–20 mg intravenously every 6 hours) or erythromycin (250 mg intravenously every 6–8 hours administered until tolerating EN for at least 24 hours); can combine metoclopramide and erythromycin, but monitor for diarrhea and tachyphylaxis.
      iii. Avoid prolonged use of promotility agents because of increased risk of adverse effects.
   c. Administering EN by a feeding tube with the tip terminating beyond the pyloric sphincter can prevent aspiration pneumonia.
   d. Prevent also by initiating EN at a slow rate (e.g., 20 mL/hour) and advance every 4–6 hours as tolerated to goal rate.
4. Diarrhea
   a. More common with elemental products because of a higher osmolarity
   b. Consider other causes of diarrhea such as antibiotic use, infection, lactose intolerance, magnesium, and sorbitol in liquid medication preparations.
5. Constipation can be prevented by adding fiber or bowel stimulation.
6. Dehydration
7. Hypernatremia occurs when patients are given insufficient water while receiving EN.
   a. Patients require about 30 mL/kg/day of water.
   b. Hypernatremia typically occurs in patients with altered mental status.
   c. Calorie-dense (i.e., 1.5 or 2 kcal/mL) EN formulas have less water than products containing 1 kcal/mL, and therefore additional water is needed to prevent hypernatremia.
8. Nasopharyngeal erosions, epistaxis, tracheoesophageal fistula
9. Sinusitis
10. Electrolyte abnormalities are most likely to occur in patients who develop refeeding syndrome (discussed later).

Patient Case

8. A 72-year-old woman (weight 65 kg) is receiving Novasource Renal, a calorie-rich tube feeding designed for patients with kidney disease. The patient's baseline and current Cr is 1.5 mg/dL, and her urine output is about 50 mL/hour. The tube feeding is infusing at a goal rate of 35 mL/hour through an NG feeding tube providing 2 kcal/mL, Na$^+$ 41 mEq/L, and 717 mL/L of water. The patient's serum sodium was 140 mEq/L when the tube feeding was initiated a few days ago, and her Na$^+$ is now 145 mEq/L. Which recommendation is the best approach for preventing hypernatremia in this patient?

   A. Change to an EN formula with a lower concentration of Na$^+$.

   B. Administer intravenous D$_5$W at 45 mL/hour.

   C. Administer 200 mL of water through a feeding tube every 4 hours.

   D. Reduce the tube feeding to 30 mL/hour.

H. EN Monitoring
1. Blood glucose concentration
2. Head of bed elevation to 30–45 degrees
3. Gastric residuals are checked, and infusion rate is generally held or reduced if the residual amount exceeds 250–500 mL (applies to gastric tube feedings only, not small bowel). According to the SCCM and ASPEN guidelines, holding EN for gastric residual volumes less than 500 mL in the absence of other signs of intolerance should be avoided.
4. GI tolerance
    a. Abdominal pain or distension
    b. Stool frequency and volume
    c. Gastric residuals
    d. Nausea, vomiting, and diarrhea
5. Prealbumin weekly. (Exception: Caution in critically ill patients because it reflects acute-phase response rather than nutritional status). See goals in the Parenteral Nutrition section.
6. Serum sodium and other electrolytes
7. Wound healing is a sign of adequate nutritional therapy.

I. Developing an EN Regimen (Table 8)

Table 8. Developing an EN Regimen

Steps	Calculation Guide	Example
Determine caloric requirements	25–35 kcal/kg/day *or* estimate energy requirements using an equation such as the Harris-Benedict equation (see more details in Parenteral Nutrition section and Critical Care chapter)	A 60-kg patient would require about 25 kcal/kg/day × 60 kg = 1500 kcal
Choose a formula and assess the calories per milliliter	Usually 1, 1.2, 1.5, or 2 kcal/mL	Ultracal provides 1 kcal/mL
Determine infusion rate	(Volume of EN)/24 hr	1500 mL/24 hr = 62.5 mL/hr
Make sure patient will receive enough protein	See product information to find protein content (see protein requirements in Parenteral Nutrition section)	Ultracal provides 45 g/L of protein; therefore, 1500 mL will provide 67.5 g of protein, or 1.1 g/kg for a patient weighing 60 kg
Make sure patient will receive about 30 mL/kg/day of water	See product information to find water content	Ultracal provides 830 mL/L of free water. A patient receiving 1500 mL/day would need about 250 mL of additional water
		This can be administered as water flushes through the feeding tube (i.e., 60–70 mL every 6 hr). It is important to consider other fluids that the patient may be receiving

EN = enteral nutrition.

J. Drug Administration Using Enteral Access
1. Liquids are preferable, and they should be diluted with 2–3 times the medication volume with water.
2. Diarrhea can occur with medications having a high osmolality (e.g., medications mixed in sorbitol).
3. Flush with 20 mL of water before and after drug administration.
4. Do not crush sustained-release or enteric-coated pills.
5. Mix crushed tablets or capsule contents with 10–15 mL of water and administer each drug separately.
6. May need to discontinue tube feedings before and after drug administration temporarily to prevent reduced bioavailability (e.g., fluoroquinolones, phenytoin, warfarin, bisphosphonates)
7. Consider feeding tube location and subsequent drug absorption (e.g., for efficacy; antacids need to be administered into the stomach, not the duodenum).

XII. PARENTERAL NUTRITION

A. PN is the administration of intravenous nutrition in patients with a nonfunctioning or inaccessible GI tract in which the duration of PN is anticipated to be at least 7 days (i.e., it is anticipated that the patient will be unable to be fed orally or enterally for at least 7 days).

B. Indications for PN
1. Severe pancreatitis in patients who cannot tolerate EN
2. Peritonitis
3. Severe inflammatory bowel disease (e.g., Crohn disease, ulcerative colitis)
4. Extensive bowel resection (e.g., short bowel syndrome) causing malabsorption or maldigestion
5. Complete bowel obstruction
6. Severe intractable vomiting or diarrhea
7. Inability to meet full nutritional needs by enteral route alone (can use PN as supplement to EN)

C. Intravenous Infusion of PN
1. PN should be administered through a central line. This includes any intravenous catheter (e.g., peripherally inserted central catheter, Hickman, Port-A-Cath) where the tip of the catheter is in the superior vena cava or adjacent to the right atrium (femoral catheters should be avoided because of higher risk of venous thrombosis and catheter-related infection).
2. Peripheral access is defined as the catheter tip position outside the central vessels or inferior or superior vena cava; if a peripheral vein is used for PN administration, the osmolarity must not exceed 900 mOsm/L. Peripheral administration can be used in patients with an appropriate indication for PN (see above) when central intravenous access is unavailable and the need for PN is expected to be less than 2 weeks.
    a. Final dextrose concentration should be 10% or less.
    b. Final AA concentration should be 2.5%–4%.
    c. Ca^{2+} concentration should be 5 mEq/L or less.
    d. K^+ concentration should be 40–60 mEq/L or less.
3. In hospitalized patients, PN is typically administered as a continuous infusion, which should be completed within 24 hours.
4. Ambulatory patients may prefer a cyclic PN in which the PN is usually infused for 12 hours.
5. Infusions are generally better tolerated by patients if they are removed from the refrigerator 30–60 minutes before infusion.

Table 9. Estimating the Osmolarity of PN

Nutrient	Estimated Osmolarity
Amino acids	10 mOsm/L
Dextrose	5 mOsm/L
Lipid emulsion 20%	1.3–1.5 mOsm/L
Sodium	2 mOsm/mEq
Potassium	2 mOsm/mEq
Calcium gluconate	1.4 mOsm/mEq
Magnesium sulfate	1 mOsm/mEq

PN = parenteral nutrition.

   D. Types of PN Admixtures
      1. 2-in-1 refers to PN in which all nutrients are mixed in the same intravenous bag, except for lipids, which are administered by a separate infusion.
         a. Lipids are infused separately, no faster than 0.1 g/kg/hour in adults.
         b. Rapid administration of lipids is associated with headache, fever, nausea, hypertriglyceridemia, dyspnea, cyanosis, flushing, sweating, and back or chest pain.
         c. Lipid infusion time should be less than 12 hours because of the potential for microbial growth after this time (growth is reduced when lipids are mixed with dextrose and AAs, as in the 3-in-1 below, because of reduced pH and increased osmolarity).
         d. Administration tubing for a 2-in-1 should be changed every 72 hours; lipid tubing should be discarded after use (no longer than 12 hours).
      2. 3-in-1 (also called total nutrient admixture) refers to PN in which all nutrients are mixed in the same intravenous bag.
         a. Stability of a 3-in-1 depends on the pH, which is determined primarily by the final AA concentration (maintain at 2.5%–4%).
         b. Do not add concentrated dextrose directly to a lipid emulsion when mixing (see order of mixing below).
         c. Avoid excessive amounts of Ca^{2+} and magnesium (see recommended doses below).
         d. Administration tubing for a 3-in-1 should be changed every 24 hours.

Table 10. 2-in-1 PN Compared with 3-in-1 PN

	Advantages	Disadvantages
2-in-1	Longer stability Visual inspection easier Filter using 0.22-micron filter (bacteria-eliminating)	Increased nursing time Requires two sets of tubing Increased bacterial growth in lipids Maximum 12-hr hang time of separate lipids
3-in-1	Time-efficient for nurses Single bag with single tube Decreased vein irritation Inhibited bacterial growth	Shorter stability (1–2 days) Complex compounding (without automated compounder) Visual inspection difficult Emulsion instability Must use 1.2-micron filter, not 0.22-micron Limited compatibility with medications Catheter occlusion more common

E. Premixed PN
   1. Products available in the United States
      a. Clinimix is a two-compartment bag containing AAs in one compartment and dextrose in the other. This product also includes electrolytes and is available without electrolytes. The seal between the two-compartment bag must be broken to mix the AAs and dextrose. Lipids can be added to the container after compartments are mixed or can be administered by Y-site.
      b. ProcalAmine is a solution containing 3% AAs, glycerin (4.3 kcal/g), and electrolytes in a single container. Not sufficient for most patients because of insufficient protein and calories
      c. Kabiven, a newer solution that has recently been approved, contains AAs, electrolytes, dextrose, and a lipid emulsion. It is available in a three-compartment bag. Perikabiven is also available for use for peripheral and central administration.
   2. Patient selection
      a. Evidence is insufficient to show that customized PN is superior to standardized premixed products.
      b. Consider in stable patients who require PN.
      c. Avoid in patients with fluid restriction or high protein needs.
   3. Premixed products require fewer manipulations and have a lower risk of contamination and compounding errors, but they may still require additives (e.g., electrolytes, vitamins, trace elements).

F. Nutritional Components of PN Formulation
   1. Dextrose used for compounding PN is usually 70% and contains 3.4 kcal/g. Glycerol (or glycerin) is another carbohydrate source. Glycerol provides 4.3 kcal/g, and it is used in premixed parenteral products (e.g., ProcalAmine).
   2. Fat emulsion is available as 10% or 20% and contains about 10 kcal/g; also available as a 30% formulation for compounding in 3-in-1 only
   3. AAs are available as 3%–20% and provide 4 kcal/g.
   4. Electrolytes are added to maintain physiologic serum concentrations.
   5. Multivitamins and trace elements are added on the basis of the recommended daily amount.

G. Developing a PN Regimen for Administration Through a Central Intravenous Line
   1. Determine caloric requirements.
      a. For patients with a body mass index (BMI) less than 30 kg/m^2, administer 25–35 kcal/kg/day based on actual body weight [BMI = (weight in kg)/(height in meters)^2].
      b. If BMI exceeds 30 kg/m^2, can administer 11–14 kcal/kg based on actual body weight or 22–25 kcal/kg based on IBW
         i. Alternatively, some practitioners advocate using adjusted body weight (ABW) rather than IBW.
         ii. ABW = [(actual weight – IBW) × 0.25] + IBW.
      c. Permissive underfeeding with high protein in EN and PN involves the administration of about 80% of caloric requirements, and it can be considered in patients with obesity (except in patients with kidney failure requiring hemodialysis and patients with hepatic failure; these patients have increased protein and caloric requirements to maintain a positive nitrogen balance).
      d. A commonly used method is to estimate basal energy expenditure (BEE) using the Harris-Benedict equation:
         i. Men: BEE = 66 + 13.7(weight in kg) + 5(height in cm) – 6.8(age in years).
         ii. Women: BEE = 655 + 9.6(weight in kg) + 1.8(height in cm) – 4.7(age in years).
      e. Energy expenditure may also be estimated through indirect calorimetry in critically ill patients (see Critical Care chapter).

2. Determine fluid requirements.
   a. Usually 30–35 mL/kg/day or 2500–3500 mL/day (for patients without fluid restrictions) to maintain urine output in the range of 0.5–2 mL/kg/hour
   b. Fluid requirements for patients with fluid restrictions (e.g., kidney or cardiac dysfunction) should be individualized.
   c. Do not use PN for fluid replacement but for maintenance fluid only.
3. Determine protein (AA) requirements.
   a. For patients with a BMI less than 30 kg/m², protein is usually in the range of 0.8–2 g/kg/day on the basis of actual body weight (may be higher in burn or trauma patients).
      i. Maintenance 0.8–1 g/kg/day
      ii. Moderate stress 1.3–1.5 g/kg/day
      iii. Severe stress 1.5–2 g/kg/day
   b. For patients with a BMI 30–40 kg/m², can give protein 2 g/kg/day based on IBW. For patients with a BMI greater than 40 kg/m², can give 2.5 g/kg/day based on IBW
   c. Patients with kidney dysfunction may need protein restriction to prevent uremia.
      i. Kidney dysfunction without dialysis, 1 g/kg/day
      ii. Kidney failure with intermittent hemodialysis, 1.2–1.5 g/kg/day (1.5–2.5 g/kg/day if continuous renal replacement)
   d. Calories from protein (4 kcal/g) should be included in the total caloric provisions to prevent overfeeding.
   e. For 3-in-1 formulations, the final AA concentration should be 4% to provide adequate buffering capacity and prevent lipid emulsion destabilization.
   f. Complete protein requirements can be provided on day 1 of PN (i.e., there is no need to slowly titrate up to recommended amount).
4. Calculate remaining non-protein calories and administer about 20%–30% of total calories as lipid and the remainder as dextrose.
   a. Make sure dextrose rate of administration does not exceed the maximum rate of hepatic oxidation rate of 4–6 mg/kg/minute (may be lower in critically ill patients, so monitor for hyperglycemia and adjust amount of dextrose provided if needed).
      i. Initial dextrose amounts can be in the range of 150–200 g/day.
      ii. May need to reduce to 100–150 g/day initially in patients with diabetes or stress-induced hyperglycemia; increase gradually during first 3–4 days to goals if blood glucose values are less than 140–180 mg/dL.
   b. A higher percentage of calories from lipid (up to 50%–60%, or 2.5 g/kg/day) can be provided for a short time in certain cases (e.g., hyperglycemia, hypercapnia).
   c. Essential fatty acid deficiency can be prevented by supplying 2%–4% of total calories as lipid (can administer lipid emulsion once every 1–2 weeks).
5. Estimate a daily maintenance amount of electrolytes, vitamins, and trace elements (see below).
   a. Electrolyte abnormalities should be addressed and corrected before PN is initiated. Avoid replacing electrolyte deficiencies using PN in acutely ill patients.
   b. Maintenance electrolytes (amounts will vary and should be individualized)
      i. Sodium 60–150 mEq/day (1–2 mEq/kg/day)
      ii. K^+ 40–80 mEq/day (1 mEq/kg/day)
      iii. Phosphate 10–40 mmol/day (or 15 mmol/1000 kcal)
      iv. Ca^{2+} 10–15 mEq/day (gluconate is preferred to prevent incompatibilities)
      v. Magnesium 8–20 mEq/day (sulfate form is preferred to Cl to prevent incompatibilities)
      vi. Cl and acetate salt forms should be used to maintain acid-base balance.

     vii. Electrolyte adjustment

       (a) Typically will need greater amounts of magnesium, phosphorus, and K^+ during the first few days of PN because of IC shifts

       (b) Cl and acetate salt forms can be adjusted as needed to maintain acid-base balance (see below under Monitoring Patients Who Are Receiving PN).

  c. Standard trace elements contain selenium, chromium, copper, manganese, and zinc (e.g., MTE-5).

     i. Patients with high-output fistulas, diarrhea, burns, or large open wounds may require additional zinc supplementation.

     ii. Patients with chronic diarrhea, malabsorption, or short-gut syndrome or those with critical illness may require additional selenium supplementation.

     iii. Patients with severe cholestasis should have copper and manganese restricted to prevent accumulation and toxicity because both undergo biliary elimination.

  d. Parenteral multivitamin should be added daily (generally contains 150 mcg of vitamin K).

     i. Additional thiamine (25–100 mg) can be supplemented in patients with a history of alcohol abuse.

     ii. During shortages of parenteral vitamins, can reduce frequency of administration to three times/week or can administer individual vitamins daily (i.e., thiamine, ascorbic acid, niacin, pyridoxine, folic acid) or monthly (i.e., vitamin B_{12})

Box 5. Central PN Calculations

Example of a central 3-in-1 PN formula for a 70-kg patient hospitalized with ischemic bowel:
1. Total calories estimated as 30 kcal/kg × 70 kg = 2100 kcal
2. Fluid requirements estimated as 1500 mL + (20 mL/kg × 50 kg) = 2500 mL/day
3. Estimated protein needs are 1.5 g/kg × 70 kg = 105 g of protein. 4 kcal/g × 105 g = 420 kcal from protein. Using 10% AA-based solution, will need 1050 mL to equal 105 g of protein (can round to 1000 mL if this makes compounding easier)
4. Determine calories from fat and dextrose. Total calories needed is 2100 kcal − 420 kcal from AAs = 1680 remaining non-protein calories needed. Administer 25%–30% of total kilocalories as lipid, or about 500 kcal from lipid. Using 10% lipid emulsion, will need 500 mL to equal 500 kcal (about 1 kcal/mL) Total calories needed is 2100 kcal − 420 kcal (AA) − 500 kcal (lipid) = 1180 kcal needed from dextrose. Assuming 3.4 kcal/g, will need about 350 g dextrose. Using a 70% base dextrose solution, will need 500 mL to equal 350 g or 1190 kcal Calculate the rate of dextrose administration in milligrams per kilogram per minute: [(350 g/24 hr) × (1000 mg/g) × (1 hr/60 min)]/70 kg = 3.5 mg/kg/min This is an appropriate rate of dextrose administration
5. Final formula will contain the following: AA 10% 1050 mL Lipid 10% 500 mL Dextrose 70% 500 mL Electrolytes, multivitamins, and trace elements (about 110 mL) Final volume of 2160 mL to infuse at 2160 mL/24 hr = 90 mL/hr (Final volume assumes patient is receiving about 350 mL of fluid from other medications to meet fluid requirements)
6. Final concentration of macronutrients in PN is: AA 105 g/2160 mL final volume = 4.9% Lipid 50 g/2160 mL = 2.3% Dextrose 350 g/2160 mL = 16%

Box 5. Central PN Calculations *(continued)*

7.   Final caloric value of PN is: AA 105 g × 4 kcal/g = 420 kcal Lipid 50 g × 10 kcal/g = 500 kcal Dextrose 350 g × 3.4 kcal/g = 1190 kcal Total calories = 420 + 500 + 1190 = 2110 kcal/70 kg = 30 kcal/kg 24% of total calories are provided as lipid

AA = amino acid; PN = parenteral nutrition.

    H.   Developing a PN Regimen for Administration Through a Peripheral Intravenous Line
        1.   Will probably not meet nutritional needs based on macronutrient and micronutrient concentration restrictions (see above)
        2.   For additional calories, increase percentage of calories administered as lipid.

Box 6. Peripheral PN Calculations

Example of a peripheral 3-in-1 PN formula for a 70-kg patient:
1.   Total calories estimated as 30 kcal/kg × 70 kg = 2100 kcal
2.   Fluid requirements estimated as 1500 mL + (20 mL/kg × 50 kg) = 2500 mL/day; prescriber wants PN to contain no more than 2000 mL
3.   Calculate amount of dextrose as 2000 mL × 10% = 200 g of maximum dextrose recommended
4.   Calculate amount of AA as 2000 mL × 3% = 60 g of maximum AA recommended
5.   Add about 500 kcal as lipid (can add more if patient tolerates). Can use 10% or 20% lipid emulsion
6.   Calculate volume so far. Using 70% dextrose, need 286 mL to equal 200 g of dextrose. Using 10% AA, will need 600 mL to equal 60 g. Using 10% lipid, will need 500 mL. Will add electrolytes, trace elements, multivitamins, and enough sterile water for a total volume of 2000 mL
7.   Final formula will contain the following: AA 10% 600 mL Lipid 10% 500 mL Dextrose 70% 286 mL Electrolytes, multivitamins, and trace elements Sterile water added for 2000 mL final volume to infuse at 2000 mL/24 hr = 83 mL/hr
8.   Final concentration of macronutrients in PN is: AA 60 g/2000 mL final volume = 3% Lipid 50 g/2000 mL = 2.5% Dextrose 200 g/2000 mL = 10%
9.   Final caloric value of peripheral PN is: AA 60 g × 4 kcal/g = 240 kcal Lipid 50 g × 10 kcal/g = 500 kcal Dextrose 200 g × 3.4 kcal/g = 680 kcal Total calories = 240 + 500 + 680 = 1420 kcal/70 kg = 20 kcal/kg 35% of total calories are provided as lipid

I. Order of Mixing (for manual compounding)
    1. Add dextrose, AAs, sterile water.
    2. Add phosphate.
    3. Add other electrolytes (except Ca) and trace minerals.
    4. Mix well to ensure phosphate is evenly distributed and to prevent precipitation with Ca.
    5. Add Ca.
    6. Observe for precipitates or contaminants.
    7. Add lipid if 3-in-1 formulation. (Note: Do not mix dextrose and lipids directly because the low pH of dextrose can destabilize the lipid emulsion.)
    8. Add vitamins last, as close to the time of PN administration as possible in acute care settings, or just before infusion in patients receiving home PN.

J. Factors Associated with Ca^{2+} and Phosphate Precipitation in PN
    1. Increasing pH (more basic) increases the risk of Ca^{2+} and phosphate precipitation.
    2. Increasing Ca^{2+} or phosphate concentration increases the risk of precipitation.
        a. If Ca^{2+} concentration is 6 mEq/L or less and phosphate concentration is 30 mmol/L or less, the risk of precipitation is low.
        b. CaCl is more likely to precipitate with phosphate than calcium gluconate; CaCl should never be used in compounding PN formulations.
    3. The final concentration of AA should be at least 2.5% or higher to prevent Ca^{2+} and phosphate precipitation.
        a. AAs form soluble complexes with Ca^{2+} and phosphate.
        b. AAs provide a buffer system to maintain a lower pH of the PN in an acceptable range to prevent Ca^{2+} or phosphate precipitation.
    4. As the temperature increases, the risk of precipitation increases.
        a. PN should be refrigerated if not administered within 24 hours of compounding.
        b. If refrigerated, PN should be administered within 24 hours of rewarming.
    5. A 1.2-micron filter (used for a 3-in-1 PN) may not prevent the embolism of a calcium phosphate precipitate, but it should be used anyway to reduce the risk.
    6. Order of mixing additives (see above)
    7. The PN should be agitated often during compounding to ensure adequate mixture into solution.

K. Medication Additives in PN
    1. In general, medications should not be added to PN.
    2. Examples of medication incompatibilities are ceftriaxone (precipitates with Ca), phenytoin (can change the pH of PN), medications containing propylene glycol or ethanol as diluents (e.g., furosemide, diazepam, lorazepam, digoxin, phenytoin, etoposide), and iron dextran (trivalent cations destabilize the lipid emulsion in 3-in-1 PN formulations).
    3. Incompatible drugs should be administered through a separate intravenous catheter or a separate lumen of a central venous catheter, if possible.
    4. If an incompatible intravenous drug is to be administered through the same intravenous catheter as the PN, the PN should be stopped, followed by a compatible flush before and after drug administration. The volume of flush should be sufficient to clear the entire catheter of PN and of drug (typically about 10 mL if flushing the port closest to the patient); for drugs requiring longer infusion times, see below for precautions to prevent rebound hyperglycemia with prolonged interruptions of PN.
    5. Only regular insulin is compatible with PN.

L. PN Complications
   1. Catheter-related infections are caused primarily by *Staphylococcus aureus* and *Candida albicans.*
   2. Catheter insertion complications (e.g., pneumothorax, incorrect placement)
   3. Peripheral venous thrombophlebitis can occur with peripheral catheter placement; risk is increased by day 4 of catheterization; therefore, site should be rotated every 3 days.
   4. Fluid imbalance
   5. Acid-base imbalances are usually related to the patient's underlying condition; however, excessive chloride salts in the PN can cause a metabolic acidosis, whereas excessive acetate salts in the PN can cause a metabolic alkalosis.
   6. Hyperglycemia can lead to nosocomial and wound infections.
   7. Gut atrophy
   8. Overfeeding can cause hepatic steatosis, hypercapnia, hyperglycemia, and azotemia.
   9. Essential fatty acid deficiency
       a. Symptoms include skin desquamation, hair loss, impaired wound healing, hepatomegaly, thrombocytopenia, fatty liver, and anemia.
       b. Can occur within 1–3 weeks of a lipid-free PN
   10. Refeeding syndrome can occur in acutely (can include critically ill patients) or chronically malnourished patients when EN or PN is initiated.
       a. Characterized by hypophosphatemia, hypokalemia, hypomagnesemia
       b. Can cause cardiac dysfunction, respiratory dysfunction, and death
       c. Prevention of refeeding syndrome:
           i. Identify patients at risk (e.g., anorexia, alcoholism, cancer, chronically ill, poor nutritional intake for 1–2 weeks, recent unintentional weight loss, malabsorption).
           ii. Initially, provide less than 50% of caloric requirements; then advance over several days to desired goal.
           iii. Supplement vitamins before initiating PN as well as K^+, phosphate, and magnesium (if needed); monitor daily for at least 1 week; and replace electrolytes as needed (many patients will need aggressive electrolyte replacement during the first week of PN).
   11. Aluminum toxicity
       a. More likely to occur in patients on long-term PN or in those with renal dysfunction (aluminum is renally eliminated)
       b. Accumulates in bone and interferes with bone Ca^{2+} uptake, causing osteopenia
       c. Neurotoxicity
       d. Aluminum contaminates many intravenous electrolytes and intravenous fluids.
       e. See drug labels for amount of aluminum content.
   12. Hepatobiliary disorders (includes steatosis, cholestasis, and gallbladder sludge or stones) can occur with long-term PN administration.
       a. Steatosis (or fatty liver) is associated with overfeeding and a transient elevation in aminotransferase concentration. Although it is usually benign, it can progress to fibrosis or cirrhosis in patients receiving long-term PN.
       b. Cholestasis usually occurs in children, but it can also occur in adults receiving long-term PN and can progress to cirrhosis and liver failure; a conjugated bilirubin concentration greater than 2 mg/dL is the primary sign.
       c. Gallbladder stasis is associated with the development of gallstones, sludge, and cholecystitis and is more attributable to a lack of EN than to PN administration.
   13. Osteoporosis and osteomalacia can occur in patients receiving long-term PN, and they are associated with higher protein doses (causes increased Ca^{2+} excretion) and chronic metabolic acidosis (because of insufficient acetate).

Patient Case

9. A 43-year-old male trauma patient (height 75 inches, weight 100 kg) was recently extubated and is receiving PN. His PN formula contains 35 kcal/kg, protein 1.2 g/kg, dextrose infusing at 4.4 mg/kg/minute, and 25% of total calories as lipid. He has gradually developed symptoms of hypercapnia and has developed a respiratory acidosis. The medical team is considering strategies to correct this to avoid reintubation. Which change to the PN formula could best correct this situation?

    A. Change PN to EN and maintain current caloric goals.

    B. Reduce dextrose amount in PN to 3 mg/kg/minute and increase lipid to maintain current caloric goal.

    C. Change electrolytes to the acetate salt in the PN to correct the acid-base imbalance.

    D. Reduce the calories to 25 kcal/kg to prevent overfeeding.

M. Monitoring Patients Who Are Receiving PN
    1. Monitor for infection (temperature, WBC, intravenous access site).
    2. Monitor for peripheral vein thrombophlebitis or infiltration (if peripheral access); symptoms include pain, erythema, and tenderness or a palpable cord at the site of the peripheral vein; treat by removing catheter.
    3. Monitor fluid status (weight, edema, vital signs, input and output, temperature).
    4. Monitor nutritional status.
        a. Prealbumin is very useful in monitoring the effects of long-term nutrition support in patients who are not critically ill (see EN Monitoring earlier) because it has a shorter half-life.
            i.   Values
                 (a) Normal range, 16–40 mg/dL
                 (b) Moderate malnutrition, 11–16 mg/dL
                 (c) Severe malnutrition, less than 11 mg/dL
            ii. Goal for malnourished patients is an increase of at least 3–5 mg/dL/week until within normal range.
        b. Serum albumin (normal 3.5–5 g/dL) is a poor predictor of nutritional status because it has a long half-life, and concentrations fluctuate during illness.
    5. Monitor for hyperglycemia and hypoglycemia.
        a. A common blood glucose goal is 150 mg/dL or less.
        b. Regular insulin (initially 0.05–0.2 unit per gram of dextrose) can be added to the PN for patients using a consistent dosage.
        c. For patients with hyperglycemia or fluctuating insulin dosages, insulin can be supplemented separately from the PN, although this practice varies by practitioner.
        d. Abrupt discontinuation of PN is usually tolerated in nondiabetic patients, but rebound hypoglycemia may occur in other patients; avoid by gradually tapering off PN over 1–2 hours; check blood glucose 30 minutes to 1 hour after discontinuing PN. If PN is discontinued abruptly, can avoid rebound hypoglycemia by administering 5% or 10% dextrose (may not be necessary if PN is administered through a peripheral catheter)
    6. Monitor for electrolyte and acid-base imbalances. The chloride and acetate salts can be adjusted on the basis of the acid-base status of the patient.
        a. For metabolic alkalosis, Na^+ and K^+ can be administered as the chloride salts.
        b. For metabolic acidosis, Na^+ and K^+ can be administered as the acetate salts (acetate is converted to bicarbonate).
        c. For respiratory acid-base disorders, correct the underlying cause or adjust the ventilator settings as needed.

7. Monitor triglyceride concentrations and withhold lipids in patients with a concentration greater than 400 mg/dL. When calculating lipid requirements, account for any drugs mixed in a lipid emulsion (e.g., propofol, clevidipine).
8. Monitor hepatic function.
9. Monitor for patient readiness for oral or EN support.
   a. Well-nourished, healthy patients can change immediately from PN to oral or EN.
   b. Older adult, debilitated, or malnourished patients may need a transition period in which oral or EN feedings are gradually increased, coinciding with a reduction in PN.

Patient Cases

10. A patient (weight 70 kg) receives propofol at 45 mcg/kg/minute. Propofol is available at a concentration of 10 mg/mL and is mixed in a 10% lipid emulsion. Assuming the patient is receiving this infusion rate for 24 hours, which best approximates the total calories provided by the propofol infusion in a 24-hour period?

   A. 200 kcal.

   B. 250 kcal.

   C. 300 kcal.

   D. 500 kcal.

11. A patient (weight 65 kg) is receiving PN after abdominal surgery. The PN contains about 1600 kcal, including 100 g of protein, 500 kcal as lipid, and 200 g of dextrose. The following additives are also included in a 24-hour infusion of PN: sodium chloride 50 mEq, sodium acetate 100 mEq, potassium acetate 60 mEq, sodium phosphate 30 mmol, magnesium sulfate 12 mEq, calcium gluconate 10 mEq/day, multivitamins 10 mL, and several trace elements 3 mL. The patient has an NG tube in place and is suctioning about 400–500 mL/day, which is being replaced with an infusion of 0.9% sodium chloride. After 48 hours of PN, the patient has the following laboratory values: Na^+ 140 mEq/L, K^+ 3.8 mEq/L, Cl^- 93 mEq/L, serum bicarbonate 35 mEq/L, pH 7.5, P_{CO_2} 47 mm Hg, and bicarbonate 36 mEq/L. Which adjustment to the PN formula is best at this time?

   A. Increase lipids to provide 750 kcal and reduce dextrose to 130 g.

   B. Increase sodium acetate to 150 mEq/day and discontinue sodium chloride.

   C. Increase sodium chloride to 150 mEq/day and discontinue sodium acetate.

   D. Add sodium bicarbonate 50 mEq to PN.

Questions 12 and 13 pertain to the following case.
A 75-year-old woman (weight 50 kg) is receiving PN after an extensive bowel resection. She is expected to require about 1 week of PN. She is receiving the following macronutrients in her formula: 70% dextrose 300 mL, 10% lipid 300 mL, and 10% AA 750 mL.

12. If these macronutrients are infused over 24 hours, which most closely approximates the total calories this patient is receiving daily?

   A. 20 kcal/kg.

   B. 26 kcal/kg.

   C. 30 kcal/kg.

   D. 35 kcal/kg.

Patient Cases *(continued)*

13. The patient has received the PN formula for 3 days. Her blood glucose concentrations have ranged from 220 to 280 mg/dL. She has orders for the following sliding scale of regular insulin: blood glucose 200–250 mg/dL, give 2 units; blood glucose 251–300 mg/dL, give 4 units; and blood glucose 301–350 mg/dL, give 6 units. She has been receiving about 14–16 units of insulin daily through the sliding-scale orders. Her medical history is significant for hypertension, diabetes, chronic obstructive pulmonary disease, and colon cancer. She was recently initiated on methylprednisolone 60 mg intravenously every 6 hours for a chronic obstructive pulmonary disease exacerbation. Today, the dose will be reduced to 40 mg intravenously every 8 hours. Which is the best recommendation to better control this patient's blood glucose?

A. Add insulin glargine 10–20 units/day to PN.

B. Change 70% dextrose in PN to D_5W.

C. Increase the sliding-scale insulin to 4 units for blood glucose 200–250 mg/dL, 8 units for blood glucose 251–300 mg/dL, and 12 units for blood glucose 301–350 mg/dL.

D. Add neutral protamine Hagedorn insulin 5 units subcutaneously every 12 hours.

REFERENCES

Fluids and Electrolytes

1. Cohn JN, Kowey PR, Whelton PK, et al. New guidelines for potassium replacement in clinical practice. A contemporary review by the National Council on Potassium in Clinical Practice. Arch Intern Med 2000;160:2429-36.

2. Dellinger RP, Levy MM, Rhodes A, et al. Surviving Sepsis Campaign: international guidelines for management of severe sepsis and septic shock. Crit Care Med 2013;41:580-637.

3. Dickerson RN, Maish GO III, Weinberg JA, et al. Safety and efficacy of intravenous hypotonic 0.225% sodium chloride infusion for the treatment of hypernatremia in critically ill patients. Nutr Clin Pract 2013;28:400-8.

4. Kellum JA, Cerda J, Kaplan LJ, et al. Fluids for prevention and management of acute kidney injury. Int J Artif Organs 2008;31:96-110.

5. Kraft MD, Btaiche IF, Sacks GS, et al. Treatment of electrolyte disorders in adult patients in the intensive care unit. Am J Health Syst Pharm 2005;62:1663-82.

6. Perel P, Roberts I, Ker K. Colloids versus crystalloids for fluid resuscitation in critically ill patients. Cochrane Database Syst Rev 2013;2:CD000567.

7. Polderman KH, Schreuder WO, Strack van Schijndel RJ, et al. Hypernatremia in the intensive care unit: an indicator of quality of care? Crit Care Med 1999;27:1105-8.

8. Rose BD, Post TW. Clinical Physiology of Acid-Base and Electrolyte Disorders, 5th ed. New York: McGraw-Hill, 2001.

9. Sterns RH. Hypernatremia in the intensive care unit: instant quality—just add water. Crit Care Med 1999;27:1041-2.

10. Verbalis JG, Goldsmith SR, Greenberg A, et al. Diagnosis, evaluation, and treatment of hyponatremia: expert panel recommendations. Am J Med 2013;126:S1-42.

11. Vincent JL, Weil MH. Fluid challenge revisited. Crit Care Med 2006;34:1333-7.

Nutrition

1. A.S.P.E.N. Board of Directors. Guidelines for the use of parenteral and enteral nutrition in adult and pediatric patients. J Parenter Enter Nutr 2002;26(suppl):1SA-138SA.

2. Bankhead R, Boullata J, Brantley S, et al. A.S.P.E.N. enteral nutrition practice recommendations. J Parenter Enter Nutr 2009;33:122.

3. Btaiche IF, Khalidi N. Metabolic complications of parenteral nutrition in adults, part 1. Am J Health Syst Pharm 2004;61:1938-49.

4. Btaiche IF, Khalidi N. Metabolic complications of parenteral nutrition in adults, part 2. Am J Health Syst Pharm 2004;61:2050-7.

5. Canada T, Crill C, Guenter P. A.S.P.E.N. Parenteral Nutrition Handbook. Silver Spring, MD: American Society of Parenteral and Enteral Nutrition, 2009.

6. Marik PE. Maximizing efficacy from parenteral nutrition in critical care: appropriate patient populations, supplemental parenteral nutrition, glucose control, parenteral glutamine, and alternative fat sources. Curr Gastroenterol Rep 2007;9:345-53.

7. Martindale RG, McClave SA, Vanek VW, et al. Guidelines for the provision and assessment of nutrition support therapy in the adult critically ill patient: Society of Critical Care Medicine and American Society for Parenteral and Enteral Nutrition: executive summary. Crit Care Med 2009;37:1757-61.

8. Miller SJ. Commercial premixed parenteral nutrition: is it right for your institution? Nutr Clin Pract 2009;24:459-69.

9. Mirtallo J, Canada T, Johnson D, et al. Task Force for the Revision of Safe Practices for Parenteral Nutrition. Safe practices for parenteral nutrition. J Parenter Enter Nutr 2004;28:S39-70.

10. Newton DW, Driscoll DF. Calcium and phosphate compatibility: revisited again. Am J Health Syst Pharm 2008;65:73-80.

11. Stapleton RD, Jones N, Heyland DK. Feeding critically ill patients: what is the optimal amount of energy? Crit Care Med 2007;35:S535-40.

ANSWERS AND EXPLANATIONS TO PATIENT CASES

1. Answer: C

Although this patient's blood pressure is not necessarily low, it is probably low compared with his baseline, considering his history of hypertension. In addition to his low blood pressure, his other signs and symptoms of intravascular volume depletion include an elevated BUN/Cr ratio and a reduced urine output. Crystalloids or colloids are appropriate fluids for resuscitation, making lactated Ringer solution (Answer C) the best option. Furosemide (Answer A) may increase his urine output but at the cost of further depleting the intravascular volume. Albumin 25% (Answer B) should be avoided for fluid resuscitation because it causes a shift of fluid from the IS space into the intravascular space, which can potentiate his dehydration. Answer D would be appropriate for a maintenance infusion; however, $D_5W/0.45\%$ sodium chloride plus potassium chloride 20 mEq/L would not provide optimal replacement of the intravascular space, given the distribution in TBF.

2. Answer: C

This patient has no current signs or symptoms of intravascular volume depletion, so he does not require fluid resuscitation. Because he is not taking adequate fluids by mouth, he should be given maintenance intravenous fluid to prevent dehydration and electrolyte imbalances. This is typically accomplished by a combination of free water and 0.45% sodium chloride with K^+ (Answer C). The infusion rate is calculated as 1500 mL + (60 kg × 20 mL/kg) = 2700 mL/24 hours, or about 110 mL/hour. Parenteral nutrition (Answer A) is inappropriate because there is no evidence that the patient's GI tract is nonfunctional. Albumin 5% (Answer B) or lactated Ringer solution (Answer D) should be reserved for fluid resuscitation in patients with signs or symptoms of intravascular volume depletion.

3. Answer: B

Although this patient has symptomatic hyponatremia, she also has signs of intravascular volume depletion. This intravascular volume depletion is a potent stimulus for ADH secretion, which will potentiate hyponatremia. In patients with hyponatremia and intravascular volume depletion, it is important to restore intravascular volume first to prevent organ hypoperfusion and inhibit ADH secretion. Fluid resuscitation should be accomplished with 0.9% sodium chloride as a fluid bolus, followed by a reevaluation of fluid status (Answer B). A slower infusion of 0.9% sodium chloride (Answer A) will not quickly restore intravascular volume. Once the intravascular volume is restored, ADH secretion will cease. This can be followed by a water diuresis, with a subsequent rise in the serum sodium concentration. Of importance, the patient should be monitored closely to prevent a rise in serum sodium greater than 10–12 mEq/L/day. If serum sodium rises too fast, 0.45% sodium chloride can be infused to slow the rate of rise of serum sodium concentration. Hypertonic saline (Answers C and D) would not be advisable unless the patient continued to have symptoms of hyponatremia after appropriate fluid resuscitation.

4. Answer: C

To prevent central pontine myelinolysis in patients with hyponatremia, it is recommended that the serum sodium concentration be raised by no more than 10–12 mEq/L in 24 hours (Answer C). Of note, the goal is not to achieve a normal serum sodium concentration in 24 hours. Rapid correction of chronic hyponatremia can cause permanent neurologic damage (Answers A and B), and because this patient is symptomatic, she should not be maintained at her current sodium concentration (Answer D).

5. Answer: D

This patient has hyponatremia and hypokalemia. In patients with hypokalemia, there is a reduction in IC K^+. To maintain cellular electroneutrality, Na^+ will shift into cells. As K^+ is replaced, Na^+ shifts out of cells, and the serum sodium concentration rises. Therefore, in this case, the hypokalemia should be corrected first, which will cause a subsequent improvement in the hyponatremia. Because this patient has no ECG changes related to the hypokalemia, oral supplementation with K^+ (Answer D) is recommended over intravenous replacement (Answer A). A dose of 60–80 mEq/day should cause an increase in the K^+ concentration by about 0.6–0.8 mEq/L. Because the patient is eating a regular diet, she should no longer require intravenous fluids (Answer B). Hypertonic saline (Answer C) is incorrect because this patient has no serious symptoms of hyponatremia.

6. Answer: D

This patient has not been given enough water, and she cannot communicate (or feel) thirst. This medical error can be prevented by administering about 1 mL of water for every calorie administered. It should also be prevented by monitoring serum sodium concentrations and adjusting water intake as needed. To correct the hypernatremia, water should be administered, preferably through the enteral feeding tube (Answer D). If this is not possible, it can be administered intravenously as D_5W (Answer B or C) but never as sterile water (Answer A). Sterile water administered intravenously can cause hemolysis and death. The patient's water deficit (in liters) can be estimated by the equation $0.4 \times LBW \times [(Na^+/140) - 1]$. Water should be replaced over several days, taking care to avoid changes in serum sodium greater than 10–12 mEq/L in 24 hours.

7. Answer: B

This patient has ECG changes consistent with hyperkalemia. Insulin (Answer B) will have the fastest onset and most predictable action of lowering serum potassium. Calcium gluconate (Answer A) should be avoided in this patient because it can potentiate digoxin toxicity and bradycardia. The efficacy of sodium bicarbonate (Answer C) is not well established. Albuterol (Answer D) can be efficacious when added to insulin, but it may not be effective in about 40% of patients and is therefore not recommended as initial therapy or as monotherapy for hyperkalemia.

8. Answer: C

This patient is receiving a calorie-dense EN formula that typically has less water than other enteral products. Therefore, although not currently hypernatremic, the patient is at risk of developing hypernatremia because of insufficient water intake. This can be prevented by administering additional water. The preferred route is enteral, if possible. The additional water needed on a daily basis can be estimated as 1 mL/kcal. Therefore, if this patient is receiving enteral feeding at 35 mL/hour × 2 kcal/mL, she is receiving 1680 kcal/day. She is receiving only 710 mL of water per liter of enteral formula, which is 596 mL/day for the 840 mL of enteral feeding daily (35 mL/hour × 24 hours = 840 mL/day). Because she is receiving 1680 kcal, she needs about 1680 mL of water per day. Subtracting the water from the feedings from the total needed, 1680 − 596 = 1084 mL is needed. This can be divided and administered through the

gastric feeding tube at about 180 mL/dose every 4 hours (Answer C). Of note, the patient should be monitored for fluid overload, especially given her chronic kidney disease. Given this patient's stable kidney disease and her adequate urine output, she should be able to tolerate this amount of free water. The amount of free water needed on a daily basis is an estimation and should be adjusted on the basis of specific patient parameters (e.g., serum sodium, input, output, daily weight, edema). Free water should not be administered as intravenous dextrose (Answer B) unless enteral administration is not feasible. Answer A is incorrect because reducing Na^+ will not prevent hypernatremia; the problem is related to too little water rather than too much Na^+. Answer D is incorrect because the caloric goals should not be sacrificed, and they would not eliminate the problem of insufficient water administered.

9. Answer: D

This patient is developing a respiratory acidosis, possibly because of overfeeding. Although dextrose is metabolized to water and CO_2, it generally will not cause a respiratory acidosis unless the patient is being overfed. Reducing the total calories to 25 kcal/kg decreases the risk of overfeeding, and reintubation can be avoided (Answer D). Answer A is incorrect because patients can be overfed with either PN or EN. Answer B is incorrect because, even if the dextrose in the PN is reduced, the patient can still develop symptoms of overfeeding. Answer C is incorrect because the underlying (overfeeding) cause should be corrected, rather than adjusting the acetate to treat a respiratory acidosis.

10. Answer: D

To determine the amount of calories provided by propofol, it must first be determined how many milliliters a day are infused. For this patient receiving propofol 45 mcg/kg/minute and weighing 70 kg, 454 mL is infused daily (assuming a constant infusion rate). Next, if a 10% lipid emulsion provides about 1.1 kcal/mL, it can be calculated that 454 mL/day of propofol provides about 500 kcal/day, making Answer D correct and Answers A–C incorrect.

11. Answer: C

This patient has developed a metabolic alkalosis, probably secondary to the loss of gastric fluid through NG suctioning. The low serum chloride and elevated serum bicarbonate concentrations support this theory.

In addition, the acid base is consistent with metabolic alkalosis with compensatory respiratory acidosis. The treatment in this circumstance is to replace the lost fluid with 0.9% sodium chloride, which is being done. In addition, Na^+ and K^+ can be administered as the chloride salt rather than the acetate salt (Answer C). For this case, only Na^+ is converted to chloride salt, and K^+ is left as the acetate salt initially. With daily monitoring, the ratio of Cl^- to acetate can be adjusted further if needed. Answer B is incorrect because it would probably worsen the metabolic alkalosis as the sodium acetate is converted to bicarbonate. Answer A is incorrect because hypercapnia is a compensatory response, not the primary acid-base disturbance. Answer D is incorrect for several reasons. First, it is never advisable to add sodium bicarbonate to PN because of incompatibility and the risk of calcium-phosphate precipitation. Second, sodium bicarbonate is the incorrect treatment for metabolic alkalosis because it can worsen alkalosis.

12. Answer: B
The total calories are calculated by adding the calories provided by dextrose, lipid, and AA. Dextrose provides 714 kcal (210 g × 3.4 kcal/g), lipid provides about 300 kcal (30 g × 10 kcal/g), and AA provides 300 kcal (75 g × 4 kcal/g). Adding these together provides calories of 1314 kcal/50 kg = 26.3 kcal/kg, making Answer B correct and Answers A, C, and D incorrect.

13. Answer: D
This patient's hyperglycemia could be attributable to either stress or corticosteroids. Because the corticosteroid dose is being tapered, the blood glucose concentrations will probably decrease with time. For patients with a fluctuating blood glucose concentration, it can be difficult to add insulin to PN because insulin cannot be adjusted in a timely manner. Regardless, Answer A is incorrect because long-acting insulin should not be added to PN. If insulin is added to PN, it should be regular insulin. Although some experts promote "permissive underfeeding," Answer B is incorrect because it would provide insufficient calories for this patient. Sliding scales of insulin can be useful when used in conjunction with a baseline of insulin in patients with a fluctuating blood glucose concentration. However, a sliding scale (Answer C) should not be used as the primary intervention for blood glucose control because it is reactive and fails to prevent hyperglycemia. In addition, the sliding scale described recommends insulin only when the blood glucose reaches 200, which is too high. Answer D is correct because it provides a baseline of insulin that can be adjusted in a timely manner as the blood glucose concentrations fluctuate according to the patient's status.

ANSWERS AND EXPLANATIONS TO SELF-ASSESSMENT QUESTIONS

1. Answer: D

This patient continues to have hypotension and tachycardia, both signs of intravascular volume depletion. The improvement in blood pressure and tachycardia after a fluid bolus also indicates intravascular volume depletion. Fluid administration should continue until there is no further improvement in vital signs. Patients with intravascular volume depletion require a rapid bolus of crystalloid (either 0.9% sodium chloride or lactated Ringer solution) of 500–1000 mL (or about 30 mL/kg), followed by reassessment (Answer D). A rapid bolus is essential to prevent organ dysfunction caused by hypoperfusion. Although the patient has poor urine output, administering furosemide (Answer A) will worsen volume depletion. As volume is replaced, urine output will probably increase. Administering 5% albumin in combination with a vasopressor (Answer B) should not be the initial treatment as long as vital signs are improving with the administration of fluid boluses with 0.9% sodium chloride. In addition, colloids are more expensive, and there is no evidence of better outcomes for fluid resuscitation with colloids than with crystalloids. Furthermore, infusion of albumin over 4 hours is incorrect because it would not restore intravascular volume rapidly enough to prevent organ dysfunction. Intravenous fluid containing D_5W (Answer C) is not appropriate for fluid resuscitation, regardless of the blood glucose concentration.

2. Answer: A

To answer this question, an alligation must first be set up using 0.9% and 23.4% sodium chloride. If 0.9% sodium chloride contains 154 mEq/L, 3% should contain about 513 mEq/L. After completing the alligation, the correct amounts can be double-checked by verifying the amount of sodium chloride in the prepared product: 907 mL of 0.9% sodium chloride contains 140 mEq of sodium chloride, and 93 mL of 23.4% sodium chloride contains 372 mEq of sodium chloride; therefore, 140 mEq + 372 mEq = 512 mEq/L of sodium chloride in the final product. The osmolarity is calculated as (3 g/100 mL) × (1 mol/58.5 g) × (2 Osm/mol) × (1000 mOsm/Osm) × (1000 mL/L) × 0.93 = 954 mOsm/L (Answer A is correct; Answer C is incorrect). Because of the osmotic coefficient (0.93), the sodium chloride does not completely dissociate in solution. Although use of the osmotic coefficient provides a more accurate osmolarity, it is probably not clinically relevant in calculating the osmolarity of intravenous sodium chloride. Therefore, it is safe to estimate the osmolarity of sodium chloride as either 954 or 1026 mOsm/L because there is no apparent clinical difference between these osmolarities. Because the osmolarity is greater than 900 mOsm/L, the infusion should be administered through a central line, if possible, to prevent pain and irritation (Answers B and D are incorrect).

3. Answer: D

In this case, hyponatremia is likely because of congestive heart failure and has probably developed over a prolonged period (not acute onset). Patients with chronic hyponatremia because of heart failure are typically asymptomatic. Rapid correction of chronic hyponatremia is associated with permanent neurologic damage caused by central pontine myelinolysis. Furthermore, hypertonic saline can worsen volume overload in patients with heart failure. Although hyponatremia is a sign of worsening heart failure, correction of hyponatremia in patients with heart failure does not improve outcomes (Answer D). For these reasons, the risks of correcting the serum sodium with hypertonic saline (Answers A–C) outweigh the potential benefits.

4. Answer: B

Patients with hyperkalemia and ECG changes should be treated first with Ca^{2+} for cardiac stability (Answer B). After Ca^{2+} administration, other measures can be taken to shift K^+ from the EC compartment to the IC compartment. Insulin (Answer A) can accomplish this; however, in this patient with hyperglycemia, insulin should be administered without glucose. Sodium polystyrene sulfonate (Kayexalate; Answer C) can be administered, but it is not effective immediately and is therefore not appropriate for first-line treatment of symptomatic hyperkalemia. Sodium bicarbonate (Answer D) is incorrect because it does not treat cardiac instability.

5. Answer: C

This patient is not taking adequate nutritional intake because of her mental status. Because her GI tract is functional, it should be used for feeding to prevent gut mucosal atrophy. An NG or nasoduodenal feeding tube is appropriate for enteral access for short-term nutritional support (Answer C). A percutaneous gastrostomy tube (Answer D), which requires a surgical procedure, is used for long-term nutritional support. The patient should receive 25–35 kcal/kg/day. The PN formulas (Answers A and B) should not be used in a patient with a functional GI tract. Although Answer B would be an appropriate PN formula for peripheral administration, PN is associated with more complications than EN.

6. Answer: C
This correct formula provides about 30 kcal/kg of calories, 1.5 g of protein per kilogram (AA), and 30% of total calories as lipid (Answer C). Answer A is incorrect because it provides 1000 calories as lipid, which is about 62% of the total calories provided. Answer B is incorrect because it contains only 0.8 g/kg of AA, an insufficient amount considering the patient's stress and apparent absence of kidney injury. Answer D is incorrect because it contains too much AA.

7. Answer: B
This patient has hypomagnesemia and hypokalemia. Correction of hypokalemia requires correction of hypomagnesemia to prevent renal loss of K^+ (Answer B). Magnesium should be administered slowly to avoid hypotension and increased renal excretion caused by rapid administration. Continued K^+ should not be given until magnesium is administered (Answers A and C). Calcium correction will not have a large effect on K^+ correction (Answer D).

8. Answer: C
Enteral nutrition prevents gut mucosal atrophy and subsequent bacterial translocation (Answer C). Bacterial translocation is the crossing of bacteria from the GI tract into the systemic circulation. Enteral nutrition is associated with fewer infectious complications than is PN, which may be partly because of a reduction in bacterial translocation (Answers A and B). Zinc does not affect atrophy and bacterial translocation (Answer D).

9. Answer: C
It is a common misconception that all patients with kidney failure need protein restriction (Answers A and B). This is true if they are not undergoing dialysis. Conversely, if they are undergoing dialysis, they do not need protein restriction and can receive AA at 1.2–1.5 g/kg/day (Answer C). Answer D is incorrect because too much protein is given.

Biostatistics: A Refresher

Kevin M. Sowinski, Pharm.D., FCCP

Purdue University College of Pharmacy
Indiana University School of Medicine
West Lafayette and Indianapolis, Indiana

BIOSTATISTICS: A REFRESHER

KEVIN M. SOWINSKI, PHARM.D., FCCP

PURDUE UNIVERSITY COLLEGE OF PHARMACY
INDIANA UNIVERSITY SCHOOL OF MEDICINE
WEST LAFAYETTE AND INDIANAPOLIS, INDIANA

Learning Objectives

1. Describe differences between descriptive and inferential statistics.
2. Identify different types of data (nominal, ordinal, continuous [ratio and interval]) to determine an appropriate type of statistical test (parametric vs. nonparametric).
3. Describe strengths and limitations of different types of measures of central tendency (mean, median, and mode) and data spread (standard deviation, standard error of the mean, range, and interquartile range).
4. Describe the concepts of normal distribution and the associated parameters that describe the distribution.
5. State the types of decision errors that can occur when using statistical tests and the conditions under which they can occur.
6. Describe hypothesis testing and state the meaning of and distinguish between p-values and confidence intervals.
7. Describe areas of misuse or misrepresentation that are associated with various statistical methods.
8. Select appropriate statistical tests on the basis of the sample distribution, data type, and study design.
9. Interpret statistical significance for results from commonly used statistical tests.
10. Describe the similarities and differences between statistical tests; state how to apply them appropriately.
11. Identify the use of survival analysis and different ways to perform and report it.

Self-Assessment Questions

Answers and explanations to these questions can be found at the end of the chapter.

1. A randomized controlled trial assesses the effects of the treatment of heart failure on global functioning in three groups of adults after 6 months of treatment. Investigators wanted to assess global functioning with the New York Heart Association (NYHA) functional classification, an ordered scale from I to IV, and to compare the patient classification after 6 months of treatment. Which statistical test is most appropriate to assess differences in functional classification between the groups?

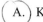

   A. Kruskal-Wallis test.
   B. Wilcoxon signed rank test.
   C. Analysis of variance (ANOVA).
   D. Analysis of covariance (ANCOVA).

2. You are evaluating a randomized, double-blind, parallel-group controlled trial that compares four antihypertensive drugs for their effect on blood pressure. The authors conclude that hydrochlorothiazide is better than atenolol (p<0.05) and that enalapril is better than hydrochlorothiazide (p<0.01), but no difference is observed between any other drugs. The investigators used an unpaired (independent samples) t-test to test the hypothesis that each drug was equal to the other. Which statement is most appropriate?

   A. Investigators used the appropriate statistical test to analyze their data.
   B. Enalapril is the most effective of these drugs.

   C. ANOVA would have been a more appropriate test.
   D. A paired t-test is a more appropriate test.

3. In the results of a randomized, double-blind, controlled clinical trial, the difference in hospital readmission rates between the intervention group and the control group is 6% (p=0.01), and it is concluded that there is a statistically significant difference between the groups. Which statement is most consistent with this finding and conclusions?
   A. The chance of making a type I error is 5 in 100.
   B. The trial does not have enough power.
   C. There is a high likelihood of having made a type II error.
   D. The chance of making a type I error is 1 in 100.

4. You are reading a manuscript that evaluates the impact of obesity on enoxaparin pharmacokinetics. The authors used an unpaired t-test to compare the baseline values of body mass index (BMI) in normal subjects and obese subjects. You are evaluating the use of an unpaired t-test to compare the BMI between the two groups. Which choice represents the most appropriate criteria to be met to use this parametric test?

A. The sample sizes in the normal and obese subjects should be equal to allow the use of a t-test.

B. A t-test is not appropriate because BMI data are ordinal.

C. The variance of the BMI data has to be similar in each group.

D. The prestudy power should be at least 90%.

5. You are evaluating the results and discussion of a journal club article to present to the pharmacy residents at your institution. The randomized, prospective, controlled trial evaluated the efficacy of a new controller drug for asthma. The primary end point was the morning forced expiratory volume in 1 second (FEV_1) in two groups of subjects (men and women). The difference in FEV_1 between the two groups was 15% (95% confidence interval [CI], 10%–21%). Which statement is most appropriate, given the results?

A. Without the reporting of a p-value, it is not possible to conclude whether these results were statistically significant.

B. There is a statistically significant difference between the men and women ($p<0.05$).

C. There is a statistically significant difference between the men and women ($p<0.01$).

D. There is no statistically significant difference between the men and women.

6. An early-phase clinical trial of 40 subjects evaluated a new drug known to increase high-density lipoprotein cholesterol (HDL-C) concentrations. The objective of the trial was to compare the new drug's ability to increase HDL-C with that of lifestyle modifications (active control group). At the beginning of the study, the mean baseline HDL-C was 37 mg/dL in the active control group and 38 mg/dL in the new drug group. At the end of the 3-month trial, the mean HDL-C for the control group was 44 mg/dL and for the new drug group, 49 mg/dL. The p-value for the comparison at 3 months was 0.08. Which statement provides the best interpretation of these results?

A. An a priori α of less than 0.10 would have made the study more clinically useful.

B. The new drug and active control appear to be equally efficacious in increasing HDL-C concentrations.

C. The new drug is better than lifestyle modifications because it increases HDL-C concentrations to a greater extent.

D. This study is potentially underpowered.

7. Researchers planned a study to evaluate the percentage of subjects who achieved less than a target blood pressure (less than 140/90 mm Hg) when initiating therapy with two different doses of amlodipine. In the study of 100 subjects, the amlodipine 5-mg group (n=50) and the amlodipine 10-mg group (n=50) were compared. The investigators used a blood pressure goal as their primary end point, defined as the percentage of subjects who successfully achieved the blood pressure goal at 3 months. Which is the most appropriate statistical test to answer such a question?

A. Independent samples t-test.

B. Chi-square or Fisher exact test.

C. Wilcoxon signed rank test.

D. One-sample t-test.

8. An investigational drug is being compared with an existing drug for the treatment of anemia in patients with chronic kidney disease. The study is designed to detect a minimum 20% difference in response rates between the groups, if one exists, with an a priori α of 0.05 or less. The investigators are unclear whether the 20% difference between response rates is too large and think a smaller difference might be more clinically meaningful. In revising their study, they decide they want to be able to detect a minimum 10% difference in response. Which change to the study parameters is most appropriate?

A. Increase the sample size.

B. Select an α of 0.001 as a cutoff for statistical significance.

C. Select an α of 0.10 as a cutoff for statistical significance.

D. Decrease the sample size.

9. You are designing a new computer alert system to investigate the impact of several factors on the risk of corrected QT interval (QTc) prolongation. You want to develop a model to predict which patients are most likely to experience QTc prolongation after the administration of certain drugs or the presence of certain conditions. You plan to assess the presence or absence of several different variables. Which technique will be most useful in completing such an analysis?

A. Correlation.
B. Kaplan-Meier curve.
C. Regression.
D. Confidence intervals.

	2 grp indep	2 gp related	>2 g indep	>2 related
m	x2 Fishers	mcNemar	x2	Cochran Q
rl	Wilcoxan mannll	signed	K w	Friedman ANOVA
nut	t test	paired t test	1 way	2 way repeated m
nut vri	ANCOVA	2 way repeatedm	2 way	2 way repeated m

I. INTRODUCTION TO STATISTICS

A. Method for Collecting, Classifying, Summarizing, and Analyzing Data

B. Useful Tool for Quantifying Clinical and Laboratory Data in a Meaningful Way

C. Assists in Determining Whether and by How Much a Treatment or Procedure Affects a Group of Patients

D. Why Pharmacists Need to Know Statistics

E. As Statistics Pertains to Most of You
   1. Pharmacotherapy Specialty Examination content outline, Domain 2: Drug Information and Evidence Based Medicine (25%)
   2. Task statements:
      a. Retrieve information that addresses pharmacotherapy-related inquiries in order to optimize patient care.
      b. Evaluate pharmacotherapy-related literature, databases, and health information in order to translate findings into practice.
      c. Conduct pharmacotherapy-related research using appropriate scientific principles in order to ensure optimal patient care.
      d. Disseminate pharmacotherapy-related information or research in order to educate health care professionals and trainees.

F. Examples of Online Statistical and Study Design Tools
   1. www.graphpad.com/quickcalcs/
   2. http://statpages.org/

G. Several Papers Have Investigated the Various Types of Statistical Tests Used in the Biomedical Literature; the data from one of these papers are illustrated below. Tables 1 and 2 modified from: Windish DM, Huot SJ, Green ML. Medicine resident's understanding of the biostatistics and results in the medical literature. JAMA 2007;298:1010-22.

Table 1. Statistical Content of Original Articles in *The New England Journal of Medicine,* 2004–2005

Statistical Procedure	% of Articles Containing Methods	Statistical Procedure	% of Articles Containing Methods
No statistics or descriptive statistics	13	Adjustment and standardization	1
t-Tests	26	Multiway tables	13
Contingency tables	53	Power analyses	39
Nonparametric tests	27	Cost-benefit analysis	<1
Epidemiologic statistics	35	Sensitivity analysis	6
Pearson correlation	3	Repeated-measures analysis	12
Simple linear regression	6	Missing-data methods	8
Analysis of variance	16	Noninferiority trials	4
Transformation	10	Receiver operating characteristics	2

Table 1. Statistical Content of Original Articles in *The New England Journal of Medicine,* 2004–2005 *(continued)*

Statistical Procedure	% of Articles Containing Methods	Statistical Procedure	% of Articles Containing Methods
Nonparametric correlation	5	Resampling	2
Survival methods	61	Principal component and cluster analyses	2
Multiple regression	51	Other methods	4
Multiple comparisons	23		

Table 2. Statistical Content of Original Articles from Six Major Medical Journals from January to March 2005 (n=239 Articles)[a]

Statistical Test	No. (%)	Statistical Test	No. (%)
Descriptive statistics (mean, median, frequency, SD, and IQR)	219 (91.6)	Others	
Simple statistics	120 (50.2)	Intention-to-treat analysis	42 (17.6)
Chi-square analysis	70 (29.3)	Incidence or prevalence	39 (16.3)
t-test	48 (20.1)	Relative risk or risk ratio	29 (12.2)
Kaplan-Meier analysis	48 (20.1)	Sensitivity analysis	21 (8.8)
Wilcoxon rank sum test	38 (15.9)	Sensitivity or specificity	15 (6.3)
Fisher exact test	33 (13.8)		
Analysis of variance	21 (8.8)		
Correlation	16 (6.7)		
Multivariate analysis	164 (68.6)		
Cox proportional hazards	64 (26.8)		
Multiple logistic regression	54 (22.6)		
Multiple linear regression	7 (2.9)		
Other regression analysis	38 (15.9)		
None	5 (2.1)		

[a]Articles published in *American Journal of Medicine, Annals of Internal Medicine, BMJ, The Journal of the American Medical Association, Lancet,* and *The New England Journal of Medicine.*

IQR = interquartile range; SD = standard deviation.

II. TYPES OF VARIABLES AND DATA

A. Definition: Random Variables—A variable with observed values that may be considered outcomes of an experiment and whose values cannot be anticipated with certainty before the experiment is conducted

B. Two Types of Random Variables
   1. Discrete variables (e.g., dichotomous, categorical)
   2. Continuous variables

C. Discrete Variables
   1. Can take only a limited number of values within a given range
   2. Nominal: Classified into groups in an unordered manner and with no indication of relative severity (e.g., male or female sex, mortality [dead or alive], disease presence [yes or no], race, marital status)
   3. Ordinal: Ranked in a specific order but with no consistent level of magnitude of difference between ranks (e.g., NYHA functional class describes the functional status of patients with heart failure, and subjects are classified in increasing order of symptoms: I, II, III, IV; Likert-type scales)
   4. Common error: Measure of central tendency—In most cases, means and standard deviations (SDs) should not be reported with ordinal data. What is a common incorrect use of means and SDs to show ordinal data?

D. Continuous Variables, Sometimes Referred to as Counting Variables
   1. Continuous variables can take on any value within a given range.
   2. Interval: Data are ranked in a specific order with a consistent change in magnitude between units; the zero point is arbitrary (e.g., degrees Fahrenheit).
   3. Ratio: Like "interval" but with an absolute zero (e.g., degrees Kelvin, heart rate, blood pressure, time, distance)

III. TYPES OF STATISTICS

A. Descriptive Statistics: Used to summarize and describe data that are collected or generated in research studies. This is done both visually and numerically.
   1. Visual methods of describing data
      a. Frequency distribution
      b. Histogram
      c. Scatterplot
      d. Boxplot
   2. Numerical methods of describing data: Measures of central tendency
      a. Arithmetic mean (i.e., average)
         i. Sum of all values divided by the total number of values
         ii. Should generally be used only for continuous and normally distributed data
         iii. Very sensitive to outliers and tend toward the tail, which has the outliers
         iv. Most commonly used and most understood measure of central tendency
         v. Geometric mean
      b. Median
         i. Midpoint of the values when placed in order from highest to lowest. Half of the observations are above and half are below. When there is an even number of observations, it is the mean of the two middle values.

        ii. Also called 50th percentile

       iii. Can be used for ordinal or continuous data (especially good for skewed populations)

       iv. Insensitive to outliers

  c. Mode

        i. Most common value in a distribution

       ii. Can be used for nominal, ordinal, or continuous data

      iii. Sometimes, there may be more than one mode (e.g., bimodal, trimodal).

      iv. Does not help describe meaningful distributions with a large range of values, each of which occurs infrequently

3. Numerical methods of describing data: Measures of data spread or variability

  a. Standard deviation

        i. Measure of the variability about the mean; most common measure used to describe the spread of data

       ii. Square root of the variance (average squared difference of each observation from the mean); returns variance back to original units (nonsquared)

      iii. Appropriately applied only to continuous data that are normally or near normally distributed or that can be transformed to be normally distributed

      iv. By the empirical rule for normal distributions, 68% of the sample values are found within ±1 SD, 95% are found within ±2 SD, and 99% are found within ±3 SD.

       v. The coefficient of variation relates the mean and the SD (SD/mean × 100%).

  b. Range

        i. Difference between the smallest and largest values in a data set does not give a tremendous amount of information by itself.

       ii. Easy to compute (simple subtraction)

      iii. Size of range is very sensitive to outliers.

      iv. Often reported as the actual values rather than the difference between the two extreme values

  c. Percentiles

        i. The point (value) in a distribution in which a value is larger than some percentage of the other values in the sample. Can be calculated by ranking all data in a data set

       ii. The 75th percentile lies at a point at which 75% of the other values are smaller.

      iii. Does not assume the population has a normal distribution (or any other distribution)

      iv. The interquartile range (IQR) is an example of the use of percentiles to describe the middle 50% values. The IQR encompasses the 25th–75th percentile.

4. Presenting data using only measures of central tendency can be misleading without some idea of data spread. Studies that report only medians or means without their accompanying measures of data spread should be closely scrutinized. What are the measures of spread that should be used with means and medians?

5. Example data set (Table 3)

Table 3. Twenty Baseline HDL-C Concentrations from an Experiment Evaluating the Impact of Green Tea on HDL-C

64	60	59	65	64	62	54
54	68	67	79	55	48	65
59	65	87	49	46	46	

HDL-C = high-density lipoprotein cholesterol.

  a. Calculate the mean, median, and mode of the above data set.

  b. Calculate the range, and SD (on examination you will not have to do this by hand).

  c. Evaluate the visual presentation of the data.

$Ca + .8(4-a(b))$

B. Inferential Statistics
1. Conclusions or generalizations made about a population (large group) from the study of a sample of that population
2. Choosing and evaluating statistical methods depend, in part, on the type of data used.
3. An educated statement about an unknown population is commonly referred to in statistics as an inference.
4. Statistical inference can be made by estimation or hypothesis testing.

IV. POPULATION DISTRIBUTIONS

A. Discrete Distributions
1. Binomial distribution
2. Poisson distribution

$SEM \dfrac{SD}{\sqrt{n}}$

B. Normal (Gaussian) Distribution
1. Most common model for population distributions
2. Symmetric or bell-shaped frequency distribution
3. Landmarks for continuous, normally distributed data
   a. μ: Population mean is equal to zero.
   b. σ: Population SD is equal to 1.
   c. x and s: These represent the sample mean and SD.
4. When a random variable is measured in a large enough sample of any population, some values will occur more often than will others.
5. A visual check of a distribution can help determine whether it is normally distributed (whether it appears symmetric and bell shaped). Need the data to perform these checks.
   a. Frequency distribution and histograms (visually look at the data; you should do this anyway)
   b. Median and mean will be about equal for normally distributed data (most practical and easiest to use).
   c. Formal test: Kolmogorov-Smirnov test
   d. More challenging to evaluate this when we do not have access to the data (when we are reading an article), because most articles do not present all data or both the mean and median
6. The parameters mean and SD define a normally distributed population.
7. Probability: The likelihood that any one event will occur given all the possible outcomes
8. Estimation and sampling variability
   a. One method that can be used to make an inference about a population parameter
   b. Separate samples (even of the same size) from a single population will give slightly different estimates.
   c. The distribution of means from random samples approximates a normal distribution.
      i. The mean of this "distribution of means" is equal to the unknown population mean, μ.
      ii. The SD of the means is estimated by the standard error of the mean (SEM).
      iii. As in any normal distribution, 95% of the sample means lie within ± 2 SEM of the population mean.
   d. The distribution of means from these random samples is about normal regardless of the underlying population distribution (central limit theorem). You will get slightly different mean and SD values each time you repeat this experiment.
   e. The SEM is estimated with a single sample by dividing the SD by the square root of the sample size (n). The SEM quantifies uncertainty in the estimate of the mean, not variability in the sample. Important for hypothesis testing and 95% CI estimation

f.   Why is all this information about the difference between the SEM and SD worth knowing?
    i.   Calculation of CIs. (95% CI is approximately the mean ± 2 times the SEM.)
    ii.   Hypothesis testing
    iii.   Deception (e.g., makes results look less "variable," especially when used in graphic format)

9.   Recall the previous example about HDL-C and green tea. From the calculated values in section III, do these data appear to be normally distributed?

V.   CONFIDENCE INTERVALS

A.   Commonly Reported as a Way to Estimate a Population Parameter

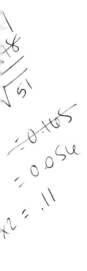

1.   In the medical literature, 95% CIs are the most commonly reported CIs. In repeated samples, 95% of all CIs include true population value (i.e., the likelihood or confidence [or probability] that the population value is contained within the interval). In some cases, 90% or 99% CIs are reported. Why are 95% CIs most often reported?

2.   Example
    a.   Assume a baseline birth weight in a group (n=51) with a mean ± SD of 1.18 ± 0.4 kg.
    b.   95% CI is about equal to the mean ± 1.96 × SEM (or 2 × SEM). In reality, it depends on the distribution being used and is a bit more complicated.
    c.   What is the 95% CI? The 95% CI is calculated to be (1.07, 1.29), meaning there is 95% certainty that the true mean of the entire population studied will be between 1.07 and 1.29 kg.
    d.   What is the 90% CI? The 90% CI is calculated to be (1.09, 1.27). Of note, the 95% CI will always be wider than the 90% CI for any given sample. Therefore, the wider the CI, the more likely it is to encompass the true population mean.

3.   The differences between the SD, SEM, and CIs should be noted when interpreting the literature because they are often used interchangeably. Although it is common for CIs to be confused with SDs, the information each provides is quite different and has to be assessed correctly.

4.   Recall the previous example about HDL-C and green tea. What is the 95% CI of the data set, and what does that mean?

B.   CIs Can Also Be Used for Any Sample Estimate. Estimates derived from categorical data such as risk, risk differences, and risk ratios are often presented with the CI and will be discussed below.

C.   CIs Instead of Hypothesis Testing
1.   Hypothesis testing and calculation of p-values tell us (ideally) whether there is or is not a statistically significant difference between groups, but they do not tell us anything about the magnitude of the difference.
2.   CIs help us determine the importance of a finding or findings, which we can apply to a situation.
3.   CIs give us an idea of the magnitude of the difference between groups and the statistical significance.
4.   CIs are a range of data, together with a point estimate of the difference.
5.   Wide CIs
    a.   Many results are possible, either larger or smaller than the point estimate provided by the study.
    b.   All values contained in the CI are statistically plausible.
6.   If the estimate is the difference between two continuous variables: A CI that includes zero (no difference between two variables) can be interpreted as not statistically significant (a p-value of 0.05 or greater). There is no need to show both the 95% CI and the p-value.
7.   The interpretation of CIs for odds ratios and relative risks is somewhat different. In that case, a value of 1 indicates no difference in risk, and if the CI includes 1, there is no statistical difference. (See the discussion of case-control/cohort in other sections for how to interpret CIs for odds ratios and relative risks.)

VI. HYPOTHESIS TESTING

A. Null and Alternative Hypotheses (see Table 4 for other types of examples)

1. Null hypothesis (H_0): Example: No difference between groups being compared (treatment A equals treatment B)

2. Alternative hypothesis (H_A): Example: Opposite of null hypothesis; states that there is a difference (treatment A does not equal treatment B)

3. The structure or the manner in which the hypothesis is written dictates which statistical test is used. Two-sample t-test: H_0: Mean 1 = Mean 2

4. Used to assist in determining whether any observed differences between groups can be explained by chance

5. Tests for statistical significance (hypothesis testing) determine whether the data are consistent with H_0 (no difference).

6. The results of the hypothesis testing will indicate whether enough evidence exists for H_0 to be rejected.
   a. If H_0 is rejected: Statistically significant difference between groups (unlikely attributable to chance)
   b. If H_0 is not rejected: No statistically significant difference between groups (any apparent differences may be attributable to chance). Note that we are not concluding that the treatments are equal.

7. Types of hypothesis testing. These are situations in which two groups are being compared. There are numerous other examples of situations these procedures could be applied to (Table 4).

Table 4. Types of Hypothesis Testing

	Question	Hypothesis	Method
Nondirectional			
Difference	Are the means different?	H_0: $Mean_1 = Mean_2$ H_A: $Mean_1 \neq Mean_2$ or H_0: $Mean_1 - Mean_2 = 0$ H_A: $Mean_1 - Mean_2 \neq 0$	Traditional 2-sided t-test Confidence intervals
Equivalence	Are the means practically equivalent?	H_0: $Mean_1 - Mean_2 \geq \Delta$ H_A: $Mean_1 - Mean_2 < \Delta$	Two 1-sided t-test (TOST) procedure Confidence intervals
Directional			
Superiority	Is mean 1 > mean 2? (or some other similarly worded question)	H_0: $Mean_1 \leq Mean_2$ H_A: $Mean_1 > Mean_2$ or H_0: $Mean_1 - Mean_2 \leq 0$ H_A: $Mean_1 - Mean_2 > 0$	Traditional 1-sided t-test Confidence intervals
Noninferiority	Is mean 1 no more than a certain amount lower than mean 2?	H_0: $Mean_1 - Mean_2 \geq \Delta$ H_A: $Mean_1 - Mean_2 < \Delta$	Confidence intervals

Δ = equivalence or noninferiority margin; H_0 = null hypothesis; H_A = alternative hypothesis.

B. To Determine What Is Sufficient Evidence to Reject H_0: Set the a priori significance level (α) and generate the decision rule.

1. Developed after the research question has been stated in hypothesis form

2. Used to determine the level of acceptable error caused by a false positive (also known as level of significance)
   a. Convention: A priori α is usually 0.05.
   b. Critical value is calculated, capturing how extreme the sample data must be to reject H_0.

C. Perform the Experiment and Estimate the Test Statistic.

1. A test statistic is calculated from the observed data in the study, which is compared with the critical value.

2. Depending on this test statistic's value, H_0 is not rejected (often referred to as fail to reject) or rejected.

3. In general, the test statistic and critical value are not presented in the literature; instead, p-values are generally reported and compared with a priori α values to assess statistical significance. p-value: Probability of obtaining a test statistic and critical value as extreme as or more extreme than the one actually obtained

4. Because computers are used in these tests, this step is often transparent; the p-value estimated in the statistical test is compared with the a priori α (usually 0.05), and the decision is made.

VII. STATISTICAL TESTS AND CHOOSING A STATISTICAL TEST

A. Which Tests Do You Need to Know?

B. Choosing the Appropriate Statistical Test Depends on the Following:

1. Type of data (nominal, ordinal, or continuous)
2. Distribution of data (e.g., normal)
3. Number of groups
4. Study design (e.g., parallel, crossover)
5. Presence of confounding variables
6. One-tailed versus two-tailed
7. Parametric versus nonparametric tests
   a. Parametric tests assume the following:
      i. Data being investigated have an underlying distribution that is normal or close to normal or, more correctly, randomly drawn from a parent population with a normal distribution. Remember how to estimate this (mean ~ median)?
      ii. Data measured are continuous data, measured on either an interval or a ratio scale.
      iii. Parametric tests assume that the data being investigated have variances that are homogeneous between the groups investigated. This is often called homoscedasticity.
   b. Nonparametric tests are used when data are not normally distributed or do not meet other criteria for parametric tests (e.g., discrete data). *ordinal/nominal*

C. Parametric Tests

1. Student t-test: Several different types
   a. One-sample test: Compares the mean of the study sample with the population mean

Group 1	Known population mean

   b. Two-sample, independent samples, or unpaired test: Compares the means of two independent samples. This is an independent samples test.

Group 1	Group 2

      i. Equal variance test
         (a) Rule for variances: If the ratio of larger variance to smaller variance is greater than 2, we generally conclude the variances are different.

        (b) Formal test for differences in variances: F test
        (c) Adjustments can be made for cases of unequal variance.
    ii. Unequal variance
  c. Paired test: Compares the mean difference of paired or matched samples. This is a related samples test.

Group 1	
Measurement 1	Measurement 2

  d. Common error: Use of multiple t-tests with more than two groups

2. Analysis of variance (ANOVA): A more generalized version of the t-test that can apply to more than two groups
  a. One-way ANOVA: Compares the means of three or more groups in a study; also known as single-factor ANOVA. This is an independent samples test.

Group 1	Group 2	Group 3

  b. Two-way ANOVA: Additional factor (e.g., age) added

Young groups	Group 1	Group 2	Group 3
Old groups	Group 1	Group 2	Group 3

  c. Repeated-measures ANOVA: This is a related samples test.

	Related Measurements		
Group 1	Measurement 1	Measurement 2	Measurement 3

  d. Several more complex factorial ANOVAs can be used.
  e. Many comparison procedures are used to determine which groups actually differ from each other. Post hoc tests: Tukey HSD (Honestly Significant Difference), Bonferroni, Scheffé, Newman-Keuls

3. Analysis of covariance (ANCOVA): Provides a method to explain the influence of a categorical variable (independent variable) on a continuous variable (dependent variable) while statistically controlling for other variables (confounding)

D. Nonparametric Tests
  1. These tests may also be used for continuous data that do not meet the assumptions of the t-test or ANOVA.
  2. Tests for independent samples
    a. Wilcoxon rank sum test, Mann-Whitney U test, or Wilcoxon Mann-Whitney test: Compare two independent samples (related to a t-test)
    b. Kruskal-Wallis one-way ANOVA by ranks
      i. Compares three or more independent groups (related to one-way ANOVA)
      ii. Post hoc testing
  3. Tests for related or paired samples
    a. Sign test and Wilcoxon signed rank test: Compares two matched or paired samples (related to a paired t-test)
    b. Friedman ANOVA by ranks: Compares three or more matched or paired groups

E. Nominal Data
1. Chi-square (χ^2) test: Compares expected and observed proportions between two or more groups
   a. Test of independence
   b. Test of goodness of fit
2. Fisher exact test: Specialized version of the chi-square test for small groups (cells) containing less than five predicted observations
3. McNemar: Paired samples
4. Mantel-Haenszel: Controls for the influence of confounders

F. Correlation and Regression (see section IX)

G. Choosing the Most Appropriate Statistical Test: Example 1
1. A trial was conducted to determine the efficacy and safety of alirocumab in reducing lipids and cardio-vascular events. Alirocumab plus statins was compared with placebo plus statins regarding their effect on low-density lipoprotein cholesterol (LDL-C) concentrations. The trial was designed such that the subjects' baseline characteristics were as comparable as possible with each other. *The intended primary end point for this trial was the difference in LDL-C between the two treatments at week 24.* The full trial is published: N Engl J Med 2015;372:1489-99. Note that only partial results are presented. The results of the trial are reported as follows:

Table 5. Baseline Characteristics and Alirocumab and Placebo Effect on LDL-C

	Alirocumab plus Statins (n=1553)	**Placebo plus Statins (n=788)**
Men/women	(63.3%) 983/570	(60.2%) 474/314
Smokers	(20.9 %) 325/1228	(20.2 %) 159/629
Baseline LDL-C, mg/dL	122.8 ± 42.7	122.0 ± 41.6
Final LDL-C, mg/dL	48.3 ± 35.2	118.9 ± 33.5

Data presented as mean ± SD. LDL-C = low-density lipoprotein cholesterol.

2. Which is the appropriate statistical test to determine baseline differences in the following:
   a. Sex distribution? Chi²
   b. LDL-C?
   c. Percentage of smokers and nonsmokers?
3. Which is the appropriate statistical test to determine the following:
   a. The effect of alirocumab plus statins on LDL-C?
   b. The primary end point?

VIII. DECISION ERRORS

Table 6. Summary of Decision Errors

	Underlying Truth or Reality	
Test Result	H_0 *is true* (no difference)	H_0 *is false* (difference)
Accept H_0 (no difference)	No error (correct decision)	Type II error (beta error)
Reject H_0 (difference)	Type I error (alpha error)	No error (correct decision)

H_0 = null hypothesis.

that doesn't exist

A. Type I Error: The probability of making this error is defined as the significance level α.
1. Convention is to set the α to 0.05, effectively meaning that, 1 in 20 times, a type I error will occur when the H_0 is rejected. So, 5.0% of the time, a researcher will conclude that there is a statistically significant difference when one does not actually exist.
2. The calculated chance that a type I error has occurred is called the p-value.
3. The p-value tells us the likelihood of obtaining a given (or a more extreme) test result if the H_0 is true. When the α level is set a priori, H_0 is rejected when p is less than α. In other words, the p-value tells us the probability of being wrong when we conclude that a true difference exists (false positive).
4. A lower p-value does not mean the result is more important or more meaningful but only that it is statistically significant and not likely to be attributable to chance.

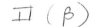 *II (β)*

B. Type II Error: The probability of making this error is called beta.
1. Concluding that no difference exists when one truly does (not rejecting H_0 when it should be rejected)
2. It has become a convention to set β between 0.20 and 0.10.

C. Power $(1 - β)$
1. The probability of making a correct decision when H_0 is false; the ability to detect differences between groups if one actually exists
2. Dependent on the following factors:
   a. Predetermined α
   b. Sample size
   c. The size of the difference between the outcomes you want to detect. Often not known before conducting the experiment, so to estimate the power of your test, you will have to specify how large a change is worth detecting
   d. The variability of the outcomes that are being measured
   e. Items c and d are generally determined from previous data or the literature.
3. Power is decreased by the following (in addition to the above criteria):
   a. Poor study design
   b. Incorrect statistical tests (use of nonparametric tests when parametric tests are appropriate)
4. Statistical power analysis and sample size calculation
   a. Related to above discussion of power and sample size
   b. Sample size estimates should be performed in all studies a priori.
   c. Necessary components for estimating appropriate sample size
      i. Acceptable type II error rate (usually 0.10–0.20)
      ii. Observed difference in predicted study outcomes that is clinically significant
      iii. The expected variability in item ii
      iv. Acceptable type I error rate (usually 0.05)
      v. Statistical test that will be used for primary end point
5. Statistical significance versus clinical significance
   a. As stated earlier, the size of the p-value is not necessarily related to the clinical importance of the result. Smaller values mean only that chance is less likely to explain observed differences.
   b. Statistically significant does not necessarily mean clinically significant.
   c. Lack of statistical significance does not mean that results are not clinically important.
   d. When considering nonsignificant findings, consider sample size, estimated power, and observed variability.

IX. CORRELATION AND REGRESSION

A. Introduction: Correlation Versus Regression
    1. Correlation examines the strength of the association between two variables. It does not necessarily assume that one variable is useful in predicting the other.
    2. Regression examines the ability of one or more variables to predict another variable.

B. Pearson Correlation
    1. The strength of the relationship between two variables that are normally distributed, ratio or interval scaled, and linearly related is measured with a correlation coefficient.
    2. Often referred to as the degree of association between the two variables
    3. Does not necessarily imply that one variable is dependent on the other (regression analysis will do that)
    4. Pearson correlation (r) ranges from −1 to +1 and can take any value in between:

−1	0	+1
Perfect negative linear relationship	No linear relationship	Perfect positive linear relationship

    5. Hypothesis testing is performed to determine whether the correlation coefficient is different from zero. This test is highly influenced by sample size.

C. Pearls About Correlation
    1. The closer the magnitude of r to 1 (either + or −), the more highly correlated the two variables. The weaker the relationship between the two variables, the closer r is to 0.
    2. There is no agreed-on or consistent interpretation of the value of the correlation coefficient. It is dependent on the environment of the investigation (laboratory vs. clinical experiment).
    3. Pay more attention to the magnitude of the correlation than to the p-value because it is influenced by sample size.
    4. Crucial to the proper use of correlation analysis is the interpretation of the graphic representation of the two variables. Before using correlation analysis, it is essential to generate a scatterplot of the two variables to visually examine the relationship.

D. Spearman Rank Correlation: Nonparametric test that quantifies the strength of an association between two variables but does not assume a normal distribution of continuous data. Can be used for ordinal data or nonnormally distributed continuous data

E. Regression
    1. A statistical technique related to correlation. There are many different types. For simple linear regression, one continuous outcome (dependent) variable and one continuous independent (causative) variable
    2. Two main purposes of regression: Development of prediction model and accuracy of prediction
    3. Prediction model: Making predictions of the dependent variable from the independent variable; $Y = mx + b$ (dependent variable = slope × independent variable + intercept)
    4. Accuracy of prediction: How well the independent variable predicts the dependent variable. Regression analysis determines the extent of variability in the dependent variable that can be explained by the independent variable.
        a. Coefficient of determination (r^2) measured describing this relationship. Values of r^2 can range from 0 to 1.
        b. An r^2 of 0.80 could be interpreted as saying that 80% of the variability in Y is explained by the variability in X.

    c.   This does not provide a mechanistic understanding of the relationship between X and Y but rather a description of how clearly such a model (linear or otherwise) describes the relationship between the two variables.

    d.   Like the interpretation of r, the interpretation of r^2 is dependent on the scientific arena (e.g., clinical research, basic research, social science research) to which it is applied.

5.   For simple linear regression, two statistical tests can be used.

    a.   To test the hypothesis that the y-intercept differs from zero

    b.   To test the hypothesis that the slope of the line is different from zero

6.   Regression is useful in constructing predictive models. The literature is full of examples of predictions. The process involves developing a formula for a regression line that best fits the observed data.

7.   Like correlation, there are many different types of regression analysis.

    a.   Multiple linear regression: One continuous independent variable and two or more continuous dependent variables

    b.   Simple logistic regression: One categorical response variable and one continuous or categorical explanatory variable

    c.   Multiple logistic regression: One categorical response variable and two or more continuous or categorical explanatory variables

    d.   Nonlinear regression: Variables are not linearly related (or cannot be transformed into a linear relationship). This is where our pharmacokinetic equations come from.

    e.   Polynomial regression: Any number of response and continuous variables with a curvilinear relationship (e.g., cubed, squared)

8.   Example of regression

    a.   The following data are taken from a study evaluating enoxaparin use. The authors were interested in predicting patient response (measured as antifactor Xa concentrations) from the enoxaparin dose in the 75 subjects who were studied.

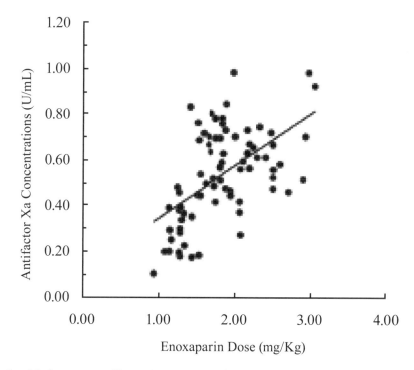

Figure 1. Relationship between antifactor Xa concentrations and enoxaparin dose.

b. The authors performed regression analysis and reported the following: Slope: 0.227, y-intercept: 0.097, $p<0.05$, $r^2 = 0.31$.

c. Answer the following questions:
i. What are the assumptions necessary to use regression analysis?
ii. Provide an interpretation of the coefficient of determination.
iii. Predict antifactor Xa concentrations at enoxaparin doses of 2 and 3.75 mg/kg.
iv. What does the $p<0.05$ value indicate?

X. SURVIVAL ANALYSIS

A. Studies the Time Between Entry in a Study and Some Event (e.g., death, myocardial infarction)
1. Censoring makes survival methods unique; considers that some subjects leave the study for reasons other than the event (e.g., lost to follow-up, end of study period)
2. Considers that all subjects do not enter the study at the same time
3. Standard methods of statistical analysis such as t-tests and linear or logistic regression may not be appropriately applied to survival data because of censoring.

B. Estimating the Survival Function
1. Kaplan-Meier method
   a. Uses survival times (or censored survival times) to estimate the proportion of people who would survive a given length of time under the same circumstances
   b. Allows the production of a table (life table) and a graph (survival curve)
   c. We can visually evaluate the curves, but we need a test to evaluate them formally.
2. Log-rank test: Compare the survival distributions between two or more groups.
   a. This test precludes an analysis of the effects of several variables or the magnitude of difference between groups or the CI (see below for Cox proportional hazards model).
   b. H_0: No difference in survival between the two populations
   c. Log-rank test uses several assumptions.
      i. Random sampling and subjects chosen independently
      ii. Consistent criteria for entry or end point
      iii. Baseline survival rate does not change as time progresses.
      iv. Censored subjects have the same average survival time as uncensored subjects.
3. Cox proportional hazards model
   a. Most popular method to evaluate the impact of covariates; reported (graphically) like Kaplan-Meier
   b. Investigates several variables at a time
   c. Actual method of construction and calculation is complex.
   d. Compares survival in two or more groups after adjusting for other variables
   e. Allows calculation of a hazard ratio (and CI)

	2 grp indep	2 grp related	>2 indep	<2 related
Nom	X2 Fishers	mcnemar	X2	Cochran Q
Ord	Wilcoxon	signed	K W	Friedman ANOVA
Cnt.	t test	paired t test	one way	rep meas 2 way
Cnt 1 Factr	ANCOVA	2 way rep meas	2 way	rep measu

XI. SELECTED REPRESENTATIVE STATISTICAL TESTS

Table 7. Representative Statistical Tests (See Reference 4 for Expanded Table)

Type of Variable	2 Groups (independent)	2 Groups (related)	>2 Groups (independent)	>2 Groups (related)
Nominal	χ^2 or Fisher exact test	McNemar test	χ^2	Cochran Q
Ordinal	Wilcoxon rank sum Mann-Whitney U test Wilcoxon−Mann-Whitney	Wilcoxon signed rank Sign test	Kruskal-Wallis (MCP)	Friedman ANOVA
Continuous No factors	Equal variance t-test Unequal variance t-test	Paired t-test	One-way ANOVA (MCP)	Repeated-measures ANOVA
1 factor	ANCOVA	Two-way repeated-measures ANOVA	Two-way ANOVA (MCP)	Two-way repeated-measures ANOVA

ANCOVA = analysis of covariance; ANOVA = analysis of variance; MCP = multiple-comparisons procedure.

REFERENCES

1. Crawford SL. Correlation and regression. Circulation 2006;114:2083-8.

2. Davis RB, Mukamal KJ. Hypothesis testing: means. Circulation 2006;114:1078-82.

3. DeYoung GR. Understanding biostatistics: an approach for the clinician. In: Zarowitz B, Shumock G, Dunsworth T, et al., eds. Pharmacotherapy Self-Assessment Program, 5th ed. Kansas City, MO: ACCP, 2005:1-20.

4. DiCenzo R, ed. Clinical Pharmacist's Guide to Biostatistics and Literature Evaluation. Lenexa, KS: ACCP, 2015.

5. Gaddis ML, Gaddis GM. Introduction to biostatistics, part 1: basic concepts. Ann Emerg Med 1990;19:86-9.

6. Gaddis ML, Gaddis GM. Introduction to biostatistics, part 2: descriptive statistics. Ann Emerg Med 1990;19:309-15.

7. Gaddis ML, Gaddis GM. Introduction to biostatistics, part 3: sensitivity, specificity, predictive value, and hypothesis testing. Ann Emerg Med 1990;19:591-7.

8. Gaddis ML, Gaddis GM. Introduction to biostatistics, part 4: statistical inference techniques in hypothesis testing. Ann Emerg Med 1990;19:820-5.

9. Gaddis ML, Gaddis GM. Introduction to biostatistics, part 5: statistical inference techniques for hypothesis testing with nonparametric data. Ann Emerg Med 1990;19:1054-9.

10. Gaddis ML, Gaddis GM. Introduction to biostatistics, part 6: correlation and regression. Ann Emerg Med 1990;19:1462-8.

11. Harper ML. Biostatistics for the clinician. In: Zarowitz B, Shumock G, Dunsworth T, et al., eds. Pharmacotherapy Self-Assessment Program, 4th ed. Kansas City, MO: ACCP, 2002:183-200.

12. Hayney MS, Meek PD. Essential clinical concepts of biostatistics. In: Carter BL, Lake KD, Raebel MA, et al., eds. Pharmacotherapy Self-Assessment Program, 3rd ed. Kansas City, MO: ACCP, 1999:19-46.

13. Jones SR, Carley S, Harrison M. An introduction to power and sample size estimation. Emerg Med J 2003;20:453-8.

14. Kier KL. Biostatistical methods in epidemiology. Pharmacotherapy 2011;31:9-22.

15. Kusuoka H, Hoffman JIE. Advice on statistical analysis for circulation research. Circ Res 2002;91:662-71.

16. Larson MG. Analysis of variance. Circulation 2008;117:115-21.

17. Larson MG. Descriptive statistics and graphical displays. Circulation 2006;114:76-81.

18. Overholser BR, Sowinski KM. Biostatistics primer, part 1. Nutr Clin Pract 2007;22:629-35.

19. Overholser BR, Sowinski KM. Biostatistics primer, part 2. Nutr Clin Pract 2008;23:76-84.

20. Rao SR, Schoenfeld DA. Survival methods. Circulation 2007;115:109-13.

21. Rector TS, Hatton RC. Statistical concepts and methods used to evaluate pharmacotherapy. In: Zarowitz B, Shumock G, Dunsworth T, et al., eds. Pharmacotherapy Self-Assessment Program, 2nd ed. Kansas City, MO: ACCP, 1997:130-61.

22. Strassels SA. Biostatistics. In: Dunsworth TS, Richardson MM, Chant C, et al., eds. Pharmacotherapy Self-Assessment Program, 6th ed. Lenexa, KS: ACCP, 2007:1-16.

23. Sullivan LM. Estimation from samples. Circulation 2006;114:445-9.

24. Tsuyuki RT, Garg S. Interpreting data in cardiovascular disease clinical trials: a biostatistical toolbox. In: Richardson MM, Chant C, Cheng JWM, et al., eds. Pharmacotherapy Self-Assessment Program, 7th ed. Lenexa, KS: ACCP, 2010:241-55.

25. Windish DM, Huot SJ, Green ML. Medicine resident's understanding of the biostatistics and results in the medical literature. JAMA 2007;298:1010-22.

ANSWERS AND EXPLANATIONS TO SELF-ASSESSMENT QUESTIONS

1. Answer: A

The NYHA functional class is an ordinal scale from I (no symptoms) to IV (severe symptoms). Neither ANOVA nor ANCOVA is appropriate for ordinal or noncontinuous data (Answer C and Answer D are incorrect). The Wilcoxon signed rank test is an appropriate nonparametric test to use for paired ordinal data, such as the change in NYHA functional class over time on the same person (Answer B is incorrect). The Kruskal-Wallis test is the nonparametric analog of a one-way ANOVA and is appropriate for this analysis (Answer A is correct).

2. Answer: C

You cannot determine which finding is more important (in this case, the best drug) on the basis of the p-value (i.e., a lower p-value does not mean more important) (Answer B is incorrect). All statistically significant results are interpreted as significant without respect to the size of the p-value. This trial had four independent samples, and use of the unpaired (independent samples) t-test is not appropriate because it requires several unnecessary tests and increases the chances of making a type I error (Answer A is incorrect). In this setting, ANOVA is the correct test (Answer C is correct), followed by a multiple-comparisons procedure to determine where the actual differences between groups lie. A paired t-test is inappropriate because this is a parallel-group trial (Answer D is incorrect). The use of ANOVA in this case assumes a normal distribution and equal variance in each of the four groups.

3. Answer: D

The typical a priori alpha error (type I) rate is 5% (i.e., when the study was designed, the error rate was designed to be 5% or less) (Answer D is correct). The actual type I error rate is reported in the question as 0.01 (1%) (Answer A is incorrect). Answer B and Answer C are related; the study did have enough power because a statistically significant difference was observed. Similarly, a type II error was not made because this error has to do with not finding a difference when one truly exists. In this question, the type I error rate is 1%, the value of the p-value.

4. Answer: C

Sample sizes need not be equal to use a t-test (Answer A is incorrect). Body mass index data are not ordinal but continuous; thus, a t-test is appropriate (Answer B is incorrect). The assumption of equal variances is required to use any parametric test (Answer C is correct). A specific value for power is not required to use a test (Answer D is incorrect).

5. Answer: B

The reporting of the mean difference and CI is thought by many to be a superior means of presenting the results from a clinical trial because it describes both precision and statistical significance, as compared with a p-value, which distills everything into one value, making Answer A incorrect. The presentation of the data in this manner clearly shows all the necessary information for making the appropriate conclusion. To assess statistical significance by use of CIs, the 95% CI (corresponding to the 5% type I error rate used in most studies) may not contain zero (signifying no difference between men and women) for the mean difference, making Answer D incorrect. Answer B is correct because the p-value of less than 0.05 corresponds to the 95% CI in that item. To evaluate Answer C, we would need to know the 99% CI.

6. Answer: D

Answer A is incorrect because it uses unconventional approaches to determine statistical significance. Although this can be done, it is unlikely to be accepted by other readers and investigators. This study observed a nonsignificant increase in HDL-C concentration between the two groups. With a small sample size, such as the one used in this study, there is always concern about adequate power to observe a difference between the two treatments. A difference may exist between these two drugs, but the number of subjects studied may be too small to detect it statistically. Answer D is correct because, with the lack of information provided in this narrative, it is not possible to estimate power; thus, more information is needed. Answer B may be correct, but without first addressing the question of adequate power, it would be an inappropriate conclusion to draw. Answer C is incorrect because even though the new drug increased HDL-C concentration more than the other treatment, it is inappropriate to conclude that it is better because, statistically, it is not.

7. Answer: B

The primary end point in this study, the percentage of subjects at or below the target blood pressure, is nominal data. Subjects at target blood pressure (less than 140/90 mm Hg) are defined as having reached the target. This type of data requires either a chi-square test or a Fisher exact test (depending on the sample size or, more accurately, the number of counts in the individual contingency table cells) (Answer B is correct). An independent samples t-test is not appropriate because actual blood pressure values are not being compared (at least not in this question or this end point) (Answer A is incorrect). If we were comparing the actual blood pressure between the two groups, the test might be appropriate if parametric assumptions were met. The Wilcoxon signed rank test is the appropriate nonparametric test for comparing paired samples (usually in a crossover trial) (Answer C is incorrect). Finally, a one-sample t-test is used to compare the mean of a single group with the mean of a reference group. This is also incorrect in this situation because two groups are being compared (Answer D is incorrect).

8. Answer: A

Detecting the smaller difference between the treatments requires more power. Power can be increased in several different ways. Answer A is correct because the most common approach is to increase the sample size, which is expensive for the researchers. Answer D is incorrect because smaller sample sizes diminish a study's ability to detect differences between groups. Power can also be increased by increasing α, but doing so increases the chances of a type I error. Answer B decreases α, thus making it more difficult to detect differences between groups. Answer C certainly makes it easier to detect a difference between the two groups, but it uses an unconventional α value and is thus not the most appropriate technique.

9. Answer: C

Regression analysis is the most effective way to develop models to predict outcomes or variables (Answer C is correct). There are many different types of regression, but all share the ability to evaluate the impact of multiple variables simultaneously on an outcome variable. Correlation analysis is used to assess the association between two (or more) variables, not to make predictions (Answer A is incorrect). Kaplan-Meier curves are used to graphically depict survival curves or time to an event (Answer B is incorrect). Confidence intervals are not used to make predictions (Answer D is incorrect).

Study Designs: Fundamentals, Interpretation, and Research Topics

Kevin M. Sowinski, Pharm.D., FCCP

Purdue University College of Pharmacy
Indiana University School of Medicine
West Lafayette and Indianapolis, Indiana

Study Designs: Fundamentals and Interpretation and Research Topics

Kevin M. Sowinski, Pharm.D., FCCP

Purdue University College of Pharmacy
Indiana University School of Medicine
West Lafayette and Indianapolis, Indiana

Learning Objectives

1. Define, compare, and contrast the concepts of internal and external validity, bias, and confounding in clinical study design.
2. Identify potential sources of bias in clinical trials; select strategies to eliminate or control for bias.
3. Outline the hierarchy of evidence generated by various study designs.
4. Compare and contrast the advantages and disadvantages of various study designs (e.g., prospective; retrospective; case-control; cohort; cross-sectional; randomized controlled clinical trials; systematic review; meta-analysis). Delineate the difference between parallel and crossover study designs.
5. Select from various biostatistical measures to appropriately compare groups or their assessments from various study designs and use their findings/output to interpret results.
6. Define and evaluate odds, odds ratio, risk/incidence rate, risk ratio/relative risks (RRs), and other risk estimates. Compute and evaluate number needed to treat and number needed to harm. Define and calculate terms such as point and period prevalence, incidence rate, prevalence rate, absolute risk difference, and RR difference.
7. Define and calculate terms such as true positive, false positive, true negative, false negative, sensitivity, specificity, positive predictive value, negative predictive value, positive likelihood ratio, and negative likelihood ratio.
8. Define research and differentiate it from quality improvement activities.
9. Define the composition, functions, and roles of the institutional review board (IRB).
10. Describe the various steps of the professional writing and peer-review processes.

Self-Assessment Questions

Answers and explanations to these questions can be found at the end of the chapter.

Questions 1 and 2 pertain to the following case.
A recently released statin is associated with less myopathy than other currently available statins. After 2 years of use, a retrospective case-control study was undertaken by the manufacturer after 20 different reports of

severe myopathy were sent to the U.S. Food and Drug Administration's (FDA's) MedWatch program. Risk factors for statin-induced myopathy were not assessed; however, both the cases and the controls of this study had identical diagnostic evaluations and were stratified according to the duration of statin use before the onset of myopathy.

1. Which type of bias is this study design most susceptible to?
   A. Confounding by indication.
   B. Recall bias.
   C. Diagnostic bias.
   D. Misclassification.

2. Which factor will be most affected by the type of bias likely to occur in this study?
   A. External validity.
   B. Internal validity.
   C. Assessment of exposure.
   D. Number of patients needed for the study.

3. When describing the results of a randomized controlled clinical trial, the investigators report using an intention-to-treat analysis to analyze their data. The results of their investigation comparing two diuretics for heart failure show no difference in the number of hospitalizations for decompensated heart failure between the treatment groups. Given their method of data analysis, which statement is most appropriate?
   A. May be susceptible to issues regarding recall bias.
   B. Provides a good measure of effectiveness under typical clinical conditions.
   C. Cannot provide an estimate of the method's effectiveness.
   D. May overestimate the actual treatment effect.

4. A prospective randomized study compared once-daily enoxaparin with twice-daily enoxaparin when treating patients with venous thromboembolism (VTE). One of the study end points was the recurrence of VTE. The following table summarizes recurrence rates in all patients.

	Once Daily	**Twice Daily**
All patients, n (%)	13/298 (4.4)	9/312 (2.9)

The 95% confidence interval (CI) for the difference in recurrence rates between the two groups was −1.5% to 4.5%. Which conclusion is most appropriate?

A. Twice-daily enoxaparin is superior to once daily

B. Superiority of twice-daily enoxaparin could not be established over once daily.

C. Once-daily enoxaparin is not inferior to twice daily.

D. No conclusion can be drawn because p-values are unavailable.

5. According to the data in the previous question and the result obtained, which best represents the number of patients who would need to be treated with twice-daily enoxaparin to prevent the recurrence of one VTE episode?

A. Number needed to treat (NNT) would be 2.

B. NNT would be 67.

C. NNT would be 152.

D. NNT should not be calculated because the result was nonsignificant.

Questions 6 and 7 pertain to the following case.
A multicenter, double-blind, placebo-controlled trial randomly assigned 4837 patients to treatment with margarine supplemented with the omega-3 fatty acid α-linolenic acid (ALA) (margarine with ALA) or a placebo margarine. The primary combined end point was the rate of cardiovascular events, defined as fatal and nonfatal cardiovascular events and percutaneous coronary interventions. Data were analyzed according to intention-to-treat analysis with the use of a Cox proportional hazards model. The hazard ratio (HR) and 95% CI for the margarine with ALA group were 0.91 and 0.78–1.05, respectively. In the prespecified subgroup of women, margarine with ALA was associated with an HR of 0.73 (95% CI, 0.51–1.03).

6. Which statement is most appropriate?

A. Margarine with ALA statistically significantly reduced the risk of cardiovascular events (p<0.05).

B. Margarine with ALA statistically significantly reduced the risk of cardiovascular events (p<0.01).

C. Margarine with ALA did not significantly reduce the risk of cardiovascular events (p>0.05).

D. Without a p-value, it is not possible to determine whether margarine with ALA affected cardiovascular events.

7. When the study was being designed, which choice describes the outcome for which the study was most likely to have been powered?

A. Differences in the rate of the composite outcome, cardiovascular events.

B. Differences in the rate of percutaneous coronary interventions.

C. Differences in the rate of the composite outcomes in women.

D. Differences in the rate of the composite outcomes in men.

8. In a meta-analysis of studies examining the effects of several antihypertensive drugs, the odds ratio (OR) for treatment with low-dose diuretics compared with calcium channel blockers for cardiovascular disease events was 0.84 (95% CI, 0.75–0.95). Which statement is the most appropriate interpretation of these findings?

A. Treatment of hypertension with low-dose diuretics was more effective in preventing cardiovascular disease events than treatment with calcium channel blockers.

B. Treatment of hypertension with calcium channel blockers was more effective in preventing cardiovascular disease events than treatment with low doses of diuretics.

C. The difference observed between treatment with calcium channel blockers and low doses of diuretics is not statistically significant.

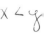

D. The odds of developing cardiovascular events when treating hypertension with low doses of diuretics are lower than when using calcium channel blockers.

9. According the Code of Federal Regulations, which statement best describes what is required of IRB membership?

A. At least one layperson must serve on the IRB.

B. The size of IRB membership changes depending on the institution size.

C. At least 10 members serve on the IRB.

D. There must be one physician on the IRB.

10. As a resident who recently completed a research project, you are writing the introduction section of the paper. Which piece of information should best be included in this section?

A. Information related to process for the selection of participants.

B. Summary of prior studies.

C. The average age of the study subjects

D. Acknowledgments to clerical staff.

I. INTRODUCTION

A. Why Do Pharmacists Need to Know About Study Design and Interpretation?
   1. Pharmacotherapy Specialty Examination content outline, Domain 2: Drug Information and Evidence Based Medicine (25%)
   2. Task Statements:
      a. Retrieve information that addresses pharmacotherapy-related inquiries in order to optimize patient care.
      b. Evaluate pharmacotherapy-related literature, databases, and health information in order to translate findings into practice.
      c. Conduct pharmacotherapy-related research using appropriate scientific principles in order to ensure optimal patient care.
      d. Disseminate pharmacotherapy-related information and/or research in order to educate health care professionals and trainees.

B. Examples of Online Statistical and Study Design Tools
   1. www.graphpad.com/quickcalcs/
   2. http://statpages.org/

II. VARIOUS ISSUES IN STUDY DESIGN

A. Research Design Classification
   1. Study purpose: Descriptive versus analytic
   2. Time orientation: Prospective versus retrospective design
      a. Prospective: Begin in the present and progress forward, collecting data from subjects whose outcomes lie in the future.
      b. Retrospective: Begin and end in the present; however, this design involves a major backward look to collect information about events that occurred in the past.
   3. Investigator orientation: Interventional versus quasi-experimental
   4. Experimental setting
      a. Randomized controlled trials
      b. Observational trials

B. Relative Strength of Evidence: Hierarchy of Study Designs

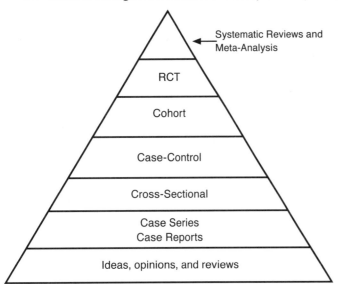

Figure 1. Hierarchy of clinical study design.

RCT = randomized controlled clinical trial.

C. Validity in Study Design
   1. Internal validity
      a. Validity within the confines of the study methods
      b. Does the study design adequately and appropriately test/measure what it purports?
      c. Does the study adequately and appropriately address bias, confounding, and measurement of end points?
   2. External validity
      a. Validity related to generalizing the study results outside the study setting
      b. Can the results be applied to other groups, patients, or systems?
      c. Addresses issues of generalizability and representativeness

D. Bias in Study Design
   1. Definition: Systematic, nonrandom variation in study methodology and conductance, ultimately introducing error in outcome interpretation. Bias can occur in all aspects of the study design.
   2. Examples of bias
      a. Selection bias: An error in the selection of or sampling of individuals for a clinical study. Classic example: subjects chosen for the case and control groups differ in one or more characteristics that alter the outcome of a study
      b. Observational or information bias: An error in the recording of individual factors of a study, such as inaccurate recording of a patient's risk factor, inaccurate recording of the timing of a blood sample
      c. Recall bias: Classic example: Studies of birth defects secondary to medications
      d. Interviewer bias: Classic example: Interviews are not conducted in a uniform manner (or by the same person) for all study participants.
      e. Misclassification bias
         i. Differential
         ii. Non-differential

3. Controlling for bias
    a. Design: For example, selection of study population
    b. Means of collecting data
    c. Sources of information (regarding disease and exposure)
    d. Analysis: May be difficult to interpret

E. Confounding in Study Design
    1. A variable that affects the independent or dependent variable, altering the ability to determine the true effect on the measured outcome. These factors may hide or exaggerate a true association.
    2. To minimize the potential for missing a confounding variable, all relevant information should be collected and evaluated.
    3. Controlling for confounding
        a. During the design of a study
            i. Randomization
            ii. Restriction
            iii. Matching
        b. Analysis
            i. Stratification
            ii. Multivariate analysis

F. Causality
    1. Temporality: Cause before effect
    2. Strength: Plausibility increases with strength of relationship
    3. Biological gradient: Dose-response?
    4. Consistency: Observations over several settings
    5. Specificity: Single cause for effect
    6. Plausibility: Biologically plausible
    7. Coherence: Consistency with existing knowledge
    8. Analogy: Preclinical expectation applied to clinical testing
    9. Experiment: Randomized controlled trials

III. CASE REPORTS/CASE SERIES

A. Document and Describe Experiences, Novel Treatments, and Unusual Events. Allows hypothesis generation that can be tested with other study designs. Note that the title does not state "study."
    1. Possible adverse drug reactions in one or more patients: QT-interval prolongation associated with fluoroquinolone antibiotics
    2. Case report: One patient
    3. Case series: More than one patient with a similar experience or many case reports combined into a descriptive review
    4. Reports should provide sufficient detail to allow readers to recognize same/similar cases at their center/practice.

B. Advantages and Disadvantages
    1. Advantages: Hypotheses are formed, which may be the first step in describing an important clinical problem. Easy to perform and inexpensive
    2. Disadvantages: Does not provide explanation other than conjecture and does not establish causality or association

IV. OBSERVATIONAL STUDY DESIGNS

A. Design Does Not Involve Investigator Intervention, Only Observation. It is essential to remember that observational study designs investigate associations—not, in most cases, causes.

B. Case-Control Study: Study Exposure in Those with and without the Outcome of Interest

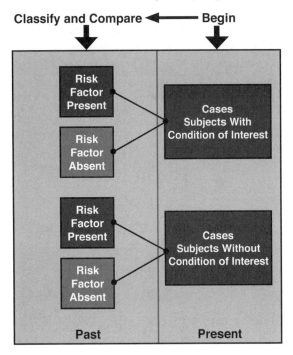

Figure 2. Case-control study design.

1. Determine the association between exposures/risk factors and disease/condition. Classic example: Aspirin use and Reye syndrome
2. Retrospective studies
3. Useful method (and perhaps the only practical way) to study exposures in rare diseases or diseases that take long periods to develop
4. Critical assumptions to minimize bias
   a. Cases are selected to be representative of those who have the disease.
   b. Controls are representative of the general population that does not have the disease and are as identical as possible to the cases, minus the presence of the disease.
   c. Information is collected from cases and controls in the same way.
5. Examples
   a. Risk of myocardial infarction associated with antihypertensive drug therapies (JAMA 1995;274:620-5)
   b. Phenylpropanolamine (PPA) and the risk of hemorrhagic stroke (N Engl J Med 2000;343:1826-32). Purpose of study:
      i. To estimate in women the association between hemorrhagic stroke and the use of appetite suppressants containing PPA
      ii. To estimate the association between any use of PPA (in appetite suppressant or cough or cold remedy) and hemorrhagic stroke
      iii. To estimate in men and women the association between hemorrhagic stroke and the type of exposure to PPA

          iv. Disease: Hemorrhagic stroke (several types). Exposure: PPA

          v. Cases: Symptomatic subarachnoid or intracerebral hemorrhage (n=702). Controls: Matched by sex, race, and age (n=1376)

          vi. Exposure assessed by structured questionnaire, product photographs, and ingredient confirmation

  6. Advantages

      a. Inexpensive and can be conducted quickly

      b. Allows investigation of several possible exposures or associations

  7. Disadvantages

      a. Confounding must be controlled for.

      b. Observational and recall bias: Looking back to recall exposures and their possible levels of exposure

      c. Selection bias: Case selection and control matching are difficult.

  8. Measure of association: OR (odds ratio): In some cases, this can be an estimate of the relative risk/risk ratio (RR). The OR is interpreted as the odds of exposure to a factor in those with a condition or disease compared with those who do not have the condition or disease. Interpretation of these concepts will be presented below.

C. Cohort Study

  1. Determines the association between exposures/factors and disease/condition development. Allows an estimation of the risk of outcome (and the RR between the exposure groups). Study outcome of interest in those with and without the exposure of interest. Classic examples follow:

      a. Framingham Study. A "cohort" of subjects from Framingham, Massachusetts, were (and are) studied over time to evaluate the relationship between a variety of conditions (exposures) on the development of cardiovascular disease.

      b. Nurses' Health Study: Investigated the potential long-term consequences of the use of oral contraceptives

  2. Describes the incidence or natural history of a disease/condition and measures it in time sequence

  3. "Retrospective" (historical): Begins and ends in the present but involves a major backward look to collect information about events that occurred in the past

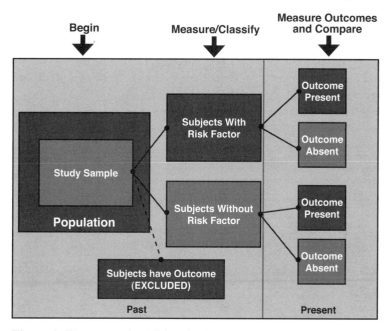

Figure 3. "Retrospective" (historical) cohort study design.

    a.   Advantages: Less expensive and time-consuming; no loss to follow-up, ability to investigate issues not amenable to a clinical trial or ethical or safety issues

    b.   Disadvantages: Only as good as the data available, little control of confounding variables through nonstatistical approaches, recall bias

  4. Prospective or longitudinal: Begin in the present and progress forward, collecting data from subjects whose outcomes lie in the future

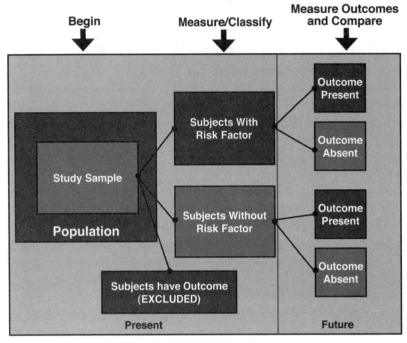

Figure 4. Prospective cohort study design.

    a.   Example: Prospective, observational study: Postmenopausal hormone use and secondary prevention of coronary events in the Nurses' Health Study (Ann Intern Med 2001;135:1-8)

    b.   Advantages: Can control for confounding factors to a greater extent, easier to plan for data collection

    c.   Disadvantages: More expensive and time-intensive, loss of subject follow-up, difficult to study rare diseases/conditions at a reasonable cost

  5. Measure of association: RR: The risk of an event or development of a condition relative to exposure; the risk of someone developing a condition when exposed compared with someone who has not been exposed

D. Cross-sectional (a.k.a. prevalence study)

  1. Identify the prevalence or characteristics of a condition in a group of individuals.

  2. Examples

    a.   Population-based, cross-sectional study: Prevalence of serious eye disease and visual impairment in a north London population (BMJ 1998;316:1643-7)

    b.   Cross-sectional analysis of data from a large cohort study: Maternal characteristics and migraine pharmacotherapy during pregnancy (Cephalgia 2009;29:1267-76)

3. Advantages: Easy design, "snapshot in time," all data collected at one time, studies are accomplished by questionnaire, interview, or other available biomedical information (e.g., laboratory values)
4. Disadvantages: Does not allow the study of a factor (or factors) in individual subjects over time, just at the time of assessment; difficult-to-study, rare conditions

OR expose > risk of dz

V. INCIDENCE, PREVALENCE, RELATIVE RISK/RISK RATIOS, AND ODDS RATIOS

A. Incidence

RR $\dfrac{dz}{exposed}$ | $\dfrac{dz}{not\ exposed}$

1. Measure of the probability of developing a disease
2. Incidence rate: Number of new cases of disease per population in a specified time
3. Calculated by dividing the number of individuals who develop a disease during a given period by the number of individuals who were at risk of developing a disease during the same period

OR $\dfrac{exposed}{dz}$ / $\dfrac{exposed}{no\ dz}$

B. Prevalence
1. Measure of the number of individuals who have a condition/disease at any given time
2. Point prevalence: Prevalence on a given date
3. Period prevalence: Prevalence in a period (e.g., year, month)

C. Interpreting RRs/ORs
1. Estimate the magnitude of association between exposure and disease. Key point: For observational studies, this is not cause and effect; it is an association.
2. The incidence of disease in the exposed group divided by the incidence of disease in the unexposed group
3. The RR (a.k.a. risk ratio) cannot be directly calculated for most case-control studies; instead, the OR is usually an estimate of the RR.
4. The RR and OR are interpreted on the basis of their difference from unity (1.0). If the 95% CI includes unity, no statistical difference is indicated. The CI also gives us an idea of the spread within which the true effect lies.
5. Interpretation of the index of risk
   a. Direction of risk

Table 1. Direction of Risk Associated with OR and RR

RR	OR	Interpretation
< 1	< 1	Negative association RR: Risk of disease is lower in the exposed group OR: Odds of exposure is lower in the diseased group
= 1	= 1	No association RR: Risk of disease in the two groups is the same OR: Odds of exposure in the two groups is the same
> 1	> 1	Positive association RR: Risk of disease is greater in the exposed group OR: Odds of exposure is greater in the diseased group

OR = odds ratio; RR = relative risk/risk ratio.

b. Magnitude of risk

Table 2. Magnitude of Risk Associated with OR and RR

RR	OR	Interpretation
0.75	0.75	25% reduction in the risk/odds
1.0	1.0	No difference in risk/odds
1.5	1.5	50% increase in the risk/odds
3.0	3.0	3-fold (or 200%) increase in the risk/odds

OR = odds ratio; RR = relative risk/risk ratio.

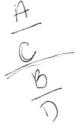

6. Calculating RR/OR/contingency tables

Table 3. Contingency Table for Estimating RR and OR

		Disease?	
		Yes	No
Exposure?	Yes	A	B
	No	C	D

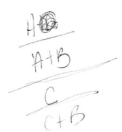

a. $RR = \dfrac{A/(A+B)}{C/(C+D)}$

b. $OR = \dfrac{\dfrac{A}{C}}{\dfrac{B}{D}}$ or = (A x D)/(B x C)

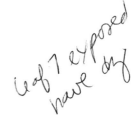

7. Example (PPA study): N Engl J Med 2000;343:1826-32

Table 4. Contingency Table

		Disease? Hemorrhagic Stroke in Women	
		Yes	No
Exposure? Appetite suppression use	Yes	6	1
	No	377	749

From: Kernan WN, Viscoli CM, Brass LM, et al. Phenylpropanolamine (PPA) and the risk of hemorrhagic stroke. N Engl J Med 2000;343:1826-32.

a. OR = (6/377)/(1/749) = 12
b. Data from the PPA study above related to appetite suppressant and development of hemorrhagic stroke

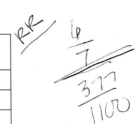

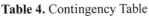

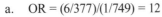

Table 5. Use of PPA and Appetite Suppressants and the Risk of Developing Hemorrhagic Stroke

	Cases (+ hemorrhagic stroke) n=383	Controls (− hemorrhagic stroke) n=750	Adjusted OR (95% CI)
Appetite suppressant: Women	6	1	16.6 (1.51–182)
Appetite suppressant: Men	0	0	—
Appetite suppressant: Either	6	1	15.9 (1.38–184)
PPA: Women	21	20	1.98 (1.00–3.90)
PPA: Men	6	13	0.62 (0.20–1.92)
PPA: Either	27	33	1.49 (0.84–2.64)

CI = confidence interval; OR = odds ratio; PPA = phenylpropanolamine.

    c.   What do these numbers mean?
    d.   Can you interpret the point estimate and 95% CI in all cases?
        i.   What does the point estimate mean?
       ii.   What does the CI mean?
      iii.   Which ones are statistically significant?

D. Causation
    1.   REMEMBER: In general, we do not prove or show causality with observational studies, but there is some general "guidance" to consider when evaluating them. It is important to recognize that, in many situations, the conduct of studies to establish causality is not possible, practical, or ethical.
    2.   Types of causality
       a.   Sufficient cause
       b.   Necessary cause
       c.   Risk factor
    3.   Questions used to evaluate causality
       a.   Was statistical significance observed?
       b.   What was the strength of the association, as measured by the OR or the RR?
       c.   Were dose-response relationships evaluated?
       d.   Was there a temporal relationship between exposure and disease/outcome?
       e.   Have the results been consistently shown?
       f.   Is there biologic plausibility to the association?
       g.   Is there any experimental (e.g., animal, in vitro) evidence?

VI. RANDOMIZED CONTROLLED TRIAL DESIGN

A. Characteristics
    1.   Experimental or interventional, investigator makes intervention and evaluates cause and effect. Examine etiology, cause, efficacy, using comparative groups.
    2.   Some previous background information or studies should exist to suggest that the intervention used will likely be beneficial.
    3.   Design allows assessment of causality.
       a.   Sufficient cause
       b.   Necessary cause
       c.   Risk factor

4. Minimizes bias through randomization and/or stratification
   a. Randomization
   b. Block randomization
   c. Stratification
   d. Cluster randomization
5. Treatment controls
   a. Placebo controlled
   b. Active controlled
   c. Historical control
6. Blinding methods
   a. Single-blind: Either subjects or investigators are unaware of subject assignment to active/control.
   b. Double-blind: Both subjects and investigators are unaware of subject assignment to active/control.
   c. Triple-blind: Both subjects and investigators are unaware of subject assignment to active/control; in addition, an analysis group is unaware.
   d. Double-dummy: Two placebos necessary to match active and control therapies
   e. Open-label: Everyone is aware of subject assignment to active/control.
7. May use parallel or crossover design (see additional information below)
   a. Crossover provides practical and statistical efficiency.
   b. Crossover is not appropriate for certain types of treatment questions (e.g., effect of treatment on a disease that worsens quickly over time or worsens during the study period).
8. Factorial design: Designed to answer two separate research questions in a single group of subjects
9. Examples
   a. Clinical trial: Comparison of two drugs, comparison of two behavioral modifications, etc.
   b. Educational intervention: Online course versus lecture class format
   c. Health care intervention: Pharmacist-based health care team versus non–pharmacist-based health care team

B. Randomized Controlled Trial: Parallel Design

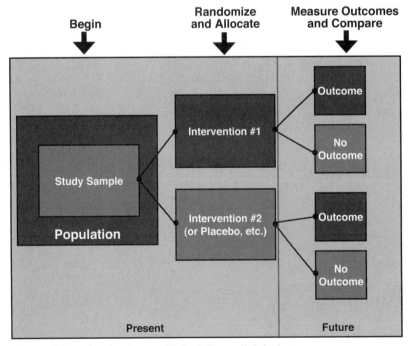

Figure 5. Randomized controlled trial: parallel design.

C. Randomized Controlled Trial: Crossover Design

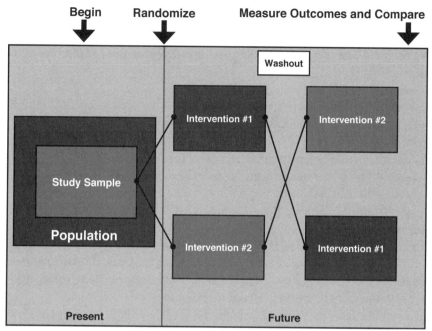

Figure 6. Randomized controlled trial: crossover design.

D. Examples of Considerations for Controlled Trials
1. Are the results of the study valid (methods)?
   a. Did the subjects undergo randomization, and what was the randomization technique? Did the randomization process result in equal baseline characteristics?
   b. Were all subjects who entered the trial accounted for? Was follow-up complete? If not, how many were lost to follow-up, from which groups did they leave, and why?
   c. Were subjects analyzed in the groups to which they were randomized? Was intention-to-treat, per-protocol, or actual treatment analysis used?
   d. How was blinding conducted (e.g., subject, investigator), if applicable?
   e. Were the inclusion and exclusion criteria appropriate, or were they too restrictive or inclusive? Were the groups similar at the start of the trial?
   f. Was the sample size sufficient, and was a power calculation included?
   g. Were the groups handled the same way, aside from the intervention(s)?
   h. Were the statistical tests appropriate and understandable?
   i. What was assessed: Surrogate markers or true outcomes? Were *a priori* subgroup analyses performed?
2. What were the results?
   a. How large was the treatment effect?
   b. How precise was the effect (based on CIs significant)?
   c. Did the authors properly interpret the results?
3. Can I apply the results of this study to my patient population? Will they help me care for my patients?
   a. Can the results of this study be applied to general practice?
   b. Was a representative population studied? Can I apply this to my setting?
   c. Do the patients I care for fulfill the enrollment criteria for this study?
   d. Do the patients I care for fulfill the subgroup criteria evaluated?
   e. Do the expected benefits outweigh the expected and/or unanticipated risks?

VII. OTHER ISSUES TO CONSIDER IN CONTROLLED TRIALS

A. Subgroup Analysis
   1. Important part of controlled clinical trials (if set *a priori*)
   2. Many times, they are overused and overinterpreted, leading to unnecessary research, misinterpretation of results, and/or suboptimal patient care.
   3. Many potential pitfalls in identifying and interpreting
      a. Failure to consider several comparisons or to adjust p-values
      b. Problems with sample size (power), classification, and lack of assessment of interaction

B. Composite End Points: Often, the impression is that this practice is not a good practice.
   1. The primary end point is one of the most important decisions to make in the design of a clinical study.
   2. A composite end point combines several end points.
      a. For example, cardiovascular death, nonfatal MI, and cardiac arrest with resuscitation
      b. Usually combines measures of morbidity and mortality
      c. What does the following statement mean? Our findings show that ramipril reduces the rates of death, MI, stroke, revascularization, cardiac arrest, heart failure, complications related to diabetes, and new cases of diabetes in a broad spectrum of high-risk patients. Treating 1000 patients with ramipril for 4 years prevents about 150 events in around 70 patients.
         i. Was there a reduction in all the end points or just in some?
         ii. Are all the outcomes just as likely to occur?
         iii. Why would the investigators of this trial have been interested in all of these outcomes?
   3. What are the positives for using composite end points?
      a. No single primary outcome
      b. To alleviate problems of multiple testing
      c. To increase number of events, which decreases sample size and cost to the investigator
   4. What are the problems?
      a. Difficulties in interpreting composite end points; consider our earlier example
      b. Misattribution of statistically beneficial effects of composite measure to each of its component end points
      c. Dilution of effects, negative results for relatively common component of composite end point "hide" real differences in other end points. Undue influence exerted on composite end point by "softer" component end points
      d. "Averaging" of overall effect: Problems when component end points move in opposite directions; a sign the composite end point should be abandoned without valid conclusions being drawn
      e. Should all end points be weighed the same, or should death "weigh" more?
   5. The results for each individual end point should be reported together with the results for the composite.

C. Surrogate End Points
   1. Parameters thought to be associated with clinical outcomes
      a. Blood pressure and stroke prevention
      b. LDL-C reduction and cardiovascular death reduction
         i. Statins: Yes
         ii. Hormone replacement therapy: No
      c. Premature ventricular contraction suppression and reduced mortality
   2. Surrogate outcomes do not always predict clinical outcomes.
   3. Short-duration studies that evaluate surrogate end points may not be large enough to detect uncommon adverse events.

D. Superiority Versus Equivalence Versus Noninferiority
  1. A superiority trial is designed to detect a difference between experimental treatments. This is the typical design in a clinical trial.
  2. An equivalence trial is designed to confirm the absence of a meaningful difference(s) between treatments, neither better nor worse (both directions). The key is the definition of the specified margin. What difference is important? One example is a bioequivalence trial.
  3. A noninferiority trial is designed to investigate whether a treatment is not clinically worse (not less effective than stated margin, or inferior) than an existing treatment.
      a. It may be the most effective, or it may have a similar effect.
      b. Useful when placebo administration is not possible for ethical reasons
      c. ONTARGET (The Ongoing Telmisartan Alone and in Combination with Ramipril Global Endpoint Trial)
          i. Designed to evaluate telmisartan, ramipril, or their combination in patients with a high risk of vascular disease
          ii. Objective was to determine whether telmisartan was noninferior to ramipril in the incidence of cardiovascular deaths.
          iii. Noninferior difference was defined as 13% or less.
      d. Essentials of noninferiority design
          i. Control group must be effective.
          ii. Current study similar to previous study with control and with equal doses, clinical conditions, and design used
          iii. Adequate power is essential, and usually, larger sample sizes are required.

VIII. CONTROLLED CLINICAL TRIALS: ANALYSIS

A. Controlled Clinical Trial: Application (JAMA 1998;280:605-13)
  1. Randomized trial of estrogen plus progestin for secondary prevention of coronary heart disease (CHD) in postmenopausal women
  2. Objective: To determine whether estrogen plus progestin therapy alters the risk of CHD in postmenopausal women with established CHD
  3. Randomized, blinded, placebo-controlled
      a. Two treatment arms: ERT-P (conjugated equine estrogen 0.625 mg/day plus medroxyprogesterone acetate 2.5 mg/day) and placebo—n=2763 with coronary artery disease, younger than 80 years; mean age 66.7 years
      b. Follow-up averaged 4.1 years; 82% of patients undergoing hormone replacement therapy still taking hormone at the end of 1 year; 75% at the end of 3 years
  4. End points
      a. Primary: Nonfatal MI or CHD death
      b. Secondary: Many, including all-cause mortality. Are these composite outcomes appropriate?
  5. Statistical analysis
      a. Baseline characteristics: t-test and c^2: Is comparing baseline characteristics necessary in this type of trial?
      b. Power analysis and sample size calculation
      c. Kaplan-Meier with Cox proportional hazards model
  6. Surrogate end point: LDL-C lowered
  7. Results:

Table 6. Death and Secondary End Points by Treatment Group (Overall)

	ERT-P	Placebo	HR (95% CI)
Primary CHD events	12.5%	12.7%	0.99 (0.80–1.22)
CHD death	5.1%	4.2%	1.24 (0.81–1.75)
Any thromboembolic event	2.5%	0.9%	2.89 (1.50–5.58)
Gallbladder disease	6.1%	4.5%	1.38 (1.00–1.92)

CHD = coronary heart disease; CI = confidence interval; ERT-P = conjugated equine estrogen 0.625 mg/day plus medroxyprogesterone acetate 2.5 mg/day; HR = hazard ratio.

8. Significant time trend: More CHD events in the treatment group than in placebo in year 1 and fewer in years 4 and 5
9. Author's conclusions
   a. During follow-up, ERT-P did not reduce overall rate of CHD events.
   b. Treatment increased rate of thromboembolic evens and gallbladder disease.

B. Questions to Consider in Evaluating and Interpreting a Clinical Trial
   1. Study design
      a. Was the studied sample representative of the population or the individual to whom the results were being applied?
      b. Were the inclusion/exclusion criteria appropriate, or were they overly restrictive or inclusive?
      c. Sufficient sample size, power, and so forth? Was a power analysis included?
      d. Was a study objective and/or hypothesis provided?
      e. Was the study blinded and to whom? (subject, investigator, study personnel, or all?)
      f. Was a run-in phase used? If so, why? Did it affect the interpretation of the trial?
      g. What type of randomization method was performed? Did the randomization process produce equal baseline characteristics between all groups?
   2. Outcomes/assessments
      a. Were the primary and/or secondary outcomes identified, were they reasonable, and did they apply to clinical practice?
      b. Was a composite outcome used, and were all the individual components identified and clearly stated in the methods and results?
      c. Were surrogate markers used instead of (or in addition to) clinically relevant outcomes?
   3. Analysis
      a. What analysis technique was used: Intention-to-treat, actual treatment, or per-protocol?
      b. Were the statistical tests appropriate?
   4. Interpretation: Was the author's interpretation appropriate and within the confines of the study design?
   5. Extrapolation
      a. Are you applying the results to similar patients in a similar setting?
      b. Are there possible additional adverse effects that were not measured in this study?

IX. COMMON APPROACHES TO ANALYZING CLINICAL TRIALS

A. Intention-to-Treat Analysis
   1. Compares outcomes on the basis of initial group assignment or "as randomized." The allocation to groups was how they were "intended to be treated," even though they may not have taken the medication for the duration of the study, dropped out, and did not comply with the protocol.

2. Determines effect of treatment under usual conditions of use. Analogous to routine clinical practice in which a patient receives a prescription but may not adhere to the prescribed drug regimen.

3. Gives a conservative estimate of differences in treatments; may underestimate treatment benefits

4. Most common approach to assessing clinical trial results

5. This is the preferred type of analysis in a superiority trial.

B. Per-Protocol Analysis

1. Subjects who do not adhere to allocated treatment are not included in the final analysis; only those who completed the trial and adhered to the protocol (based on some predetermined definition [e.g., 80% adherence])

2. Provides additional information about treatment efficacy and provides more generous estimates of differences between treatments

3. Subject to several issues because of factors such as lower sample size and definitions of adherence. Results are more difficult to interpret and would be validly applied only to adherent patients like those in the trial; not necessarily generalizable to all patients

C. As-Treated Analysis

1. Subjects are analyzed by the actual intervention received. If subjects were in the active treatment group but did not take active treatment, the data would be analyzed as if they were in the placebo group.

2. This analysis essentially ignores/destroys the randomization process for those who did not adhere to the study design. Results should be interpreted with caution.

X. SYSTEMATIC REVIEW/META-ANALYSIS

A. Introduction

1. Dramatic increase in the number of these types of papers

2. First meta-analysis probably published in 1904: Assessment of typhoid vaccine effectiveness

B. Systematic Review

1. Summary that uses explicit methods to perform a comprehensive literature search, critically appraise it, and synthesize the world literature on a specific topic

2. Differs from a standard literature review: The study results are more comprehensively synthesized and reviewed.

3. As with a controlled clinical trial (or other studies), the key is a well-documented and well-described systematic review.

4. Some systematic reviews will attempt to statistically combine results from many studies.

5. Differs from other reviews, which combine evaluation with opinions

C. Meta-analysis

1. Systematic review that uses mathematical/statistical techniques to summarize the results of the evaluated studies

2. These techniques may improve on the following:

a. Calculation of effect size

b. Increase in statistical power

c. Interpretation of disparate results

d. Reduction in bias

e. Answers to questions that may not be addressable with individual studies

3. Reliant on criteria for inclusion of previous studies and statistical methods to ensure validity. Details of included studies are essential.
4. Elements of trial methodology
    a. Research question
    b. Identification of available studies
    c. Criteria for trial inclusion/exclusion
    d. Data collection and presentation of findings
    e. Calculation of summary estimate: Ideally with Forest plot (Figure 7)
    f. Assessment of heterogeneity
        i. Statistical heterogeneity
        ii. χ^2 and Cochran Q are common tests for heterogeneity.
    g. Assessment of publication bias: Funnel plot
    h. Sensitivity analysis

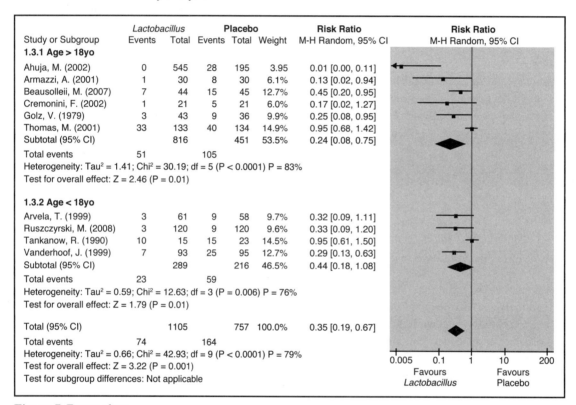

Figure 7. Forest plots.

CI = confidence interval; yo = years old.

From: Kale-Pradhan PB, Jassal HK, Wilhelm SM. Role of Lactobacillus in the prevention of antibiotic-associated diarrhea: a meta-analysis. Pharmacotherapy 2010;30:119-26.

D. Meta-analysis: Additional example (Arch Intern Med 2008;168:687-94)

XI. SUMMARY MEASURES OF EFFECT

A. Absolute and Relative Differences
1. Absolute differences or absolute changes
2. Relative differences or relative changes
3. Absolute differences are more important than relative differences, although the authors of many clinical studies highlight the differences observed in trials with relative differences because they are numerically larger. Why? Larger numbers are more convincing to practitioners and patients. Most drug advertisements (both directly to patients and to health care professionals) quote relative differences.

B. Number Needed to Treat (NNT)
1. Characteristics
   a. Another means to characterize changes or differences in absolute risk
   b. Definition: The reciprocal of the absolute risk reduction (ARR)
      i. NNT = 1/(ARR).
      ii. Rounded to the next highest whole number is the most conservative approach
   c. Applied to clinical outcomes with dichotomous data (e.g., yes/no, alive/dead, MI/no MI)
   d. Caution: Assumes the baseline risk is the same for all patients (or that it is unrelated to RR)
   e. Extrapolation beyond studied time points
   f. NNTs should be provided only for statistically significant effects.
   g. Number needed to harm
2. NNT application
   a. HOPE (Heart Outcomes Prevention Evaluation) study (N Engl J Med 2000;342:145-53)
   b. Study evaluated the effect of ramipril on cardiovascular events in high-risk patients.
   c. Prospective randomized double-blind study
      i. 9297 high-risk patients received ramipril or matching placebo once daily for an average follow-up of 5 years.
      ii. Primary outcome: Composite of MI, stroke, or death from cardiovascular causes
   d. Results (data taken from above-referenced article). NNTs = 1/(0.178 − 0.140) = 1/0.038 = 26.3, rounded up to 27.

Table 7. Risk of Primary and Secondary End Points by Treatment Group

Outcome	Ramipril, %	Placebo, %	Relative Risk	RRR	ARR	NNT
Combined	14.0	17.8	0.79	0.21	0.038	27
Death from CV causes	6.1	8.1	0.74	0.25	0.02	50
Myocardial infarction	9.9	12.3	0.80	0.20	0.024	42
Stroke	3.4	4.9	0.68	0.31	0.015	67

ARR = absolute risk reduction; CV = cardiovascular; NNT = number needed to treat; RRR = relative risk reduction.

   e. Online calculator: http://araw.mede.uic.edu/cgi-bin/nntcalc.pl

C. OR to NNT calculator: http://ktclearinghouse.ca/cebm/practise/ca/calculators/

XII. REPORTING GUIDELINES FOR CLINICAL STUDIES

A. The Consolidated Standards of Reporting Trials (CONSORT)
1. Initially published in 1996 and updated several times since—most recently, in 2010
2. Created in an effort to improve, standardize, and increase the transparency of the reporting of clinical trials and to facilitate the improvement of literature evaluation
3. Available at www.consort-statement.org/
4. The CONSORT statement has been endorsed by several publications and published in these journals.
5. The CONSORT statement
   a. The checklist: 25-item checklist pertaining to the content of the following:
      i. Title
      ii. Abstract
      iii. Introduction
      iv. Methods
      v. Results
      vi. Discussion
      vii. Other information
   b. The flow diagram: Intended to depict the passage of study participants through the randomized controlled trial
6. Extensions of the CONSORT statement
   a. Design extensions
      i. Cluster trials
      ii. Noninferiority and equivalence trials
      iii. Pragmatic trials
   b. Intervention extension
      i. Herbal medicinal interventions
      ii. Nonpharmacologic interventions
      iii. Acupuncture interventions
   c. Data extensions
      i. Patient-reported outcomes
      ii. Harms
      iii. Abstracts

B. Strengthening the Reporting of Observational Studies in Epidemiology (STROBE) Statement
1. Initially published in 2007
2. "An international, collaborative initiative of epidemiologists, methodologists, statisticians, researchers and journal editors involved in the conduct and dissemination of observational studies"
3. Available at www.strobe-statement.org
4. Endorsed by several publications and published in these journals
5. The STROBE checklist: 22-item checklist, same basic concepts as the CONSORT checklist, with alterations germane to observational trials

C. Preferred Reporting Items for Systematic Reviews and Meta-analyses (PRISMA)
1. Established in 1996 (as QUOROM), renamed in 2009
2. Evidence-based minimum set of items for reporting systematic reviews and meta-analyses
3. Available at www.prisma-statement.org/
   a. The PRISMA checklist: 27-item checklist with alterations germane to systematic reviews and meta-analyses

    b.   The PRISMA flow diagram: Four-stage diagram, depicting the flow of information through the systematic review

    c.   The PRISMA explanation and elaboration document: Intended to enhance the use and understanding of the PRISMA statement

D.   Enhancing the Quality and Transparency of Health Research (EQUATOR) Network
1.   International initiative to improve the reliability and value of medical research literature by promoting transparent and accurate reporting of research studies
2.   Does not have its own statements, but promotes the use of key reporting guidelines
3.   Many other statements regarding study types not addressed in the discussion related to CONSORT, STROBE, and PRISMA are listed on the EQUATOR network Web site (www.equator-network.org).

XIII. PHARMACOECONOMIC STUDIES

A.   Cost-Minimization Analysis
1.   Differences in cost among comparable therapies are evaluated
2.   Only useful to compare therapies that have similar outcomes

B.   Cost-Effectiveness Analysis
1.   Outcome: Clinical units or cost per unit health outcome (outcome examples: years of life saved, number of symptom free days, blood glucose, blood pressure, etc.)
2.   Useful to measure the cost impact when health outcomes are improved

C.   Cost-Utility Analysis
1.   Assigns utility weights to outcomes so the impact can be measured in relation to cost (outcome example: quality-adjusted life-years)
2.   Compares outcomes related to mortality when mortality may not be the most important outcome

D.   Cost-Benefit Analysis
1.   Monetary value is placed on both therapy costs and beneficial health outcomes.
2.   Allows analysis of both the cost of treatment and the costs saved with beneficial outcomes

XIV. SENSITIVITY/SPECIFICITY/PREDICTIVE VALUES

A.   Sensitivity: Proportion of True Positives That Are Correctly Identified by a Test; a test with a high sensitivity means that a negative test can rule OUT the disorder

B.   Specificity: Proportion of True Negatives That Are Correctly Identified by a Test; a test with high specificity means that a positive test can rule IN the disorder

C.   Positive Predictive Value: Proportion of Patients with a Positive Test Result Who Actually HAVE the Disease

D.   Negative Predictive Value: Proportion of Patients with a Negative Test Result Who Actually DO NOT HAVE the Disease

E.   Example: Tables 8 and 9

Table 8. Relationship Between Test and Correct Diagnosis Identified by Disease

Test	Disease		Total
	Disease Present	**Disease Absent**	**Total**
Test positive	True positive (TP)	False positive (FP)	TP + FP
Test negative	False negative (FN)	True negative (TN)	TN + FN
Total	TP + FN	FP + TN	Total

Sensitivity = TP/(TP + FN)

Specificity = TN/(TN + FP)

Positive predictive value = TP/(TP + FP)

Negative predictive value = TN/(TN + FN)

Positive likelihood ratio = sensitivity/(1 − specificity)

Negative likelihood ratio = specificity/(1 − sensitivity)

Table 9. Relationship Between Test and Correct Diagnosis Identified by Disease in a Published Study

Test	Disease		Total
	Positive disease	**Negative disease**	**Total**
Positive	231 (true positive)	32 (false positive)	263
Negative	27 (false negative)	54 (true negative)	81
Total	258	86	344

From: Drum DE, Christacapoulos JS. Hepatic scintigraphy in clinical decision making. J Nucl Med 1972;13:908-15.

XV. INSTITUTIONAL REVIEW BOARD/HUMAN SUBJECTS' RESEARCH

A. Definitions
1. Research: "Systematic investigation (i.e., research development, testing, and evaluation) designed to develop or contribute to generalizable knowledge"
2. Human subject: "Living individual about whom an investigator obtains data through intervention or interaction with the individual OR identifiable private information"
3. Quality improvement versus research
    a. In general, if the results of a project are presented outside an organization (i.e., contributes to generalized knowledge), either as a publication or a presentation, it is defined as research.
    b. If the results of a project are to be used internally and are not meant to contribute to generalized knowledge, the activities will fall under quality improvement. Ideally, the IRB makes this decision.

B. History and Development of Research Ethics
1. Nuremberg Code (1948)
    a. Subjects should give informed voluntary consent.
    b. The benefits of research must outweigh the risks.
2. Declaration of Helsinki (1964)
    a. Governs international research ethics
    b. Defines rules for "research combined with clinical care" and "nontherapeutic research"
    c. Basis for good clinical practices used today

3. Tuskegee Syphilis Study (1972)
   a. The study did not minimize risks to human subjects. In fact, it increased their risks.
   b. These issues heightened awareness of the need to protect human subjects and to ensure their informed voluntary consent.
4. Belmont Report (1978): Prepared by the National Commission for the Protection of Human Subjects of Biomedical and Behavioral Research
   a. Summarizes the basic ethical principles identified in its deliberations
   b. Serves as a statement of basic ethical principles and guidelines that assist in resolving the ethical problems that surround the conduct of research with human subjects
5. Code of Federal Regulations (CFR) (1981): The Department of Health and Human Services (DHHS) and the U.S. Food and Drug Administration (FDA) issued regulations according to the Belmont Report:
   a. DHHS: CFR Title 45 (public welfare), Part 46 (protection of human subjects)
   b. FDA: CFR Title 21 (food and drugs), Parts 50 (protection of human subjects) and 56 (IRBs)
6. Common Rule (1991)
   a. Obtaining and documenting informed consent
   b. IRB membership, function, operations, review of research, and recordkeeping
   c. Additional protections for certain vulnerable research subjects: Pregnant women, prisoners, children, individuals with impaired capacity
   d. Ensuring compliance by research institutions
      i. All institutions that conduct federally sponsored research must provide the federal government "assurance" that states the institution's principles for protecting the rights and welfare of human subjects.
      ii. Multiple project assurance is the most common approach to this.
7. IRB review of studies: Reviewed at one of three levels, depending on the level of risk to the human subjects. The federal guidelines that define the categories of review, which are as follows:
   a. Exemption from full IRB review
      i. Categories
         (a) Research conducted in established or commonly accepted educational settings
         (b) Research involving the use of educational tests (cognitive, diagnostic, aptitude, achievement), survey procedures, interview procedures, or observation of public behavior
         (c) Research involving the collection or study of existing data, documents, records, pathologic specimens, or diagnostic specimens if these sources are publicly available or if the information is recorded by the investigator in such a manner that subjects cannot be identified, directly or through identifiers linked to the subjects
         (d) Research and demonstration projects that are conducted by or subject to the approval of department or agency heads
      ii. Projects are not assigned an expiration date.
      iii. The IRB makes the final decision on exemption; a staff member usually reviews the proposal.
      iv. Review usually takes a few days.
   b. Expedited IRB review
      i. Minimal risk to participant
      ii. Minor change to previously approved study
      iii. Chairperson or designee reviews the proposal.
      iv. Review usually takes a few weeks.
   c. Full IRB review: More than minimal risk
      i. Review protocol and supporting documents.
      ii. Lengthy process, usually months
      iii. Full IRB reviews the proposal.

Table 10. Examples of IRB Review Categories

Type of Review	Examples
Exemption from review	Epidemiologic study with NHANES data Study of changes in the number of days requiring antibiotics, using de-identified institutional data
Expedited review	Cross-sectional study of patients with heart failure measuring a biomarker, requiring a single blood sample Case-control study of the relationship between admission to the hospital and drug use
Full review	Randomized controlled trial of a new drug or device for heart failure therapy Cross-sectional study requiring bronchoscopy after administration of methacholine

IRB = institutional review board; NHANES = National Health and Nutrition Examination Survey.

8. IRB composition
   a. At least five members
      i. Chairperson
      ii. Scientific member
      iii. Nonscientific member
      iv. Layperson unaffiliated with the institution
      v. Practitioner
   b. Sufficient qualifications through the experience, expertise, and diversity of its members and backgrounds, including considerations of their racial and cultural heritage and their sensitivity to issues such as community attitudes, to promote respect for its advice and counsel in safeguarding the rights and welfare of human subjects
   c. Membership must be able to ensure protection of vulnerable populations.
   d. Membership must come from more than one profession.
9. Informed consent
   a. Informed consent is a process, not a form. Information must be presented to the individual (or representative) to enable that person to make a voluntary decision to participate as a research subject.
   b. Components
      i. Description of any reasonably foreseeable risks or discomforts
      ii. Description of any benefits to the subject or to others that may reasonably be expected
      iii. Disclosure of appropriate alternative procedures or courses of treatment, if any
      iv. Statement describing the extent, if any, to which confidentiality of records identifying the subject will be maintained
      v. For research involving more than minimal risk, an explanation about whether any compensation and an explanation about whether any medical treatments are available if injury occurs
      vi. Contact information for answers to questions about the research and research subjects' rights; whom to contact if the subject has a research-related injury
      vii. A statement that participation is voluntary; refusal to participate will involve no penalty or loss of benefits, and the subject may discontinue participation at any time without penalty

    c. Waiver or alteration of consent: An IRB may waive/alter informed consent if the following are met:
       i. No more than minimal risk
       ii. Will not adversely affect the rights and welfare of the subjects
       iii. The research could not practicably be carried out without waiver.
       iv. Subjects will be provided additional pertinent information after participation.
    d. An IRB may also waive informed consent in a limited class of research in emergency settings.

XVI. PROFESSIONAL WRITING: THE PUBLICATION PROCESS

A. Primary Literature
    1. Experimental studies
    2. Observational studies
    3. Descriptive reports

B. Publication Process
    1. Journal selection
       a. Topic
       b. Journal quality
          i. Impact factor
          ii. Immediacy index
       c. Open access
    2. Preparation of submission: Paper parts
       a. Title page
       b. Abstract
       c. Introduction/background
       d. Methods
       e. Results
       f. Discussion
    3. Editorial and peer review
       a. Types of reviews
          i. Single-blind review: The reviewer's identity is hidden from the author, but the reviewer knows the author.
          ii. Double-blind review: Both reviewer and author are blinded.
          iii. Open review: Reviewer and author are known to each other.
          iv. Published review: Reviewers' comments are published together with the paper.
       b. Role of reviewer
          i. Does the scientific content have value and originality?
          ii. Is the paper consistent with journal guidelines?
          iii. Are the methods appropriate?
          iv. What changes should be made or additional experiments conducted?
          v. Make a recommendation (accept, revise, reject) to the editor.
    4. Revision process
    5. Poor-quality research, why?
       a. Academic scientists need to publish.
       b. Poor training or investigators/writers
       c. Lack of reviewers with sufficient knowledge or time to review

    d.   Least publishable unit: Several publications from same study

    e.   Other influences

        i.   Current political issues and hot topics

       ii.   Industry

            (a)   Design and funding of studies

            (b)   Comments during publication stage

            (c)   Ghost writers

            (d)   Promotional activities

REFERENCES

1. Altman DG, Bland JM. Diagnostic tests 1: sensitivity and specificity. BMJ 1994;308:1552.

2. Altman DG, Bland JM. Diagnostic tests 2: predictive values. BMJ 1994;309:102.

3. Clancy MJ. Overview of research designs. Emerg Med J 2002;19:546-9.

4. Dasgupta A, Lawson KA, Wilson JP. Evaluating equivalence and noninferiority trials. Am J Health Syst Pharm 2010;67:1337-43.

5. DiCenzo R, ed. Clinical Pharmacist's Guide to Biostatistics and Literature Evaluation. Lenexa, KS: ACCP, 2015.

6. DiPietro NA. Methods in epidemiology: observational study designs. Pharmacotherapy 2010;30:973-84.

7. Koretz RL. Methods of meta-analysis: an analysis. Curr Opin Clin Nutr Metab Care 2002;5:467-74.

8. Lagakos SW. The challenge of subgroup analyses – reporting without distorting. N Engl J Med 2006;354:1667-9.

9. Lesaffre E. Superiority, equivalence and non-inferiority trials. Bull NYU Hosp Jt Dis 2008;66:150-4.

10. Mann CJ. Observational research methods: research design II: cohort, cross sectional and case-control studies. Emerg Med J 2003;20:54-60.

11. Moher D, Liberati A, Tetzlaff J, et al.; The PRISMA Group. Preferred reporting items for systematic reviews and meta-analyses: the PRISMA statement. Ann Intern Med 2009;151:264-9.

12. Neely JG, Magit AE, Rich JT, et al. A practical guide to understanding systematic reviews and meta-analysis. Otolaryngol Head Neck Surg 2010;142:6-14.

13. Piaggio G, Elbourne DR, Altman DG, et al.; CONSORT Group. Reporting of noninferiority and equivalence randomized trials, an extension of the CONSORT statement. JAMA 2006;295:1152-60.

14. Quilliam BJ, Barbour MM. Evaluating drug-induced cardiovascular disease: a pharmacoepidemiologic perspective. In: Richardson MM, Chant C, Cheng JWM, et al., eds. Pharmacotherapy Self-Assessment Program, 7th ed. Lenexa, KS: ACCP, 2010:225-39.

15. Schulz KF, Altman DG, Moher D; CONSORT Group. CONSORT 2010 statement: updated guidelines for reporting parallel group randomized trials. Ann Intern Med 2010;152:726-32.

16. Shermock KM. Secondary data analysis/observational research. In: Dunsworth TS, Richardson MM, Chant C, et al., eds. Pharmacotherapy Self-Assessment Program, 5th ed. Kansas City, MO: ACCP, 2005:43-63.

17. Shields KM, DiPietro NA, Kier KL. Principles of drug literature evaluation for observational study designs. Pharmacotherapy 2011;31:115-27.

18. Smith GH, Mays DA. Clinical study design and literature evaluation. In: Zarowitz B, Shumock G, Dunsworth T, et al., eds. Pharmacotherapy Self-Assessment Program, 4th ed. Kansas City, MO: ACCP, 2002:203-31.

19. Strassels SA, Wilson JP. Pharmacoepidemiology. In: Dunsworth TS, Richardson MM, Chant C, et al., eds. Pharmacotherapy Self-Assessment Program, 6th ed. Lenexa, KS: ACCP, 2007:17-31.

20. Tomlinson G, Detsky AS. Composite endpoints in randomized trials: there is no free lunch. JAMA 2010;303:267-8.

21. Tsuyuki RT, Garg S. Interpreting data in cardiovascular disease clinical trials: a biostatistical toolbox. In: Richardson MM, Chant C, Cheng JWM, et al., eds. Pharmacotherapy Self-Assessment Program, 7th ed. Lenexa, KS: ACCP, 2010:241-55.

22. von Elm E, Altman DG, Egger M, et al. Strengthening the Reporting of Observational Studies in Epidemiology (STROBE) statement: guidelines for reporting observational studies. Ann Intern Med 2007;147:573-7.

23. Windish DM, Huot SJ, Green ML. Medicine resident's understanding of the biostatistics and results in the medical literature. JAMA 2007;298:1010-22.

24. Byerly WG. Working with the institutional review board. Am J Health Syst Pharm 2009;66:176-84.

25. Enfield KB, Truwit JD. The purpose, composition, and function of an institutional review board: balancing priorities. Respir Care 2008;53:1330-6.

26. Hamilton CW. How to write and publish scientific papers: scribing information for pharmacists. Am J Hosp Pharm 1992;49:2477-84.

27. Ness RB; for the Joint Policy Committee, Societies of Epidemiology. Influence of the HIPAA privacy rule on health research. JAMA 2007;298:2164-70.

28. Van Way CW III. Writing a scientific paper. Nutr Clin Pract 2002;22:636-40.

ANSWERS AND EXPLANATIONS TO SELF-ASSESSMENT QUESTIONS

1. Answer: B

Recall bias is always a potential concern for case-control studies because of the amount of time that passes between the study and the drug "ingestion." Because risk factors were not included in the study design, this is of concern (Answer B is correct). Although a study may be susceptible to many types of bias, the other choices would not pose as much risk (if any) compared with recall bias (Answers A, C, and D are incorrect).

2. Answer: B

Internal validity is greatly jeopardized because the study is not designed to protect against this possible bias. In a sense, this design flaw jeopardizes external validity (how well does a study apply to other patients with this condition/disease?), but a lack of internal validity is most affected (Answer B is correct). The other answers can be adequately controlled for in the design and conduct of the study (Answers A, C, and D are incorrect).

3. Answer: B

Intention-to-treat analysis generally considers the approach, which gives the best estimate of use effectiveness (use under typical clinical trial conditions), whereas per-protocol analysis gives a better estimate of method effectiveness (use under ideal conditions) (Answer B is correct; Answer C is incorrect). Intention-to-treat analysis is the most common approach to data analysis for randomized controlled trials and may underestimate the treatment effect (Answer D is incorrect). Recall bias is not a concern with randomized controlled trials (Answer A is incorrect).

4. Answer: B

The CI of the difference in recurrence rate between the two groups includes zero; thus, there is no statistically significant difference between the two groups (Answer B is correct). Answer A is incorrect because the 95% CI contains zero and is therefore not statistically significant. Answer C is incorrect because not enough information is provided. Answer D is incorrect because all the above information can be determined without the benefit of reported p-values.

5. Answer: D

Answers A and C are incorrect calculations. Calculating the NNT to prevent one recurrence using twice-daily therapy is as follows: $0.044 - 0.029 = 0.015$ and $1/0.015 = 66.7...67$; however, the NNT should not be calculated when the end point of interest is nonsignificant (Answer B is incorrect; Answer D is correct).

6. Answer: C

Answers A and B are incorrect because the margarine with ALA did not significantly reduce the risk of cardiovascular events (the 95% CI includes 1 [no difference in risk]). Answer D is incorrect because the p-value is not required for interpreting statistical significance when the 95% CI is provided. Answer C is correct because the p-value corresponds to the 95% CI.

7. Answer: A

Clinical trials are usually adequately powered to compare primary end points (Answer A is correct). Because Answer B is part of the composite outcomes, the study was likely not powered to detect this outcome independently. Similarly, even though the subgroup analysis was determined a priori, the study is not typically designed to have sufficient power to make this comparison (Answers C and D are incorrect).

8. Answer: D

Answers A and B are incorrect because each implies that one drug is more effective than the other. In this type of study design, neither drug is more/less effective. Answer C is incorrect because the CI of the OR does not include 1; thus, the finding is statistically significant at the 5% level, making Answer D correct.

9. Answer: A

Federal law guidance for IRB membership simply states that membership must include at least five individuals: a chairperson, a scientific member, a nonscientific member, a layperson unaffiliated with the institution, and a practitioner (Answer A is correct). There is no requirement for size of membership or a certain number of individuals (Answers B and C are incorrect) or for a physician (Answer D is incorrect).

10. Answer: B

Answer A is incorrect because information related to how the selection of research participants occurred should be in the methods. The results/summary of previous studies (Answer B) are found in the introduction to the study to frame the objective of the current study or in the discussion to relate the results of the current study to the results of other studies. Answer C is incorrect because this information should be in the results section. Answer D is incorrect because acknowledgments should be contained in the acknowledgment section.

Oncology Supportive Care

LeAnn B. Norris, Pharm.D., BCPS, BCOP

South Carolina College of Pharmacy
Columbia, South Carolina

ONCOLOGY SUPPORTIVE CARE

LeAnn B. Norris, Pharm.D., BCPS, BCOP

South Carolina College of Pharmacy
Columbia, South Carolina

Learning Objectives

1. Identify, assess, and recommend appropriate pharmacotherapy for managing common complications of cancer chemotherapy, including nausea and vomiting, myelosuppression and the appropriate use of growth factors, infection, anemia and fatigue, cardiotoxicity, and extravasation injury.

2. Assess and recommend appropriate pharmacotherapy for managing cancer-related pain.

3. Assess and recommend appropriate pharmacotherapy for managing oncologic emergencies, including hypercalcemia, tumor lysis syndrome, and spinal cord compression.

Self-Assessment Questions

Answers and explanations to these questions can be found at the end of this chapter.

1. A 50-year-old man is in the clinic to receive his third cycle of R-CHOP (rituximab, cyclophosphamide, doxorubicin, vincristine, and prednisone) for non-Hodgkin lymphoma. He is very anxious, with nausea and vomiting lasting for about 12 hours after his previous cycle of chemotherapy. The antiemetic regimen he received for his previous cycle of chemotherapy was granisetron 1 dose plus dexamethasone 1 dose administered 30 minutes before chemotherapy. Which regimen is most appropriate for the patient to receive on day 1 of the next cycle of chemotherapy?

   A. Granisetron 1 dose plus dexamethasone 1 dose administered 30 minutes before chemotherapy.

   B. Dolasetron 1 dose plus dexamethasone 1 dose plus aprepitant 1 dose administered 30 minutes before chemotherapy.

   C. Palonosetron 1 dose plus dexamethasone 1 dose plus lorazepam 1 dose administered 30 minutes before chemotherapy.

   D. Metoclopramide 1 dose plus dexamethasone 1 dose plus aprepitant 1 dose administered 30 minutes before chemotherapy.

2. A 65-year-old man with metastatic non–small cell lung cancer is brought to the clinic by his family because of alterations in his mental status. Pertinent laboratory values include a serum calcium concentration of 12 mg/dL and an albumin concentration of 2 g/dL. Which therapy is best for this patient's altered mental status due to hypercalcemia of malignancy?

   A. Calcitonin 4 units/kg every 12 hours.

   B. Furosemide 20 mg orally.

   C. Dexamethasone 10 mg orally two times a day.

   D. Zoledronic acid 4 mg intravenously.

3. A 20-year-old man was recently given a diagnosis of acute myeloid leukemia. He has an elevated white blood cell count (WBC), and he will receive chemotherapy tomorrow. Which is the best prevention strategy for tumor lysis syndrome (TLS)?

   A. Hydration with 5% dextrose (D_5W), 1 L before chemotherapy, plus allopurinol 300 mg/day.

   B. Hydration with D_5W, 100 mL/hour starting at least 24 hours before chemotherapy, plus allopurinol 300 mg/day.

   C. Hydration with normal saline 250 mL/hour starting at least 24 hours before chemotherapy plus allopurinol 300 mg/day.

   D. Hydration with normal saline 100 mL/hour starting at least 24 hours before chemotherapy plus sodium bicarbonate 500 mg orally every 6 hours.

4. An 18-year-old man is about to begin chemotherapy for acute lymphoblastic leukemia. On today's complete blood cell count (CBC), his hemoglobin is 7g/dL, and he is experiencing fatigue. Which is the best treatment recommendation?

   A. Initiate epoetin.

   B. Administer transfusion of packed red blood cells (RBCs).

   C. Delay chemotherapy treatment until hemoglobin recovers.

   D. Reduce chemotherapy dosages to prevent further decreases in hemoglobin.

5. A patient received her fourth cycle of chemotherapy with paclitaxel/carboplatin for ovarian cancer 12 days ago. She reports to the clinic this morning with a temperature of 103°F. Her CBC is WBC 500 cells/mm³, segmented neutrophils 55%, band neutrophils 5%, basophils 15%, eosinophils 5%, monocytes 15%, and platelet count 99,000 cells/mm³. She denies any signs or symptoms of infection. Her blood pressure (BP) is 115/60 mm Hg, heart rate is 80 beats/minute, and respiratory rate is 15 breaths/minute. Which best represents the patient's absolute neutrophil count (ANC)?

   A. 275 cells/mm³.
   B. 300 cells/mm³.
   C. 25 cells/mm³.
   D. 500 cells/mm³.

6. Which is the best course of action for the patient in the previous question?

   A. Admit to the hospital for intravenous antibiotic drugs.
   B. Treat as an outpatient with antibiotic drugs.
   C. Initiate a colony-stimulating factor (CSF).
   D. Discontinue chemotherapy.

7. Which statement about the above patient is most accurate?

   A. Given her monocyte count, her neutropenia is expected to last for another week.
   B. This is a nadir neutrophil count, and neutrophils would be expected to start increasing soon.
   C. The elevated absolute eosinophil count indicates an allergic reaction to carboplatin.
   D. It is unusual for the ANC to be this low in the setting of an elevated platelet count.

8. A 60-year-old man has head and neck cancer with extensive involvement of facial nerves. His pain medications include transdermal fentanyl 100 mcg/hour every 72 hours and oral morphine solution 40 mg every 4 hours as needed. He is still having problems with neuropathic pain. Which treatment is best to recommend?

   A. Begin gabapentin and decrease the dosage of fentanyl.

   B. Increase the dosages of fentanyl and morphine.
   C. Begin diazepam and increase the dosage of fentanyl.
   D. Begin gabapentin and continue fentanyl and morphine at the same dosage.

9. A patient is receiving chemotherapy for limited-stage small cell lung carcinoma. After the third cycle of chemotherapy, she is hospitalized with febrile neutropenia. She recovers, and today she is scheduled to receive the fourth cycle of chemotherapy. Which statement is the best treatment course for this patient?

   A. The patient should receive filgrastim 250 mcg/m²/day subcutaneously for 10 days, given at least 24 hours after chemotherapy.
   B. The patient should receive filgrastim 5 mcg/kg/day subcutaneously, starting today.
   C. The patient should receive pegfilgrastim 1 mg/day subcutaneously for 6 days, given at least 24 hours after chemotherapy.
   D. The patient should receive filgrastim 5 mcg/kg/day subcutaneously for 7 days, given at least 24 hours after chemotherapy.

10. A 60-year-old woman with breast cancer is to begin chemotherapy with AC (doxorubicin and cyclophosphamide). Laboratory values today include sodium 140 mEq/L, potassium 3.8 mEq/L, glucose 100 mg/dL, serum creatinine 1.1 mg/dL, aspartate aminotransferase 6 IU/L, alanine aminotransferase 35 IU/L, and total bilirubin 2 mg/dL. Which statement is most appropriate?

   A. The dosage of doxorubicin should be decreased.
   B. The dosage of cyclophosphamide should be decreased.
   C. Both chemotherapy drugs should be given at standard dosages.
   D. Both chemotherapy drugs should be given at decreased dosages.

11. Large cell lymphoma is considered intermediate (between indolent and highly aggressive) in tumor growth and biology. Large cell lymphoma is sensitive to chemotherapy and potentially curable.

Metastatic colorectal cancer is considered slow growing. Although responses to chemotherapy commonly occur and chemotherapy can prolong survival (by months), metastatic colorectal cancer is not generally considered curable with chemotherapy. Given these differences between large cell lymphoma and metastatic colorectal cancer, which one of the following statements is correct?

A. Patients with large cell lymphoma should receive allopurinol before the first cycle of chemotherapy because they are at an elevated risk of developing TLS.

B. Patients with metastatic colorectal cancer should receive allopurinol before the first cycle of chemotherapy because they are at an elevated risk of developing TLS.

C. Patients with large cell lymphoma should receive pamidronate before the first cycle of chemotherapy because they are at an elevated risk of developing hypercalcemia.

D. Patients with metastatic colorectal cancer should receive pamidronate before the first cycle of chemotherapy because they are at an elevated risk of developing hypercalcemia.

12. Consider the information provided above about large cell lymphoma and metastatic colorectal cancer. Patient 1 with large cell lymphoma is receiving CHOP-R (cyclophosphamide, doxorubicin [hydroxydaunomycin], vincristine [Oncovin], prednisone, and rituximab) chemotherapy. Patient 2 with metastatic colorectal cancer is receiving FOLFIRI (5-fluorouracil-leucovorin, irinotecan) chemotherapy. On the day cycle 2 is due, both patients have an ANC of 800 cells/mm³. Which statement is most appropriate given the ANC?

A. Patient 1 should get chemotherapy to keep him on schedule because he has a curable disease.

B. Patient 2 should get chemotherapy to keep him on schedule because he has a curable disease.

C. The chemotherapy for patient 1 should be held for now, and he should receive filgrastim after the next time he has chemotherapy.

D. The chemotherapy for patient 2 should be held for now, and he should receive filgrastim after the next time he has chemotherapy.

13. Sometimes, extravasation is not immediately evident when it occurs. Immediately after patient 1 receives CHOP-R, an extravasation is suspected. Which is the best treatment recommendation for the patient's extravasation?

A. Application of a warm pack for suspected extravasation of doxorubicin.

B. Application of a cold pack for suspected extravasation of vincristine.

C. Application of dimethyl sulfoxide and intravenous dexrazoxane for suspected extravasation of doxorubicin.

D. Application of sodium thiosulfate for suspected extravasation of vincristine.

BPS Pharmacotherapy Specialty Examination Content Outline
This chapter covers the following sections of the Pharmacotherapy Specialty Examination Content Outline:
1.   Domain 1: Patient-Centered Pharmacotherapy
     a.   Tasks 1, 4
     b.   Systems and Patient-Care Problems:
          i.   Antiemetics
          ii.   Pain Management
          iii. Treatment of Febrile Neutropenia
          iv.   Use of CSFs in Neutropenia and Febrile Neutropenia
          v.   Thrombocytopenia
          vi.   Anemia/Fatigue
          vii. Chemoprotectants
          viii. Oncology Emergencies
          ix.   Miscellaneous Antineoplastic Pharmacotherapy
          x.   Parathyroid disorders
2.   Domain 3: System-Based Standards and Population-Based Pharmacotherapy
     a.   Tasks 1, 3, 6

I. ANTIEMETICS

A. Important Definitions Pertaining to Chemotherapy-Induced Nausea and Vomiting (CINV)

1. Nausea is described as an awareness of discomfort that may or may not precede vomiting; nausea is accompanied by decreased gastric tone and decreased peristalsis.

2. Retching is the labored movement of abdominal and thoracic muscles associated with vomiting without the expulsion of vomitus and is also called dry heaves.

3. Vomiting (emesis) is the ejection or expulsion of gastric contents through the mouth.

   a. Acute onset: Occurs 0–24 hours after chemotherapy administration and commonly resolves within 24 hours (intensity peaks after 5–6 hours)

   b. Delayed onset: Occurs more than 24 hours after chemotherapy administration

      i. Delayed symptoms are best described with cisplatin, although they are commonly reported in association with other agents as well (carboplatin or doxorubicin).

      ii. The distinction between acute and delayed symptoms with respect to time of onset is somewhat arbitrary, and it becomes blurred when chemotherapy is administered for many days.

      iii. The importance of the distinction between acute and delayed (and anticipatory) symptoms is that they probably have different mechanisms and therefore different management strategies.

4. Anticipatory vomiting (or nausea) is triggered by sights, smells, or sounds and is a conditioned response; it is more likely to occur in patients whose previous postchemotherapy nausea and vomiting was not well controlled.

5. Breakthrough emesis occurs despite prophylactic treatment or necessitates additional rescue medications.

6. Refractory emesis is emesis that occurs during treatment cycles when antiemetic prophylaxis or rescue therapy has failed in previous cycles.

B. Risk Factors for CINV

1. Patient-related risk factors

   a. Patient's age (younger than 50 years)

   b. Female sex

   c. History of motion sickness

   d. History of nausea or vomiting during pregnancy

   e. Poor control of nausea or vomiting in previous chemotherapy cycles

   f. History of chronic alcoholism (decreases incidence of emesis)

2. Emetogenicity of chemotherapy agents: Several schemes for assessing emetogenicity have been proposed.

   a. Originally, emetogenic risk was classified as "none," "mild," "moderate," or "severe."

   b. The Hesketh model, proposed in 1997, classified emetogenic risk as levels ranging from level 1 (less than 10% frequency of emesis) to level 5 (more than 90% frequency of emesis).

   c. Current model includes four levels for intravenous chemotherapy and two levels for oral chemotherapy.

   d. Levels for intravenous chemotherapy (e.g., minimal, low, moderate, high emetogenic risk) are defined by the percentage of patients expected to experience emesis when not receiving antiemetic prophylaxis.

   e. Levels for oral chemotherapy (prophylaxis recommended and as needed)

3. Radiation therapy can also cause nausea and vomiting. The incidence and severity of radiation-induced nausea and vomiting vary by site of radiation and size of radiation field.

   a. Mildly emetogenic: Radiation to the head and neck or to the extremities

   b. Moderately emetogenic: Radiation to the upper abdomen or pelvis or craniospinal radiation

   c. Highly emetogenic: Total body irradiation, total nodal irradiation, and upper-half-body irradiation

C. General Principles for Managing CINV and Radiation-Induced Nausea and Vomiting

    1. Prevention is the key. Prophylactic antiemetics should be administered before moderately or highly emetogenic agents and before moderately and highly emetogenic radiation.

    2. Antiemetics should be scheduled for delayed nausea and vomiting for select chemotherapy regimens (e.g., cisplatin, doxorubicin/cyclophosphamide (AC)), and rescue antiemetics should be available if prolonged acute symptoms or ineffective antiemetic prophylaxis occurs.

    3. Begin with an appropriate antiemetic regimen based on the emetogenicity of the chemotherapy drugs.

        a. The most common antiemetic regimen for highly emetogenic chemotherapy and radiation is the combination of a neurokinin 1 (NK1) receptor antagonist, a serotonin receptor antagonist, and dexamethasone. Adding a corticosteroid to a serotonin receptor antagonist for highly (or moderately) emetogenic anticancer therapy increases efficacy by 10%–20%. Based on randomized clinical trial data, the AC regimen (see Table 1) should always include a three-drug regimen with an NK1 receptor antagonist, a serotonin receptor antagonist, and dexamethasone.

        b. For moderately emetogenic chemotherapy, the most common antiemetic regimen now includes a serotonin receptor antagonist and dexamethasone. The use of an NK1 receptor antagonist may be considered after risk stratification.

        c. The combination of high-dose metoclopramide and dexamethasone was the most common regimen to prevent delayed nausea and vomiting before the availability of aprepitant. This combination is still used when aprepitant has not been incorporated into the initial regimen for CINV.

        d. Single-agent phenothiazine, butyrophenone, or steroids are used for mildly to moderately emetogenic regimens and are given on either a scheduled or an as-needed basis for prolonged symptoms (i.e., breakthrough symptoms).

        e. Consider using a histamine-2 blocker or proton pump inhibitor (PPI) for dyspepsia (which can mimic nausea).

        f. Cannabinoids are generally used after other regimens have failed or to stimulate appetite.

        g. Agents whose primary indication is other than treatment of nausea and vomiting are being investigated (e.g., olanzapine). Clinically, these agents may be used for patients whose symptoms do not respond to standard antiemetics.

        h. Potential drug interactions between antineoplastic agents or antiemetics and other drugs should always be considered.

        i. Follow-up is essential. The response to the emetogenic regimen should always guide the choice of antiemetic regimen for subsequent therapy courses.

D. Emetogenic Potential of Intravenous Chemotherapy Agents

Table 1. Emetogenic Potential of Intravenous Chemotherapy Agents

High Emetic Risk (>90% frequency of emesis)	
AC (combination defined as either doxorubicin or epirubicin with cyclophosphamide)	Doxorubicin >60 mg/m^2
Carmustine >250 mg/m^2	Epirubicin >90 mg/m^2
Cisplatin[a]	Ifosfamide ≥2 g/m^2/dose
Cyclophosphamide >1500 mg/m^2	Mechlorethamine
Dacarbazine	Streptozocin

Moderate Emetic Risk (30%–90% frequency of emesis)	
Aldesleukin >12–15 million IU/m^2	Dactinomycin
Amifostine >300 mg/m^2	Daunorubicin
Arsenic trioxide	Doxorubicin <60 mg/m^2
Azacitidine	Epirubicin ≤90 mg/m^2
Bendamustine	Idarubicin
Busulfan	Ifosfamide <2 g/m^2/dose
Carboplatin	Interferon alfa ≥10 million IU/m^2
Carmustine ≤250 mg/m^2	Irinotecan
Clofarabine	Melphalan
Cyclophosphamide ≤1500 mg/m^{2a}	Methotrexate ≥250 mg/m^2
Cytarabine >200 mg/m^2	Oxaliplatin
	Temozolomide

Low Emetic Risk (10%–30% frequency of emesis)	
Ado-trastuzumab emtansine	Interferon alfa >5 million IU/m^2 to <10 million IU/m^2
Aldesleukin ≤12 million IU/m^2	Ixabepilone
Amifostine ≤300 mg/m^2	Methotrexate >50 mg/m^2 to <250 mg/m^2
Belinostat	Mitomycin
Blinatumomab	Mitoxantrone
Brentuximab vedotin	Omacetaxine
Cabazitaxel	Paclitaxel
Carfilzomib	Paclitaxel/albumin
Cytarabine (low dose) 100–200 mg/m^2	Pemetrexed
Docetaxel	Pentostatin
Doxorubicin (liposomal)	Pralatrexate
Eribulin	Romidepsin
Etoposide	Thiotepa
Floxuridine	Topotecan
Fluorouracil	Ziv-aflibercept
Gemcitabine	

Table 1. Emetogenic Potential of Intravenous Chemotherapy Agents *(continued)*

Minimal Emetic Risk (<10% frequency of emesis)	
Alemtuzumab	Obinutuzumab
Asparaginase	Ofatumumab
Bevacizumab	Panitumumab
Bleomycin	Pegaspargase
Bortezomib	Peginterferon
Cetuximab	Pembrolizumab
Cladribine (2-chlorodeoxyadenosine)	Pertuzumab
Cytarabine <100 mg/m^2	Ramucirumab
Decitabine	Rituximab
Denileukin diftitox	Siltuximab
Dexrazoxane	Temsirolimus
Fludarabine	Trastuzumab
Interferon alfa ≤5 million IU/m^2	Valrubicin
Ipilimumab	Vinblastine
Methotrexate ≤50 mg/m^2	Vincristine
Nelarabine	Vincristine (liposomal)
Nivolumab	Vinorelbine

[a]Causes delayed emesis.

E. Emetogenic Potential of Oral Chemotherapy Agents (Table 2)

Table 2. Emetogenic Potential of Oral Chemotherapy Agents

Moderate to High Emetic Risk; Prophylaxis Recommended	
Altretamine	Lomustine (single day)
Busulfan ≥4 mg/day	Mitotane
Ceritinib	Olaparib
Crizotinib	Panobinostat
Cyclophosphamide ≥100 mg/m^2/day	Procarbazine
Estramustine	Temozolomide >75 mg/m^2/day
Etoposide	Vismodegib
Lenvatinib	

Table 2. Emetogenic Potential of Oral Chemotherapy Agents *(continued)*

Moderate to Low Emetic Risk; As Needed	
Afatinib	Melphalan
Axitinib	Mercaptopurine
Bexarotene	Methotrexate
Bosutinib	Nilotinib
Busulfan <4 mg/day	Palbociclib
Cabozantinib	Pazopanib
Capecitabine	Pomalidomide
Chlorambucil	Ponatinib
Cyclophosphamide <100 mg/m^2/day	Regorafenib
Dabrafenib	Ruxolitinib
Dasatinib	Sorafenib
Erlotinib	Sunitinib
Everolimus	Temozolomide ≤75 mg/m^2/day
Fludarabine	Thalidomide
Gefitinib	Thioguanine
Hydroxyurea	Topotecan
Ibrutinib	Trametinib
Idelalisib	Tretinoin
Imatinib	Vandetanib
Lapatinib	Vemurafenib
Lenalidomide	Vorinostat

F.   Antiemetics
   1.   Serotonin-3 (5-HT3) receptor antagonists (dolasetron, granisetron, ondansetron, and palonosetron)
      a.   Mechanism of action (MOA): Block serotonin receptors peripherally in the gastrointestinal tract and centrally in the medulla
      b.   Adverse events: Headache and constipation, occurring in 10%–15% of patients. May increase liver function tests and cause QT prolongation (especially with high dosages or intravenous push administration).
      c.   Dolasetron, granisetron, ondansetron, and palonosetron are considered equally efficacious at equivalent dosages. Therefore, the antiemetic drug of choice is often based on cost and organizational contract.
      d.   Dosage forms: Granisetron and ondansetron are available in oral and intravenous forms (including an orally disintegrating tablet for ondansetron). Dolasetron is now indicated only in CINV in its oral form. Granisetron is also available in a transdermal patch (34.3 mg applied about 24–48 hours before the first dose of chemotherapy; maximal duration of patch is 7 days).
      e.   Palonosetron is indicated to prevent acute CINV for highly emetogenic chemotherapy and acute and delayed CINV for moderately emetogenic chemotherapy.
         i.   Half-life: About 40 hours (longer compared with other serotonin antagonists)
         ii.   Dosage: 0.25 mg intravenous push 30 minutes before chemotherapy administration
         iii.   May be used before the start of a 3-day chemotherapy regimen instead of several daily doses of oral or intravenous serotonin-3 receptor antagonists
         iv.   Adverse events: Headache and constipation (same as other serotonin antagonists)

2. Corticosteroids (dexamethasone, methylprednisolone)
   a. MOA: Unknown; thought to act by inhibiting prostaglandin synthesis in the cortex
   b. Adverse effects associated with single doses and short courses of steroids are infrequent; they may include euphoria, anxiety, insomnia, increased appetite, and mild fluid retention; rapid intravenous administration may be associated with transient and intense perineal, vaginal, or anal burning.
   c. Dexamethasone has been studied more often in clinical trials than methylprednisolone.
3. NK1 receptor antagonists (aprepitant, fosaprepitant, rolapitant)
   a. MOA: Aprepitant is a selective high-affinity antagonist of human substance P/NK1.
   b. Aprepitant is approved for use in combination with other antiemetic drugs for preventing acute and delayed nausea and vomiting associated with initial and repeat courses of chemotherapy known to cause these problems, including high-dose cisplatin.
   c. Aprepitant improved the overall complete response (defined as no emetic episodes and no use of rescue therapy) by about 20% when added to a serotonin receptor antagonist and dexamethasone.
   d. Aprepitant dosage: 125 mg on day 1, then 80 mg on day 2 and 80 mg on day 3
   e. Fosaprepitant dosage (prodrug): 150 mg intravenously on day 1 only (intravenous formulation)
   f. Metabolized primarily by cytochrome P450 (CYP) 3A4 with minor metabolism by CYP1A2 and CYP2C19
      i. Oral contraceptives: May reduce the effectiveness of oral contraceptives. Would recommend another form of birth control for women of childbearing age when taking with aprepitant
      ii. Warfarin: May decrease international normalized ratio (clinically significant). After completing a 3-day course of aprepitant, patients should have their international normalized ratios checked within 7–10 days.
      iii. Dexamethasone: May increase area under the curve of dexamethasone. Decrease dosage by about 40% on day 2 or 3 if dexamethasone given orally (not necessary if given intravenously because of first-pass metabolism).
      iv. Caution use in patients with lymphoma: Studies suggest neuropathy is more common in patients on R-CHOP receiving aprepitant, because of aprepitant's CYP3A4 inhibition.
   g. Adverse events: Asthenia, dizziness, and hiccups
   h. MOA: Rolapitant substance P/NK1 receptor antagonist indicated in combination with other antiemetic agents in adults with cancer for the prevention of delayed nausea and vomiting associated with initial and repeat courses of emetogenic cancer chemotherapy, including highly emetogenic chemotherapy.
   i. Rolapitant dosage: 180 mg orally on day 1 only in combination with dexamethasone on days 2 and 3
   j. Adverse events: Loss of appetite, neutropenia, and hiccups
4. NK1 receptor antagonist/serotonin 5-HT3 combination netupitant/palonosetron
   a. MOA: Fixed combination of netupitant, a substance P/NK1 receptor antagonist, and palonosetron, a serotonin-3 (5-HT3) receptor antagonist indicated for the prevention of acute and delayed nausea and vomiting associated with initial and repeat courses of cancer chemotherapy, including highly emetogenic chemotherapy. Oral palonosetron prevents nausea and vomiting during the acute phase, and netupitant prevents nausea and vomiting during both the acute and delayed phases after cancer chemotherapy.
   b. Netupitant/palonosetron dosage: 1 capsule once on day 1 (capsule contains 300 mg of netupitant/palonosetron 0.5 mg)
   c. Adverse effects: Headache, asthenia, dyspepsia, fatigue, constipation, and erythema
   d. Caution in patients with hepatic dysfunction, severe renal impairment, or end-stage renal disease

5. Benzamide analogs (metoclopramide)
   a. MOA: Blockade of dopamine receptors in the chemoreceptor trigger zone; stimulation of cholinergic activity in the gut, increasing (forward) gut motility; and antagonism of peripheral serotonin receptors in the intestines. These effects are dose related.
   b. Adverse events: Mild sedation and diarrhea, as well as extrapyramidal reactions (e.g., dystonia, akathisia), which may be mitigated by diphenhydramine or lorazepam.
   c. High dosages of metoclopramide are used for desired results (1–2 mg/kg intravenously)
6. Phenothiazines (prochlorperazine, chlorpromazine, promethazine)
   a. MOA: Block dopamine receptors in the chemoreceptor trigger zone
   b. Adverse events: Drowsiness, hypotension, akathisia, and dystonia
   c. Chlorpromazine is often preferred in children because it is associated with fewer extrapyramidal reactions than prochlorperazine.
7. Butyrophenones (haloperidol, droperidol)
   a. MOA: Similar to phenothiazines
   b. They are at least as effective as the phenothiazines, and some studies indicate they are superior; they offer a different chemical structure that may bind differently to the dopamine receptor and offer an initial alternative when a phenothiazine fails.
   c. Adverse events: Sedation; hypotension is less common than with phenothiazines; extrapyramidal symptoms are also seen.
   d. The use of droperidol as an antiemetic has fallen out of favor because of the risk of QT prolongation or torsades de pointes.
8. Benzodiazepines (lorazepam)
   a. Lorazepam as a single agent has minimal antiemetic activity. However, several properties make lorazepam useful in combination with or as an adjunct to other antiemetics.
      i. Anterograde amnesia helps prevent anticipatory nausea and vomiting.
      ii. Relief of anxiety
      iii. Management of akathisia caused by phenothiazines, butyrophenones, or metoclopramide
   b. Adverse events: Amnesia, sedation, hypotension, perceptual disturbances, and urinary incontinence. Note that amnesia and sedation may, in fact, be desirable.
9. Atypical antipsychotic (olanzapine)
   a. Approved by the U.S. Food and Drug Administration (FDA) to treat schizophrenia and bipolar disorder, this thienobenzodiazepine is used off label as an alternative agent for preventing nausea and vomiting in highly emetogenic regimens and may be used as an option for breakthrough nausea and vomiting.
   b. MOA: Blocks multiple neurotransmitters, including dopamine, serotonin, catecholamines, acetylcholine, and histamine
   c. Adverse effects: Sedation, dry mouth, increased appetite, weight gain, postural hypotension, QTc prolongation, and dizziness
   d. Olanzapine has been associated with an elevated risk of hyperlipidemia, hyperglycemia, and new-onset diabetes. Use with caution in older adults because olanzapine use in this patient population has been associated with an elevated risk of death and an elevated incidence of cerebrovascular adverse events in patients with dementia-related psychosis (black box warning)
   e. Recently, a phase III study was conducted comparing olanzapine with aprepitant in highly emetogenic chemotherapy regimens. Overall response rates were similar in both groups for acute and delayed nausea and vomiting. The proportion of patients without nausea was similar between the two groups in the acute period but was higher in the olanzapine arm in the delay period, resulting in a higher rate of nausea control. As an alternative to aprepitant, an olanzapine-based regimen may be an option in highly or moderately emetogenic regimens according to the most recent National Comprehensive Cancer Network (NCCN) guidelines.

10. Cannabinoids (dronabinol, nabilone)
    a. MOA: Cannabinoid receptors may mediate at least some of the antiemetic activity of this class of agents. Additional antiemetic mechanisms that have been proposed include inhibition of prostaglandins and blockade of adrenergic activity.
    b. Adverse events: Drowsiness, dizziness, euphoria, dysphoria, orthostatic hypotension, ataxia, hallucinations, and time disorientation. Appetite stimulation is also seen with cannabinoids and may, in fact, be desirable.

G. Emesis Prevention Algorithms (Tables 3 and 4)

Table 3. Emesis Prevention Algorithm for Intravenous Chemotherapy (per NCCN Guidelines)

Level of Emetogenicity	Emesis Treatment Day 1	Emesis Treatment Days 2, 3, and 4

High	Neurokinin-1 antagonist
	  - Aprepitant 125 mg PO
	  - Fosaprepitant 150 mg IV once
	  - Rolapitent 180 mg PO
	
	AND
	
	Serotonin 5-HT3 antagonist
	
	AND
	
	Steroid
	± Lorazepam
	± Histamine-2 blocker or proton pump inhibitor
		- If aprepitant PO given day 1, aprepitant 80 mg PO daily on days 2 and 3
		- If fosaprepitant given on day 1, no further aprepitant needed on days 2 and 3. Dexamethasone dosage is twice daily on days 3 and 4.
		
		AND steroid until day 4

	OR
	
	Netupitant-containing regimen
	  - Netupitant 300 mg/palonosetron 0.5 mg PO once
	  - Dexamethasone 12 mg PO/IV
	± Lorazepam
	± Histamine-2 blocker or proton pump inhibitor
		OR
		
		Dexamethasone 8 mg PO/IV daily on days 2 and 3

	OR
	
	Olanzapine-containing regimen:
	  1. Olanzapine 10 mg PO day 1
	  2. Palonosetron 0.25 mg IV day 1
	  3. Dexamethasone 20 mg IV day 1
	± Lorazepam
	± Histamine-2 blocker or proton pump inhibitor
		OR
		
		Olanzapine-containing regimen:
		Olanzapine 10 mg PO days 2–4
		  (if given day 1)

Table 3. Emesis Prevention Algorithm for Intravenous Chemotherapy (per NCCN Guidelines) *(continued)*

Level of Emetogenicity	Emesis Treatment Day 1	Emesis Treatment Days 2, 3, and 4

Moderate	Serotonin 5-HT3 antagonist
	
	AND
	
	Steroid
	
	WITH/WITHOUT
	
	Neurokinin-1 antagonist
	± Lorazepam
	± Histamine-2 blocker or proton pump inhibitor
	
	OR
	
	Netupitant-containing regimen
	  - Netupitant 300 mg/palonosetron 0.5 mg PO once
	  - Dexamethasone 12 mg PO/IV
	± Lorazepam
	± Histamine-2 blocker or proton pump inhibitor
	
	OR
	
	Olanzapine-containing regimen:
	  1. Olanzapine 10 mg PO day 1
	  2. Palonosetron 0.25 mg IV day 1
	  3. Dexamethasone 20 mg IV day 1
	± Lorazepam
	± Histamine-2 blocker or proton pump inhibitor
		Serotonin 5-HT3 antagonist
		
		OR
		
		Steroid monotherapy daily on days 2 and 3
		
		OR
		
		Neurokinin-1 antagonist
		
		OR
		
		Dexamethasone 8 mg PO/IV daily on days 2 and 3
		
		OR
		
		Olanzapine-containing regimen:
		Olanzapine 10 mg PO days 2–4 (if given day 1)

Level of Emetogenicity	Emesis Treatment Day 1	Emesis Treatment Days 2–3
Low	Steroid OR Metoclopramide as needed OR Prochlorperazine as needed OR Serotonin-3 antagonists (oral therapy) daily ± Lorazepam ± Histamine-2 blocker or proton pump inhibitor	Steroid OR Metoclopramide as needed OR Prochlorperazine as needed OR Serotonin-3 antagonists (oral therapy) daily ± Lorazepam ± Histamine-2 blocker or proton pump inhibitor
Minimal	No routine prophylaxis	No routine prophylaxis

IV = intravenous(ly); PO = by mouth

Table 4. Emesis Prevention Algorithm for Oral Chemotherapy per NCCN Guidelines

Level of Emetogenicity	Emesis Treatment (start before chemotherapy and continue daily)
High to moderate emetic risk	Serotonin-3 antagonist (choose one): Dolasetron 100 mg daily Granisetron 2 mg PO daily or 1 mg PO BID Ondansetron 16–24 mg PO daily ± Lorazepam ± Histamine-2 blocker or proton pump inhibitor
Low to minimal emetic risk	Metoclopramide 10–40 mg PO and then q4h or q6h PRN Prochlorperazine 10 mg PO or IV and then q6h PRN (maximum 40 mg/day) OR Haloperidol 1–2 mg PO and then q4h or q6h PRN OR Serotonin-3 antagonist (choose one): Dolasetron 100 mg daily Granisetron 2 mg PO daily or 1 mg PO BID Ondansetron 16–24 mg PO daily ± Lorazepam ± Histamine-2 blocker or proton pump inhibitor

BID = twice daily; h = hours; IV = intravenous; PO = by mouth; PRN = as needed; q4h = every 4 hours; q6h = every 6 hours.

Patient Cases

1. A 60-year-old woman was recently given a diagnosis of advanced non–small cell lung cancer. She will begin treatment with cisplatin 100 mg/m^2 plus vinorelbine 30 mg/m^2. Which is the most appropriate antiemetic regimen for preventing acute emesis?

    A. Aprepitant plus palonosetron plus dexamethasone.

    B. Aprepitant plus prochlorperazine plus dexamethasone.

    C. Aprepitant plus granisetron plus ondansetron.

    D. Lorazepam plus ondansetron plus metoclopramide.

2. Which is the most appropriate regimen for anticipatory nausea and vomiting?

    A. Aprepitant plus dexamethasone.

    B. Aprepitant plus metoclopramide.

    C. Ondansetron plus dexamethasone.

    D. Aprepitant plus ondansetron plus dexamethasone plus lorazepam.

II. PAIN MANAGEMENT

A. Principles of Cancer Pain Management
   1. The most important step in treating pain is the assessment.
   2. The oral route is preferred when available. Although the ratio of oral to parenteral potency of morphine is commonly noted to be 6:1, clinical observation of chronic morphine use indicates that this ratio is closer to 3:1.
   3. Choose the analgesic drug and dosage to match the patient's degree of pain.
   4. For persistent severe pain, use a product with a long duration of action. Pain medications should always be administered on a scheduled basis or around the clock, not as needed.
      a. It is always easier to prevent pain from recurring than to treat it once it has recurred.
      b. As-needed dosing should be used for breakthrough pain, which is pain that "breaks through" the regularly scheduled opioid; an immediate-release, short-acting opioid should always accompany a long-acting opioid.
   5. Reevaluate pain and pain relief often, especially when initiating pain therapy; if more than two as-needed doses are necessary for breakthrough pain in a 24-hour period, consider modifying the regimen. Before adding or changing to another drug, maximize the dosage and schedule of the current analgesic drug.
   6. Provide medications to prevent other potential side effects from opioid therapy (e.g., constipation).
   7. Use appropriate adjuvant analgesics and nondrug measures to maximize pain control.

B. Diagnosis and Assessment of Pain
   1. Best addressed by proper pain assessment including comprehensive history and physical examination
   2. Evaluation of pain management: Pain intensity, pain relief, and medication adverse effects or allergies must be assessed and reassessed.
   3. Objective observations such as grimacing, limping, or tachycardia may be helpful in assessment.
   4. Clinicians must accept the patient's report of pain.

C. Pain Rating Scales
   1. Use pain assessment tools to evaluate pain intensity at baseline and to assess how well a pain medication regimen is working.
      a. Numeric rating scale of 0–10, with 0 = no pain and 10 = worst pain imaginable
      b. Pediatric patients: Faces-of-Pain Scale, poker chip method
   2. Because pain is subjective, it is best evaluated by the patient (i.e., not a caregiver and not the health professional).

D. Treatment of Pain: The Analgesic Ladder
   1. For mild to moderate pain (pain rating of 1–3 on a 10-point scale), the first step is a nonopioid analgesic drug: Nonsteroidal anti-inflammatory drug (NSAID), aspirin, or acetaminophen (APAP), or consider slow titration of short-acting opioids either as needed or as scheduled.
   2. For persistent or moderate to severe pain (pain rating of 4–6 on a 10-point scale), add a weak opioid: Codeine or hydrocodone, available in combination with nonopioid analgesic drugs. Slow titration of a short-acting opioid may also be considered.
   3. For persistent or for severe pain (pain rating of 7–10 on a 10-point scale), replace the weak opioid with a strong opioid: Morphine, oxycodone, or similar drug. In opioid-naive patients experiencing severe pain, short-acting opioids should be rapidly titrated. Once a patient with persistent pain is taking stable dosages of short-acting opioids, the drug should be changed to an extended-release or long-acting formulation with breakthrough short-acting opioids.

E. Nonopioid Analgesics: NSAIDs
   1. MOA: Act peripherally to inhibit the activity of prostaglandins in the pain pathway
   2. There is a ceiling effect to the analgesia provided by NSAIDs.
   3. Adverse events: Consider inhibition of platelet aggregation and the effects of inhibition of renal prostaglandins. NSAIDs in patients with hematologic disorders are not recommended because of platelet inhibition. In addition, there are concerns about the possibility that NSAIDs will mask fever in a patient with neutropenia who is potentially febrile.
   4. Remember, NSAIDs are generally used in addition to, not instead of, opioids.
   5. NSAIDs are often used for patients with cancer and metastatic bone pain.

F. Nonopioid/Opioid Combinations
   1. Aspirin or APAP or ibuprofen plus codeine or hydrocodone or oxycodone is the most commonly used combination.
   2. Be aware of the risk of APAP overdose with these products. As with any combination product, dosage escalation of one component necessitates escalation of the others. For patients needing high dosages, pure opioids are preferred.
   3. Oxycodone/APAP is available in several strengths; however, the amount of APAP increases with increasing oxycodone.

G. Opioid Analgesics
   1. Mechanism: Opioids act centrally in the brain (periaqueductal gray region) and at the level of the spinal cord (dorsal horn) at specific opioid receptors.
   2. The opioids have no analgesic ceiling.
   3. Morphine
      a. Morphine is the standard with which all other drugs are compared; opioids may differ in duration of action, relative potency, oral effectiveness, and adverse event profiles, but none is clinically superior to morphine.
      b. Flexibility in dosage forms and administration routes: Oral (sustained release, immediate release), sublingual, intravenous, intrathecal/epidural, subcutaneous, and rectal
      c. Long duration of action: Sustained-release products last 8–12 hours or, for some preparations, 24 hours.
      d. Morphine is one of the least expensive opioids but should be used with caution in patients with renal dysfunction because of the metabolite.
   4. Oxycodone
      a. Available in oral formulation only
      b. Available as a single drug (i.e., not in combination) in both long- and short-acting formulations
      c. Alternative to morphine in the setting of renal dysfunction
   5. Fentanyl
      a. Fentanyl is available as an intravenous formulation; a sublingual, intranasal, or transdermal preparation; an oral transmucosal preparation; and a buccal tablet. Transmucosal and buccal fentanyl are used for breakthrough pain.
      b. Each transdermal patch provides sustained release of drug and can provide pain relief for 48–72 hours. These should not be used in opioid-naive patients.
      c. Consider the implications for dosing transdermal fentanyl in cachectic patients: Fentanyl initially forms a depot in subcutaneous tissue, and patients with little or no fat may not achieve pain relief.
      d. Slow onset and long elimination after patch application and removal, respectively
      e. Bioavailability is greater with buccal tablets than with the transmucosal preparation; thus, equivalent dosages are higher for transmucosal and lower for buccal tablets.

6. Hydromorphone
   a. Available in intravenous and oral formulations (short- and long-acting)
   b. Considered a semisynthetic compound
   c. Alternative to morphine with higher potency
   d. Alterative option in patients with renal dysfunction
7. Oxymorphone
   a. Semisynthetic opioid analgesic
   b. Most commonly seen as immediate- and extended-release tablets
   c. Used for moderate to severe pain
   d. Should not be implemented in patients who are not currently on an opioid regimen
8. Methadone
   a. Semisynthetic used in maintenance treatment for opioid-dependent patients and as an effective analgesic in patients taking opioids long term for moderate to severe pain
   b. Has activity not only at the opioid receptors but also at the N-methyl-D-aspartate receptor, which may confer benefit to patients with neuropathic pain
   c. Complex pharmacokinetics with extended half-life (8–59 hours), which creates difficulties in dosing and transitioning from one opioid to another
   d. Associated with QT prolongation and torsades de pointes
   e. Effective long-acting agent also used for neuropathic pain
   f. Start low and titrate slowly (only escalating after 3–5 days) because of the changing conversion ratios with increasing morphine equivalents.

H. Adverse Events
   1. Sedation: Tolerance usually develops within several days; remember that more sedation may be expected in a patient who has been unable to sleep because of uncontrolled pain. For patients who do not develop tolerance to sedation and have good pain control, a dosage reduction may be considered. If dosage reduction compromises pain control, adding a stimulant (e.g., dextroamphetamine, methylphenidate) may be considered. Other central nervous system adverse events include dysphoria and hallucinations.
   2. Constipation is very common, and tolerance does not develop to this effect. Decreased intestinal peristalsis is caused by decreased intestinal tone; delayed gastric emptying may also occur. Regular use of stool softeners in addition to a stimulant laxatives is imperative to manage constipation.
   3. Nausea and vomiting are common. As seen with sedation, tolerance develops within about a week. Nausea and vomiting may have a vestibular component, developing as pain relief promotes increased mobility. Antivertigo agents (e.g., meclizine, dimenhydrinate) may be useful in managing the vestibular component, although these agents should be used with caution because combination use with opioids may increase sedation. Nausea and vomiting may also occur because of stimulation of the chemoreceptor trigger zone. Drugs that block dopamine receptors (e.g., phenothiazines) provide relief of this component of nausea and vomiting until tolerance develops.
   4. Urinary retention and bladder spasm are more common in older adults and in patients taking long-acting formulations.

I. Bisphosphonates
   1. Bisphosphonates decrease the worsening of pain by preventing disease progression in the bone and the number of skeletal-related events in patients with breast cancer and multiple myeloma when given for 1 year. Skeletal-related events include pathologic fracture, need for radiation therapy to bone, surgery to bone, and spinal cord compression.

2. In 2000, the American Society of Clinical Oncology published initial guidelines for the use of bisphosphonates in breast cancer (updated in November 2003).

   a. It is recommended that patients with breast cancer who have evidence of bone metastases on plain radiographs receive either pamidronate 90 mg delivered over 2 hours or zoledronic acid 4 mg over 15 minutes every 3–4 weeks. Dosage adjustments for renal dysfunction are necessary according to package insert recommendations.

   b. Women with abnormal bone scan and abnormal computed tomographic scan or magnetic resonance imaging showing bone destruction but a normal radiograph should also receive the above-recommended bisphosphonates.

   c. Therapy should continue until there is evidence of a substantial decline in a patient's performance status.

   d. Bisphosphonates may be used in combination with other pain therapies in patients with pain caused by osteolytic disease.

3. In 2002, the American Society of Clinical Oncology published guidelines for the use of bisphosphonates in multiple myeloma.

   a. Patients with lytic bone destruction seen on plain radiographs should receive either pamidronate 90 mg intravenously over at least 2 hours or zoledronic acid 4 mg over 15 minutes every 3–4 weeks.

   b. Therapy should continue until there is evidence of substantial decline in a patient's performance status.

   c. Patients with osteopenia but no radiologic evidence of bone metastases can receive bisphosphonates.

   d. Bisphosphonates are not recommended for patients with solitary plasmacytoma, smoldering or indolent myeloma, or monoclonal gammopathy of undetermined significance.

   e. Bisphosphonates may be used in patients with pain caused by osteolytic disease.

4. Adverse events: Low-grade fevers, nausea, anorexia, vomiting, hypomagnesemia, hypocalcemia, hypokalemia, and nephrotoxicity

   a. Serum creatinine should be monitored before each dose (see package insert for specific recommendations).

   b. Package insert recommends initiating patients on oral calcium 500 mg plus vitamin D 400 IU/day to prevent hypocalcemia.

   c. Several reports of osteonecrosis of the jaw occurring in patients receiving bisphosphonates have appeared in the literature. Osteonecrosis of the jaw usually follows a dental or dental disorder. The long half-life of bisphosphonates in bone makes this adverse event difficult to prevent and manage. Patient education and education of dentists are important. Patients should have a dental examination with preventive dentistry before treatment with bisphosphonates.

J. Receptor Activator of NF-κB Ligand (RANKL) Inhibitor

   1. Denosumab: Fully human monoclonal antibody that targets and inhibits RANKL, a protein that acts as the primary signal to promote bone removal

   2. Indication: Prevention of skeletal-related events in patients with bone metastases from solid tumors

   3. Dosage: 120 mg subcutaneously every 4 weeks

   4. Adverse events: Urinary and respiratory tract infections, cataracts, constipation, rashes, hypocalcemia (especially in patients with CrCl less than 30 mL/minute), and joint pain

   5. Contraindications: Hypocalcemia. Patients should be taking calcium and vitamin D.

   6. No adjustment for hepatic or renal dysfunction is needed.

K. Adjuvant analgesics are drugs whose primary indication is other than pain; they are used to manage specific pain syndromes. Most often, adjuvant analgesics are used in addition to, rather than instead of, opioids.

1. Antidepressants (e.g., amitriptyline, duloxetine) and anticonvulsants (e.g., gabapentin, carbamazepine, pregabalin) are used for neuropathic pain (e.g., phantom limb pain, nerve compression caused by tumor).

2. Transdermal lidocaine is useful in localized neuropathic pain.

3. Corticosteroids are useful in pain caused by nerve compression or inflammation, lymphedema, bone pain, or elevated intracranial pressure.

4. Benzodiazepines: Diazepam, lorazepam. Useful for muscle spasms; baclofen is another alternative for intractable muscle spasms.

5. Strontium-89: Radionuclide for treatment of bone pain caused by osteoblastic lesions; a single dose may provide relief for several weeks or even months; however, it is myelosuppressive.

6. NSAIDs are recommended for treating pain caused by bone metastases. Prostaglandins sensitize nociceptors (pain receptors) to painful stimuli, thus providing a rationale for using NSAIDs.

L. Risk Evaluation and Mitigation Strategy (REMS) for Extended-Release/Long-Acting Opioid Analgesics

1. On June 9, 2012, the FDA announced it would require manufacturers of extended-release and long-acting opioid analgesics to provide training for health care professionals who prescribe these agents.

2. Components of the REMS program

   a. Prescriber education: Information on extended-release or long-acting opioid analgesics; information on assessing patients for treatment with these drugs; initiating therapy, modifying dosing, and discontinuing use of extended-release or long-acting opioid analgesics; managing therapy and monitoring patients; and counseling patients and caregivers about the safe use of these drugs. Prescribers will also learn how to recognize evidence of potential opioid misuse, abuse, and addiction.

   b. Patient counseling: Patient counseling documents for providers will be developed to assist prescribers in counseling patients about their responsibilities for using these medications safely. Patients will receive an updated medication guide, together with their prescription, that contains information on the safe use and disposal of extended-release or long-acting opioid analgesics from their pharmacist. Guide will include instructions for patients to consult their health care professional before changing dosages, signs of potential overdose and emergency contact instructions, and advice on safe storage to prevent accidental exposure of family members.

   c. Short-acting opioid products are not included in this program.

Patient Cases

3. A 75-year-old man has metastatic prostate cancer. The main sites of metastatic disease are regional lymph nodes and bone (several hip lesions). He experiences aching pain with occasional shooting pains. The latter are thought to be the result of nerve compression by enlarged lymph nodes. He has been taking oxycodone/APAP 5 mg 2 tablets every 4 hours and ibuprofen 400 mg every 8 hours. His current pain rating is 8/10, and he states that his pain cannot be controlled. Which is the best recommendation to manage his pain at this time?

   A. Increase oxycodone/APAP to 7.5 mg/325 mg, 2 tablets every 4 hours.

   B. Increase oxycodone/APAP to 10 mg/325 mg, 2 tablets every 4 hours.

   C. Discontinue oxycodone/APAP, discontinue ibuprofen, and add morphine sustained release every 12 hours.

   D. Discontinue oxycodone/APAP and add morphine sustained release every 12 hours.

4. Which is the most appropriate adjunctive medication for this patient's pain?

   A. Naproxen.

   B. Single-agent (single ingredient) APAP.

   C. Gabapentin.

   D. Baclofen.

III. TREATMENT OF FEBRILE NEUTROPENIA

A. Principles of Chemotherapy-Induced Bone Marrow Suppression

   1. Bone marrow suppression is the most common dose-limiting toxicity associated with traditional cytotoxic chemotherapy.

   2. WBC = a normal range of $4.8-10.8 \times 100$ cells/mm^3 with a circulating life span of 6–12 hours; decreased WBC = neutropenia, leucopenia, or granulocytopenia; the risk is life-threatening infections; the risk increases with absolute neutrophil count (ANC) less than 500 cells/mm^3, and the risk is greatest with ANC less than 100 cells/mm^3. Because neutrophils have the fastest turnover, the effects of cytotoxic chemotherapy are greatest on neutrophils (compared with platelets or red blood cells [RBCs]).

      a. The nadir (usually described by the ANC) is the lowest value to which the blood count falls after cytotoxic chemotherapy. Usually occurs 10–14 days after chemotherapy administration, with counts usually recovering by 3–4 weeks after chemotherapy; exceptions include mitomycin, decitabine, and nitrosoureas (carmustine and lomustine), which have nadirs of 28–42 days after chemotherapy and recovery of neutrophils 6–8 weeks after treatment

      b. ANC = WBC × percentage granulocytes or neutrophils (segmented neutrophils plus band neutrophils). Example: A patient's WBC = 4500 cells/mm^3 with 10% segmented neutrophils and 5% band neutrophils. What is the ANC? $4500 \times (0.1 + 0.05) = 675$ cells/m^3.

      c. To receive chemotherapy, a patient should have a WBC greater than 3000 cells/mm^3 or an ANC greater than 1500 cells/mm^3 and a platelet count of 100,000 cells/mm^3 or more. These are general guidelines; some protocols and FDA labels or package inserts specify different (lower) thresholds for administering chemotherapy; if cytopenia is attributable to disease in the bone marrow, chemotherapy (full dose) may cause improvement; some drugs are nonmyelosuppressive (e.g., vincristine, bleomycin, monoclonal antibodies).

      d. The potential curability of the disease influences what action will be taken during the next cycle of chemotherapy, either dosage reduction of myelosuppressive chemotherapy or support with a CSF.

---

3. Other factors affecting myelosuppression include previous chemotherapy, previous radiation therapy, and direct bone marrow involvement by tumor.

B. Neutropenia and Febrile Neutropenia
   1. Infectious Diseases Society of America guidelines for antibiotic use were updated in 2010.
   2. Neutropenia is defined as an ANC of 500 cells/mm^3 or less or a count of less than 1000 cells/mm^3, with a predicted decrease to less than 500 cells/mm^3 during the next 48 hours.
   3. Febrile neutropenia is defined as neutropenia and a single oral temperature of 101°F or more or a temperature of 100.4°F or more for at least 1 hour.
   4. Neutropenic patients are at an elevated risk of developing serious and life-threatening infections.
   5. The usual signs and symptoms of infection (e.g., abscess, pus, infiltrates on chest radiograph) are absent, with fever often being the only indicator. In addition, cultures are negative more often than not. Therefore, prompt investigation and treatment of febrile neutropenia are essential.
   6. The initial assessment of patients with febrile neutropenia includes a risk assessment for complications and severe infection.
      a. Characteristics of low-risk neutropenia include the following: ANC of 100 cells/mm^3 or more and absolute monocyte count of 100 cells/mm^3 or more, normal chest radiograph, almost normal renal and hepatic function, neutropenia for less than 7 days and resolution expected in less than 10 days, no intravenous access site or catheter site infection, early evidence of bone marrow recovery, malignancy in remission, peak oral temperature of less than 102°F, no neurologic or mental status changes, no appearance of illness, absence of abdominal pain, and no comorbid complications (e.g., shock, hypoxia, pneumonia, other deep organ infection, vomiting, diarrhea).
      b. The Multinational Association for Supportive Care in Cancer has developed a scoring index to help identify patients with low-risk febrile neutropenia. Scores are assessed on the basis of factors such as those listed above.
      c. Febrile neutropenia that is considered to carry a low risk of complications may be treated with either oral or intravenous antibiotics in an outpatient or inpatient setting.
      d. Patients with high-risk febrile neutropenia (i.e., patients who do not have low-risk characteristics as noted above) should receive intravenous antibiotics in the hospital.
   7. Considerations in the initial selection of an antibiotic include the potential infecting organism, potential sites and source of infection, local antimicrobial susceptibilities, organ dysfunction potentially affecting antibiotic clearance or toxicity, and drug allergy. The most common source of infection is endogenous flora, which could be gram-negative or gram-positive bacteria; the more prolonged the neutropenia (and the more prolonged the administration of antibacterial antibiotics), the greater chance of fungi playing a role in the infection.
   8. All patients should be reassessed after 3–5 days of antibiotic therapy, and antibiotics should be adjusted accordingly.
   9. Prophylactic antibiotics (fluoroquinolones, TMP/SMX) may be considered for patients who are receiving chemotherapy who are expected to be profoundly neutropenic for more than 7 days.

IV. USE OF COLONY-STIMULATING FACTORS IN NEUTROPENIA AND FEBRILE NEUTROPENIA

A. CSFs improve both the production and function of their target cells. Four products and one biosimilar are currently available in the United States: Granulocyte colony-stimulating factor (G-CSF, or filgrastim [Neupogen]) or tbo-filgrastim (Granix), pegylated granulocyte colony-stimulating factor (pegfilgrastim, or PEG G-CSF) granulocyte-macrophage colony-stimulating factor (GM-CSF, sargramostim [Leukine]), and filgrastim-sndz (Zarxio).

B. Pegfilgrastim, the long-acting agent, is approved for use in patients with nonmyeloid malignancies who are receiving myelosuppressive chemotherapy associated with a high incidence of febrile neutropenia.

C. Studies have shown that G-CSF and GM-CSF reduce the incidence, magnitude, and duration of neutropenia after chemotherapy and bone marrow transplantation.

D. Guidelines for the use of CSFs were established by the American Society of Clinical Oncology in 1994; the most recent update was published in 2006.

E. CSFs are recommended with chemotherapy regimens associated with a 20% or greater risk of febrile neutropenia.
   1. G-CSF, tbo-filgrastim, GM-CSF, and filgrastim-sndz are given by daily subcutaneous injection.
   2. To date, no large trials have compared G-CSF and GM-CSF. Therefore, although it cannot be stated unequivocally that the two are therapeutically equivalent, they are often used interchangeably. However, they have varying adverse effect profiles (increased in fluid retention and fevers with GM-CSF).
   3. A meta-analysis of tbo-filgrastim and filgrastim resulted in tbo-filgrastim being noninferior to filgrastim for reducing the incidence of febrile neutropenia. Toxicities are considered similar between the two agents.
   4. Pegfilgrastim is given as a single 6-mg subcutaneous dose, generally administered 24 hours after chemotherapy. Pegfilgrastim on-body injector is also available for administration in the outpatient setting.
   5. A single dose of pegfilgrastim is as effective as 11 daily doses of G-CSF 5 mcg/kg in reducing the frequency and duration of severe neutropenia, promoting neutrophil recovery, and reducing the frequency of febrile neutropenia.
   6. Tbo-filgrastim was approved in an original biologics license application by the FDA in 2012. The FDA has not approved tbo-filgrastim as a biosimilar to Neupogen (filgrastim). Tbo-filgrastim is administered at 5 mcg/kg daily.
   7. Filgrastim-sndz was the first biosimilar approved by the FDA (March 2015). Filgrastim-sndz is also administered at 5 mcg/kg daily.
   8. The choice of CSF (pegfilgrastim vs. filgrastim) should be based on the expected duration of neutropenia and the specific anticancer regimen (e.g., short courses of a daily CSF rather than one dose of pegfilgrastim) with chemotherapy administration on a weekly schedule.
   9. Adverse events associated with all three preparations appear similar; they include bone pain (most common) and fever.
   10. The CSF should be initiated between 24 and 72 hours after the completion of chemotherapy.
   11. The package literature recommends continued administration of G-CSF until the postnadir ANC is greater than 10,000 cells/mm³; however, both G-CSF and GM-CSF are usually discontinued when adequate neutrophil recovery is evident. To decrease cost without compromising patient outcome, many centers continue the CSF until ANC is greater than 2000–5000 cells/mm³. Note that the ANC will decrease about 50% per day after the CSF is discontinued if the marrow has not recovered (i.e., if the CSF is discontinued before the ANC nadir is reached).
   12. Avoid the concomitant use of CSF in patients receiving chemotherapy and radiation therapy; the potential exists for worsening myelosuppression.

F. Refer to the American Society of Clinical Oncology Guidelines for the following indications: increasing chemotherapy dosage intensity, using as adjuncts to progenitor cell transplantation, administering to patients with myeloid malignancies, and using in pediatric populations.

G. American Society of Clinical Oncology Guidelines for Secondary CSF Administration
   1. If chemotherapy administration has been delayed or the dosage reduced because of prolonged neutropenia, then CSF use can be considered for subsequent chemotherapy cycles; administering CSF in this setting is considered secondary prophylaxis.
   2. Dosage reduction of chemotherapy should be considered the first option (i.e., instead of a CSF) after an episode of neutropenia in patients being treated with the intent to palliate (i.e., not a curative intent).

H. Use of CSFs for Treatment of Established Neutropenia
   1. Administering CSFs in patients who are neutropenic but not febrile is not recommended.
   2. Administering CSFs in patients who are neutropenic and febrile may be considered in the presence of risk factors for complications (e.g., ANC less than 100 cells/mm^3, pneumonia, hypotension, multiorgan dysfunction, invasive fungal infection); CSFs may be used in addition to antibiotics to treat neutropenia in patients with these risk factors.

Patient Cases

5. A 50-year-old woman is receiving adjuvant chemotherapy for stage II breast cancer. She received her third cycle of AC 10 days ago. Her CBC today includes WBC 600 cells/mm^3, segmented neutrophils 60%, band neutrophils 10%, monocytes 12%, basophils 8%, and eosinophils 10%. She is afebrile. Which best represents this patient's ANC?

   A. 600 cells/mm^3.
   B. 360 cells/mm^3.
   C. 240 cells/mm^3.
   D. 420 cells/mm^3.

6. Given this ANC, which statement is most appropriate?

   A. The patient should be initiated on a CSF.
   B. The patient should begin prophylactic treatment with either a quinolone antibiotic or trimethoprim/sulfamethoxazole.
   C. The patient, who is neutropenic, should be monitored closely for signs and symptoms of infection.
   D. Decrease the dosages of AC with the next cycle of treatment.

V. THROMBOCYTOPENIA

A. Megakaryocytes (platelets) = a normal range of 140,000–440,000 cells/mm^3 with a circulating life span of 5–10 days.

B. Thrombocytopenia is defined as a platelet count less than 100,000 cells/mm^3; however, the risk of bleeding is not substantially elevated until the platelet count is 20,000 cells/mm^3 or less. Practices for platelet transfusion vary widely from institution to institution. Many institutions do not transfuse platelets until the patient becomes symptomatic (ecchymosis, petechiae, hemoptysis, or hematemesis). Other institutions transfuse when the platelet count is 10,000 cells/mm^3 or less, even in the absence of bleeding.

C. Oprelvekin (interleukin-11) is approved to prevent severe thrombocytopenia in patients undergoing chemotherapy for nonmyeloid malignancies.

1. Oprelvekin is administered as a daily subcutaneous injection, beginning 6–24 hours after completion of myelosuppressive chemotherapy.

2. Treatment is continued until a postnadir platelet count of 50,000 cells/mm^3 or greater is achieved; dosing beyond 21 days is not recommended, and oprelvekin must be discontinued at least 2 days before (the next cycle of) chemotherapy.

3. The current role of oprelvekin is to maintain the dosage intensity of chemotherapy, although it is not nearly as widely used as the CSFs for neutrophils. A pharmacoeconomic analysis (from the payer's perspective) did not show oprelvekin to be a cost-saving strategy compared with routine platelet transfusions for patients with severe chemotherapy-induced thrombocytopenia.

4. Common adverse events associated with oprelvekin include edema, shortness of breath, tachycardia or arrhythmias, and conjunctival redness.

5. Although commercially available, oprelvekin is not currently used in clinical practice.

VI. ANEMIA AND FATIGUE

A. Overview of Anemia

1. Occurs in 3.4 million Americans each year and most common in women, African Americans, and older adults

2. Defined as hemoglobin (Hgb) less than 13 g/dL in men or 12 g/dL in women

3. Anemia defined as a reduction of RBC mass, number of RBCs, and Hgb concentration of RBCs

4. Caused by a deficiency, impaired bone marrow function, and peripheral causes.

5. Signs and symptoms of anemia include weakness and fatigue, irritability, tachycardia and palpitations, shortness of breath, chest pain, pale appearance, dizziness, decreased mental acuity, ecchymoses, blood in urine or stool, and hematomas.

6. There are several types of anemia, including microcytic (iron deficiency anemia), macrocytic/megaloblastic anemia (vitamin B$_{12}$ deficiency, folic acid deficiency), anemia of chronic disease (including chemotherapy-induced anemia), anemia of critical illness, hemolytic anemias, and drug-induced anemias.

7. Hematologic laboratory values:

Table 5. Hematologic Laboratory Values

Test	Reference Range	Definition
Hgb	M 13.5 - 17.5 g/dL F 12 - 16 g/dL	Hemoglobin per volume of whole blood
Hct	M 41%–53% F 36%–46%	Percentage of total blood volume composed of RBCs (3 × Hgb)
MCV	80–96 fL	Average volume of RBCs (Hct/RBC)
MCHC	31%–37%	Weight of Hgb per volume (Hgb/Hct)
MCH	26–34 pg	Percentage volume of Hgb in RBC (Hgb/RBC)
RBC	4.5–5.9 million/m3	RBCs per unit blood
Reticulocyte count	0.5%–1.5%	Immature RBCs
RDW	11%–16%	RBC distribution width
EPO	0–19 mU/mL	Endogenous erythropoietin
Serum iron	M 50–160 mcg/dL F 12–150 mcg/dL	Concentration of iron bound to transferrin
TIBC	250–400 mcg/dL	Iron binding capacity of transferrin
Ferritin	M 15–200 ng/mL F 12–150 ng/mL	Stored iron concentration
Folate	1.8–1.6 ng/mL	Serum folic acid
Vitamin B12	100–900 pg/mL	Serum vitamin B12
Transferrin saturation	>30%	Serum iron divided by TIBC

EPO = erythropoietin; F = female; Hct = hematocrit; Hgb = hemoglobin; M = male; MCH = mean corpuscular hemoglobin; MCHC = mean corpuscular hemoglobin concentration; MCV = mean corpuscular volume; RBC = red blood cells; RDW = RBC distribution width; TIBC = iron binding capacity of transferrin.

B. Microcytic Anemia
  1. Iron deficiency is the most common nutritional deficiency, with laboratory values reflecting a decreased RBC, Hgb/Hct, mean corpuscular volume (MCV), mean corpuscular hemoglobin concentration (MCHC), iron, ferritin, and transferrin. Total iron binding capacity (TIBC) and RBC distribution width (RDW) are increased.
  2. Treatment includes oral iron supplementation: 200 mg elemental iron divided twice daily or three times daily for 3–6 months.
  3. Available oral iron products (multiple branded agents):

Table 6. Available Oral Iron Products (multiple branded agents):

Product	% Elemental	Elemental Iron
Ferrous sulfate 325 mg tablet	20%	65 mg
Ferrous gluconate 325 mg tablet	12%	39 mg
Ferrous fumarate 100 mg tablet	33%	33 mg
Polysaccharide iron complex 150 mg capsule	100%	150 mg
Carbonyl iron 50 mg caplet	100%	50 mg

4. Iron side effects include constipation and nausea or vomiting.
5. Iron products should be taken with food to avoid gastrointestinal discomfort (but absorption will be decreased). Vitamin C may increase the absorption of iron and is often used to increase the efficacy of iron products. Iron therapy may cause dark stools.
6. Parental iron products:

Table 7. Parental Iron Products

	Iron Dextran	**Sodium Ferric Gluconate**	**Iron Sucrose**	**Ferumoxytol**
Elemental iron	50 mg/mL	62.5 mg/5 mL	20 mg/mL	30 mg/mL
Preservative	None	Benzyl alcohol 9 mg/5 mL 20%	None	None
Indication	IDA where PO not an option	IDA in patients on chronic HD receiving EPO	IDA in patients on chronic HD receiving EPO	IDA with CKD
Warning	Boxed warning: anaphylactic type reactions	Hypersensitivity reactions	Boxed warning: anaphylactic type reactions	Hypersensitivity reactions
IM injection	Yes	No	Yes	No
Usual dosage	100 mg IV push (no faster than 50 mg/min)	125 mg diluted in 100 ml NS over 60 min (IV injection at 12.5 mg/min)	100 mg at 1 mL undiluted solution/ min into dialysis line	510 mg IV injection repeated 3–8 days later
Test dose	Yes	No	No	No
Common adverse events	Pain, stinging at injection site (brown), hypotension, flushing, chills, fever, myalgia, anaphylaxis	Cramps, nausea or vomiting, flushing, hypotension, rash, pruritus	Leg cramps and hypotension	Diarrhea, constipation, nausea, dizziness, hypotension, peripheral edema

CKD = chronic kidney disease; EPO = erythropoietin; HD = hemodialysis; IDA = iron deficiency anemia; IM = intramuscular; IV = intravenous; NS = normal saline; PO = by mouth.

C. Macrocytic Anemia
1. Vitamin B_{12} and folate deficiency are the most common causes of macrocytic anemia. Causes of B_{12} deficiency include inadequate intake, malabsorption, and inadequate utilization. Folate deficiency is caused by inadequate intake, decreased absorption, hyperutilization, and inadequate utilization.
2. In B_{12} deficiency RBC, Hgb and Hct, and serum B_{12} are decreased, with an increase in MCV, MCH, methylmalonic acid, and homocysteine. Hypersegmented polymorphonuclear leukocytes may also be present on the peripheral smear.
3. In folate deficiency, RBC, Hgb and Hct, and serum folic acid are decreased, with an increase in MCV and MCH. B_{12} will be normal (will need to rule out this deficiency).
4. In B_{12} deficiency, patients may experience neurological changes, glossitis, weakness, loss of appetite, and possibly thrombocytopenia, leucopenia, and pancytopenia. Folate deficiency also presents with glossitis and other central nervous system symptoms including weakness, forgetfulness, headache, syncope, and loss of appetite.

     5.   Treatment options for vitamin B$_{12}$ deficiency include oral replacement daily or intramuscular replacement weekly for 1 month, then monthly.

     6.   Folate deficiency anemia should be treated with 1 mg of folate daily for 4 months. Women who are pregnant should take supplements to prevent neural tube defects in the fetus.

D. Anemia of Chronic Disease (Specifically Chemotherapy-Induced Anemia): Causes of Anemia and Fatigue in Adult Patients with Cancer

     1.   Unmanaged pain or other symptoms can increase fatigue.

     2.   Decreased RBC production because of anticancer therapy, either radiation or chemotherapy

     3.   Decreased or inappropriate endogenous erythropoietin production or decreased responsiveness to endogenous erythropoietin

     4.   Decreased body stores of vitamin B$_{12}$, iron, or folic acid

     5.   Increased destruction of RBCs

     6.   Blood loss

     7.   Although anemia can certainly contribute to or worsen fatigue, there are probably other (perhaps many) mechanisms of fatigue (e.g., cytokines) that are independent of hemoglobin concentration.

E. Principles of Anemia and Fatigue

     1.   Fatigue is estimated to affect 60%–80% of all patients with cancer.

     2.   Fatigue may be caused by the disease or treatment.

     3.   Fatigue can be assessed with a numeric rating scale, 0 = no fatigue and 10 = worst fatigue imaginable, or with any of several questionnaires (e.g., FACT-An).

     4.   Drugs used in the treatment of anemia and fatigue

         a.   Epoetin and darbepoetin alfa (erythropoiesis-stimulating agents [ESAs]) are approved for treating chemotherapy-induced anemia, the end point of treatment being a decreased need for transfusion. Darbepoetin has additional carboxy chains, resulting in a longer half-life compared with epoetin.

         b.   In recent years, reports of a detrimental effect of ESAs (e.g., increased deaths, poorer chemotherapy outcomes) have led to changes in practice guidelines and reimbursement for these agents. Hemoglobin targets are lower than they were previously, and hemoglobin is carefully monitored. According to the most recent guidelines, ESAs are initiated once a patient's hemoglobin drops below 10 g/dL.

         c.   It is important to distinguish between the use of these agents for chemotherapy-associated anemia and cancer-associated anemia. The latter is not an approved use. These agents should be used only in the noncurative setting.

         d.   Adverse events: Hypertension and seizures, venous thromboembolism, and pure red cell aplasia (rare)

         e.   The use of these agents requires baseline and follow-up monitoring to determine whether agents need titration or discontinuation.

     5.   Transfusions are an option if patients are symptomatic. Transfusion goal is to maintain hemoglobin between 8 g/dL and 10 g/dL.

F. Dosing of Erythropoiesis-Stimulating Agents

Table 8. Dosing of Erythropoiesis-Stimulating Agents

Agent	Starting Dosage	Dosage Increase	Dosing Parameters
Erythropoietin (Procrit, Epogen)	150 units/kg subcutaneously 3 times/week 40,000 units subcutaneously weekly	300 units/kg subcutaneously 3 times/week 60,000 units subcutaneously weekly	Hemoglobin must be <10 to initiate and continue therapy Evaluate after 4 weeks and increase dosage if rise is <1 g/dL Decrease by ~25% if rapid rise in hemoglobin Discontinue therapy if no response after 8 weeks
Darbepoetin (Aranesp)	2.25 mcg/kg subcutaneously weekly 500 mcg every 3 weeks	4.5 mcg/kg subcutaneously weekly Not applicable	Hemoglobin must be <10 to initiate and continue therapy Evaluate after 6 weeks and increase dosage if rise is <1 g/dL Decrease by ~40% if rapid rise in hemoglobin Discontinue therapy if no response after 8 weeks

G. REMS for ESAs
1. The FDA requires these agents to be prescribed and monitored under a risk management program to ensure their safety.
2. Requirements of the REMS program
   a. All patients who are prescribed and receive ESAs must be provided with a medication guide on therapy initiation and with each dose, explaining the risks and benefits of these agents. Patients will also be asked to sign an acknowledgment form that confirms they have talked with their health care professional about the risks of ESAs (may cause tumors to grow faster, may cause patients to die sooner, and may cause patients to develop blood clots or heart problems).
   b. Health care providers prescribing ESAs to patients with cancer must be enrolled in the ESA APPRISE (Assisting Providers and Cancer Patients with Risk Information for the Safe Use of ESAs).

Patient Case

7. A 45-year-old woman is beginning her third cycle of chemotherapy for the adjuvant treatment of breast cancer. At diagnosis, her hemoglobin was 10 g/dL; however, today her hemoglobin is less than 10 g/dL. The patient has fatigue that is interfering with her activities of daily living. Which is the most appropriate treatment option?

   A. Treatment with epoetin should be considered.
   B. Treatment with darbepoetin should be considered when hemoglobin decreases to less than 9 g/dL.
   C. The patient is being treated in the curative setting and therefore is not eligible to receive an ESA.
   D. The patient should not receive RBC transfusions because she is symptomatic.

VII. CHEMOPROTECTANTS

A. Properties of an Ideal Protectant Drug for Chemotherapy- and Radiation-Induced Toxicities
   1. Easy to administer
   2. No adverse events
   3. Prevents all toxicities, including non–life-threatening (alopecia) toxicities, irreversible morbidities (neuropathies, ototoxicity), and mortality (severe myelosuppression, cardiotoxicity)
   4. Does not interfere with the efficacy of the cancer treatment
   5. To date, no such drug has been identified.

B. Dexrazoxane
   1. The anthracyclines (daunorubicin, doxorubicin, idarubicin, and epirubicin), anthracenedione, and mitoxantrone can cause cardiomyopathy that is related to the total lifetime cumulative dosage.
   2. Dexrazoxane acts as an intracellular chelating agent; iron chelation leads to a decrease in anthracycline-induced free radical damage.
      a. Dexrazoxane is approved for use in patients with metastatic breast cancer. It may be considered for patients who have received doxorubicin 300 mg/m^2 or more and who may benefit from continued doxorubicin, considering the patient's risk of cardiotoxicity with continued doxorubicin use.
      b. Dexrazoxane may increase the hematologic toxicity of chemotherapy.
      c. An early study suggested that dexrazoxane decreases the response rate to chemotherapy. More recent data suggest this is not the case, but dexrazoxane is still not indicated for patients with early (curable) breast cancer.
   3. Dexrazoxane is also approved for use as an antidote for the extravasation of anthracycline chemotherapy.

C. Amifostine
   1. Amifostine is used to prevent nephrotoxicity from cisplatin.
   2. It is also used to decrease the incidence of both acute and late xerostomia in patients with head and neck cancer who are undergoing fractionated radiation therapy.
   3. Adverse events associated with amifostine include sneezing, allergic reactions, warm or flushed feeling, metallic taste in mouth during infusion, nausea and vomiting, and hypotension. The latter is the most clinically significant toxicity. Prevention of hypotension includes withholding antihypertensive medications, using hydration, and close monitoring of BP. Because of the problems with nausea and vomiting and the incidence of hypotension, this agent is not used very often.

D. Mesna (sodium-2-mercaptoethane sulfonate)
   1. The metabolite acrolein is produced from both cyclophosphamide and ifosfamide, and it has been implicated in sterile hemorrhagic cystitis.
   2. Mesna detoxifies acrolein by binding to the compound and preventing its interaction with host cells.
   3. Mesna is always used with ifosfamide and may be used with cyclophosphamide (in dosages of 1500 mg/m^2 or greater), although this is not a label indication.
   4. Mesna may be given intravenously or orally. Several dosing schedules may be used. With any schedule, mesna must begin concurrently with or before ifosfamide or cyclophosphamide and end after ifosfamide or cyclophosphamide because of its short half-life (i.e., mesna must be present in the bladder when acrolein is present in the bladder).

Patient Cases

8. A 38-year-old woman has a history of Hodgkin lymphoma. Two years ago, she completed six cycles of ABVD chemotherapy (i.e., doxorubicin, bleomycin, vinblastine, and dacarbazine). Each cycle included doxorubicin 50 mg/m². Recently, she was given a diagnosis of stage IV breast cancer. She will be initiated on doxorubicin 50 mg/m² and cyclophosphamide 500 mg/m² for four cycles. Which statement is most applicable?

    A. The patient has not reached the appropriate cumulative dosage of doxorubicin to consider dexrazoxane.

    B. The patient has reached the appropriate cumulative dosage of doxorubicin to consider dexrazoxane.

    C. The patient should not receive any more doxorubicin because she is at an elevated risk of cardiotoxicity.

    D. The patient should not receive dexrazoxane because of the possibility of increased myelosuppression.

9. Which is the best sequence for administering mesna and ifosfamide?

    A. Mesna before ifosfamide and then at 4 and 8 hours after ifosfamide.

    B. Ifosfamide before mesna and then at 4 and 8 hours after mesna.

    C. Mesna and ifosfamide beginning and ending at the same time.

    D. Mesna on day 1 and ifosfamide on days 2–5.

VIII. ONCOLOGIC EMERGENCIES

A. Hypercalcemia
    1. The most common tumors associated with hypercalcemia are lung (metastatic non–small cell lung cancer more than small cell lung cancer), breast, multiple myeloma, head and neck, renal cell, and non-Hodgkin lymphoma.
    2. Cancer-associated hypercalcemia results from increased bone resorption with calcium release into the extracellular fluid; in addition, renal clearance of calcium is decreased.
        a. Some tumors cause direct bone destruction, resulting in osteolytic hypercalcemia.
        b. Other tumors release parathyroid hormone–related protein (i.e., humoral hypercalcemia).
        c. Immobile patients are also at an elevated risk of hypercalcemia because of increased resorption of calcium.
        d. Medications (e.g., hormonal therapy, thiazide diuretics) may precipitate or exacerbate hypercalcemia.
        e. Corrected Ca (mg/dL) = (4 – plasma albumin in g/dL) × 0.8 + serum calcium.
        f. Symptoms of hypercalcemia: Lethargy, confusion, anorexia, nausea, constipation, polyuria, and polydipsia
    3. Management of hypercalcemia
        a. Mild hypercalcemia (corrected calcium less than 12 mg/dL) may not warrant aggressive treatment. Hydration with normal saline followed by observation is an option in asymptomatic patients with chemotherapy-sensitive tumors (e.g., lymphoma, breast cancer).
        b. Moderate hypercalcemia (corrected calcium 12–14 mg/dL) requires basic treatment of clinical symptoms with aggressive hydration.

   c. Severe hypercalcemia (corrected calcium greater than 14 mg/dL; symptomatic) requires aggressive inpatient treatment.

      i. Hydration with normal saline about 3–6 L in 24 hours

      ii. Loop diuretics may be administered after volume status has been corrected or to prevent fluid overload during hydration.

      iii. Thiazide diuretics are contraindicated in hypercalcemia because of the increase in renal tubular calcium absorption.

      iv. Bisphosphonates bind to hydroxyapatite in calcified bone, which prevents dissolution by phosphatases and inhibits both normal and abnormal bone resorption. The onset of action is 3–4 days.

      v. Calcitonin (intramuscular formulation) inhibits the effects of parathyroid hormone and has a rapid-onset (though short-lived) hypocalcemic effect.

      vi. Steroids may be used to lower calcium in patients with steroid-responsive tumors (lymphoma and myeloma).

      vii. Phosphate is reserved for patients who are both hypophosphatemic and hypercalcemic. Phosphate is seldom used because of the possibility of calcium and phosphate precipitation in soft tissue.

      viii. Dialysis may be needed in patients with hypercalcemia and renal failure.

B. Spinal Cord Compression

   1. Signs and symptoms include back pain, weakness, paresthesias, and loss of bowel and bladder function.

   2. Treatment consists of dexamethasone and radiation therapy or surgery.

C. Tumor Lysis Syndrome

   1. Occurs secondary to the rapid cell death that follows the administration of chemotherapy in patients with leukemia or lymphoma or in patients with high tumor burdens from other diseases that are also highly chemosensitive. Tumor lysis syndrome (TLS) can occur spontaneously in hematologic malignancies, without being triggered by the administration of chemotherapy (i.e., some patients present in tumor lysis).

   2. Manifestations include hyperuricemia, hyperkalemia, hyperphosphatemia, and secondary hypocalcemia. Uric acid and calcium/phosphorus may precipitate in the kidney and can lead to renal failure.

   3. The primary management strategy is prevention with intravenous hydration (with normal saline) and allopurinol.

   4. Rasburicase is a recombinant urate oxidase that converts uric acid into allantoin, which is 5–10 times more soluble in urine than uric acid. Rasburicase should be considered for patients at high risk of developing TLS, such as those with a serum uric acid concentration greater than 8 mg/dL, a large tumor burden, preexisting renal dysfunction, or an inability to take allopurinol. The drug is expensive, and currently it is not recommended for prophylaxis in all patients but may be used together with hydration for treatment of TLS. The approved dosage is 0.2 mg/kg intravenously for 5 doses. There is now increasing evidence for the use of an off-label, low, fixed, single dose of rasburicase for chemotherapy-induced hyperuricemia in adults. The FDA indication is management of uric acid levels. Rasburicase causes enzymatic degradation of the uric acid in blood, plasma, and serum samples, potentially resulting in spuriously low plasma uric acid assay readings. Blood must be collected in prechilled tubes containing heparin anticoagulant; immediately immerse plasma samples for uric acid measurement in an ice water bath.

IX. MISCELLANEOUS ANTINEOPLASTIC PHARMACOTHERAPY

A. Leucovorin rescue may be used after methotrexate doses greater than 100 mg/m²; in general, methotrexate doses greater than 500 mg/m² require leucovorin rescue.

B. Factors that increase the likelihood of methotrexate toxicity include renal dysfunction (causing delayed elimination), third-space fluid (e.g., pleural effusion, ascites), and administration of other drugs that may delay methotrexate elimination (penicillin, NSAIDs, PPIs). Toxic reactions include mucous membrane toxicity (e.g., oral mucositis), renal and hepatic toxicity, central nervous system toxicity, and myelosuppression.

C. The dosage of leucovorin depends on the methotrexate dosage or level and the time since the completion of methotrexate. Methotrexate levels are usually obtained 24–48 hours after intermediate- or high-dose methotrexate, and leucovorin is continued until the methotrexate level falls to less than 0.1 mM (less than 1×10^{-7} M). This regimen is typically protocol driven.

D. In contrast to its use with methotrexate, leucovorin is given in combination with fluorouracil in colorectal cancer to improve activity, not to rescue normal cells.

E. Glucarpidase, a carboxypeptidase enzyme, is now approved and indicated for treating toxic methotrexate concentrations (greater than 1 μmol/L) in patients with delayed methotrexate clearance due to renal function. Administered as a single intravenous dose of 50 units/kg. Continue leucovorin until the methotrexate concentration has been maintained below the leucovorin treatment threshold for a minimum of 3 days. However, caution must be used with administering leucovorin in conjunction with glucarpidase. Leucovorin should not be administered within 2 hours before or after a dose of glucarpidase.

F. Extravasation Injuries
   1. A vesicant is an agent that, on extravasation, can cause tissue necrosis. Vesicant antineoplastic drugs include doxorubicin, daunorubicin, epirubicin, mechlorethamine, mitomycin, vincristine, vinblastine, vinorelbine, and streptozocin.
   2. Anthracyclines cause the most severe tissue damage on extravasation.
   3. The literature generally recommends administering vesicants by intravenous injection rather than infusion, but some exceptions exist.
      a. Some institutional policies require infusions for every drug or approved protocols.
      b. Vincristine has been incorrectly administered by intrathecal injection, with fatal consequences. Dilution of vincristine for administration as a short intravenous infusion has been recommended to prevent this error from occurring.
      c. Paclitaxel is administered as an infusion (1, 3, or 24 hours, depending on the protocol).
   4. Management of extravasation
      a. Cold for doxorubicin, daunorubicin, and epirubicin
      b. Heat for vincristine, vinblastine, and vinorelbine
      c. Sodium thiosulfate for mechlorethamine
      d. Topical dimethyl sulfoxide has been recommended for anthracyclines. Its use is not as well established as that of the antidotes above. Hyaluronidase is recommended for vinca alkaloids, but hyaluronidase is of limited availability. Antidotes for mitomycin, streptozocin, paclitaxel, and oxaliplatin are not well documented in the literature.

    e.   Dexrazoxane (Totect) for doxorubicin, daunorubicin, idarubicin, and epirubicin. Cold compress should be removed 15 minutes before dexrazoxane treatment.

    f.   Many institutions do not allow the administration of vesicants through a peripheral vein but instead require that vesicants be administered through a central line with a venous access device. Although administering vesicants through a central line minimizes the likelihood of an extravasation injury, extravasation may still occur. Management of extravasation is intended for suspected or actual extravasation from a peripheral or central vein.

G.   Management of Diarrhea

    1.   Intensive loperamide therapy using dosages higher than recommended was initially described for irinotecan-induced diarrhea. Atropine is used to prevent cholinergic activity of acute irinotecan-induced diarrhea. There is no maximal dosage of loperamide when used for delayed diarrhea in this setting. The recommended dosing regimen of loperamide is 4 mg by mouth, followed by 2 mg every 2 hours until diarrhea free.

    2.   Intensive antidiarrhea treatment is also used for other agents (e.g., fluorouracil, epidermal growth factor receptor inhibitors).

H.   Dosage Adjustment for Organ Dysfunction

    1.   Conflicting recommendations for dosage adjustment have been reported. Many drugs have not been studied in patients with organ dysfunction. Consultation of oncology-specific drug information resources may be useful.

    2.   Dosage adjustment for renal dysfunction may be considered for methotrexate, carboplatin, cisplatin, etoposide, bleomycin, topotecan, capecitabine, and lenalidomide.

    3.   Dosage adjustment for hepatic dysfunction is often based on total bilirubin concentrations.

REFERENCES

Antiemetics

1. Gralla RJ, Raftopoulos H. Progress in the control of chemotherapy-induced emesis: new agents and new studies. J Oncol Pract 2009;5:130-3.

2. Grunberg SM, Warr D, Gralla RJ, et al. Evaluation of new antiemetic agents and definition of antineoplastic agent emetogenicity: state of the art. Support Care Cancer 2010;19:S43-47.

3. Herrstedt J, Dombernowsky P. Anti-emetic therapy in cancer chemotherapy: current status. Basic Clin Pharmacol Toxicol 2007;101:143-50.

4. Hesketh PJ, Kris MG, Grunberg SM, et al. Proposal for classifying the acute emetogenicity of cancer chemotherapy. J Clin Oncol 1997;15:103-9.

5. Multinational Association for Supportive Care in Cancer. MASCC/ESMO Antiemetic Guideline 2010. Available at www.mascc.org. Accessed October 10, 2012.

6. Naeim A, Dy SM, Lorenz KA, et al. Evidence-based recommendations for cancer nausea and vomiting. J Clin Oncol 2008;26:3903-10.

7. National Comprehensive Cancer Network (NCCN). Clinical Practice Guidelines in Oncology: Antiemesis, version 2. 2015. Available at www.nccn.org/professionals/physician_gls/pdf/antiemesis.pdr. Accessed October 12, 2015.

8. Navari RM, Gray SE, Kerr AC. Olanzapine versus aprepitant for the prevention of chemotherapy-induced nausea and vomiting: a randomized phase III trial. J Support Oncol 2011;9:188-95.

9. Navari RM, Nagy CK, Gray SE. Olanzapine versus metoclopramide for the treatment of breakthrough chemotherapy-induced nausea and vomiting in patients receiving highly emetogenic chemotherapy. Support Care Cancer 2013;21:1655-63.

Pain Management

1. Berenson JR, Hillner BE, Kyle RA, et al. American Society of Clinical Oncology clinical practice guidelines: the role of bisphosphonates in multiple myeloma. J Clin Oncol 2002;20:3719-36.

2. Foley KM. The treatment of cancer pain. N Engl J Med 1985;313:84-95.

3. Hillner BE, Ingle JN, Chlebowski RT, et al. American Society of Clinical Oncology 2003 update on the role of bisphosphonates and bone health issues in women with breast cancer. J Clin Oncol 2003;21:4042-57.

4. National Comprehensive Cancer Network (NCCN). Clinical Practice Guidelines in Oncology: Adult Cancer Pain, version 2.2015. Available at www.nccn.org/professionals/physician_gls/f_guidelines.asp. Accessed October 10, 2015.

5. U.S. Department of Health and Human Services (DHHS). Public Health Service Agency for Health Care Policy and Research (AHCPR). Clinical Practice Guideline, No. 9. Management of Cancer Pain. AHCPR Publication 94-0592, March 1994. Washington, DC: DHHS, 1994.

6. U.S. Food and Drug Administration Web site. FDA Approves a Risk Evaluation and Mitigation Strategy (REMS). Available at www.fda.gov/Drugs/DrugSafety/InformationbyDrugClass/ucm309742.htm#Q7. Accessed October 10, 2012.

Febrile Neutropenia and CSFs

1. Freifeld AG, Bow EJ, Sepkowitz KA, et al. The Infectious Diseases Society of America 2010 guidelines for the use of antimicrobial agents in patients with cancer and neutropenia: salient features and comments. Clin Infect Dis 2011;52:e56-93.

2. Hughes WT, Armstrong D, Bodey GP, et al. 2002 guidelines for the use of antimicrobial agents in neutropenic patients with unexplained fever. Clin Infect Dis 2002;34:730-51.

3. Klastersky J, Paesmans M. Risk-adapted strategy for the management of febrile neutropenia in cancer patients. Support Care Cancer 2007;15:477-82.

4. National Comprehensive Cancer Network (NCCN). Clinical Practice Guidelines in Oncology: Myeloid Growth Factors, version 1.2015. Available at www.nccn.org/professionals/physician_gls/f_guidelines.asp. Accessed October 12, 2015.

5. National Comprehensive Cancer Network (NCCN). Clinical Practice Guidelines in Oncology: Prevention and Treatment of Cancer-Related Infections, version 2.2015. Available at www.nccn.org/professionals/physician_gls/f_guidelines.asp. Accessed October 10, 2015.

6. Smith TJ, Khatcheressian J, Lyman GH, et al. 2006 Update of recommendations for the use of white blood cell growth factors: an evidence-based clinical practice guideline. J Clin Oncol 2006;24:1-19.

Thrombocytopenia

1. Adams VR, Brenner TL. Oprelvekin (Neumega). J Oncol Pharm Pract 1999;5:117-24.

2. Cantor SB, Elting LS, Hudson DV, et al. Pharmacoeconomic analysis of oprelvekin for secondary prophylaxis of thrombocytopenia for solid tumor patients receiving chemotherapy. Cancer 2003;97:3099-106.

3. Schiffer CA, Anderson KC, Bennett CL, et al. Platelet transfusions for patients with cancer: clinical practice guidelines of the American Society of Clinical Oncology. J Clin Oncol 2001;19:1519-38.

Anemia and Fatigue

1. National Comprehensive Cancer Network (NCCN). Practice Guidelines in Oncology: Cancer- and Chemotherapy-Induced Anemia, version 1.2016. Available at www.nccn.org/professionals/physician_gls/f_guidelines.asp. Accessed October 12, 2015.

2. Rizzo JD, Somerfield MR, Hagerty KL, et al. Use of epoetin and darbepoetin inpatients with cancer: 2007 American Society of Clinical Oncology/American Society of Hematology clinical practice guideline update [published correction appears in J Clin Oncol 2008;26:1192]. J Clin Oncol 2008;26:132-49.

Chemoprotectants

1. Bukowsi R. Cytoprotection in the treatment of pediatric cancer: review of current strategies in adults and their application to children. Med Pediatr Oncol 1999;32:124-34.

2. Hensley ML, Hagerty KL, Kewalramani T, et al. American Society of Clinical Oncology 2008 clinical practice guideline update: use of chemotherapy and radiation therapy protectants. J Clin Oncol 2009;27:127-45.

3. Links M, Lewis C. Chemoprotectants: a review of their clinical pharmacology and therapeutic efficacy. Drugs 1999;57:293-308.

4. Schuchter LM, Hensley ML, Meropol NJ, et al. 2002 update of recommendations for the use of chemotherapy and radiotherapy protectants: clinical practice guidelines of the American Society of Clinical Oncology. J Clin Oncol 2002;20:2895-903.

Oncologic Emergencies

1. Abrahm JL. Management of pain and spinal cord compression in patients with advanced cancer. Ann Intern Med 1999;131:37-46.

2. Brigden ML. Hematologic and oncologic emergencies. Doing the most good in the least time. Postgrad Med 2001;109:143-63.

3. Coiffler B, Altman A, Pui CH, et al. Guidelines for the management of pediatric and adult tumor lysis syndrome: an evidence-based review. J Clin Oncol 2008;26:2767-78.

4. Holdsworth MT, Nguyen P. Role of i.v. allopurinol and rasburicase in tumor lysis syndrome. Am J Health Syst Pharm 2003;60:2213-24.

5. Krimsky WS, Behrens RJ, Kerkvliet GJ. Oncology emergencies for the internist. Cleve Clin J Med 2002;69:209-22.

6. Nakshima L. Guidelines for the treatment of hypercalcemia associated with malignancy. J Oncol Pharm Pract 1997;3:31-7.

7. Nicolin G. Paediatric update. Emergencies and their management. Eur J Cancer 2002;38:1365-77.

8. Vadhan-Raj S, Fayad LE, Fanale MA, et al. A randomized trial of single-dose rasburicase versus five-daily doses in patients at risk for tumor lysis syndrome. Ann Oncol 2012;23:1640-5.

9. Yim BT, Sims-McCallum RP, Chong PH. Rasburicase for the treatment and prevention of hyperuricemia. Ann Pharmacother 2003;37:1047-54.

ANSWERS AND EXPLANATIONS TO PATIENT CASES

1. Answer: A

This is a highly emetogenic regimen that is associated with delayed nausea and vomiting. The best choice is a serotonin receptor antagonist with dexamethasone and aprepitant for prophylaxis against nausea and vomiting. Prochlorperazine is not effective against a highly emetogenic stimulus. Granisetron and ondansetron are both serotonin receptor antagonists, and no rationale exists for combining them. Lorazepam may be a useful addition, but it does not replace dexamethasone or aprepitant for highly emetogenic chemotherapy.

2. Answer: D

Lorazepam is recommended for use in combination with the standard antiemetic regimen based on chemotherapy emetogenicity to prevent anticipatory nausea and vomiting. Aprepitant and dexamethasone should and can be used together to prevent acute and delayed emesis. Metoclopramide would not be appropriate for anticipatory nausea and vomiting. Serotonin receptor antagonists are generally thought not to be effective alone in preventing anticipatory nausea and vomiting.

3. Answer: D

The patient is taking oxycodone/APAP 5 mg/325 mg, which provides 60 mg of oxycodone per day and 3900 mg of APAP. We should not increase his current drugs because of concerns about APAP toxicity. If he is changed to a higher strength of the combination product, APAP toxicity is still a concern, which eliminates the choices of increasing to oxycodone/APAP 7.5 mg 2 tablets every 4 hours. Adding sustained-release morphine is a good option. Continuing the ibuprofen might be helpful for bone pain. Oxycodone/APAP, which is short acting, could be continued for breakthrough pain, but he is already getting a lot of APAP without good pain relief.

4. Answer: C

Gabapentin might help the neuropathic component (i.e., the shooting pains) of his pain. He is already receiving an NSAID, so there is no need to add naproxen. There is no point to adding APAP, and the case does not mention muscle spasms.

5. Answer: D

To calculate the ANC, multiply the WBC by the segmented neutrophils and the band neutrophils: 600 cells/mm^3 × (0.6 + 0.1) = 420 cells/mm^3.

6. Answer: C

The patient is neutropenic; however, she should not begin a CSF. Her ANC is greater than 100 cells/mm^3, and she has no signs or symptoms of active infection. Prophylactic treatment with antibiotic drugs is not necessary and can increase the risk of resistant organisms. At this time, the patient should be monitored for evidence of infection (e.g., she should be instructed to take her temperature and return to the clinic or emergency department if she has a single oral temperature of 101°F or more or of 100.4°F or more for at least 1 hour or if she develops any signs or symptoms of infection). Because the disease is potentially curable, dosages should not be reduced on the next cycle.

7. Answer: C

Recent literature and subsequent changes in guidelines and Centers for Medicare & Medicaid Services reimbursement suggest that an erythropoiesis-stimulating protein be considered when hemoglobin is less than 10 g/dL. However, this patient is being treated potentially for a cure; therefore, she would not be eligible for an ESA. Transfusions are an option if patients are symptomatic. Transfusion goal is to maintain hemoglobin between 8 and 10 g/dL.

8. Answer: B

The patient has received a cumulative dose of 300 mg/m^2 of doxorubicin (50 mg/m^2 × 6 cycles). This is the appropriate cumulative dosage of doxorubicin to consider dexrazoxane. She is at an elevated risk of cardiotoxicity; however, dexrazoxane protects the heart from this toxicity. Dexrazoxane may increase the myelosuppression from chemotherapy, but that does not represent a contraindication.

9. Answer: A

Several different schedules of ifosfamide and mesna administration exist (e.g., ifosfamide short infusion, followed by intermittent infusions of mesna and continuous infusion of both ifosfamide and mesna). But mesna should always be continued longer than ifosfamide.

ANSWERS AND EXPLANATIONS TO SELF-ASSESSMENT QUESTIONS

1. Answer: C

Patients who have had poor control of nausea and vomiting on previous cycles of chemotherapy are at an elevated risk of anticipatory emesis. Anxious patients are also at an elevated risk of CINV. Benzodiazepines help decrease anxiety and, by causing anterograde amnesia, may minimize anticipatory symptoms. Although it is unclear whether patients who do not respond to one serotonin receptor antagonist will respond to another, a change in regimen is needed. Substituting dolasetron for granisetron would be acceptable, but adding lorazepam is essential. Palonosetron is the preferred serotonin receptor antagonist in some guidelines, but this is not universally agreed on. For this patient, the palonosetron option also includes lorazepam. Metoclopramide is another option, but an effective dose might be difficult to administer orally (especially as tablets), and again, adding lorazepam would be preferred over adding aprepitant in this patient.

2. Answer: D

This patient's altered mental status is probably caused by hypercalcemia. The corrected calcium is 13.6 mg/dL. Corrected calcium concentrations greater than 12 g/dL should be treated with a bisphosphonate (either pamidronate or zoledronic acid) in addition to hydration with normal saline. Furosemide may be needed during hydration but not before hydration because the patient is probably dehydrated. This patient does not need rapid reversal of hypercalcemia; therefore, calcitonin is not needed. Dexamethasone may be used in patients with lymphoma or myeloma, but it will have no effect on metastatic non–small cell lung cancer.

3. Answer: C

The patient is at risk of TLS because he has a chemosensitive tumor and a high tumor burden (elevated WBC). Prevention is the key in TLS, which includes adequate saline hydration and the use of allopurinol. Dextrose 5% is not an appropriate intravenous fluid for hydration because it does not contain saline. The value of alkalinization with sodium bicarbonate is somewhat controversial, and alkalinization is not a replacement for allopurinol.

4. Answer: B

This anemia is not attributable to treatment because chemotherapy has not yet begun. Epoetin and darbepoetin are indicated only for noncurative chemotherapy-associated anemia. Chemotherapy should not be delayed, nor should chemotherapy dosages be reduced in the setting of a potentially curable malignancy. Therefore, the patient should receive a transfusion of packed RBCs.

5. Answer: B

$(55\% + 5\%) \times 500 = 300$.

6. Answer: A

The patient is neutropenic (ANC 300 cells/mm^3). Temperature of 103°F places the febrile neutropenia outside the definition of low-risk febrile neutropenia. Therefore, the patient should be hospitalized for intravenous antibiotics and an infection workup. She does not have any of the appropriate reasons to administer CSFs (i.e., documented pneumonia, hypotension, sepsis syndrome, or fungal infection). Her chemotherapy may need to be delayed, but it should be continued. She should receive a CSF with the next cycle of chemotherapy.

7. Answer: B

Febrile neutropenia developed at the time of the expected neutrophil nadir, 12 days after chemotherapy. Marrow recovery would be expected to follow. The percentage of eosinophils may be slightly elevated, but the absolute count is low. The platelet count is also low, not elevated. Neutrophils are often affected by myelosuppressive chemotherapy to a greater degree than platelets.

8. Answer: D

Opioids may provide some relief from neuropathic pain, but often the response to opioids is less than optimal. In general, higher dosages of opioids provide greater pain relief; therefore, increasing the dosage of fentanyl and morphine is an option for this patient. Nothing in the history suggests that the patient is deriving much, if any, benefit at the present opioid dosages. Adjuvant analgesic drugs, including tricyclic antidepressants and anticonvulsants, are used to help manage neuropathic pain. Gabapentin, with a good adverse event profile, is a reasonable option. However, adjuvant analgesic drugs should not be given to decrease the opioid dosage or discontinue the use of opioid drugs. (It may be possible to decrease the dosage later if gabapentin provides adequate pain relief.) Diazepam is more effective for muscle spasms than for neuropathic pain, and this option includes decreasing the fentanyl dosage at the same time the new drug is initiated.

9. Answer: D

Limited-stage small cell lung cancer is potentially curable; therefore, the patient should continue on the planned dosages of chemotherapy. The correct dosage of filgrastim is 5 mcg/kg/day subcutaneously, not 250 mcg/m^2 (this is the dose for sargramostim). The correct dosage for pegfilgrastim is a single 6-mg injection. Filgrastim should not be given on the same day as chemotherapy; therefore, Answer D is correct.

10. Answer: A

Doxorubicin undergoes hepatic clearance, and there are recommendations for dosage reduction based on bilirubin. There is no reason to reduce the dosage of cyclophosphamide.

11. Answer: A

Large cell lymphoma is faster growing and more chemosensitive than metastatic colorectal cancer. Therefore, patients with large cell lymphoma are more likely to develop hyperuricemia or TLS from rapid cell turnover, both before treatment and after chemotherapy. Hypercalcemia is not a common complication of either of these diseases. Some aggressive lymphomas may be associated with hypercalcemia, but pamidronate is used to treat, not prevent, this complication.

12. Answer: C

Neither patient should undergo chemotherapy with an ANC of 800 cells/mm^3. Both can be treated when neutropenia resolves (probably within 1 week). It is important to keep patient 1 on schedule because his disease is potentially curable; therefore, patient 1 should receive filgrastim after the next chemotherapy treatment to prevent another dose delay. When patient 2 resumes chemotherapy, his dosages can be decreased to prevent a recurrence of neutropenia. The dosage decrease is not likely to have a substantially negative effect on the treatment outcome because the treatment goal is usually not cure.

13. Answer: C

Injury after extravasation of an anthracycline is potentially the most severe. Therefore, when the recommended antidotes for different vesicants conflict (e.g., heat vs. cold), treatment should be directed at the anthracycline. Dexrazoxane is now indicated for doxorubicin extravasation. Cold rather than heat would also be appropriate. Although vincristine is considered a vesicant, sodium thiosulfate is not the recommended antidote..

CRITICAL CARE

CHRISTOPHER A. PACIULLO, PHARM.D., BCCCP, FCCM

EMORY UNIVERSITY HOSPITAL
ATLANTA, GEORGIA

CRITICAL CARE

CHRISTOPHER A. PACIULLO, PHARM.D., BCCCP, FCCM

EMORY UNIVERSITY HOSPITAL
ATLANTA, GEORGIA

Learning Objectives

1. Interpret hemodynamic parameters and acid-base status in critically ill patients.
2. Differentiate between presentation of and treatment strategies for hypovolemic, obstructive, and distributive shock.
3. Discuss the appropriate use of fluids, vasopressors, antibiotics, and corticosteroids in patients with sepsis, severe sepsis, or septic shock.
4. Discuss strategies to optimize the safety and efficacy of therapeutic hypothermia for patients after cardiac arrest.
5. Recommend therapeutic options to minimize delirium and provide optimal analgesia, sedation, neuromuscular blockade, and nutritional support in critically ill patients.
6. Recommend therapeutic options to prevent stress ulcers, venous thromboembolism, hyperglycemia, and ventilator-associated pneumonia in critically ill patients.
7. Recommend treatment options for acute intracranial hemorrhage.

-7\13

Self-Assessment Questions

Answers and explanations to these questions can be found at the end of this chapter.

1. A 58-year-old woman remains intubated in the intensive care unit (ICU) after a recent abdominal operation. In the operating room, she receives more than 10 L of fluid and blood products but has received aggressive diuresis with furosemide postoperatively. In the past 3 days, she has generated 12 L of urine output, and her blood urea nitrogen (BUN) and serum creatinine (SCr) have steadily increased to 40 and 1.5 mg/dL, respectively. Her urine chloride (Cl) concentration was 9 mEq/L (24 hours after her last dose of furosemide). This morning, her arterial blood gas (ABG) reveals pH 7.50, $Paco_2$ 46 mm Hg, and bicarbonate (HCO_3^-) 34 mEq/L. Her vital signs include a blood pressure (BP) of 85/40 mm Hg and a heart rate (HR) of 110 beats/minute. Which action is best to improve her acid-base status?
    A. 0.9% sodium chloride (NaCl) bolus.
    B. 5% dextrose (D_5W) bolus.

C. Hydrochloric acid infusion.
D. Acetazolamide intravenously.

2. A 21-year-old, 80-kg man admitted 1 day ago after a gunshot wound to the abdomen is receiving mechanical ventilation and is thrashing around in bed and pulling at his endotracheal tube. On the Richmond Agitation-Sedation Scale (RASS), he is rated a +3. The patient is negative for delirium according to the Confusion Assessment Method for the ICU (CAM-ICU). His pulmonary status precludes extubation, and the attending physician estimates that he will remain intubated for at least 48 more hours. The medical team has decided that his RASS goal should be −1. He is receiving a morphine 4-mg/hour infusion for pain control, which has been adequately controlling his pain (pain scores less than 3 for 24 hours). Vital signs include BP 110/70 mm Hg and HR 110 beats/minute. His baseline QTc interval is 480 milliseconds. In addition to nonpharmacologic interventions to treat delirium, which is the best intervention for achieving this patient's RASS goal?
    A. Initiate a dexmedetomidine 1-mcg/kg loading dose over 10 minutes, followed by 0.2 mcg/kg/hour.
    B. Initiate lorazepam 3-mg intravenous load, followed by a lorazepam 3-mg/hour infusion.
    C. Initiate propofol at 5 mcg/kg/minute and titrate by 5 mcg/kg/minute every 5 minutes as needed.
    D. Initiate haloperidol 1 mg intravenously and double the dose every 20 minutes as needed.

3. A patient is admitted to the ICU after a motor vehicle accident for traumatic brain injury and several abdominal injuries. He is initiated on propofol, morphine, and vecuronium for sedation, analgesia, and neuromuscular blockade to help control his intracranial pressure. On day 3 of hospitalization, the patient develops peritonitis with severe sepsis and is treated with vancomycin, piperacillin/tazobactam, and tobramycin. His train-of-four (TOF) is 0/4. Which intervention would be best to recommend at this time?
    A. Sedation should be assessed with the RASS.
    B. Change tobramycin to levofloxacin because it can enhance the effects of vecuronium.

C. The patient should be initiated on parenteral nutrition.

D. Morphine can be discontinued because the patient is sedated with propofol.

4. A 62-year-old woman is admitted to your ICU for respiratory dysfunction necessitating mechanical ventilation. Her medical history is nonsignificant, and she is taking no medications at home. Her chest radiograph shows bilateral lower lobe infiltrates, her white blood cell count (WBC) is 21×10^3 cells/m^3, her temperature is 39.6°C, her BP is 82/45 mm Hg (normal for her is 115/70 mm Hg), and her HR is 110 beats/minute. After she receives a diagnosis of community-acquired pneumonia, she is empirically initiated on ceftriaxone 2 g/day and levofloxacin 750 mg/day intravenously. After fluid resuscitation with 6 L of lactated Ringer's solution, her BP is unchanged. Dopamine is initiated and titrated to 9 mcg/kg/minute, with a resulting BP of 96/58 mm Hg, and her HR is 138 beats/minute. She has made less than 100 mL of urine during the past 6 hours, and her creatinine (Cr) has increased from 0.9 mg/dL to 1.3 mg/dL. Her serum albumin concentration is 2.1 g/dL. Which therapy is best for this patient at this time?

A. Administer 5% albumin 500 mL intravenously over 1 hour and reassess mean arterial pressure (MAP).

B. Initiate hydrocortisone 50 mg intravenously every 6 hours.

C. Change dopamine to norepinephrine 0.01 mcg/kg/minute to maintain an MAP greater than 65 mm Hg.

D. Reduce the dopamine infusion to 1 mcg/kg/minute to maintain urine output of at least 1 mL/kg/hour.

5. A 92-year-old woman is admitted to the ICU with urosepsis and septic shock. She lives in a long-term care facility and has a medical history significant for coronary artery disease and hypertension. Her BP is 72/44 mm Hg, central venous pressure (CVP) is 5 mm Hg, HR 120 beats/minute, and oxygen saturation is 99%; her laboratory values arc normal, except for a BUN of 74 mg/dL and Cr of 2.7 mg/dL (baseline of 1.5 mg/dL). Her urine output is about 20 mL/hour. Appropriate empiric antibiotics were initiated. Which therapy is most appropriate to initiate next?

A. Norepinephrine 0.05 mcg/kg/minute.

B. Lactated Ringer's 500-mL bolus.

C. Normal saline 500-mL bolus.

D. Albumin 5% 500-mL bolus.

6. A 46-year-old man had a witnessed cardiac arrest in an airport terminal. After about 5 minutes, emergency medical services arrived, and defibrillator pads were applied. The cardiac monitor showed ventricular tachycardia (VT), and the patient had no discernible pulse. He was defibrillated with 200 J without return of spontaneous circulation. He received an additional two shocks of 200 J with no improvement. Between shocks, the patient received cardiopulmonary resuscitation (CPR). An intravenous line was obtained, and an epinephrine 1-mg intravenous push was given; chest compressions and artificial respirations were initiated. Within 1 minute, the patient was reassessed. The cardiac monitor still showed VT, and he remained pulseless; therefore, another shock of 200 J, followed by an amiodarone 300-mg intravenous push, was administered. After this, the patient was converted to a normal sinus rhythm with an HR of 100 beats/minute. The patient was then transported to the hospital, intubated and unresponsive. Which recommendation is most likely to improve this patient's outcomes?

A. Administer sodium bicarbonate intravenously.

B. Administer vasopressin 40 units intravenously.

C. Administer a continuous infusion of heparin.

D. Initiate a targeted temperature management protocol.

7. A 22-year-old man is admitted to the trauma ICU after a motor vehicle accident. He has several rib fractures, a ruptured spleen, and a small brain contusion. He is rushed to the operating room for an emergency splenectomy, and the trauma team places an orogastric feeding tube (OGT) before returning to the ICU. The patient is unresponsive and mechanically ventilated, with no plans for extubation. Which is most cost-effective for stress ulcer prophylaxis (SUP)?

A. Pantoprazole intravenous push.

B. Famotidine by OGT.

C. Sucralfate by OGT.

D. No SUP indicated.

8. A 45-year-old man is admitted to the ICU with H1N1 causing respiratory failure. He is intubated and sedated with fentanyl 200 mcg/hour and propofol 25 mcg/kg/minute. He has received 4 L of plasmalyte and 1 L of albumin and is currently receiving norepinephrine 0.15 mcg/kg/minute and vasopressin 0.03 units/minute for hemodynamic support. His current vital signs are BP 85/58 mm Hg, HR 99 beats/minute, and respiratory rate (RR) 18 breaths/minute. Which of the following is the best plan for steroid therapy in this patient?

A. Begin hydrocortisone 50 mg every 6 hours intravenously.

B. Perform a cosyntropin stimulation test and begin hydrocortisone 50 mg every 6 hours intravenously if the patient does not have an increase greater than 9 mcg/dL from baseline.

C. Check a random cortisol and begin hydrocortisone 50 mg every 6 hours intravenously if the result is less than 10 mcg/dL.

D. Steroids are not indicated at this time.

9. The patient in question 8 continued to decline and was placed on cisatracurium overnight for hypoxemia. He is currently on cisatracurium 3 mcg/kg/minute, fentanyl 500 mcg/hour, propofol 40 mcg/kg/minute, and ketamine 10 mg/hour. His ABG shows a pH of 7.32, P_{CO_2} of 45 mm Hg, Pa_{O_2} of 60 mm Hg (O_2 saturation 93%), and HCO_3 of 27 mEq/L on 70% Fi_{O_2}. All laboratory values are normal except for a sodium of 148 mEq/L and creatinine of 1.4 mg/dL. His vasopressor doses have increased to norepinephrine 1 mcg/kg/minute and vasopressin 0.03 units/minute. An Scv_{O_2} is measured and found to be 45%. His skin is mottled, and urine output has decreased to 0.1 mL/kg/hour for the last 12 hours. Other pertinent vital signs are BP 100/64 mm Hg, HR 95 beats/minute, and RR 26 breaths/minute. Which of the following is the best recommendation to optimize the patient's hemodynamics?

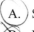

A. Start dobutamine 5 mcg/kg/minute.

B. Decrease norepinephrine to 0.5 mcg/kg/minute.

C. Decrease propofol to 20 mcg/kg/minute.

D. Start epinephrine 0.05 mcg/kg/minute.

10. A 69-year-old man has a seizure on postoperative day (POD) 0 after four-vessel coronary bypass and maze procedure. On POD 2, he develops hypotension and an increase in lactate to 3.5 mmol/L. His pulmonary artery catheter shows a cardiac index of 1.5 L/minute/m^2, pulmonary capillary wedge pressure 34 mm Hg, CVP 24 mm Hg, and systemic vascular resistance of 1240 dynes/s/cm^5. Other vital signs are HR 110 beats/minute and BP 95/45 mm Hg. Which of the following is the best intervention for the patient's shock?

A. Administer 500 mL of 5% albumin.

B. Start dobutamine 5 mcg/kg/minute.

C. Call surgical attending for immediate pericardiocentesis.

D. Start norepinephrine at 0.05 mcg/kg/minute.

11. A 19-year-old man is admitted to the ICU after ingesting an unknown quantity of acetaminophen. He is 180 cm tall and weighs 68 kg. After initial resuscitation and treatment with acetylcysteine, the patient remains unresponsive and intubated. The intensivist would like to start enteral nutrition as soon as possible. Which of the following is the best way to calculate the patient's caloric and protein needs?

A. Calculate caloric needs based on the modified Penn State equation and estimate protein needs at 1.2 g/kg.

B. Perform indirect calorimetry to estimate caloric and protein needs.

C. Estimate caloric needs at 14 kcal/kg and protein at 2 g/kg.

D. Calculate caloric needs based on the Mifflin equation and order a prealbumin level to assess protein needs.

12. A 57-year-old woman is admitted to the ICU with injuries sustained after a fall from 12 feet. She has traumatic brain injury and has been intubated for airway protection. Which of the following is the

best intervention to prevent ventilator-associated pneumonia in this patient?

A. Initiate pantoprazole 40 mg intravenously daily.

B. Perform selective digestive decontamination with enteral polymyxin B sulfate, neomycin sulfate, and vancomycin hydrochloride.

C. Maintain head of bed elevation at 20° at all times.

D. Start chlorhexidine 0.12% oral swabs twice daily.

13. You are the critical care pharmacist for a 300-bed hospital. The critical care committee wants to institute an evidence-based glucose control protocol for the ICU. Which of the following goals should be implemented for patients who present with septic shock?

A. Check blood glucose every 6 hours and treat with sliding scale protocol when greater than 180 mg/dL.

B. Initiate insulin infusion with a target of 110–140 mg/dL for two blood glucose values greater than 140 mg/dL.

C. Initiate insulin infusion with a target of 110–180 mg/dL for two blood glucose values greater than 180 mg/dL.

D. Initiate insulin infusion with a target blood glucose of 80–110 mg/dL for two blood glucose values greater than 150 mg/dL.

BPS Pharmacotherapy Specialty Examination Content Outline

This chapter covers the following sections of the Pharmacotherapy Specialty Examination Content Outline:

1. Domain 1: Patient-Centered Pharmacotherapy
   a. Tasks 1, 4, 5
   b. Systems and Patient-Care Problems
      i. Interpreting Hemodynamic Parameters
      ii. Shock
      iii. Acute Respiratory Failure
      iv. Cardiac Arrest
      v. Analgesics, Sedatives, Antipsychotics, and Paralytics
      vi. Preventing Hyperglycemia and Hypoglycemia
      vii. Preventing Stress Ulcer
      viii. Pharmacologic Therapy for Preventing Venous Thromboembolism (VTE) or Pulmonary Embolism
      ix. Preventing Ventilator-Associated Pneumonia
      x. Optimizing Nutrition Support
      xi. Intracranial Hemorrhage

I. INTERPRETATION OF HEMODYNAMIC PARAMETERS

A. Hemodynamics (Table 1)
1. Arterial blood pressure is the product of cardiac output and resistance to flow (systemic vascular resistance [SVR]).
   a. Cardiac output (milliliters of blood pumped per minute) consists of stroke volume (milliliters of blood ejected from the left ventricle per beat) and heart rate (HR).
   b. Stroke volume is determined by preload (amount of blood available to eject), afterload (resistance to ejection), and contractility (amount of force generated by the heart). These will be discussed in more detail below.
2. Arterial blood pressure can be described by systolic blood pressure (SBP), diastolic blood pressure (DBP), or mean arterial pressure (MAP). This is the driving pressure for organ perfusion and oxygen delivery. MAP = [SBP + (2 × DBP)]/3. Note that MAP is based largely on DBP because most of the cardiac cycle is spent in diastole.
   a. Normal MAP is 70–100 mm Hg.
   b. MAP is an indication of global perfusion pressure; a MAP of at least 60 mm Hg is necessary for adequate cerebral perfusion.
   c. MAP can be calculated using the above equation, but direct measurement from an arterial line provides more timely and accurate measurements.
3. Preload is defined as ventricular end diastolic volume, and it increases proportionally with stroke volume (Frank-Starling mechanism). Commonly used measures of preload include central venous pressure (CVP), pulmonary capillary wedge pressure (PCWP) or pulmonary artery occlusion pressure (PAOP), and newer measures such as stroke volume variation (SVV) and pulse pressure variation (PPV).
   a. CVP is the pressure in the vena cava at the point of blood returning to the right atrium and may reflect volume status, although its utility in assessing volume responsiveness (whether or not a patient's low blood pressure will improve with an increase in intravascular volume) is poor. A CVP of 8–12 mm Hg (12–16 mm Hg if mechanically ventilated due to increases in thoracic pressure) has been suggested as being optimal for a patient with hypoperfusion from sepsis, but data on the use of CVP are lacking. CVP values at the extremes usually reflect hypovolemia (less than 2 mm Hg) and hypervolemia (greater than 18 mm Hg).
   b. PCWP or PAOP is the pressure when a balloon is inflated (wedged) in one of the pulmonary artery branches. Because the measurement is taken closer to the left ventricle than CVP, it may be a more accurate marker of volume status, but controversy remains. Its utility is diminished because the use of pulmonary artery catheters has severely declined.
   c. Dynamic markers (SVV, PPV) are increasingly used to determine a patient's volume responsiveness to a fluid challenge. These measurements consider other variables and provide a better assessment of an individual patient's position on the Starling curve. Further information about dynamic markers can be found in the references.

B. Indicators of Oxygen Delivery
1. Assessment of end organ function is perhaps the simplest measurement of adequate oxygen delivery. Changes in mental status, decreased urine output (less than 0.5 mL/kg/hour), and cold extremities may be the first markers of organ hypoperfusion.
2. Blood pressure is the driving force behind oxygen delivery. Every organ is able to autoregulate blood flow, but this ability is generally lost at MAP values lower than 65 mm Hg.
3. Lactic acid
   a. Lactic acid is formed during anaerobic metabolism.
   b. During states of hypoperfusion, the tissues receive less blood and therefore less oxygen.

    c.   If there is less oxygen for the tissues, they will use anaerobic metabolism, with the subsequent production of lactic acid.

    d.   Lactate clearance may be used as a therapeutic end point in shock states.

4.   Venous oxygen saturation

    a.   The oxyhemoglobin saturation of venous blood returning to the right atrium is normally 70%–75% (with a normal [99%–100%] arterial oxygen saturation, Sao_2), indicating that the normal oxygen extraction ratio is approximately 25%–30%.

    b.   In times of decreased oxygen delivery (caused by anemia, a decrease in Sao_2, CO, or tissue perfusion), more oxygen is extracted from the blood that is being perfused to tissues, causing an increased extraction ratio and thus a decrease in venous oxygen saturation.

    c.   Central venous oxygen saturation ($Scvo_2$) and mixed venous oxygen saturation (Svo_2) are measurements of venous oxygen saturation. These values are similar, but $Scvo_2$ is slightly higher than Svo_2 because it has not mixed with venous blood from the coronary sinus. $Scvo_2$ is measured in the superior vena cava, and Svo_2 is measured from the pulmonary artery (therefore, Svo_2 is about 5% lower than $Scvo_2$).

    d.   A normal Svo_2 does not rule out hypoperfusion in patients with impaired extraction (e.g., sepsis). An elevated lactate concentration may indicate hypoperfusion in this scenario.

Table 1. Hemodynamic Parameters and Normal Values

Parameter	Calculation (if applicable)	Normal Range
Systolic blood pressure (SBP)		90–140 mm Hg
Diastolic blood pressure (DBP)		60–90 mm Hg
Mean arterial blood pressure (MAP)	[SBP + (2·DBP)]/3	70–100 mm Hg
Systemic vascular resistance (SVR)	80 [(MAP − CVP)/CO]	800–1200 dynes/s/cm^5
Heart rate (HR)		60–80 beats/minute
Cardiac output (CO)	HR·SV	4–7 L/minute
Cardiac index (CI)	CO/BSA	2.5–4.2 L/minute/m^2
Stroke volume (SV)	CO/HR	60–130 mL/beat
Pulmonary capillary wedge pressure (PCWP) or pulmonary arterial occlusion pressure (PAOP)		5–12 mm Hg
Central venous pressure (CVP)		2–6 mm Hg
Lactic acid		<1 mmol/L
Central venous oxygen saturation ($Scvo_2$)		70%–75%

BSA = body surface area.

II. TREATMENT OF SHOCK

A. Diagnosis of Shock Based on Hemodynamic Parameters. Many patients have more than one type of shock (Table 2).

Table 2. Definitions of Shock

Hemodynamic Subset	CI	CVP/PCWP	SVR	Description
Distributive or vasodilatory	High (early) Low (late)	Low (early) Normal to high (late)	Low (early and late)	Patients with distributive shock are typically hyperdynamic (high CI), with vasodilation (low SVR) and increased vascular permeability ("leaky capillaries"), causing intravascular fluid to shift into the interstitial spaces (thus, low PCWP) The vasodilation and vascular permeability are attributable to cytokines and inflammatory mediators
Hypovolemic	Low	Low	High	To understand why patients with hypovolemia have a low CI, the Starling curve illustrates reduced cardiac function as intravascular volume is reduced The reduced intravascular volume is indicated by a low PCWP, with a reflex increase in SVR to maintain tissue perfusion Remember that resistance (SVR) is inversely related to flow (CI)
Obstructive	Low	Low (impaired ejection) High (impaired filling)	High	Impairment in diastolic filling (caused by tamponade) or systolic contraction (massive pulmonary embolus, aortic stenosis) lead to the same hemodynamic status Differentiation can usually be made by patient history
Cardiogenic	Low	High	High	Patients with cardiogenic shock have acute heart failure (low CI) The insufficient forward flow of blood causes venous congestion (high PCWP) and an underfilled arterial blood volume The subsequent reduced tissue perfusion causes a reflex vasoconstriction (which, although it can improve blood flow to vital organs, can worsen heart function by increasing afterload) and reduced renal excretion of Na^+ and water

CI = cardiac index; CVP = central venous pressure; Na^+ = sodium; PCWP = pulmonary capillary wedge pressure; SVR = systemic vascular resistance.

B. Treatment of Hypovolemic Shock
  1. Treatment centers on restoring intravascular volume and oxygen-carrying capacity. Crystalloids and colloids are discussed in Chapter 7, "Fluids, Electrolytes, and Nutrition."
  2. Blood products (packed red blood cells and coagulation factors) should be administered in hypovolemic shock, if clinically indicated.
     a. A hemoglobin less than 7 g/dL is defined as a transfusion threshold in patients in the general ICU. It is reasonable to have higher hemoglobin targets in selected patients (e.g., symptomatic cardiovascular disease).
     b. Actively bleeding patients should have blood products administered regardless of hemoglobin level in conjunction with interventions to stop the source of bleeding.
  3. Patients may need vasopressors if hypotension is not rapidly reversed with fluid resuscitation. See below for vasopressor options.
     a. The efficacy of vasopressors is reduced in patients who have not received adequate intravascular volume resuscitation.
     b. The risk associated with vasopressors (e.g., arrhythmias, ischemia) are greater in patients who have not received adequate fluid resuscitation.

C. Treatment of Obstructive Shock
  1. Fluids and vasopressors may be used temporarily to improve end organ perfusion but may not improve outcomes.
  2. Treatment of the actual obstruction is the only way to reverse the shock state.
     a. Massive pulmonary embolism: Thrombectomy or administration of systemic or catheter-directed thrombolytics may be indicated if the patient has a high risk of death.
     b. Cardiac tamponade: Drainage or removal of fluid in the pericardial sac is the only definitive treatment.

Table 3. Classification of Sepsis Syndromes

	Definition	Criteria
Sepsis	Documented or suspected infection plus some of the criteria on the right	Temperature >38.3°C or <36°C[a] Heart rate >90 beats/minute[a] Respiratory rate >20 breaths/minute or $Paco_2$ <32 mm Hg[a] WBC >12 × 10^3 cells/m^3 or <4 × 10^3 cells/mm^3[a] Altered mental status Hyperglycemia (BG >120 mg/dL without diabetes) Immature leukocytes (bands) >10% Significant edema or positive fluid balance (>20 mL/kg over 24 hours)

Table 3. Classification of Sepsis Syndromes *(continued)*

	Definition	Criteria
Sepsis	Documented or suspected infection plus some of the criteria on the right	Temperature >38.3°C or <36°C[a] Heart rate >90 beats/minute[a] Respiratory rate >20 breaths/minute or $Paco_2$ <32 mm Hg[a] WBC >12 × 10³ cells/m³ or <4 × 10³ cells/mm³[a] Altered mental status Hyperglycemia (BG >120 mg/dL without diabetes) Immature leukocytes (bands) >10% Significant edema or positive fluid balance (>20 mL/kg over 24 hours)
Severe sepsis	Sepsis complicated by organ dysfunction (Table 4) or hypoperfusion	SBP <90 mm Hg (or a >40–mm Hg drop) or MAP <70 mm Hg Venous saturation (Svo_2) <70% Need for mechanical ventilation Hypoxemia (Pao_2/Fio_2 <300) CI >3.5 Lactate >1 mmol/L Decreased capillary refill (press finger until turns white; time for color to return is refill time and normally <2 seconds) Mottling Creatinine increase >0.5 mg/dL Urine output <0.5 mL/kg/hour for ≥2 hours Coagulopathy (INR >1.5 or aPTT >60 seconds) Thrombocytopenia (platelet count <100,000/mm³) Ileus Hyperbilirubinemia (total bilirubin >4 mg/dL)
Septic shock	Sepsis-induced hypotension	Persistent hypotension or a requirement for vasopressors after the administration of an intravenous fluid bolus

[a]Criteria including temperature, heart rate, respiratory rate, and WBC make up the original definition of systemic inflammatory response syndrome.

aPTT = activated partial thromboplastin time; BG = blood glucose; CI = cardiac index; INR = international normalized ratio; MAP = mean arterial pressure; SBP = systolic blood pressure; WBC = white blood cell count.

Table 4. Organ Dysfunction

Organ System	Signs of Dysfunction
Central nervous system	Altered mental status (Glasgow coma score <15)
Cardiovascular	SBP <90 or MAP <70 mm Hg Positive biomarkers (troponin, CK MB) Persistently hypotensive despite adequate fluid resuscitation Metabolic acidosis
Pulmonary	Need for mechanical ventilation because of respiratory failure
Kidney	Abrupt decrease in urine output (i.e., <0.5 mL/kg/hour for at least 2 hours) or increased creatinine
Liver	Elevated liver function tests, prothrombin time, INR, bilirubin
Hematologic or coagulation	Reduced platelet count or white blood cell count or an increase in INR

CK MB = creatinine kinase myocardial band; INR = international normalized ratio; MAP = mean arterial pressure; SBP = systolic blood pressure.

D. Treatment of Vasodilatory and Distributive Shock

1. Septic shock is the most common cause of vasodilatory shock (Table 3). Other causes such as anaphylaxis, vasoplegia, intoxication, pancreatitis, and neurogenic and endocrine causes will not be discussed in this section.

2. The hallmark treatment of septic shock is rapid antibiotic administration, ideally within the first hour of hypotension.

3. The Surviving Sepsis Campaign (SSC) is an initiative to reduce mortality from severe sepsis and septic shock.

4. SSC "bundles"

   a. The SSC bundles are selected elements of care taken from evidence-based practice guidelines that, when implemented as a group, have a greater effect on outcomes than any individual element. In 2015, after publication of three trials on early goal directed therapy, the SSC bundles (specifically the 6 hours bundles) were updated.

   b. The SSC recommends the following bundle for patients presenting with severe sepsis or septic shock.

      i. To be completed within 3 hours

         (a) Measure lactate level.

         (b) Obtain blood cultures before administering antibiotics.

         (c) Administer broad-spectrum antibiotics.

         (d) Administer 30 mL/kg crystalloid for hypotension or lactate 4 mmol/L or greater.

            (1) Albumin can be considered when patients need a substantial amount of crystalloids. There is no evidence that colloids are superior to crystalloids in improving outcomes, and they are more expensive.

            (2) Hydroxyethyl starches (e.g., hetastarch) are not recommended for fluid resuscitation because of an increased risk of acute kidney injury.

            (3) Administration of large volumes of chloride-rich solutions leads to metabolic acidosis and acute kidney injury. The use of "balanced crystalloids" (solutions with electrolyte concentrations similar to those of extracellular fluid, such as lactated Ringer's, PlasmaLyte) for volume replacement may lead to less acute kidney injury than the use of other fluids (normal saline or 5% albumin). This is probably a dose-dependent phenomenon.

      ii. To be completed within 6 hours

         (a) Apply vasopressors (for hypotension that does not respond to initial fluid resuscitation) to maintain MAP 65 mm Hg or greater (Table 5).

            (1) The goal MAP of 65 mm Hg should be individualized. A higher goal may be appropriate in patients with atherosclerosis or a history of hypertension. The individualized target MAP should correlate with improvement in other clinical parameters (e.g., lactate level, mental status, urine output, capillary refill).

            (2) Ideally, vasopressors should be used after restoration of intravascular volume, but in patients with septic shock and hypoperfusion, vasopressors may be necessary during fluid resuscitation to optimize perfusion of vital organs. Once intravascular volume is optimized with fluid resuscitation, vasopressors should be weaned if possible.

            (3) Vasopressors improve tissue perfusion by increasing BP or CO. Very few studies have evaluated an improvement in clinical outcomes, but differences in safety profile have been observed. Therefore, drug selection is based largely on expert opinion, practitioner experience, and patient response.

            (4) Norepinephrine is the initial vasopressor of choice.

            (5) Epinephrine can be added to or substituted for norepinephrine if needed.

(6) Vasopressin (0.03 unit/minute) can be added to norepinephrine if needed. The efficacy of vasopressin when added to norepinephrine is similar to that of norepinephrine alone. Vasopressin can have a vasopressor-sparing effect, although mortality is not improved with the combination. The addition of vasopressin earlier (at norepinephrine doses of less than 15 mcg/minute) may be associated with an improvement in outcomes.

(7) Dopamine is an alternative to norepinephrine, but it is associated with a higher incidence of arrhythmias compared with norepinephrine. Dopamine use should be limited to patients with a low risk of tachyarrhythmias and absolute or relative bradycardia. Low-dose dopamine should not be used for renal protection.

(8) Phenylephrine is an alternative to consider in patients with vasopressor-induced serious tachyarrhythmias or persistent hypotension.

(9) Use of an arterial catheter for BP measurements is preferred in patients needing vasopressors because it is a more accurate measurement of arterial pressure (compared with a BP cuff) and allows continuous monitoring.

(10) Vasopressors should be administered through a central line as soon as possible to reduce the risk of extravasation and subsequent tissue ischemia. If extravasation occurs, phentolamine (an α-receptor antagonist) can be used to reduce tissue necrosis. In a phentolamine shortage, other options include nitroglycerin ointment (applied around the site of extravasation every 6 hours) or subcutaneous terbutaline (peripheral vasodilation is mediated through β_2-receptors).

(b) In the event of persistent arterial hypotension despite volume resuscitation or initial lactate 4 mmol/L or more, volume status and tissue perfusion should be reassessed by either of the following:

(1) Repeat focused examination including vital signs, cardiopulmonary examination, capillary refill, pulse, and skin findings.

(2) Two of the following:

(A) CVP measurement

(B) $Scvo_2$ measurement

(C) Bedside cardiovascular ultrasound

(D) Dynamic assessment of fluid responsiveness with passive leg raise or fluid challenge

Table 5. Vasopressors and Inotropes

Drug	Dose	α_1	β_1	β_2	DA	Notes
Norepinephrine	0.01–3 mcg/kg/minute	++++	+++	0	0	↓ Renal perfusion ↑ SVR, ↑ BP 0 – ↓ CO (at high doses) Peripheral ischemia Can induce tachyarrhythmias and myocardial ischemia
Epinephrine	0.04–1 mcg/kg/minute for refractory hypotension	+++	+++	++	0	Positive inotropic and chronotropic effects can induce arrhythmias and myocardial ischemia Low doses primarily β-adrenergic; escalating doses primarily α-adrenergic Some evidence of reduced splanchnic circulation, which can lead to gut ischemia Increases blood glucose and lactate concentrations (type B lactic acidosis)
Vasopressin	0.03–0.04 unit/minute (physiologic replacement dose)	0	0	0	0	Direct stimulation of smooth muscle V1 vasopressin receptors; peripheral vasoconstriction, no adrenergic activity Theoretically beneficial because of an apparent relative vasopressin deficiency in septic shock but no evidence of efficacy over other vasopressors Effective during acidosis and hypoxia because it does not rely on adrenergic receptors Doses ≥0.04 unit/minute are associated with coronary vasoconstriction and peripheral necrosis Not titrated like traditional vasopressors Prone to dosing errors because of "unit/minute"
Phenylephrine	0.5–8 mcg/kg/minute for septic shock (or a common maximum amount is 300 mcg/minute)	++++	0	0	0	↓ Renal perfusion Pure α-adrenergic agonist with minimal cardiac activity Rapid ↑ SBP and DBP can cause a reflex bradycardia and reduction in CO Can be administered as a rapid bolus for acute hypotension (e.g., intraoperative) or as a continuous infusion. Extravasation produces ischemic necrosis and sloughing

Table 5. Vasopressors and Inotropes *(continued)*

Drug	Dose	α_1	β_1	β_2	DA	Notes
Dopamine	1–3 mcg/kg/minute	+/–	++	+/–	++++	Lower doses cause renal, coronary, mesenteric, and cerebral arterial vasodilation and a natriuretic response Lower "inotropic" doses can complement the vasoconstrictive effects of norepinephrine Do not use low-dose dopamine for renal protection because evidence does not support this practice Moderate doses can ↑ contractility and SVR
	3–10 mcg/kg/minute	++	+++	+	++	Any dose can induce arrhythmias
	10–20 mcg/kg/minute	++++	+++	0	+	Any dose can cause endocrine changes (e.g., decreased prolactin, growth hormone, thyroid hormone); however, the clinical significance is unknown Immediate precursor of norepinephrine Prolonged infusions can deplete endogenous norepinephrine stores, resulting in a loss of vasopressor response Effects on renal blood flow may be lost at higher doses because of predominant α_1-vasoconstrictive effects
Dobutamine	2–20 mcg/kg/minute	+	+++	+	0	Positive inotrope to ↑ CO Can cause hypotension because of β_2-stimulation Higher doses can cause tachyarrhythmias and changes in BP, which can lead to myocardial ischemia
Milrinone	50-mcg/kg load over 10 minutes, followed by 0.375–0.75 mcg/kg/minute	0	0	0	0	Noncatecholamine, phosphodiesterase inhibitor Positive inotrope Vasodilation or hypotension, arrhythmias possible Use lower doses in renal failure Loading doses often omitted especially if patient hypotensive

BP = blood pressure; CO = cardiac output; DA = dopamine; DBP = diastolic blood pressure; SBP = systolic blood pressure; SVR = systemic vascular resistance.

E. Appropriate Use of Antimicrobials in Patients with Sepsis

1. Empiric antimicrobials should cover likely pathogens according to suspected location of infection and risk of multidrug-resistant pathogens. Common sources of infection are lung, abdomen, blood, and urinary tract. Please refer to the infectious diseases chapter for discussion of specific agents.

2. Consider empiric fungal therapy with either triazoles such as fluconazole, an echinocandin, or a lipid formulation of amphotericin B if patients have several risk factors, including recent abdominal surgery, chronic parenteral nutrition, indwelling central venous catheters, or recent treatment with broad-spectrum antibiotics or if patients are immunocompromised (e.g., chronic corticosteroids or other immunosuppressants, neutropenia, malignancy, organ transplant). An echinocandin is preferred in patients recently treated with antifungal agents or if *Candida glabrata* or *krusei* infection is suspected.

3. Other considerations in choosing appropriate antimicrobials include the patient's history of drug allergy or intolerance, recent antibiotic use, comorbidities, and antimicrobial susceptibility patterns in the community and hospital.

4. Begin intravenous antimicrobials as early as possible, at least within the first hour but preferably after at least two sets of blood cultures (one drawn percutaneously) are obtained. Quantitative cultures of other potential sites of infection (e.g., urine, sputum) should also be obtained before antimicrobials are administered if possible.

5. If several antibiotics are prescribed, administer the broadest coverage first and infuse as quickly as possible.

6. Mortality increases by 7.9% for each 1-hour delay in administering appropriate antimicrobials.

7. Appropriate antimicrobials do not reduce the importance of emergency source control by drainage, debridement, or device removal as needed.

8. De-escalation should occur with respect to culture data or clinical judgment. Empiric use of combination therapy should not be administered for longer than 3–5 days if de-escalation to a single agent is appropriate.

9. Consider discontinuing antimicrobials in 7–10 days unless there is slow response, undrainable foci, immunosuppression, or multidrug-resistant pathogens. Blood cultures will be negative in most patients, despite a bacterial or fungal origin of sepsis. Clinical judgment is needed when considering discontinuation of antimicrobials.

10. Procalcitonin, a biomarker for bacterial infections, can be used as a guide for antibiotic therapy.

11. Discontinue antimicrobials if no infectious cause is found.

12. Consider empiric antiviral therapy with oseltamivir for patients presenting with flulike symptoms during flu season.

F. Indication for and Use of Corticosteroids

1. Adrenal function in critically ill patients may be suppressed by endotoxins produced by bacteria and by the body's immune response to stress.

2. Early studies showed a relationship between vasopressor responsiveness and glucocorticoid administration.

3. To determine a patient's adrenal function during critical illness, a corticotropin stimulation test ("stim test") may be performed, although it is no longer recommended.

   a. A corticotropin stimulation test is performed by administering 250 mcg of cosyntropin (synthetic adrenocorticotropic hormone) and measuring cortisol levels at baseline, 30 minutes, and 60 minutes after.

   b. A cortisol increase of more than 9 mcg/dL is said to be an appropriate response (responders), perhaps indicating appropriate adrenal function. Changes of less than 9 mcg/dL may indicate corticosteroid insufficiency. A random cortisol level of less than 10 mcg/dL may also indicate corticosteroid insufficiency.

c. The corticotropin stimulation test has come under criticism because of the high dose of cosyntropin administered, the inability to measure free (active) cortisol, and lack of data on outcomes of responders versus nonresponders. It is not indicated for use in the general ICU population.

4. Clinical trials of steroids in septic shock

a. In a study published in 2002, adult patients with septic shock were given a corticotropin stimulation test and then randomly assigned to intravenous hydrocortisone combined with oral fludrocortisone or placebo, regardless of stimulation test results. In the entire patient population, steroid therapy improved 28-day survival; however, this occurred because of a marked improvement in nonresponders to the corticotropin stimulation test. Responders showed no improvement with steroid therapy.

b. The CORTICUS trial, published in 2008, had a similar method to the study above but omitted fludrocortisone. In this study, corticosteroids were not associated with a mortality benefit; however, they were associated with a higher risk of hyperglycemia, new sepsis, or septic shock. For this reason, corticosteroids are not recommended in patients with septic shock who have been stabilized with fluid and vasopressor therapy.

5. Evidence-based guidelines

a. SSC guidelines

i. The SSC recommends against using hydrocortisone to treat adults with septic shock if adequate fluid resuscitation and vasopressor therapy are able to restore hemodynamic stability. If this is not achievable, the SSC suggests intravenous hydrocortisone alone at a dose of 200 mg per day.

ii. The SSC recommends against using the corticotropin stimulation test to identify the subset of adults with septic shock who should receive hydrocortisone.

b. American College of Critical Care Medicine corticosteroid insufficiency guidelines recognize that although hypothalamic-pituitary-adrenal (HPA) axis dysfunction is common in some critically ill patients (sepsis), diagnosis and management of this disorder are complicated.

i. The expert panel's recommendations for septic shock are similar to the SSC guidelines, that hydrocortisone should be considered in the management strategy for patients with septic shock, particularly those who have responded poorly to fluid resuscitation and vasopressor agents.

ii. Furthermore, the corticotropin stimulation test should not be used to identify patients with septic shock or acute respiratory distress syndrome (ARDS) who should receive glucocorticoids.

iii. Patients should be weaned off steroid therapy once vasopressors are no longer necessary.

III. INTERPRETATION OF ACID-BASE DISTURBANCES

A. Normal Arterial Blood Gas Values

pH	7.40 (range 7.35–7.45)
Pco_2	35–45 mm Hg
Po_2	80–100 mm Hg
HCO_3^-	22–26 mEq/L (or mmol/L)
Sao_2	95%–100%

B. Acidosis: Any pH less than 7.35 indicates a primary acidosis.

C. Alkalosis: Any pH greater than 7.45 indicates a primary alkalosis.

D. Metabolic Disorders
1. Acidosis: Decreased HCO_3^-
2. Alkalosis: Increased HCO_3^-

E. Respiratory Disorders
1. Acidosis: Increased Pco_2
2. Alkalosis: Decreased Pco_2

F. Compensation: Occurs in an attempt to normalize the pH in response to the primary problem (Table 6)
1. Respiratory compensation occurs immediately with changes in respiratory rate.
   a. The compensation for metabolic acidosis is respiratory alkalosis (i.e., decrease in Pco_2). This is achieved by increasing the respiratory rate to eliminate more CO_2, thus making pH more basic (i.e., higher pH).
   b. The compensation for metabolic alkalosis is a respiratory acidosis (i.e., increase in Pco_2). This is achieved by slowing the respiratory rate to retain more CO_2, thus making pH more acidic (i.e., lower pH).
2. Metabolic compensation occurs slowly in the kidneys by regulating the excretion and reabsorption of HCO_3^- and H^+.
   a. The compensation for a respiratory acidosis is metabolic alkalosis (i.e., an increase in HCO_3^-).
   b. The compensation for a respiratory alkalosis is metabolic acidosis (i.e., a decrease in HCO_3^-).

Table 6. Predicted Degrees of Compensation in Acid-Base Disturbances

Normal Values $HCO_3^- = 24$ mmol/L $Pco_2 = 40$ mm Hg	Primary Disturbance	Compensation
Metabolic acidosis	↓ HCO_3^- by 1 mmol/L	↓ Pco_2 by 1.2 mm Hg
Metabolic alkalosis	↑ HCO_3^- by 1 mmol/L	↑ Pco_2 by 0.7 mm Hg
Respiratory acidosis Chronic (>3 days) Acute	↑ Pco_2 by 10 mm Hg ↑ Pco_2 by 10 mm Hg	↑ HCO_3^- by 3.5 mmol/L ↑ HCO_3^- by 1 mmol/L
Respiratory alkalosis Chronic (>3 days) Acute	↓ Pco_2 by 10 mm Hg ↓ Pco_2 by 10 mm Hg	↓ $HCO_3^- = 4$ mmol/L ↓ $HCO_3^- = 2$ mmol/L

G. Steps to Evaluate Acid-Base Disorders (Table 7)
1. Assess pH, Pco_2, and HCO_3^-.
   a. Acidosis if pH less than 7.35
      i. If Pco_2 is elevated, the primary disorder is respiratory acidosis.
      ii. If HCO_3^- is decreased, the primary disorder is metabolic acidosis.
   b. Alkalosis if pH is greater than 7.45
      i. If Pco_2 is decreased, the primary disorder is respiratory alkalosis.
      ii. If HCO_3^- is elevated, the primary disorder is metabolic alkalosis.
2. Calculate the anion gap (AG) = $[Na+] - [Cl^- + HCO_3^-]$.
   a. Normal range is 6–12 mEq/L.
   b. If AG is more than 12, there is a primary metabolic acidosis regardless of pH or HCO_3^-. Some patients have a mixed acid-base disorder in which they have more than one primary disorder.
   c. Hypoalbuminemia decreases the AG by 2.5–3 mEq/L for every 1-g/dL decrease in serum albumin less than 4 g/dL.

3. Calculate the excess AG = total AG − normal AG. Add excess AG to serum bicarbonate.
   a. If the sum is greater than a normal serum bicarbonate (i.e., more than 30 mEq/L), there is also an AG metabolic alkalosis (this can occur in addition to other primary disorders).
   b. If the sum is less than a normal serum bicarbonate (i.e., less than 23 mEq/L), there is an underlying non-AG metabolic acidosis.

Table 7. Causes of Acid-Base Disturbances

	Respiratory Acidosis	Respiratory Alkalosis	Metabolic Acidosis	Metabolic Alkalosis
Etiology	Pulmonary edema Cardiac arrest CNS depression Stroke Pulmonary embolus Pneumonia Bronchospasm Spinal cord injury Sedatives	Anxiety Pain CNS tumor Stroke Head injury Hypoxia Stimulant drugs Reduced oxygen-carrying capacity Reduced alveolar oxygen extraction Respiratory rate stimulation Extracorporeal removal	**Anion gap** (MUDPILES) Methanol Uremia DKA Propylene glycol Intoxication or infection Lactic acidosis Ethylene glycol Salicylate **Non–anion gap** (F-USED CARS) Fistula (pancreatic) Uteroenteric conduits Saline excess Endocrine (hyperparathyroid) Diarrhea Carbonic anhydrase inhibitors Arginine, lysine, Cl⁻ Renal tubular acidosis Spironolactone	**Urine Cl⁻ >25** (Chloride resistant) Hyperaldosteronism ↑ Mineralocorticoid **Urine Cl⁻ <25** (Chloride responsive) Vomiting NG suction Diuretic
Treatment	Correct cause Invasive/ noninvasive ventilation	Correct cause Oxygen supplementation Invasive/ noninvasive ventilation Hypoventilation Sedation	Correct cause Use of bases (sodium bicarbonate or THAM) may be considered in non-AG metabolic acidosis Base use in AG metabolic acidosis is controversial (Sodium bicarbonate and THAM have traditionally been used, but evidence of clinical benefit is lacking)	Correct cause **If urine Cl⁻ < 25** 0.9% NaCl Consider HCl (if severe) Consider acetazolamide **If urine Cl⁻ > 25** Potassium Aldosterone antagonist Acetazolamide

AG = anion gap; Cl⁻ = chloride; CNS = central nervous system; DKA = diabetic ketoacidosis; HCl = hydrochloric acid; NaCl = sodium chloride; NG = nasogastric; THAM = tromethamine or tris-hydroxymethyl aminomethane.

Patient Cases

1. A 62-year-old woman has been hospitalized in the ICU for several weeks. Her hospital stay has been complicated by aspiration pneumonia and sepsis, necessitating prolonged courses of antibiotics. For the past few days, she has been having high temperatures again, and her stool output has increased dramatically. Her most recent stool samples have tested positive for *Clostridium difficile* toxin, and her laboratory tests reveal serum sodium 138 mEq/L, potassium (K) 3.5 mEq/L, Cl 115 mEq/L, HCO_3^- 15 mEq/L, albumin 4.4 g/dL, pH 7.32, $Paco_2$ 30 mm Hg, and HCO_3^- 15 mEq/L. Which is most consistent with this patient's primary acid-base disturbance?

    A. AG metabolic acidosis.

    B. Non-AG metabolic acidosis.

    C. Chloride-responsive metabolic alkalosis.

    D. Acute respiratory acidosis.

2. A 27-year-old man with no medical history is admitted to the hospital after being "found down" at a party, where he reportedly ingested a handle of whiskey during a 60-minute period. On arrival at the emergency department, he was neurologically unresponsive, with the following ABG values: pH 7.23, $Paco_2$ 58 mm Hg, Pao_2 111 mm Hg, HCO_3^- 24 mEq/L, and Sao_2 88% on 2 L/minute of oxygen by nasal cannula. Which action is most appropriate?

    A. Administer tromethamine 500 mL over 30 minutes.

    B. Administer 100% oxygen by face mask.

    C. Give $NaHCO_3^-$ 100 mEq intravenous push.

    D. Urgent intubation.

3. A 55-year-old woman is admitted to the hospital after several days of worsening shortness of breath. Recently, she was discharged from the hospital after a similar episode and was doing fine until 3 days before admission, when she developed a productive cough, necessitating an increase in her home oxygen and more frequent use of her metered dose inhalers. On admission to the medical ICU, she was anxious and markedly distressed, with rapid, shallow breaths. She was hypertensive (160/80 mm Hg), tachycardic (140 beats/minute), and tachypneic (respiratory rate 28 breaths/minute). Her ABG showed a pH of 7.30, $Paco_2$ 59 mm Hg, Pao_2 50 mm Hg, HCO_3^- 28 mEq/L, and Sao_2 83% on 6 L/minute of oxygen by face mask, and she was immediately intubated. Which primary acid-base disturbance is most consistent with this patient's presentation and laboratory data?

    A. Metabolic acidosis.

    B. Metabolic alkalosis.

    C. Respiratory acidosis.

    D. Respiratory alkalosis.

Patient Cases

4. A 65-year-old woman is admitted to the cardiac surgery after an aortic valve replacement. On the fourth day of hospitalization, she is hypotensive (BP 80/50 mm Hg), tachycardic (HR 125 beats/minute), tachypneic (respiratory rate 30 breaths/minute), hypoxemic (Pao_2 40 mm Hg), febrile (39.5°C), and confused. The patient is given two 1000-mL boluses of normal saline and then is reintubated and initiated on piperacillin/tazobactam 4.5 g intravenous piggyback every 6 hours and vancomycin 1000 mg intravenous piggyback every 12 hours for possible nosocomial pneumonia. After fluid boluses fail to improve her hemodynamic and clinical status, a pulmonary artery catheter is placed, which reveals a PCWP of 18 mm Hg, CI of 4.8 L/minute/m², and SVR of 515 dynes/second/cm². Her chest radiograph shows a left lower lobe consolidation, and she still needs 100% Fio_2. Which action is best?

   A. Add clindamycin 600 mg intravenous piggyback every 8 hours.

   B. Administer dobutamine infusion titrated to achieve an MAP of at least 65 mm Hg.

   C. Administer norepinephrine infusion titrated to achieve an MAP of at least 65 mm Hg.

   D. Administer hydrocortisone 50 mg intravenously every 6 hours.

5. A 70-kg patient is to be started on a continuous infusion of epinephrine for BP support after return of spontaneous circulation after a cardiac arrest. The nurse has a 250-mL bag of D_5W containing 4 mg of epinephrine. Which rate is most appropriate to infuse the epinephrine drip at a dose of 0.03 mcg/kg/minute?

   A. 8 mL/hour.

   B. 13 mL/hour.

   C. 31.5 mL/hour.

   D. 79 mL/hour.

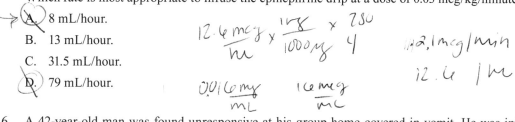

6. A 42-year-old man was found unresponsive at his group home covered in vomit. He was intubated by the paramedics. On arrival at the emergency department, his BP is 72/30 mm Hg and HR is 122 beats/minute. During the next few hours, he receives 5 L of normal saline, 500 mL of 5% albumin, and norepinephrine infusing at 20 mcg/minute. With these interventions, his BP is 87/56 mm Hg, and his HR is 95 beats/minute. Pertinent laboratory values include a WBC of 20×10^3 cells/mm³, lactic acid 1.5 mmol/L, aspartate aminotransferase 78 units/L, Cr 2.2 (baseline 1) mg/dL, platelet count 118,000 cells/mm³, INR 1.4, and urine output about 45 mL/hour since arrival. Which is most appropriate intervention at this time?

   A. Add hydrocortisone 50 mg intravenously every 6 hours.

   B. Add enoxaparin 40 mg subcutaneously every 24 hours.

   C. Add low-dose dopamine.

   D. Add heparin 5000 units subcutaneously every 8 hours.

IV. ACUTE RESPIRATORY FAILURE

A. Causes of Respiratory Failure (Table 8)

Table 8. Respiratory Failure

Indication for Mechanical Ventilation	Examples
Hypoventilation (hypercapnic respiratory failure)	Drug overdose Neuromuscular disease Cardiopulmonary resuscitation Central nervous system injury or disease
Hypoxemia (hypoxic respiratory failure)	Pulmonary injury or disease Pneumonia Pulmonary edema Pulmonary embolus Acute respiratory distress syndrome
Inability to maintain airway	Loss of airway patency (mechanical obstruction, tracheal or chest wall injury) Loss of gag or cough reflex with large-volume aspiration risk (e.g., central nervous system injury, central nervous system depression, cardiovascular accident, seizures, cardiac arrest)

B. Complications Associated with Mechanical Ventilation (see individual sections later in text for prevention of these complications)
   1. Ventilator-associated pneumonia
   2. Stress ulcers
   3. Venous thrombosis

V. CARDIAC ARREST

A. Training: Any pharmacist who participates in codes should complete basic life support (BLS) and advanced cardiac life support (ACLS) training. In general, BLS training takes 3–5 hours to complete, and ACLS training takes 2 days. The information presented in this section consists of selected highlights from these training sessions; it should not be used in place of a comprehensive training program.

B. 2015 American Heart Association (AHA) Guidelines
   1. Medications used during ACLS: See "Cardiology I" chapter for information on drugs, indications, and dosages.
   2. CAB (compressions, airway, breathing): In an unresponsive patient or patient who is not breathing, one rescuer should initiate a cycle of 30 chest compressions as soon as possible, followed immediately by 2 rescue breaths.
   3. Emphasis is on high-quality cardiopulmonary resuscitation (CPR), with a compression rate of at 100–120/minute at a depth of at least 2 inches but not to exceed 2.4 inches.
   4. Electrical therapy (via an automated external defibrillator [AED] or defibrillator) should be initiated as soon as it is available.
   5. Interruptions in chest compressions should be minimal and be as short as possible. Chest compressions and defibrillation should not be interrupted for vascular access, medication administration, or airway placement.

6. Medication administration
   a. Central venous administration is preferred.
   b. Intraosseous administration is preferred to endotracheal administration if intravenous administration is not possible because of its more predictable drug delivery and pharmacologic effect.
   c. Endotracheal drug administration can be performed by administering 2–2.5 times the standard intravenous dose and diluting in 5–10 mL of sterile water. The following drugs can be administered through an endotracheal tube: naloxone, atropine, vasopressin, epinephrine, lidocaine (NAVEL).
   d. If medications are administered through a peripheral vein, it is important to follow the medication with 20 mL of intravenous fluid to facilitate drug flow from the extremity to the central circulation.

C. Post–Cardiac Arrest Care
   1. After return of spontaneous circulation (ROSC), systematic postarrest care can improve survival and quality of life.
   2. Initial therapy should be to optimize ventilation, oxygenation, and blood pressure.
      a. Oxygen saturation should be maintained at 94% or higher.
         i. Insertion of an advanced airway may be necessary.
         ii. Hyperventilation and excess oxygen delivery are harmful and should be avoided, especially after ROSC.
      b. Hypotension (SBP 90 mm Hg or lower) should be treated with fluid boluses and vasopressors if necessary.
   3. Target temperature management (therapeutic hypothermia)
      a. Induction of hypothermia (32°C–36°C) for 12–24 hours beginning as soon as possible after ROSC can improve neurologic recovery and mortality. The AHA Guidelines recommend that all comatose adult patients with ROSC should have targeted temperature management. One study has shown that a standard target temperature (33°C) did not confer a benefit over a higher target temperature (36°C). The AHA guidelines allow the clinician to select the exact target temperature.
      b. Consider hypothermia in patients who have been successfully resuscitated after a cardiac arrest but who remain comatose (usually defined as a lack of meaningful response to verbal commands). Cooling should be continued for a period of at least 24 hours.
      c. No single method for inducing hypothermia is recommended over another. Surface cooling devices, endovascular catheters, cooling blankets, ice packs, and cold intravenous fluids may be used.
      d. Core temperature should be continuously monitored.
      e. Many patients will need sedation and analgesia during periods of hypothermia.
      f. Rewarming should be done slowly (0.3–0.5°C every hour).
      g. Complications
         i. Shivering
            (a) Shivering causes excess heat production, increased oxygen consumption, and a general stress response and thus should be treated and prevented.
            (b) Shivering can be treated with sedatives (dexmedetomidine, ketamine), anesthetics, analgesics (e.g., meperidine, fentanyl, tramadol), dexamethasone, clonidine, magnesium (Mg), ondansetron, buspirone, and paralytics (please see Crit Care Med 2012;40:3070–82 for individual drugs and doses).
            (c) Note that shivering can be treated without the use of paralytics in many patients. Therefore, paralytics are not mandatory and should be avoided if possible (see disadvantages of paralytics below). Paralytics may be most beneficial during the induction of hypothermia and during rewarming (when risk of shivering is greatest); however, they should be continually reevaluated and discontinued, if possible, once goal temperature is achieved.

    ii. Altered drug metabolism

       (a) Drug clearance is typically reduced during hypothermia, including a depressed activity of cytochrome P450 (CYP) 3A4 and 3A5 hepatic enzymes. Hypothermia can also affect the distribution of drugs to their site of action (e.g., propofol).

       (b) Use bolus dosing during the induction of hypothermia.

       (c) Reduce maintenance doses of sedatives (e.g., midazolam, propofol), opiates (fentanyl, remifentanil), phenobarbital, phenytoin, paralytics, and other drugs as needed (see review article Tortorici MA, Kochanek PM, Poloyac SM. Effects of hypothermia on drug disposition, metabolism, and response: a focus of hypothermia-mediated alterations on the cytochrome P450 enzyme system. Crit Care Med 2007;35:2196–204).

    iii. Coagulopathy

    iv. Increased renal excretion of water and subsequent volume depletion

    v. Arrhythmia and hypotension

       (a) Usually bradycardia

       (b) Discontinue or slightly warm patient if life-threatening arrhythmias or persistent hemodynamic instability develops.

    vi. Hyperglycemia and hypoglycemia

       (a) Hyperglycemia during hypothermia, hypoglycemia during rewarming.

       (b) Monitor blood glucose frequently (i.e., every 1–2 hours) and adjust insulin accordingly.

    vii. Infection

    viii. Electrolyte disturbances

       (a) Reductions in K, Mg, and phosphate during cooling

       (b) Hyperkalemia during rewarming

       (c) Special electrolyte replacement protocols should be used to ensure patients do not receive too much potassium during cooling such that they are hyperkalemic during rewarming.

Patient Case

7. A 61-year-old woman collapsed in front of her family, who called 911 and began CPR. The paramedics arrive and find the victim unresponsive, with an electrocardiogram showing ventricular fibrillation, and administer two additional rounds of CPR and two defibrillations, which are successful. In the emergency department, the patient's MAP is 68 mm Hg after fluids and norepinephrine, but the patient remains unresponsive. She is initiated on the hypothermia protocol. After 24 hours of hypothermia (temperature 33°C), the patient is in the ICU, and the rewarming process has recently begun. The pharmacist arrives in the ICU about 30 minutes into the rewarming process. The patient has been receiving a continuous infusion of insulin throughout the period of hypothermia at an average rate of 4 units/hour, with blood glucose testing every 3 hours. The patient has been sedated with a continuous infusion of propofol and fentanyl and is on cisatracurium for neuromuscular blockade. The patient's vital signs are stable, and her laboratory values are normal. Which pharmacist recommendation is most appropriate at this time?

  A. Increase BG testing to now and every 1–2 hours during rewarming.

  B. Adjust cisatracurium infusion to achieve a train-of-four (TOF) of 0/4 impulses.

  C. Discontinue propofol infusion to facilitate extubation.

  D. Increase insulin infusion to prevent hyperkalemia.

VI. PAIN, AGITATION, DELIRIUM, AND NEUROMUSCULAR BLOCKADE

A. General Considerations
  1. Nonpharmacologic strategies to improve patient comfort include lighting, music, massage, verbal reassurance, avoidance of sleep deprivation, and patient positioning based on patient preferences.
  2. Determine patient goals using validated scales and routinely assess pain and sedation.
    a. Routine assessment of pain and sedation should be performed in every patient in the ICU.
      i. Self-reporting is preferred to pain scales for assessing pain in patients who are able to communicate.
      ii. To assess pain in patients unable to communicate, the Behavioral Pain Scale (BPS; Table 9) and the Critical-Care Pain Observation Tool (CPOT; Table 10) are recommended because, compared with other scores, they are more valid and reliable for monitoring pain in adult patients in the ICU (except those with brain injury).
        (a) The total BPS score can range from 3 (no pain) to 12 (maximum pain). A score of 6 or higher is generally considered to reflect unacceptable pain.
        (b) The total CPOT score can range from 0 to 8.

Table 9. The Behavioral Pain Scale

Item	Description	Score
Facial expression	Relaxed	1
	Partially tightened (e.g., brow lowering)	2
	Fully tightened (e.g., eyelid closing)	3
	Grimacing	4
Upper limb movements	No movement	1
	Partially bent	2
	Fully bent with finger flexion	3
	Permanently retracted	4
Compliance with mechanical ventilation	Tolerating movement	1
	Coughing but tolerating ventilation for most of the time	2
	Fighting ventilator	3
	Unable to control ventilation	4

Adapted from Payen JF, Bru O, Bosson JL, et al. Assessing pain in critically ill sedated patients by using a behavioral pain scale. Crit Care Med 2001;29(12):2258-63.

Table 10. Critical Care Pain Observation Tool

Indicator	Description	Score
Facial expression	No muscular tension observed	Relaxed, neutral: 0
	Presence of frowning, brow lowering, orbit tightening, and levator contraction	Tense: 1
	All the above facial movements plus eyelids tightly closed	Grimacing: 2
Body movements	Does not move at all (does not necessarily mean absence of pain)	Absence of movement: 0
	Slow, cautious movements; touching or rubbing the pain site; seeking attention through movements	Protection: 1
	Pulling tube, attempting to sit up, moving limbs or thrashing, not following commands, striking at staff, trying to climb out of bed	Restlessness: 2
Muscle tension	No resistance to passive movements	Relaxed: 0
	Resistance to passive movements	Tense, rigid: 1
	Strong resistance to passive movements, inability to complete them	Very tense or rigid: 2
Compliance with the ventilator	Alarms not activated, easy ventilation	Tolerating ventilator or movement: 0
or	Alarms stop spontaneously	Coughing but tolerating: 1
	Asynchrony: blocking ventilation, alarms frequently activated	Fighting ventilator: 2
Vocalization (extubated patients)	Talking in normal tone or no sound	Talking in normal tone or no sound: 0
	Sighing, moaning	Sighing, moaning: 1
	Crying out, sobbing	Crying out, sobbing: 2

Adapted from Gélinas C, Fillion L, Puntillo KA, et al. Validation of the critical-care pain observation tool in adult patients. Am J Crit Care 2006;15(4):420-7.

    iii. Vital signs (e.g., elevated HR or BP) are cues that indicate further assessment of pain is necessary (using a scale described earlier).

    iv. To assess sedation, the Richmond Agitation-Sedation Scale (RASS; Table 11) and Sedation-Agitation Scale (SAS; Table 12) are recommended because, compared with other sedation scores, they are more valid and reliable for monitoring the quality and depth of sedation in adult ICU patients. Goal sedation scores should be individualized for each patient, but generally an SAS score of 3 to 4 or a RASS score of 0 to –1 is recommended.

Table 11. Richmond Agitation-Sedation Scale (RASS)

Scale	Term	Description
+4	Combative	Combative, violent, immediate danger to staff
+3	Very agitated	Pulls to remove tubes or catheters; aggressive
+2	Agitated	Frequent nonpurposeful movement, fights ventilator
+1	Restless	Anxious but movements not aggressive
0	Alert and calm	Spontaneously pays attention to caregiver
−1	Drowsy	Not fully alert but has sustained awakening to voice (eye opening and eye contact for ≥10 seconds)
−2	Light sedation	Briefly (<10 seconds) awakens with eye contact to voice
−3	Moderate sedation	Movement or eye opening to voice but no eye contact
−4	Deep sedation	No response to voice but movement or eye opening to physical stimulation
−5	Unarousable	No response to voice or physical stimulation

Table 12. Sedation-Agitation Scale (SAS)

Score	Term	Description
7	Dangerous agitation	Pulling at endotracheal tube, trying to remove catheters, climbing over bedrail, striking at staff, thrashing side to side
6	Very agitated	Requiring restraint and frequent verbal reminding of limits, biting endotracheal tube
5	Agitated	Anxious or physically agitated, calms to verbal instructions
4	Calm and cooperative	Calm, easily roused, follows commands
3	Sedated	Difficult to arouse but awakens to verbal stimuli or gentle shaking, follows simple commands but drifts off again
2	Very sedated	Arouses to physical stimuli but does not communicate or follow commands, may move spontaneously
1	Unarousable	Minimal or no response to noxious stimuli, does not communicate or follow commands

    b. Pain and discomfort are primary causes of agitation; therefore, treat pain first and add a sedative if needed.

        i. Use bolus dose analgesics or nonpharmacologic interventions before potentially painful procedures.

        ii. Opioid analgesics are considered first line for the treatment of nonneuropathic pain (gabapentin or carbamazepine can be considered for neuropathic pain).

        iii. Nonopioid analgesics (e.g., acetaminophen, ketamine) can be used in conjunction with opioids to optimize pain control and avoid dose-related adverse effects.

        iv. Nonsteroidal anti-inflammatory drugs are usually avoided because of the risk of bleeding and kidney injury in critically ill patients.

        v. Nonbenzodiazepine sedatives may be preferred to benzodiazepines to improve clinical outcomes in mechanically ventilated patients.

c. Dosing strategies for analgesics and sedatives
   i. Analgesics and sedatives should be dosed to achieve pain and sedation goals. Adjust sedative medications to achieve a light level of sedation (RASS 0 to –1). Light sedation is needed for evaluating pain and delirium and for early patient mobility.
   ii. Goals may be achieved using intermittent dosing administered routinely or as needed.
   iii. If unable to achieve goals with intermittent dosing, use a combination of bolus dosing with a continuous infusion.
      (a) In patients receiving a continuous infusion, use a bolus dose before or instead of increasing the infusion rate (a bolus dose has a faster onset and can eliminate the need for an increase in the infusion rate). Exception is with drugs such as propofol or dexmedetomidine, which can cause hypotension or bradycardia when bolused.
      (b) Use bolus dosing proactively (e.g., before dressing changes, suctioning, repositioning).
   iv. Daily awakening involves an interruption of continuous infusion opioid or sedatives until the patient is awake (SAS at least 4 or RASS at least 0) or shows discomfort or pain necessitating reinitiation. Although evidence is mixed, a scheduled daily interruption of continuous infusions is associated with several important benefits.
      (a) Assess the patient's neurologic function.
      (b) Reevaluate lowest effective opioid or sedative dose.
      (c) Prevent drug accumulation and overdose.
      (d) Reduce time on the ventilator (although one randomized study contradicts this by finding no reduction in the duration of mechanical ventilation or ICU stay with sedation interruption; Mehta S, Burry L, Cook D, et al. Daily sedation interruption in mechanically ventilated critically ill patients cared for with a sedation protocol: a randomized controlled trial. JAMA 2012;308(19):1985-92.).
      (e) Reduce mortality and ICU length of stay when combined with a spontaneous breathing trial.
      (f) Reduce symptoms of posttraumatic stress disorder and post-ICU syndrome.

B. Analgesics (Table 13)

Table 13. Analgesics

	Morphine	**Fentanyl**	**Hydromorphone**
Pharmacokinetics			
Onset (minutes)	5–10	1–2	5–10
Duration of effect (hours)	2–4	1–5	2–6
Prolonged in renal failure	Yes	No	No
Prolonged in hepatic failure	Yes	Yes	Yes
Elimination half-life (hours)	1–4	2–5	2–3
Active metabolites	Yes	No	No
Adverse effects			
Hypotension	Yes	No	Yes
Flushing	Yes	No	Yes
Bronchospasm	Yes	No	No
Constipation	Yes	Yes	Yes

C. Sedatives
  1. Benzodiazepines should be titrated or avoided to prevent adverse outcomes, including prolonged duration of mechanical ventilation, increased ICU length of stay, and development of delirium (Table 14).
  2. Lorazepam
     a. Intermittent dosing 1–4 mg every 2–6 hours
     b. Continuous infusion: Start at 1 mg/hour and titrate to goal (e.g., RASS, SAS). Total daily doses as low as 1 mg/kg can cause propylene glycol toxicity. Monitor for an osmolal gap greater than 10–12 mOsm/L, indicating propylene glycol toxicity.
     c. Lorazepam is the preferred benzodiazepine in severe hepatic dysfunction because of its metabolism.
     d. Midazolam
        i. Intermittent dosing 1–4 mg every 15 minutes to 1 hour
        ii. Continuous infusion: Start at 1 mg/hour and titrate to goal (e.g., RASS, SAS).
        iii. Often used for procedural sedation or daily dressing changes because of its rapid onset and short duration
        iv. Prolonged infusions of midazolam may accumulate because of its greater lipophilicity compared with lorazepam, especially in patients with renal dysfunction.

Table 14. Benzodiazepines

	Diazepam	**Lorazepam**	**Midazolam**
Pharmacokinetics			
Onset (minutes)	2–5	5–20	2–5
Duration of effect (hours)	2–4	4–6	1–2
Prolonged in renal failure	Yes	No	Yes
Prolonged in hepatic failure	Yes	No	Yes
Elimination half-life (hours)	24–120	10–20	1–10
Active metabolite	Yes	No	Yes
CYP3A4 interactions	Yes	No	Yes
Adverse effects	Yes	No	No
Hypotension	Yes	Maybe	No
Thrombophlebitis	No	Yes	No
Propylene glycol toxicity			

CYP = cytochrome P450.

  3. Propofol
     a. Rapid onset (1–2 minutes) and short duration (3–5 minutes or longer if prolonged infusion)
     b. Initiate at 5 mcg/kg/minute and titrate to achieve sedation goals by 5 mcg/kg/minute every 5 minutes. Avoid prolonged infusions greater than 50 mcg/kg/minute.
     c. Avoid loading doses because of the risk of hypotension.
     d. In general, used in intubated patients because of the risk of respiratory depression
     e. Propofol has no significant analgesic activity. If a patient has pain, propofol must be combined with an analgesic.
     f. Monitoring
        i. Blood pressure
        ii. Triglycerides
        iii. Calories provided from 10% lipid emulsion (1 kcal/mL). May need to adjust lipid or calories provided by nutrition support (i.e., enteral nutrition [EN] or parenteral nutrition [PN])

       iv. Propofol-related infusion syndrome is more likely to occur with prolonged infusions greater than 50 mcg/kg/minute and is associated with metabolic acidosis, cardiac failure, arrhythmias (e.g., bradycardia), cardiac arrest, rhabdomyolysis, hyperkalemia, and kidney failure.

    g. Propofol is more commonly used than benzodiazepines because of its shorter duration, easy titration, and predictability.

  4. Dexmedetomidine

    a. Sedative properties through central and peripheral α_2-receptor agonist activity

    b. Extent of analgesic activity in patients in the ICU is not well described.

    c. Does not cause respiratory depression

    d. Rapid onset (5–15 minutes if bolus, longer without bolus) and short duration (2-hour half-life). Longer duration in patients with severe hepatic dysfunction

    e. A loading dose is suggested for patients undergoing surgery; however, loading doses are *not* recommended for patients in the ICU because of the risk of bradycardia and hypotension.

    f. Maintenance dose of 0.2–0.7 mcg/kg/hour is approved by the U.S. Food and Drug Administration for a maximum of 24 hours; however, there is evidence showing the safety and efficacy of prolonged infusions at doses of up to 1.5 mcg/kg/hour, and this is most commonly used in practice.

    g. Compared with benzodiazepines, dexmedetomidine is associated with a lower prevalence of ICU delirium in some studies.

    h. Results from the MIDEX and PRODEX studies show that dexmedetomidine is noninferior to midazolam and propofol in maintaining light to moderate sedation. Dexmedetomidine reduced the duration of mechanical ventilation compared with midazolam (Jakob SM, Ruokonen E, Grounds R, et al. Dexmedetomidine vs midazolam or propofol for sedation during prolonged mechanical ventilation: two randomized controlled trials. JAMA 2012;307(11):1151-60).

    i. Monitoring: Primary adverse effects are dose-related bradycardia and hypotension.

    j. Does not cause drug dependency, but withdrawal symptoms (e.g., nausea, vomiting, agitation) have occurred after prolonged use (1 week).

D. Assessment and Management of Delirium

  1. Delirium is an acute change in cognitive function characterized by disorganized thought, altered level of consciousness, and inattentiveness.

  2. Delirium is associated with increased mortality and prolonged length of stay in the ICU.

  3. Validated tools to proactively identify and assess delirium include the Confusion Assessment Method for the ICU (CAM-ICU) and the Intensive Care Delirium Screening Checklist (ICDSC). The CAM-ICU is designed to detect delirium at the time of testing, whereas the ICDSC detects delirium during a nursing shift. For a detailed description of delirium monitoring tools, see http://icudelirium.org/delirium/monitoring.html.

  4. Nonpharmacologic interventions are preferred to pharmacologic treatment. These include maintaining communication with the patient, reorienting the patient (to person, place, and time), maximizing uninterrupted sleep (e.g., control light and noise, cluster patient care activities, decrease stimuli at night), providing access to natural lighting (rooms with windows), removing unnecessary equipment from room, correcting sensory deficits (e.g., hearing aids, glasses), removing unneeded invasive devices (e.g., urinary catheters, intravenous lines, endotracheal tubes, enteral feeding tubes), minimizing physical restraint, and encouraging patient autonomy and early mobility.

  5. Correctable causes of delirium include hypotension, hypoxia, and electrolyte disturbances.

  6. Few interventions have been shown to improve delirium-related outcomes, so a strong focus should be put on minimizing or treating reversible risk factors such as avoiding or minimizing the dose of benzodiazepines and other medications that may cause delirium (e.g., opioids, anticholinergic medications).

E. Pharmacologic Treatment of Delirium (Table 15)
  1. Haloperidol
     a. Although commonly used, there is no evidence that haloperidol reduces the duration of delirium.
     b. Monitoring
        i. Hypotension
        ii. Assess QTc interval at baseline and daily during haloperidol administration. In addition, monitor for other drugs that could prolong QTc interval.
        iii. Extrapyramidal effects, including laryngeal dystonia and dysphagia, are more common with chronic oral administration than with intravenous administration.
     c. Lower initial doses of haloperidol (1–2.5 mg) should be used in older adults. Doses of haloperidol for acute agitation may be doubled every 20 minutes until an effective dose is reached.
  2. Atypical antipsychotics
     a. Atypical or second-generation antipsychotics may reduce the duration of delirium in critically ill patients.
     b. Atypical antipsychotics are associated with a lower incidence of extrapyramidal side effects (EPSs) compared with haloperidol.
     c. Differences between agents are half-life, the risk of QTc prolongation, sedation, and risk of EPSs.
        i. Sedative effects may or may not be beneficial (e.g., hyperactive vs. hypoactive delirium).
        ii. Agents with a shorter half-life (quetiapine) generally act faster and can be quickly titrated.
        iii. Olanzapine and risperidone have less risk of QTc prolongation but should still be monitored.

Table 15. Medications Used to Treat Delirium

Medication	Initial Dosing	Dosage Forms	Half-life	Side Effects
Haloperidol	2.5 mg every 6 hours	Tablet, IM, IV	18 hours	QTc prolongation EPSs
Quetiapine	25 mg twice daily	Tablet	6 hours	Sedation QTc prolongation
Olanzapine	5 mg daily	Tablet, ODT, IM	33 hours	Sedation
Risperidone	0.5 mg twice daily	Tablet, ODT, solution, IM[a]	24 hours	EPSs (doses >6 mg/day)
Ziprasidone	5 mg daily	Oral, IM	7 hours	QTc prolongation

[a]IM formulation of risperidone is a long-acting formulation that is not indicated for acute delirium management.

EPS = extrapyramidal side effect; IM = intramuscular; IV = intravenous; ODT = orally disintegrating tablet.

F. Neuromuscular Blockade in Patients in the ICU (Table 16)
  1. Neuromuscular blockade is typically indicated for intubated patients with severe respiratory failure (e.g., ARDS, status asthmaticus) despite optimization of analgesia, sedation, and ventilator management. Recent data suggest that early empiric neuromuscular blockade in patients with severe ARDS may be beneficial. Neuromuscular blockers are also used as adjunctive agents to control severe intracranial hypertension in patients with neurologic injury (e.g., traumatic brain injury). A 48-hour infusion of cisatracurium (15-mg bolus followed by 37.5 mg/hour for 48 hours) in patients with severe ARDS (defined as Pao_2/Fio_2 less than 150) decreased the adjusted 90-day mortality. Note that in this study, the cisatracurium infusion was a fixed dose and was not adjusted on the basis of the monitoring parameters described later (e.g., train-of-four [TOF]).
  2. Neuromuscular blockers are typically used once efforts to facilitate ventilation have failed (e.g., poor oxygenation, dyssynchrony, high intrathoracic pressures that put the patient at risk for barotrauma) and a combination of high-dose opioids and sedatives have failed (i.e., patient continues to have poor oxygenation).

3. *Never* use neuromuscular blockers in a patient who is not completely sedated or does not have adequate pain control.

4. Neuromuscular blockers should be used only in conjunction with a continuously infused sedative. Sedatives should have amnestic properties (e.g., benzodiazepines, propofol). Analgesics can also be used as needed in patients with pain. Many practitioners insist on the combination of a sedative and an analgesic in paralyzed patients. Patients should be provided with lubricating eye drops while paralyzed.

5. Neuromuscular blockade in the ICU may be used in cases of elevated ICP, tetanus, or intubation and to decrease movement during procedures.

Table 16. Neuromuscular Blocking Agents

Recommendation	Pancuronium	Vecuronium	Atracurium	Cisatracurium
Duration of effect (hours)	0.75–1.5	0.5–0.75	0.25–0.5	0.5–1
Prolonged in renal failure	Yes	Yes	No	No
Prolonged in hepatic failure	Yes	Yes	No	No
Loading dose	0.08 mg/kg	0.1 mg/kg	0.4 mg/kg	0.1 mg/kg
Maintenance dose	0.02–0.04 mg/kg/hour	0.02–0.04 mg/kg/hour	0.4 mg/kg/hour	2–10 mcg/kg/minute
Adverse effects				
Tachycardia	Yes	No	No	No
Hypotension	No	No	Dose dependent	No

6. Concerns with neuromuscular blockade
   a. May mask seizure activity
   b. Prolonged use is associated with critical illness polyneuromyopathy, characterized by prolonged muscle weakness.
   c. Can mask insufficient analgesia and sedation
   d. Increased risk of venous thromboembolism (VTE)
   e. Increased risk of skin breakdown and decubitus
   f. Corneal abrasions caused by eye dryness and lack of blinking; prevent by applying ophthalmic ointment or drops to eyes every 6–8 hours

7. Monitoring
   a. Neuromuscular blockers must be monitored to prevent an excessive degree of blockade and prolonged paralysis.
   b. The goal of neuromuscular blockade is to facilitate safe and optimal mechanical ventilation strategies using the minimal degree of neuromuscular blockade needed.
   c. Even with appropriate individualized dosing and monitoring of neuromuscular blockade, a principal adverse effect is prolonged muscle weakness after discontinuation. This can dramatically slow patient recovery, increasing the need for health care resources (e.g., physical therapy, rehabilitation). For this reason, it must be emphasized that the need for therapeutic paralysis must be carefully considered and reevaluated every day.
   d. A simple way to assess the appropriateness of the paralytic is as follows: Regularly (e.g., once daily) but temporarily discontinue the drug to determine the time needed for the patient to move or breathe spontaneously. Although not applicable to all patients, this "drug holiday" can be useful for the following reasons:
      i. Assess sedation and adjust sedatives as needed (e.g., if the patient is agitated after the drug is discontinued, he or she is not receiving adequate sedation or analgesia).
      ii. Assess the need for continued blockade (e.g., if the patient is able to maintain oxygenation, then perhaps the drug is no longer necessary).

        iii. Assess the dose of the paralytic (e.g., determine whether the paralysis wore off within the expected time according to the expected drug duration); this is especially important for drugs such as vecuronium and pancuronium because of the long half-life and dependence on end organ clearance.

        iv. Note: The study listed above used cisatracurium continuously (without a holiday) for 48 hours without an increased incidence of prolonged weakness.

    e. A peripheral nerve stimulator can be used in conjunction with drug holidays to assess the level of neuromuscular blockade and guide drug dosing.

    f. The TOF refers to peripheral nerve stimulation using four electrical impulses, usually applied to the ulnar or facial nerves.

    g. Obtain a baseline TOF before initiation to determine patient sensitivity to impulses. Patients who are not blocked should exhibit 1 twitch for each impulse (for 4/4 twitches).

    h. During neuromuscular blockade infusions for respiratory failure, patients should typically be maintained at 1 or 2 twitches, which indicate the extent of receptor blockade.

    i. Technical problems that limit the accuracy of TOF monitoring include the presence of perspiration or tissue edema.

8. In addition to the monitoring described, clinical assessment involves adjusting the neuromuscular blocker dose to prevent patient-ventilator dyssynchrony (e.g., "bucking" the ventilator, elevated peak airway pressures).

9. Avoid other medications or electrolyte abnormalities that can potentiate or inhibit paralysis (Table 17).

Table 17. Interactions with Neuromuscular Blockers

	Potentiate Block	**Antagonize Block**
Drugs	Corticosteroids Aminoglycosides Clindamycin Tetracyclines Polymyxins Calcium channel blockers Type Ia antiarrhythmics Furosemide Lithium	Aminophylline Theophylline Carbamazepine Phenytoin (chronic)
Electrolyte disorders	Hypermagnesemia Hypocalcemia Hypokalemia	Hypercalcemia Hyperkalemia

Patient Cases

8. An older woman is admitted to the ICU for acute decompensated heart failure and acute kidney injury with an ejection fraction of less than 30%. She is administered a continuous infusion of bumetanide; however, the benefit is limited because of her acute on chronic kidney disease. She is intubated on ICU day 2 because of worsening pulmonary edema and hypoxia. After intubation, she scores a zero on the RASS, but her CAM-ICU is positive for delirium. Her BPS score is 4. Her BP is 120/70 mm Hg, and HR is 88 beats/minute. Which is the best recommendation for achieving her analgesia, sedation, and delirium goals?

    A. Initiate propofol at 5 mcg/kg/minute and titrate as needed.

    B. Administer haloperidol 5 mg intravenously and double the dose every 20 minutes as needed.

    C. Initiate morphine 4 mg intravenously every 4 hours as needed.

    D. Offer the patient verbal reassurance.

Questions 9–11 pertain to the following case.
A 42-year-old woman with acute respiratory distress syndrome and a significant history of alcohol and tobacco abuse is transferred to the medical ICU from an outside hospital. She presented to the outside hospital after 1 week of productive cough, fever, chills, and increased shortness of breath. On admission to the medical ICU, she is hypotensive (80/60 mm Hg), tachycardic (130 beats/minute), and febrile (39.0°C). Her ABG shows pH 7.1, $Paco_2$ 56 mm Hg, Pao_2 49 mm Hg, HCO_3^- 16 mEq/L, and Sao_2 76% on 100% Fio_2. The only other significant laboratory results are an SCr of 2.1 mg/dL and a WBC of 16×10^3 cells/mm³. She is achieving her sedation goals with continuous infusions of midazolam 3 mg/hour and fentanyl 250 mcg/hour.

9. After several nonpharmacologic attempts to improve her oxygenation fail, she is paralyzed, and her ventilator settings are adjusted accordingly. Which statement about neuromuscular blockade in this patient is most appropriate?

    A. Opioids should be discontinued to avoid prolonged neuromuscular weakness.

    B. Vecuronium is the agent of choice.

    C. Sedatives should be titrated to maintain an RASS goal of 0 to –2 during neuromuscular blockade.

    D. Neuromuscular blockers should be titrated to the minimal dose necessary to achieve ventilator synchrony.

10. The patient was initiated on neuromuscular blockade as instructed and appeared to being doing well until about 8 hours later, when she began to move around violently in her bed. At this time, she was tachycardic (120 beats/minute) and appeared very agitated; her Sao_2 dropped to 80%. Which action is best?

    A. Double the rate of the neuromuscular blocker every 5 minutes as needed until the patient stops moving.

    B. Administer a midazolam bolus and increase the infusion rate as needed to achieve sedation goals.

    C. Increase the fentanyl infusion rate as needed to achieve sedation goals.

    D. Check the TOF.

Patient Cases

11. After that event, the patient did poorly the rest of the night. The patient was initiated on a norepinephrine infusion at 0.02 mcg/kg/minute to maintain an adequate BP. Other medications initiated overnight included piperacillin/tazobactam, vancomycin, and gentamicin. By morning, her SCr has increased to 2.8 mg/dL, and the night shift nurse reports that the patient has had 0/4 twitches on TOF for the past 8 hours. Pertinent electrolyte values include K^+ 4.9 mEq/L, calcium (Ca^{++}) 9 mg/dL, and Mg^{++} 2 mg/dL. Which is most likely to potentiate the effects of cisatracurium?

    A. Piperacillin/tazobactam.

    B. Gentamicin.

    C. Norepinephrine.

    D. K value of 4.9 mEq/L.

VII. GLUCOSE CONTROL

  A. History of Blood Glucose Control
    1. 2001: Study by van den Berghe et al. of surgical ICU patients showed a significant morbidity and mortality benefit of maintaining blood glucose in the range of 80–110 mg/dL, despite an increased risk of hypoglycemia (5.1% vs. 0.8%).
    2. 2006: Study by van den Berghe et al. of primarily medical ICU patients showed no mortality benefit associated with maintaining blood glucose in the range of 80–110 mg/dL in the entire study population. The study did show a reduction in ventilator time and length of stay, as well as a reduction in mortality in patients with an ICU length of stay of 3 days or more. The incidence of hypoglycemia (18%) was higher than previously reported.
    3. Subsequent investigations of tight glycemic control (80–110 mg/dL) never replicated the mortality benefit seen in the 2001 study. Studies did show much higher rates of hypoglycemia with tight glycemic control.
    4. 2009: Results of a large, international, randomized study (NICE-SUGAR) involving more than 6000 critically ill medical and surgical patients showed higher mortality and higher risk of hypoglycemia in patients receiving intensive blood glucose control (goal glucose 81–108 mg/dL) compared with patients having a goal of 180 mg/dL or less (mean blood glucose 142 mg/dL).
    5. The 2012 SSC guidelines recommend initiating insulin when two consecutive blood glucose readings are greater than 180 mg/dL. The target blood glucose concentration is 180 mg/dL or less for patients with sepsis.
    6. The 2012 Society of Critical Care Medicine guidelines for using an insulin infusion to manage hyperglycemia in general critically ill patients suggest using a blood glucose of 150 mg/dL or higher as a trigger for insulin therapy, adjusted to keep blood glucose less than 150 mg/dL, and maintaining values less than 180 mg/dL using an insulin protocol that achieves a low rate of hypoglycemia (blood glucose 70 mg/dL or less).
  B. Treatment Strategies to Achieve Glycemic Control in Critically Ill Patients
    1. For a continuous insulin infusion approach, use a validated dosing protocol that considers blood glucose concentration, rate of change, and insulin infusion rate.
    2. Intravenous insulin is preferred for patients with type 1 diabetes mellitus, for patients with hyperglycemia who are hemodynamically unstable, and for patients in whom long-acting basal insulin should not be initiated because of changing clinical status. Once stable, patients can be considered for transitioning to a protocol-driven subcutaneous insulin regimen.

3. Regularly scheduled subcutaneous administration of basal or rapid-acting insulin can prevent hyperglycemia in clinically stable patients who do not need an intravenous infusion of insulin. The use of subcutaneous insulin is not recommended in patients on vasopressors, patients with significant peripheral edema, or patients for whom rapid correction of blood glucose is warranted.

4. A sliding-scale or correctional insulin regimen can be used in conjunction with the regularly scheduled subcutaneous doses; however, the baseline of insulin administered should be adjusted daily to prevent hyperglycemia and the need for additional doses of insulin. Subcutaneous sliding-scale or correctional insulin should not be the sole method of glucose control in critically ill patients.

C. Monitoring Blood Glucose
1. For a continuous insulin infusion approach, monitoring blood glucose every 1–2 hours is typically needed to provide safe and effective therapy.

2. Interpret point-of-care testing of capillary blood with caution because it can overestimate plasma glucose values. Overestimation of blood glucose is more common in patients with anemia, hypotension, or hypoperfusion. It is also more common when blood glucose is in the hypoglycemic or hyperglycemic range.

3. Arterial or venous whole blood sampling is recommended instead of fingerstick capillary blood glucose testing in patients with shock or severe peripheral edema and for patients on a prolonged insulin infusion.

VIII. PREVENTING STRESS ULCERS

A. Mucosal Bleeding in Critically Ill Adults
1. The incidence of stress-related mucosal bleeding in critically ill adults is estimated to be about 6%.

2. Signs and symptoms of stress ulcers include hematemesis, gross blood in gastric tube aspirates, coffee ground emesis or aspiration from gastric tube, and melena. Clinically significant stress ulcers are defined as those that cause hemodynamic compromise or necessitate blood transfusion.

B. Prophylactic Therapy for Stress Ulcers
1. Prophylactic medications are recommended for any one of the following major risk factors:
    a. Respiratory failure necessitating mechanical ventilation (for more than 48 hours)
    b. Coagulopathy, defined as platelet count less than 50,000/mm³, international normalized ratio (INR) greater than 1.5, or activated partial thromboplastin time more than 2 times control. (Note: Prophylactic or treatment doses of anticoagulants do not constitute coagulopathy.)

2. Prophylactic medications or continuing home acid suppressive regimens are also recommended for any patient with a history of gastrointestinal (GI) ulceration or bleeding within 1 year before ICU admission.

3. Prophylactic medications are recommended for patients with two or more of the following risk factors (although data on this approach are lacking):
   a. Head or spinal cord injury
   b. Severe burn (more than 35% of body surface area)
   c. Hypoperfusion
   d. Acute organ dysfunction
   e. High doses of corticosteroids (more than 250 mg/day of hydrocortisone or equivalent)
   f. Liver failure with associated coagulopathy
   g. Transplantation
   h. Acute kidney injury
   i. Major surgery
   j. Multiple trauma

C. Strategies for Stress Ulcer Prophylaxis (see Table 18 for specific medications)
   1. Efficacy of intravenous histamine-2 (H_2)-blockers in preventing stress-related upper GI bleeding has been shown in multiple clinical trials. These are commonly administered enterally when possible because of excellent bioavailability; however, evidence of efficacy is primarily with the intravenous administration of H_2-blockers.
   2. Despite limited evidence in preventing stress-related mucosal bleeding, intravenous or enterally administered proton pump inhibitors (PPIs) are often used.
   3. Regardless of the drug choice or route, it is important to discontinue therapy when risk factors are no longer present to avoid unnecessary drug interactions, adverse effects (pneumonia), and increased costs. This step is easily overlooked, with the result that patients are discharged from hospitals and continued on acid suppressive therapy with no indication.
   4. Not recommended for prevention
      a. Antacids are not used to prevent stress ulcers.
      b. Sucralfate has been found to be inferior to H_2-blockers and is therefore not recommended for preventing stress ulcers. In addition, it can cause obstruction of enteral feeding tubes and aluminum toxicity in patients with renal failure.
      c. Safety: The benefits of preventing stress ulcers by increasing the stomach pH must be weighed against an increased risk of infection, including *Clostridium difficile,* hospital-acquired pneumonia, and community-acquired pneumonia (for patients discharged on a PPI).

Table 18. Medications for Stress Ulcer Prophylaxis

Class	Examples and Dosing	Adverse Effects	Notes
H$_2$-receptor blockers	Ranitidine 150 mg PO every 12 hours or 50 mg IV every 8 hours Famotidine 20 mg IV or PO every 12 hours Nizatidine 150 mg PO every 12 hours Cimetidine 300 mg PO or IV every 6 hours or continuous infusion 37.5–50 mg/hour	Mental status changes, thrombocytopenia (cimetidine)	Excellent bioavailability Low cost Potential for reduced efficacy over time (tachyphylaxis) Dose adjustment for renal dysfunction Low risk of nosocomial pneumonia Cimetidine not routinely used because of drug interactions (strong P450 inhibitor) and side effects
Proton pump inhibitors	Omeprazole 20 mg PO daily Powder for oral suspension available Esomeprazole 20–40 mg PO or IV daily Lansoprazole 30 mg PO or IV daily Delayed-release orally disintegrating tablets and oral suspension available Pantoprazole 40 mg PO or IV daily Granules available for oral or tube administration	Headache, diarrhea, constipation, abdominal pain, nausea	Solutions of certain PPIs may be compounded; refer to individual package inserts for instructions No adjustment needed for renal or liver dysfunction Higher cost than H$_2$-blockers Administration problems when given via NG tube Risk of ventilator-associated pneumonia increased Risk of *Clostridium difficile* infection (nosocomial or community acquired)

H$_2$ = histamine-2; IV = intravenously; PO = orally; NG = nasogastric; PPI = proton pump inhibitor.

Patient Cases

Questions 12 and 13 pertain to the following case.

A 73-year-old woman weighing 84 kg is admitted to the ICU after a pneumonectomy. Her BP is 104/65 mm Hg, HR is 88 beats/minute, and oxygen saturations are 98% on 40% F_{IO_2} and PEEP 5; her Glasgow Coma Scale score is 11. Other laboratory values are normal. A small-bore feeding tube is in place, she is being fed enterally at goal rate, and she has no gastric residuals. Her medications include simvastatin 20 mg every night, aspirin 81 mg/day, metoprolol 25 mg twice daily, heparin 5000 units subcutaneously every 8 hours, and 0.9% NaCl intravenously at 75 mL/hour.

12. The surgeon would like to initiate stress ulcer prophylaxis (SUP). Which of the following is the best recommendation for this patient?
    A. Famotidine 20 mg per tube every 12 hours.
    B. Esomeprazole 40 mg intravenously daily.
    C. Sucralfate 1 g per tube four times daily.
    D. Ranitidine 50 mg intravenously every 8 hours.

13. One week later, the patient is extubated but still in the ICU. Her Glasgow Coma Scale score is 15, BP 112/70 mm Hg, and HR 75 beats/minute, but her appetite is poor. Which statement is most appropriate regarding SUP for this patient?
    A. SUP should continue until the patient is discharged from the ICU.
    B. SUP should be discontinued now.
    C. Continue SUP until patient is eating.
    D. SUP should be discontinued at hospital discharge.

IX. PHARMACOLOGIC THERAPY FOR PREVENTING VENOUS THROMBOEMBOLISM

A. General Overview: VTE is a common complication of critical illness, with an incidence of deep vein thrombosis (DVT) of 8%–40% and pulmonary embolism (PE) of up to 12%.

B. Risk Factors for VTE
    1. Critically ill patients are usually at high risk of VTE.
    2. Additional risk factors include surgery, major trauma, lower extremity injury, immobility, malignancy, sepsis, heart failure, respiratory failure, venous compression, previous VTE, increasing age, pregnancy, erythropoiesis-stimulating agents, obesity, and central venous catheterization.

C. Nonpharmacologic Prevention of VTE
    1. Early mobility is the ideal nonpharmacologic therapy.
    2. Mechanical prophylaxis with intermittent pneumatic compression or graduated compression stockings is recommended for medical patients at risk of VTE who have a contraindication to pharmacologic anticoagulation (e.g., thrombocytopenia, severe coagulopathy, active bleeding, recent intracerebral hemorrhage).
    3. Mechanical prophylaxis can be used in combination with pharmacologic treatment.

D. Recommendations for Critically Ill Patients
   1. American College of Chest Physicians Ninth Edition
      a. Recommends low-molecular-weight heparin (LMWH) or low-dose unfractionated heparin over no prophylaxis
      b. For patients who are bleeding or at high risk for major bleeding, the guidelines recommend mechanical thromboprophylaxis and institution of pharmacologic prophylaxis when the bleeding risk decreases.
      c. The guidelines provide separate postoperative recommendations. A detailed assessment is beyond the scope of this text, and readers are encouraged to see the guideline for more information.
   2. SSC also provides recommendations that are identical to those above.

E. Pharmacologic Prophylaxis (see Table 19 for dosage)
   1. Unfractionated heparin
      a. Low cost
      b. Twice- versus three-times-daily administration: No head-to-head comparison has been completed. Two meta-analyses have been completed on the subject. The first, in 2007, concluded that there was no difference in efficacy, but three-times-daily administration was associated with a slightly higher risk of bleeding. The second, in 2011, found no difference in efficacy or safety with either regimen.
      c. Risk of heparin-induced thrombocytopenia (HIT) lower than that of full anticoagulation doses
   2. LMWHs
      a. All considered therapeutically equivalent
      b. Dalteparin is renally eliminated but may be considered in patients with CrCl less than 30 mL/minute because of its low accumulation.
      c. Low risk of HIT
   3. Fondaparinux
      a. May be safe in patients with a history of HIT
      b. Data on reversal of fondaparinux are lacking.
      c. Contraindicated for CrCl less than 30 mL/minute
      d. Very limited data in critically ill patients
   4. New oral anticoagulants
      a. Rivaroxaban was evaluated against enoxaparin in a study of acutely ill medical patients needing hospitalization. Although rivaroxaban was as efficacious as enoxaparin at study day 10, there was an excess risk of bleeding in the rivaroxaban group. Of note, patients with cardiogenic or septic shock with the need for vasopressors were excluded. Rivaroxaban is renally eliminated and is not recommended in patients with renal insufficiency.
      b. Apixaban was evaluated against enoxaparin in a study of acutely ill medical patients needing hospitalization. There were no difference in rates of VTE but a higher bleeding rate with apixaban. Patients with septic shock were also excluded from this trial.
      c. Compared with heparins, there is limited experience in reversal of anti-Xa inhibitors in clinical practice.
      d. At this time, new oral anticoagulants cannot be recommended for routine use in VTE prophylaxis in critically ill patients.

F. Special Populations
    1. Impaired kidney function
        a. If estimated CrCl is less than 30 mL/minute, LMWH dosage reduction is usually necessary. If creatinine clearance is less than 20 mL/minute or patient is on dialysis, dosing information is limited for LMWH; anti-Xa monitoring may not be reliable in patients on dialysis.
        b. Alternatively, if estimated CrCl is less than 30 mL/minute, dalteparin can be used because it has minimal renal metabolism.
        c. Fondaparinux is contraindicated in patients with an estimated creatinine clearance less than 30 mL/minute.
        d. Low-dose unfractionated heparin is minimally renally eliminated and is safe to use in patients with reduced kidney function.
    2. Overweight or underweight adults: For obese patients, some experts recommend increasing unfractionated heparin dose to 7500 units and LMWH prophylaxis doses by 30%–100% if body mass index (BMI) is greater than 40 kg/m^2; a peak (4 hours postdose) anti-Xa of 0.2–0.4 IU/mL is recommended. Note that these recommendations have not been validated in controlled trials and are considered expert opinion only (see Nutescu EA et al. Low-molecular-weight heparins in renal impairment and obesity: available evidence and clinical practice recommendations across medical and surgical settings. Ann Pharmacother 2009;43(6):1064-83).

G. Antithrombotic Therapy and Regional Anesthesia
    1. Critically ill patients often have their spinal meninges accessed for either therapeutic (epidural anesthesia, lumbar drains) or diagnostic (lumbar puncture) purposes.
    2. The combination of antithrombotic medications with these techniques is associated with an elevated risk of spinal or epidural hematoma, which may lead to ischemia and paralysis.
    3. The American Society of Regional Anesthesia and Pain Medicine has released guidelines on regional anesthesia in the patient receiving antithrombotic or thrombolytic therapy.
        a. There is no contraindication to low-dose unfractionated heparin at daily doses of less than 10,000 units (i.e., 5,000 units every 12 hours). It is unknown whether subcutaneous heparin at doses greater than 10,000 units daily (i.e., 5,000 units every 8 hours) carries a higher risk of complication than lower doses. If patients receive subcutaneous heparin at doses greater than 10,000 units daily, enhanced monitoring for neurodeficits should take place.
        b. For patients receiving LMWH, needle placement should occur 10–12 hours after the last LMWH dose (longer in patients with renal disease).
        c. Indwelling catheters should be removed before initiation of twice-daily LMWH postoperatively but may be maintained for patients on once-daily regimens.
            i.   The first dose of LMWH should be at least 2 hours after catheter removal.
            ii. Catheter removal should be at least 10–12 hours after the last LMWH dose (longer in patients with renal disease).
        d. Because of a lack of data and early clinical trial data, the use of fondaparinux should be avoided.

H. Prevention of VTE: Pharmacologic Options in Critically Ill Patients

Table 19. Prevention of VTE Pharmacologic Options

Medication	Mechanism	Dosing	Adjustment for Renal Dysfunction
Unfractionated heparin	Factor Xa and indirect thrombin inhibition	5000 units SC 2 or 3 times daily	None
Low-molecular-weight heparins	Factor Xa inhibition and some indirect thrombin inhibition	Enoxaparin 40 mg SC daily Dalteparin 5000 units SC daily	CrCl <30: enoxaparin 30 mg SC daily
Fondaparinux	Factor Xa inhibition	2.5 mg SC daily	Contraindicated for CrCl <30 mL/minute

SC = subcutaneously.

X. PREVENTING VENTILATOR-ASSOCIATED PNEUMONIA

A. The Institute for Healthcare Improvement has developed a ventilator bundle with the following elements that directly target ventilator-associated pneumonia (VAP) and complications arising from VAP.
   1. Head of the bed elevation: Maintain the head of the bed elevated (about 30–45°).
   2. Daily sedation interruptions and assessment of readiness to extubate
   3. Stress ulcer prophylaxis
   4. VTE prophylaxis
   5. Daily oral care with chlorhexidine (0.12% oral rinse)

B. Additional Methods
   1. Selective decontamination of the digestive tract (SDD)
      a. SDD is a short course of antimicrobial therapy aimed at eradicating potential pathogens to minimize ICU-acquired infections.
      b. Despite three decades of research, SDD is still not routinely performed.
   2. Endotracheal tubes coated in an antimicrobial (silver) reduce infection but are cost prohibitive in many centers.

XI. NUTRITION SUPPORT IN CRITICALLY ILL PATIENTS

A. General Overview
   1. Many critically ill patients have increased caloric and protein needs, and caloric deficit in these patients leads to excess morbidity (length of stay, infection) and mortality.
   2. Skeletal muscle wasting and weakness occurring during critical illness may lead to prolonged mechanical ventilation and rehabilitation.
   3. Ideally, nutrition should be provided within 24–48 hours of admission to the ICU.
   4. Route of delivery (EN vs. PN)
      a. In general, EN is preferred to PN in patients with a functional GI tract who are not malnourished.
      b. American and Canadian guidelines allow hypocaloric feeding during the first 7 days in previously well-nourished patients before consideration of PN.

      c.   The SSC guidelines recommend intravenous glucose and EN rather than total PN alone or PN in conjunction with EN in the first 7 days after a diagnosis of severe sepsis or septic shock.

      d.   PN is recommended for patients who have extensive small bowel resection, chronic malabsorption, high-output enterocutaneous fistulas, severe malnutrition at baseline, suspected or confirmed GI ischemia, mechanical bowel obstruction, or persistent, severe hemodynamic instability.

B.   Estimating Nutrition Needs

    1.   Traditional biomarkers of nutrition (albumin, prealbumin, nitrogen balance) are not well validated in critically ill patients.

    2.   Indirect calorimetry and predictive equations may be used to determine energy needs in critically ill patients.

      a.   Indirect calorimetry measures the metabolic rate, but it requires special equipment and trained staff and is subject to inaccuracies in some patient populations. Indirect calorimetry also provides a respiratory quotient (RQ), indicating substrate metabolism and allowing modification of macronutrient delivery (e.g., carbohydrates, fats, protein).

         i.   RQ 1.0–1.3: Lipogenesis (overfeeding), hyperventilation, or system "leak"

         ii.   RQ 0.9–1.0: Primary carbohydrate oxidation, metabolic acidosis

         iii.   RQ 0.82–0.85: Normal, "mixed" substrate oxidation

         iv.   RQ 0.80: Primary protein oxidation

         v.   RQ 0.70: Primary fat oxidation, systemic inflammatory response syndrome , metabolic alkalosis, or ethanol oxidation

         vi.   RQ less than 0.67 or greater than 1.3: Outside range; question test validity

      b.   Several predictive equations for determining caloric goals have been used (e.g., Harris-Benedict, Penn State and modified Penn State, Ireton-Jones, Mifflin, and Swinamer equations).

      c.   The modified Penn State equation has shown closer association to indirect calorimetry in critically ill patients.

      d.   Some guidelines recommend a 25-kcal/kg actual body weight target, but this approach may be too simplistic for the majority of critically ill patients.

      e.   See the references for a review of the usefulness of predictive equations in critically ill patients.

    3.   Hypocaloric feeding

      a.   The SSC recommends avoiding mandatory full caloric feeding in the first week but rather suggests low-dose feeding (i.e., up to 500 kcal per day), advancing only as tolerated.

      b.   One study showed that intentional underfeeding (60%–70% of target) of critically ill patients while providing 90%–100% of protein needs showed a significant reduction in hospital mortality.

      c.   It is recommended that obese patients (BMI greater than 30) can be fed at 60%–70% of target energy requirements or 11–14 kcal/kg actual body weight per day. Protein should be delivered in the range of 2–2.5 g/kg ideal body weight per day.

    4.   Protein needs

      a.   The stress response in critical illness increases gluconeogenesis, which cannot be fully suppressed by exogenous glucose.

      b.   Protein intake of 1.2–2 g/kg of actual body weight is recommended in most critically ill patients.

         i.   Patients on continuous renal replacement therapy may need up to 2.5 g/kg per day.

         ii.   Patients with acute kidney injury who are not on renal replacement may need as little as 0.6–0.8 g/kg per day.

         iii.   Patients with extensive burn injury may need up to 3 g/kg per day.

C. Enteral Nutrition
    1. It is important to recognize that the prescribed dose of enteral nutrition is often not delivered to patients because of interruptions, intolerance, or many other reasons. Use of an enteral nutrition protocol with guidance on initiation, advancement, and interruptions is essential.
    2. "Trophic" feeding, or low-dose enteral feeding with the intent of maintaining GI tract function, is commonly used despite limited evidence.
    3. EN may be safely delivered to patients on low-dose vasopressors.
    4. Gastric versus small bowel (postpyloric) feeding delivery
        a. Delivery of EN directly into the small bowel may be associated with a reduction in pneumonia.
        b. In units where small bowel access is readily available, routine use of small bowel feeding is recommended.
        c. If small bowel access is not readily available, then small bowel feedings should be considered only for patients at high risk of intolerance to EN (on inotropes, continuous infusion of sedatives, or paralytic agents, or patients with high nasogastric drainage) or at high risk for regurgitation and aspiration (nursed in supine position) or who have repeatedly demonstrated intolerance of gastric feeds.
    5. Gastric residual volumes
        a. There are no data indicating that interruption of gastric feeding for a specific residual volume prevents morbidity (aspiration pneumonia) in critically ill patients.
        b. A residual volume of 250–500 mL is recommended as a point where intervention (prokinetic agents, tube feeding interruption, small bowel tube placement) should take place.

D. Parenteral Nutrition
    1. PN should be administered by central vein whenever possible. Peripheral administration is possible but must be dilute and may cause problems with the volume of the solution.
    2. Intravenous catheters intended for PN should not be used for any other purpose.
    3. Blood glucose measurements should be taken at least every 4–6 hours for patients on PN during initiation and changes in carbohydrate content.

E. Supplemental Antioxidants and Immunomodulation: Supplemental antioxidants and immunomodulating micronutrients (vitamin E, selenium, fish oils, arginine, glutamine, zinc) are not recommended for general critically ill patients.

F. Further Guidance: See the "Fluids, Electrolytes, and Nutrition." chapter.

Patient Cases

Questions 14 and 15 pertain to the following case.

A 75-year-old woman (height 165 cm, weight 68 kg) who is intubated needs mechanical ventilation for an acute exacerbation of chronic obstructive pulmonary disease. She has a past medical history of heart failure and hypertension. Her laboratory values are normal except for a Cr of 1.9 mg/dL.

14. Which is the most appropriate recommendation to prevent VTE in this patient?

    A. Initiate intermittent pneumatic compression.

    B. Administer fondaparinux 2.5 mg subcutaneously once daily.

    C. Administer enoxaparin 30 mg subcutaneously once daily.

    D. Administer heparin continuous intravenous infusion to maintain an aPTT of 40–60 seconds.

15. Three days later, the patient continues to need mechanical ventilation. Enteral nutrition has been initiated through her nasogastric feeding tube and gradually increased to 45 mL/hour. Her gastric residuals are consistently 150–200 mL. Which statement is most appropriate to optimize nutrition support for this patient?

    A. Switch to PN.

    B. Add metoclopramide 5 mg intravenously every 6 hours.

    C. Switch feeds to a more concentrated formula.

    D. Continue tube feedings at the current infusion rate.

XII. INTRACRANIAL HEMORRHAGE

A. General Overview
   1. Intracranial hemorrhage (ICH) is a broad term that encompasses a number of clinical scenarios. Goals of care are to minimize hemorrhage expansion and to treat associated organ dysfunction, thereby decreasing mortality and improving quality of life.
   2. ICH is classified by the anatomical location of the bleed.
      a. Intraparenchymal hemorrhage (IPH)—Nontraumatic bleeding into the brain parenchyma.
      b. Subarachnoid hemorrhage (SAH)—Bleeding into the space between the pia and arachnoid membranes. May be caused by rupture of a cerebral aneurysm, bleeding from arteriovenous malformations, tumors, amyloid angiopathy, or vasculopathy. Patients may present early on with the classic "worst headache of my life."
      c. Subdural hematoma (SDH)—Bleeding between the dura and arachnoid space
      d. Epidural hematoma (EDH)—Bleeding between the dura and the bone
   3. SDH and EDH are usually caused by traumatic injury.
   4. Severity of ICH and resulting neurologic injury guide diagnostic tests, treatment, and prognosis. Commonly used scales include the Glasgow Coma Scale (GCS; Table 20) to assess the level of consciousness and the National Institutes of Health Stroke Scale.
      - Disease-specific scales are also used for SAH and IPH. The Hunt and Hess Scale is a qualitative scale that rates patients with SAH from 1 (no symptoms) to 5 (deeply comatose). Because the etiologies of IPH and SAH are different, the ICH score is used for IPH. The ICH score is a composite score consisting of hemorrhage size, age, site of hemorrhage, and GCS and rates patients from 0 (best) to 6 (worst).

Table 20. Glasgow Coma Scale

Axes	Score
Eye Opening	
Does not open eyes	1
Opens eyes in response to painful stimuli	2
Opens eyes in response to voice	3
Opens eyes spontaneously	4
Motor Response	
Makes no movements	1
Extension to painful stimuli	2
Abnormal flexion to painful stimuli	3
Flexion or withdrawal to painful stimuli	4
Localizes painful stimuli	5
Obeys commands	6
Verbal Response	
Makes no sounds	1
Incomprehensible sounds	2
Utters appropriate words	3
Confused, disoriented	4
Oriented, converses normally	5

B. Risk Factors
   1. Hypertension is the most common risk factor.
   2. Use of fibrinolytic (e.g., alteplase), anticoagulant, and antiplatelet medications
   3. Amyloid angiopathy
   4. Intracranial aneurysm
      a. Rupture may be spontaneous or may result from exertion or hypertension.
      b. Risk factors for rupture include tobacco use, hypertension, cocaine use, a history of prior SAH, familial history of SAH, large aneurysm size, female sex, connective tissue disease, and older age.
   5. Liver failure–induced coagulopathy
   6. Mycotic aneurysms

C. Management
   1. Blood pressure control
      a. Acute hypertension should be controlled after the diagnosis of SAH. The goal blood pressure has not been definitively established. The American Heart Association (AHA) Guidelines for the Management of Aneurysmal Subarachnoid Hemorrhage recommend balancing the risk of stroke, rebleeding due to hypertension, and maintenance of cerebral perfusion pressure in determining a patients goal blood pressure. They further state that a goal systolic blood pressure less than 160 mm Hg is reasonable.
      b. Blood pressure should be controlled with an intravenous, titratable agent such as nicardipine or clevidipine.
   2. Antifibrinolytic therapy
      a. For patients who will have a delay in surgical intervention, short-term (less than 72 hours or until angiography) treatment with tranexamic acid or aminocaproic acid is reasonable.
      b. Many different dosing protocols exist for aminocaproic acid and transexamic acid. Typically, aminocaproic acid is administered as a 4- to 5-g load followed by 1 g/hour.
      c. Patients who receive antifibrinolytic therapy should be monitored for the development of a VTE.

3. Coagulation factors—In a study of ICH not due to anticoagulant therapy, recombinant activated factor VII has been shown to decrease the size of ICH but did not improve outcomes.

4. Seizure prophylaxis in aneurysmal SAH

   a. The incidence of seizures after SAH may reach 20%, seen mostly at the time of rupture, with the incidence decreasing after treatment. The use of antiepileptic drugs (AEDs) is controversial and may stem from earlier studies that used primarily phenytoin for prophylaxis. Current guidelines state that prophylaxis may be considered in the immediate post-hemorrhage period.

   b. Phenytoin is subject to drug interactions, notably with nimodipine (decreasing nimodipine serum concentrations). Both the AHA and the Neurocritical Care Society guidelines recommend against the use of phenytoin because of adverse outcomes.

   c. Levetiracetam is generally considered a safer AED, but data supporting its use is limited.

5. Seizure prophylaxis in ICH—Compared with SAH, the incidence of seizures is estimated to be the same or slightly higher. However, seizures may present at the onset or may occur late in therapy because of scarring. The current AHA guidelines on ICH recommend against prophylactic anticonvulsants; however, this may be because of early studies that used primarily phenytoin.

6. Vasospasm

   a. Vasospasm is the acute narrowing of the cerebral arteries after aneurysmal SAH. It is most common during the first 7–10 days after aneurysm rupture and resolves after 21 days. Untreated, vasospasm leads to delayed cerebral ischemia, a major cause of death and disability.

   b. Oral nimodipine 60 mg every 4 hours for 21 days should be administered in all patients with aneurysmal SAH.

   c. Euvolemia should be maintained in all patients. Large volumes of hypotonic fluids should be avoided.

7. Microsurgical clip obliteration via craniotomy and endovascular coiling are both surgical interventions for aneurysmal SAH that should be performed as early as possible. Determination of which procedure yields better outcomes is ongoing. Advancements in both approaches have improved the rate of survival and lowered the rate of disability.

REFERENCES

Acid Base

1. Adrogue HJ, Madias NE. Management of life-threatening acid-base disorders. Part I. N Engl J Med 1998;338:26-34.

2. Adrogue HJ, Madias NE. Management of life-threatening acid-base disorders. Part II. N Engl J Med 1998;338:107-11.

3. Haber RJ. A practical approach to acid-base disorders. West J Med 1991;155:146-51.

4. Berend K, de Vries AP, Gans RO. Physiological approach to assessment of acid-base disturbances. N Engl J Med 2014;371:1434-45.

Shock and Sepsis

1. Dellinger RP, Levy MM, Rhodes A, et al. Surviving Sepsis Campaign: international guidelines for management of severe sepsis and septic shock: 2012. Crit Care Med 2013;41:580-637.

2. Rivers E, Nguyen B, Havstad S, et al. Early goal-directed therapy in the treatment of severe sepsis and septic shock. N Engl J Med 2001;345:1368-77.

3. Russell JA. Management of sepsis. N Engl J Med 2006;355:1699-713.

4. Angus DC, van der Poll T. Severe sepsis and septic shock. N Engl J Med 2013;369:840-51.

5. The ARISE Investigators and the ANZICS Clinical Trials Group. Goal-directed resuscitation for patients with early septic shock. N Engl J Med 2014;371:1496-506.

6. Surviving Sepsis Campaign Bundles. Available at www.survivingsepsis.org/Bundles/Pages/default.aspx. Accessed October 2015.

Steroids

1. Annane D, Sebille V, Charpentier C, et al. Effect of treatment with low doses of hydrocortisone and fludrocortisone on mortality in patients with septic shock. JAMA 2002;288:862-70.

2. Sprung CL, Annane D, Keh D, et al. Hydrocortisone therapy for patients with septic shock. N Engl J Med 2008;358:111-4.

3. Sprung CL, Brezis M, Goodman S, et al. Corticosteroid therapy for patients in septic shock: some progress in a difficult decision. Crit Care Med 2011;39:571-4.

4. Marik PE, Pastores SM, Annane D, et al. Recommendations for the diagnosis and management of corticosteroid insufficiency in critically ill adult patients: consensus statements from an international task force by the American College of Critical Care Medicine. Crit Care Med 2008;36(6):1937-49.

Volume Replacement and Vasopressors

1. Vincent JL, De Backer D. Circulatory shock. N Engl J Med 2013;369:1726-34.

2. DeBacker D, Biston P, Devriendt J, et al. Comparison of dopamine and norepinephrine in the treatment of shock. N Engl J Med 2010;362:779-89.

3. Finfer S, Bellomo R, Boyce N, et al. A comparison of albumin and saline for fluid resuscitation in the intensive care unit. N Engl J Med 2004;350:2247-56.

4. Russell JA, Walley KR, Singer J, et al. Vasopressin versus norepinephrine infusion in patients with septic shock. N Engl J Med 2008;358:877-87.

5. Zarychanski R, Abou-Setta AM, Turgeon AF, et al. Association of hydroxyethyl starch administration with mortality and acute kidney injury in critically ill patients requiring volume resuscitation: a systematic review and meta-analysis. JAMA 2013;309(7):678-88.

6. Yunos N, Bellomo R, Hegarty C, et al. Association between a chloride-liberal vs chloride-restrictive intravenous fluid administration strategy and kidney injury in critically ill adults. JAMA 2012;308(15):1566-72.

7. Chew MS, Åneman A. Haemodynamic monitoring using arterial waveform analysis. Curr Opin Crit Care 2013;19(3):234-41.

8. Young P, Bailey M, Beasley R, et al; for the SPLIT investigators and the ANZICS CTG. Effect of a buffered crystalloid solution vs saline on acute kidney injury among patients in the intensive care unit: the SPLIT randomized clinical trial. JAMA. doi:10.1001/jama.2015.12334.

Cardiac Arrest

1. American Heart Association. American Heart Association guidelines for cardiopulmonary resuscitation and emergency cardiovascular care. Circulation 2015;132:S315-S367

2. Nunnally ME, Jaeschke R, Bellingan GJ, et al. Targeted temperature management in critical care: a report and recommendations from five professional societies. Crit Care Med 2011;39:1113-25.

3. Nielsen N, Wetterslev J, Cronberg T, et al. Targeted temperature management at 33°C versus 36°C after cardiac arrest. N Engl J Med 2013;369:2197-206.

Sedation

1. Barr J, Fraser GL, Puntillo K, et al. Clinical practice guidelines for the management of pain, agitation, and delirium in adult patients in the intensive care unit. Crit Care Med 2013;41:263-306.

2. Kress JP, Pohlman AS, O'Connor MF, et al. Daily interruption of sedative infusions in critically ill patients undergoing mechanical ventilation. N Engl J Med 2000;342:1471-7.

3. Pun B, Dunn J. The sedation of critically ill adults: part 1. Assessment. Am J Nurs 2007;107:40-8.

4. Sessler CN, Varney K. Patient-focused sedation and analgesia in the ICU. Chest 2008;133:552-65.

Delirium

1. Ely EW, Shintani A, Truman B, et al. Delirium as a predictor of mortality in mechanically ventilated patients in the intensive care unit. JAMA 2004;291:1753-62.

2. ICU Delirium and Cognitive Impairment Study Group. Brain dysfunction in critically ill patients. Vanderbilt Medical Center. Available at www.icudelirium.org/delirium. Accessed September 30, 2009.

3. Gilchrist NA, Asoh I, Greenberg B. Atypical antipsychotics for the treatment of ICU delirium. J Intensive Care Med 2012;27:354-61.

Neuromuscular Blockade

1. Baumann MH, McAlpin BW, Brown K, et al. A prospective randomized comparison of train-of-four monitoring and clinical assessment during continuous ICU cisatracurium paralysis. Chest 2004;126:1267-73.

2. Murray MJ, Cowen J, DeBlock H, et al. Clinical practice guidelines for sustained neuromuscular blockade in the adult critically ill patient. Crit Care Med 2002;30:142-56.

3. Papazian L, Forel JM, Gacouin A, et al. Neuromuscular blockers in early acute respiratory distress syndrome. N Engl J Med 2010;363:1107-16.

Glucose Control

1. Jacobi J, Bircher N, Krinsley J, et al. Guidelines for the use of an insulin infusion for the management of hyperglycemia in critically ill patients. Crit Care Med 2012;40:3251-76.

2. NICE-SUGAR Study Investigators; Finfer S, Chittock DR, Su SY, et al. Intensive versus conventional glucose control in critically ill patients. N Engl J Med 2009;360:1283-97.

3. Kavanagh BP, McCowen KC. Glycemic control in the ICU. N Engl J Med 2010;363:2540-6.

Stress Ulcer Prophylaxis

1. Allen ME, Kopp BJ, Erstad BL. Stress ulcer prophylaxis in the postoperative period. Am J Health Syst Pharm 2004;61:588-96.

2. ASHP Commission on Therapeutics. ASHP therapeutic guidelines on stress ulcer prophylaxis. Am J Health Syst Pharm 1999;56:347-79.

3. Cook D, Guyatt G, Marshall J, et al. A comparison of sucralfate and ranitidine for the prevention of upper gastrointestinal bleeding in patients requiring mechanical ventilation. N Engl J Med 1998;338:791-7.

4. Herzig SJ, Howell MD, Ngo LH, et al. Acid-suppressive medication use and the risk for hospital-acquired pneumonia. JAMA 2009;301:2120-8.

5. Sessler JM. Stress-related mucosal disease in the intensive care unit: an update on prophylaxis. AACN Adv Crit Care 2007;18:199-26.

6. Stevens AM, Thomas Z. The case against stress ulcer prophylaxis in 2007. Hosp Pharm 2007;42:995-1002.

Preventing VTE

1. Alhazzani W, Lim W, Jaeschke RZ, et al. Heparin thromboprophylaxis in medical-surgical critically ill patients: a systematic review and meta-analysis of randomized trials. Crit Care Med 2013;41:2088-98.

2. Cook D, Meade M, Guyatt G, et al. Dalteparin versus unfractionated heparin in critically ill patients. N Engl J Med 2011;364:1305-14.

3. Guyatt GH, Akl EA, Crowther DD, et al. Executive summary: antithrombotic therapy and prevention of thrombosis, 9th ed. American College of Chest Physicians evidence-based clinical practice guidelines. Chest 2012;141(2 suppl):7S-47S.

4. Nutescu EA. Assessing, preventing, and treating venous thromboembolism: evidence-based approaches. Am J Health Syst Pharm 2007;64 (suppl 7):5-13.

5. Gould MK, Garcia DA, Wren SM, et al. Prevention of VTE in nonorthopedic surgical patients. Chest 2012;141(2 suppl):e227S-77S.

6. Cohen AT, Spiro TE, Buller HR, et al. Rivaroxaban for thromboprophylaxis in acutely ill medical patients. N Engl J Med 2013;368:513-23.

7. Phung OJ, Kahn SR, Cook DJ, et al. Dosing frequency of unfractionated heparin thromboprophylaxis. Chest 2011;140(2):374-81.

Prevention of Ventilator-Associated Pneumonia

1. IHI ventilator bundle. Available at www.ihi.org/resources/Pages/Changes/ImplementtheVentilatorBundle.aspx. Accessed November 21, 2014.

Nutrition

1. Casaer MP, Mesotten D, Hermans G, et al. Early versus late parenteral nutrition in critically ill adults. N Engl J Med 2011;365:506-17.

2. Martindale RG, McClave SA, Vanek VW, et al. Guidelines for the provision and assessment of nutrition support therapy in the adult critically ill patient: Society of Critical Care Medicine and American Society for Parenteral and Enteral Nutrition: executive summary. Crit Care Med 2009;37:1757-61.

3. Walker RN, Heuberger RA. Predictive equations for energy needs for the critically ill. Respir Care 2009;54:509-21.

4. Ziegler TR. Parenteral nutrition in the critically ill patient. N Engl J Med 2009;361:1088-97.

5. Casaer MP, Van den Berghe G. Nutrition in the acute phase of critical illness. N Engl J Med 2014;370:1227-36.

6. Arabi YM, Tamim HM, Dhar GS, et al. Permissive underfeeding and intensive insulin therapy in critically ill patients: a randomized controlled trial. Am J Clin Nutr 2011;93(3):569-77.

7. Dickerson RN, Boschert KJ, Kudsk KA, et al. Hypocaloric enteral tube feeding in critically ill obese patients. Nutrition 2002;18:241-6.

8. Dhaliwal R, Cahill N, Lemieux M, et al. The Canadian critical care nutrition guidelines in 2013: an update on current recommendations and implementation strategies. Nutr Clin Pract 2014;29(1):29-43.

Intracranial Hemorrhage

1. Naidech AM. Intracranial hemorrhage. Am J Respir Crit Care Med 2011;184:998-1006.

2. Connolly ES, Rabinstein AA, Carhuapoma JR, et al. Guidelines for the management of aneurysmal subarachnoid hemorrhage. Stroke 2012:43.

3. Rowe SA, Goodwin H, Brophy GM, et al. Seizure prophylaxis in neurocritical care: evidence-based support. Pharmacotherapy 2014;34(4):396-409.

4. Diringer MN, Bleck TP, Hemphill JC, et al. Critical care management of patients following aneurysmal subarachnoid hemorrhage: recommendations from the Neurocritical Care Society's Multidisciplinary Consensus Conference. Neurocrit Care 2011;15:211-40.

5. Hemphill JC, Greenberg SM, Anderson CS, et al. Guidelines for the management of spontaneous intracerebral hemorrhage: a guideline for healthcare professionals from the American Heart Association/American Stroke Association. Stroke 2015. doi:10.1161/STR.0000000000000069

6. FAST Trial Investigators. Efficacy and safety of recombinant activated factor VII for acute intracerebral hemorrhage. N Engl J Med 2008;358:2127-37

ANSWERS AND EXPLANATIONS TO PATIENT CASES

1. Answer: B

This ABG is consistent with metabolic acidosis. The pH is less than 7.40 (indicating primary acidosis), and the HCO_3^- and $Paco_2$ are lower than normal. In metabolic acidosis, the decrease in HCO_3^- is the primary disorder. When metabolic acidosis is present, the AG should be calculated to provide additional insight about the potential cause of the disorder. The AG is calculated by subtracting the sum of measured anions (Cl^- and HCO_3^-) from cations (Na^+). This patient's AG (8 mEq/L) is within the reference range of 6–12 mEq/L; therefore, it is referred to as a normal anion gap metabolic acidosis or non–anion gap metabolic acidosis. *C. difficile*–induced diarrhea is the most likely cause of this patient's acid-base disorder.

2. Answer: D

Given this patient's neurologic status and his elevated $Paco_2$, he should be intubated and transferred to the ICU. In patients without chronic obstructive pulmonary disease, a $Paco_2$ greater than 50 mm Hg is usually an indication for mechanical ventilation, regardless of oxygenation status (this patient was oxygenating well: Pao_2 111 mm Hg, Sao_2 100%). Oxygen (Answer B) therapy alone is unlikely to correct this patient's cause of respiratory failure (i.e., hypoventilation). Likewise, his acid-base disturbance is consistent with a pure acute respiratory acidosis (elevated $Paco_2$, normal HCO_3^-) and is therefore unlikely to respond to HCO_3^- (Answer C), or tromethamine (Answer A), which is usually reserved for a severe metabolic acidosis.

3. Answer: C

This ABG is consistent with respiratory acidosis. The pH is below 7.40 (indicating acidosis), and the $Paco_2$ is higher than normal (about 40 mm Hg). In chronic respiratory acidosis, the kidneys conserve HCO_3^- (a base) in an attempt to maintain a normal pH. This compensatory metabolic alkalosis is obvious in this patient, whose serum HCO_3^- is 28 mEq/L (which is about 4 mEq/L higher than normal). The elevated HCO_3^- concentration in this patient confirms the diagnosis of respiratory acidosis (because the HCO_3^- would be expected to be less than 24 mEq/L if the acidemia were attributable to a metabolic cause).

4. Answer: C

This patient's hemodynamic profile is most consistent with sepsis (i.e., high CI, low SVR). Her PCWP is consistent with an adequate volume challenge. Because she remains hypotensive despite receiving an adequate fluid load, an α-adrenergic agent such as norepinephrine (Answer C) should be initiated. The goals of treatment are to improve BP (typically MAP) and restore adequate organ perfusion. Norepinephrine is a more potent vasoconstrictor than phenylephrine and provides less β-stimulation than dopamine. If she became more tachycardic while receiving norepinephrine, phenylephrine could be tried. Dobutamine (Answer B) is an inotropic agent that increases CI, which is adequate in this patient. Piperacillin/tazobactam and vancomycin will provide adequate gram-positive, gram-negative, and anaerobic coverage for nosocomial pneumonia, eliminating the need for clindamycin (Answer A). If the patient continues to be hypotensive despite adequate fluid resuscitation and use of vasopressors, then hydrocortisone (Answer D) can be considered.

5. Answer: A

Calculating an infusion rate is a very important role for the pharmacist in code situations. The infusion pump is set to run in milliliters per hour, so the answer should always be in these units. To determine the rate (in milliliters per hour) needed to achieve a 0.03-mcg/kg/minute dose, use the following calculation:

Concentration of epinephrine drip: 4 mg/250 mL = 0.016 mg/mL or 16 mcg/mL

Therefore, 70 kg × 0.03 mcg/kg/minute × 60 minutes/1 hour × 1 mL/16 mcg = 7.875 mL/hour, which is then rounded to 8 mL/hour.

6. Answer: D

This patient is at high risk of developing a VTE and should receive prophylaxis with unfractionated heparin (Answer D). An elevated INR of 1.4, probably caused by temporary hypoperfusion of the liver, is no reason to withhold prophylaxis for VTE. Hydrocortisone (Answer A) is not necessary in this case because the patient is responding to fluid resuscitation and the infusion of norepinephrine, as evidenced by the increase in MAP from 44 mm Hg on arrival to the emergency department to 66 mm Hg after initial resuscitation. Enoxaparin is appropriate for DVT prophylaxis (Answer B), but his serum creatinine has more than doubled, and because enoxaparin is renally cleared it would not be the preferred answer in this case. Adding dopamine (Answer C) is not necessary at this time because the MAP is greater than 65 mm Hg, thus allowing global organ perfusion. In addition, there is no evidence that a low dose of dopamine will prevent acute kidney injury, and it increases the risk of arrhythmias compared with norepinephrine.

7. Answer: A

During rewarming, patients can become hypoglycemic. Therefore, a reduction in the insulin infusion is likely, and BG should be monitored more often (Answer A). Neuromuscular blockade assessment can include titrating to a TOF goal; however, a more applicable goal would be the absence of shivering in this patient when the paralytic is briefly interrupted. If the patient is not shivering, consideration should be given to discontinuing the paralytic. Of note, the TOF goal is 2/4 twitches, rather than 0/4 (Answer B), to avoid overparalysis. Although discontinuing propofol (Answer C) can facilitate extubation, this should not be done until the patient is no longer paralyzed, is at a normal body temperature, and is ready for ventilator weaning. Finally, although rewarming can cause hyperkalemia, it is appropriate to monitor K concentrations and treat as needed. It is not appropriate to increase the infusion of insulin (Answer D) to prevent hyperkalemia because this could precipitate hypoglycemia during rewarming.

8. Answer: D

Using a nonpharmacologic approach such as offering verbal reassurance to the patient is the most logical starting point for this patient with delirium. Although propofol (Answer A) is an effective sedative that does not worsen delirium, a sedative is not needed in this patient with a RASS of 0 (alert and calm). Haloperidol (Answer B) is an option; however, nonpharmacologic strategies should be tried first. Morphine (Answer C) is incorrect because her BPS score is 4. This score ranges from 3 (no pain) to 12 (maximum pain). Furthermore, although opioids can be effective sedatives, morphine should be avoided, if possible, in patients with kidney injury because of active metabolites that are renally eliminated.

9. Answer: D

Neuromuscular blocking agents should be titrated to the minimal effective dose. Although a peripheral nerve stimulator may provide information on the level of blockade, the true therapeutic end point in all patients is ventilator synchrony (Answer D). Clinicians must recognize that neuromuscular blocking agents do not cross the blood-brain barrier and are not useful as sedatives or analgesics. For this reason, sedatives and analgesics should be optimized before initiation of neuromuscular blockade, because titrating to an RASS goal while on neuromuscular blockers is not possible (Answer C). Adequate sedation and analgesia must be achieved before initiating a neuromuscular blocker and should continue throughout the treatment. Vecuronium, though inexpensive, accumulates in renal disease and should be avoided (Answer B). Answer A is incorrect because analgesics and sedatives should be continued during paralysis.

10. Answer: B

Although this patient is no longer paralyzed, it would be inappropriate to reparalyze an obviously agitated patient (Answer A) because he or she should first be adequately sedated. Likewise, performing a TOF test using a peripheral nerve stimulator (Answer D) is unnecessary because it is obvious from the patient's movement that she is not adequately blocked. It is possible that the patient is agitated and tachycardic because she was on neuromuscular blockers without adequate sedation or analgesia. Before the paralytic is adjusted, the patient should be given a sedative bolus (Answer B). In patients on neuromuscular blockade, it is generally better to err on the side of oversedation than undersedation, so an increase in the sedative drip rates would also be appropriate in this patient. Answer C is incorrect because increasing the infusion rate of fentanyl will not have an immediate effect. It would be an acceptable option if the increased infusion rate were accompanied by a fentanyl bolus.

11. Answer: B

Gentamicin (Answer B) has pharmacodynamic effects (i.e., inhibits the release of acetylcholine at the nicotinic receptor), which may potentiate the action of neuromuscular-blocking agents. Piperacillin/tazobactam and norepinephrine (Answer A and Answer C) will not prolong the effects of cisatracurium. Although hypokalemia can prolong the effects of neuromuscular blocking agents, a K level of 4.9 mEq/L (Answer D) will not.

12. Answer: A
Although this patient had hypotensive episodes during her resuscitation period, she currently has a functioning GI system, as noted by her tolerance of tube feeds. Therefore, SUP should be administered via her feeding tube, making the best choice for this patient famotidine administered enterally (Answer A). Ranitidine (Answer D) is incorrect because it is administered intravenously. Esomeprazole (Answer B) is incorrect because no data show a benefit of PPIs over histamine receptor antagonists; they are usually more expensive and may have more side effects. Sucralfate (Answer C) is incorrect because it has been shown to be inferior to histamine receptor antagonists.

13. Answer: B
This patient's risk factors for SUP (mechanical ventilation and hypoperfusion) are no longer present, so SUP should be discontinued (Answer B). There is no reason to continue SUP until ICU (Answer A) or hospital (Answer D) discharge, and this practice just increases the risk of continuing the SUP in an outpatient without an appropriate indication. Answer C is incorrect because a poor appetite is not a risk factor for developing stress-related mucosal disease (SRMD).

14. Answer: C
This patient has several risk factors for VTE, including age, respiratory failure, and a history of heart failure. For this reason, intermittent pneumatic compression (Answer A) is insufficient prophylaxis. Fondaparinux (Answer B) is contraindicated in patients with an estimated creatinine clearance less than 30 mL/minute. Enoxaparin 30 mg subcutaneously once daily (Answer C) is an appropriate dose for this patient, considering her reduced kidney function. A continuous infusion of heparin (Answer D) is not an appropriate administration method for preventing a VTE, but it would be appropriate as a treatment strategy for a known or suspected VTE.

15. Answer D
The EN can be continued (Answer D) unless gastric residuals exceed 250 mL. Parenteral nutrition (Answer A) is not indicated in patients with a functional GI tract. Metoclopramide (Answer B) could be considered if gastric residuals increase or if the patient experiences abdominal distension. Switching to a more concentrated feed would not be indicated unless the patient is volume overloaded (Answer C).

ANSWERS AND EXPLANATIONS TO SELF-ASSESSMENT QUESTIONS

1. Answer: A
This patient's ABG and urine Cl are consistent with a saline-responsive metabolic alkalosis. In critically ill patients, the most common cause of metabolic alkalosis is volume contraction. In this case, the volume contraction is probably caused by overly aggressive diuresis. In patients receiving diuretics, the urine Cl should be measured at least 12–24 hours after the last dose. Additionally, the patient is hypotensive with an elevated heart rate, which probably represents hypovolemia. This patient should receive a normal saline infusion. Hydrochloric acid infusions (Answer C) are typically reserved for more severe alkalosis (pH more than 7.55) that is not responding to conventional therapy. Administering D_5W (Answer B) will provide hydration but will not correct intravascular volume depletion. Acetazolamide (Answer D) would be a consideration if the metabolic alkalosis persisted after correcting the underlying problem (i.e., volume contraction).

2. Answer: C
Assuming that analgesia with morphine is adequate, this patient needs a sedative to achieve the RASS goal. Propofol is a sedative that is easily titrated and cost-effective. Dexmedetomidine (Answer A) is another option that is safe and effective, even when used for longer than 24 hours, but it has not been shown superior to propofol in randomized controlled trials. Furthermore, dexmedetomidine is more expensive than propofol. Lorazepam (Answer B) should be avoided in patients with (or at high risk of) delirium. Use of benzodiazepines is associated with an increased risk of delirium. Haloperidol (Answer D) is incorrect because the patient is CAM-ICU negative. Haloperidol can cause further prolongation of the QTc interval and could lead to torsades.

3. Answer: B
Aminoglycosides can potentiate the effect of neuromuscular blockers; therefore, they should be avoided if possible (Answer B). This could be the reason for the TOF score of 0/4, which can indicate overparalysis. A reasonable goal for the TOF is 2/4 twitches. It is important to note that the study of untitrated neuromuscular blockade was with cisatracurium in ARDS, which does not fit this patient case. The level of sedation cannot

be assessed with the RASS (Answer A) or other sedation scales because the patient is under neuromuscular blockade. Parenteral nutrition (Answer C) can be withheld until the patient is hemodynamically stable. Furthermore, late initiation (after 1 week) of PN support is associated with improved outcomes. Opioids such as morphine (Answer D) should not be withheld in paralyzed trauma patients. Propofol has minimal analgesic properties and will not be sufficient in a trauma patient with several injuries.

4. Answer: C
This patient meets the criteria for severe sepsis. Treatment with 5% albumin (Answer A) is unlikely to offer additional benefit because the patient's MAP is at goal (more than 65 mm Hg). Furthermore, colloids are no more effective than crystalloids for fluid resuscitation, and a serum albumin concentration does not predict the efficacy of albumin administration. Hydrocortisone (Answer B) is incorrect because the patient is not persistently hypotensive after receiving fluids and vasopressors. Although this patient's BP is responding to the infusion of dopamine, the HR has increased. Norepinephrine (Answer C) is correct because it has similar efficacy but with fewer tachyarrhythmias than dopamine. The dopamine should not be reduced (Answer D) because lower doses are not renal protective.

5. Answer: B
The Surviving Sepsis Campaign guidelines recommend adequate fluid resuscitation with either crystalloids or colloids before the addition of vasopressor agents in patients with severe sepsis. This patient's CVP, BP, HR, and BUN/Cr ratio indicate that she has intravascular volume depletion and needs immediate volume replacement. Therefore, intravenous fluids with either crystalloid or colloid should be the next therapy added to this patient's regimen. Answer A is incorrect because fluid resuscitation should be attempted before addition of vasopressors. When deciding between a balanced crystalloid such as lactated Ringer's and a hyperchloremic fluid such as normal saline, many experts would choose Answer B (lactated Ringer's) because of a slight improvement in renal morbidity when used compared with Answer C (normal saline), especially in

a patient who already has acute kidney injury. There are no data that favor colloids over crystalloids, and the substantial increase in cost associated with colloids precludes it from being first line, so Answer D (albumin) is incorrect.

6. Answer: D
Targeted temperature management (i.e., therapeutic hypothermia) improves neurologic recovery and mortality in patients who have had a cardiac arrest. Although the patient probably has a metabolic acidosis, administering sodium bicarbonate (Answer A) does not improve outcomes. Vasopressin (Answer B) is an acceptable option during a cardiac arrest for patients with ventricular fibrillation or pulseless VT, but it has no role after cardiac arrest or in a patient who has returned to normal sinus rhythm. Although acute coronary syndrome is a common cause of cardiac arrest, anticoagulation with heparin (Answer C) would be a consideration after initiation of targeted temperature management. A continuous infusion of heparin does not improve mortality in patients with an acute coronary syndrome. Of note, the induction of hypothermia does not necessarily interfere with treatment plans for acute coronary syndrome (e.g., percutaneous coronary intervention).

7. Answer: B
Mechanical ventilation for more than 48 hours and coagulopathy are independent risk factors for stress ulcers; therefore, Answer D is incorrect because the patient has a high risk of developing a stress ulcer. This patient is critically ill and may be intubated for an extended time; therefore, he is at risk of stress ulcers, and he will need SUP. The patient has an OGT, meaning that EN and medications administered by the tube will go directly into the stomach. Sucralfate (Answer C) was inferior to H$_2$-receptor antagonists in preventing clinically significant bleeding from SRMD in a large randomized controlled trial, and it is generally not recommended for SUP. Proton pump inhibitors such as intravenous pantoprazole (Answer A) do not prevent SRMD better than H$_2$-receptor antagonists and have been associated with an increased risk of hospital-acquired pneumonia. Therefore, famotidine (Answer B) administered enterally is the most cost-effective agent for SUP in this patient.

8. Answer: A
The SSC suggests hydrocortisone at a dose of 200 mg per day if fluids and vasopressors cannot restore hemodynamic stability (Answer A, so Answer D is incorrect). Although low random cortisol concentrations predict worse outcomes, there are no data supporting treatment of low cortisol levels (Answer C). Because of the results of the most recent clinical trial and increased health care costs, a cosyntropin stimulation test is no longer recommended for patients with septic shock (Answer B).

9. Answer: A
The patient has an adequate MAP but has poor oxygen delivery to peripheral tissues. Because the MAP is at goal (more than 65 mm Hg), norepinephrine should be continued at the current dose (Answer B). Although decreasing propofol may increase blood pressure and allow a reduction in norepinephrine, this would not be recommended while the patient is on neuromuscular blockade, and the patient is not having problems maintaining an adequate blood pressure (Answer C). The patient needs an increase in oxygen delivery. The arterial oxygen saturation and hemoglobin are adequate, meaning that cardiac output is low. This can be achieved by addition of an inotrope. Dobutamine is the preferred inotrope in septic patients (Answer A) over epinephrine (Answer D), which may cause an unwanted increase in MAP, as well as hyperglycemia and lactic acidosis.

10. Answer: C
The patient's hemodynamics are most consistent with obstructive shock due to tamponade and an inability to properly fill the ventricles, as evidenced by high filling pressures (pulmonary capillary wedge pressure and CVP with a low cardiac index). Prompt drainage of fluid surrounding the heart is the only definitive therapy (Answer C). Fluid boluses would worsen this condition (Answer A). An intrope may temporize the reduction in cardiac output but will not correct the underlying cause (Answer B). The patient's MAP and SVR are high, so vasopressors would not be indicated (Answer D).

11. Answer: A
There are a number of ways to estimate nutritional needs in critically ill patients. The modified Penn State equation has been found to closely predict caloric needs. The

recommended protein intake for medically ill patients in the ICU is 1.2–1.5 g/kg (Answer A). Indirect calorimetry will most closely calculate caloric needs but does not provide information on the amount of protein needed (Answer B). Feeding at 11–14 kcal/kg is recommended for obese patients, but this patient's BMI is less than 30 kg/m^2 (Answer C). Prealbumin levels have not shown good correlation with nutritional deficits in critically ill patients and are not recommended (Answer D).

12. Answer: D
PPIs have been associated with an increase in ventilator-associated pneumonia (Answer A). Selective digestive decontamination has been shown effective, but because of its side effects and increases in resistant bacteria it is not in widespread use, and it is not part of the Institute for Healthcare Improvement ventilator bundle (Answer B). Head elevation prevents ventilator-associated pneumonia but should be between 30° and 45° (Answer C). Chlorhexidine is inexpensive, carries few side effects, is easy to administer, and has been shown effective in the prevention of ventilator-associated pneumonia (Answer D).

13. Answer: C
Sliding scale protocol is inappropriate as the sole therapy for hyperglycemia in the ICU (Answer A). The Surviving Sepsis Campaign recommends an insulin infusion for two blood glucose values greater than 180 mg/dL (Answer C). The ideal blood glucose range for critically ill adults has yet to be determined, but a goal of 80–110 mg/dL has not been found to improve outcomes and may increase mortality (Answer D). A target of 110–180 mg/dL prevents hyperglycemia but without an excess risk of hypoglycemia (Answer C).

Pharmacokinetics: A Refresher

Curtis L. Smith, Pharm.D., BCPS

Ferris State University
Lansing, Michigan

Pharmacokinetics: A Refresher

Curtis L. Smith, Pharm.D., BCPS

Ferris State University
Lansing, Michigan

Learning Objectives

1. Identify and solve pharmacotherapy problems using basic pharmacokinetic concepts, including bioavailability, volume of distribution, clearance, and the elimination rate constant.
2. Describe specific pharmacokinetic characteristics of commonly used therapeutic agents, including aminoglycosides, vancomycin, phenytoin, and digoxin, as well as pharmacokinetic alterations in patients with renal and hepatic disease.
3. Define important issues as they pertain to drug concentration sampling and interpretation.

Self-Assessment Questions

Answers and explanations to these questions can be found at the end of this chapter.

-4\13

1. J.H., a 65-year-old woman (65 kg), was recently initiated on tobramycin and piperacillin/tazobactam for the treatment of hospital-acquired pneumonia. After the first tobramycin dose of 120 mg (infused from noon to 1:00 p.m.), serum tobramycin concentrations are drawn. They are 4.4 mg/L at 3:00 p.m. and 1.2 mg/L at 7:00 p.m. Which is the best assessment regarding the calculation of tobramycin pharmacokinetic parameters in this patient?

    A. Data are sufficient to determine the half-life but not the volume of distribution (Vd).
    B. Data are sufficient to determine both the half-life and the Vd.
    C. Data are insufficient to determine either the half-life or the Vd.
    D. Data are sufficient to determine the Vd but not the half-life.

2. P.L. is a 60-year-old woman (60 kg) recently initiated on gentamicin and clindamycin. After the first gentamicin dose of 110 mg (infused from 6:00 p.m. to 6:30 p.m.), serum gentamicin concentrations are drawn. They are 3.6 mg/L at 7:30 p.m. and 0.9 mg/L at 11:30 p.m. Which is the best assessment of this patient's gentamicin pharmacokinetic parameters?

    A. The half-life is about 2 hours.
    B. The half-life is about 3 hours.

$\frac{3.6}{.9}$, Δt

$\ln \frac{3.6 - 0.9}{4}$

$t'_{1/2} = 1.77$

$\ln(0.675) = 0.39$

C. The maximum concentration (Cmax) is about 3.8 mg/L.
D. The Vd is about 11.6 L.

3. R.O. is a 74-year-old woman initiated on gentamicin 100 mg intravenously every 24 hours for pyelonephritis. On admission, her serum creatinine (SCr) is 1.8 mg/dL. She also has congestive heart failure and is fluid overloaded because of her diminished renal function, and she is nonadherent to her angiotensin-converting enzyme inhibitor and diuretic. A few days into her hospitalization, her SCr is down to 1.1 mg/dL, and she is reinitiated on furosemide and enalapril. Which probably happened to the gentamicin half-life in R.O. during her hospitalization?

    A. Her clearance increased, which increased her Vd and decreased her half-life.
    B. Her clearance increased, which increased her elimination rate constant and decreased her half-life.
    C. Her Vd decreased, which increased her clearance and decreased her half-life.
    D. Her Vd decreased, which increased her elimination rate constant and increased her half-life.

4. A patient receives vancomycin 1000 mg intravenously every 24 hours and has a trough concentration, drawn 30 minutes before the next dose, of 6 mg/L. Which regimen is best for this patient if the goal trough concentration is 10–15 mg/L?

    A. Maintain the dosage at 1000 mg intravenously every 24 hours.
    B. Lower the dosage to 500 mg but keep the interval at every 24 hours.
    C. Keep the dosage at 1000 mg but shorten the interval to every 12 hours.
    D. Lower the dosage to 500 mg and shorten the interval to every 12 hours.

5. R.K., a 39-year-old man who is human immunodeficiency virus (HIV)-positive, receives a diagnosis of cryptococcal meningitis and begins taking amphotericin B and flucytosine. You want to keep flucytosine peak concentrations between 50 and 100 mcg/mL. Assuming a trough concentration of

25 mcg/ mL, dosing every 6 hours, and 100% bio-availability, which is the best dosage to achieve a peak concentration within the desired range (flucytosine volume of distribution of 0.7 L/kg and half-life of 3 hours)?

A. 12.5 mg/kg.

B. 37.5 mg/kg.

C. 75 mg/kg.

D. 150 mg/kg.

6. L.R. is a 49-year-old patient with diabetes mellitus and renal failure. He was recently in a car accident and sustained a head trauma. He currently receives phenytoin 100 mg intravenously three times a day, and his most recent concentration was 5.6 mcg/mL. You are asked to suggest a new dosage to achieve a concentration within the therapeutic range. Laboratory results include sodium 145 mEq/L, potassium 3.9 mEq/L, chloride 101 mEq/L, carbon dioxide 26 mEq/L, blood urea nitrogen (BUN) 95 mg/dL, SCr 5.4 mg/dL, glucose 230 mg/dL, and albumin (Alb) 2.8 g/dL. Which is the best recommendation?

A. Increase the dosage to 200 mg intravenously three times a day.

B. Increase the dosage to 200 mg intravenously two times a day.

C. Decrease the dosage to 100 mg intravenously two times a day.

D. Keep the dosage the same.

7. You are asked how the fluorescence polarization immunoassay (TDx) and enzyme multiplied immunoassay technique (EMIT) assays compare with each other. Which statement is most accurate?

A. Although both are immunoassays, one labels antibody, whereas the other labels antigen.

B. Although both are immunoassays, one uses antibody as a marker, whereas the other uses a radioisotope.

C. Although both are immunoassays, one uses an enzyme label, whereas the other uses a fluorescent label.

D. They are both names for the same assay technique.

8. An older adult is seen in the morning medicine clinic for a routine follow-up. Medication history includes digoxin 0.25 mg/day by mouth, furosemide 40 mg/day by mouth, and potassium chloride 10 mEq/day by mouth. All doses were last taken at 8:00 a.m. today at home. The patient has vague complaints of stomach upset, which began 2 days ago, but is otherwise in no apparent distress. A serum digoxin concentration drawn today at 10:00 a.m. is 2.5 mcg/L. Which statement best describes what should be done next?

A. Admit the patient for administration of digoxin Fab.

B. Tell the patient to skip tomorrow's dose of digoxin and begin 0.125 mg/day by mouth.

C. Administer a dose of activated charcoal.

D. Do nothing today about the digoxin.

9. A research group is analyzing the relationship between various independent patient demographics (e.g., age, height, weight, Alb, creatinine clearance [CrCl]) and phenytoin pharmacokinetics. Which is the best statistical test to use in assessing the relationship?

A. One-way analysis of variance.

B. Analysis of covariance.

C. Multiple regression.

D. Spearman rank correlation.

10. N.T. is a 24-year-old woman receiving valproic acid for tonic-clonic seizures. Her most recent trough valproic acid concentration was 22 mg/L. Her most recent Alb concentration was 4.1 g/dL. Given this Alb, which recommendation is best regarding her dosage?

A. Continue with the current dosage; the concentration is close enough to the therapeutic range.

B. Assess adherence and increase her dosage; the concentration is below the therapeutic range.

C. Decrease her dosage; the concentration is slightly above the therapeutic range.

D. Assess adherence and then check a free valproic acid concentration and adjust accordingly.

11. N.G. is a 54-year-old woman with a recent head injury. She comes to your pharmacy complaining about the prescription for acetaminophen with codeine you dispensed to her yesterday. She says that it does not seem any stronger than when she uses acetaminophen alone. On her profile you notice results from pharmacogenomics testing performed 3 years ago that shows she is a CYP2D6 poor metabolizer. Besides the acetaminophen and codeine she is also receiving aspirin, clopidogrel, omeprazole, lisinopril, citalopram, metoprolol succinate, docusate, and trazodone. What is the best explanation why N.G. does not seem to benefit from codeine?

   A. Omeprazole inhibited CYP2C19, causing less codeine activation.

   B. Codeine is not as active in N.G. because of her genetic profile.

   C. Codeine is metabolized faster in N.G., leading to lower concentrations.

   D. Metoprolol inhibited CYP2C9, causing less codeine activation.

12. At your hospital you are responsible for making dosing adjustments in patients with poor renal function. While working with you, a student asks why you are using the Cockcroft and Gault method for estimating creatinine clearance instead of the newer Modification of Diet in Renal Disease (MDRD) or Chronic Kidney Disease Epidemiology Collaboration (CKD-Epi) equations. What is the best response to provide to this student?

   A. MDRD and CKD-Epi are not as good estimates of renal function and may lead to inappropriate changes in drug dosing.

   B. MDRD and CKD-Epi were developed in an ambulatory care population and cannot be used for hospitalized patients.

   C. The Cockcroft and Gault estimate of creatinine clearance has units that are different from the glomerular filtration rate estimates calculated using the MDRD and CKD-Epi equations.

   D. Recommendations for renal dosing adjustments in package inserts are based on creatinine clearance estimates using the Cockcroft and Gault equation.

13. An assay used for therapeutic drug monitoring at your institution has a low sensitivity and low precision. What is the best statement about the impact of this assay on drug monitoring?

   A. The assay may not be able to detect concentrations that are therapeutic, and it will report highly variable values when repeatedly run on the same sample.

   B. The assay may not be able to detect concentrations that are therapeutic, and it will consistently over- or under-measure the true concentration.

   C. The assay will not be able to differentiate between like substances, and it will consistently over- or under-measure the true concentration.

   D. The assay will not be able to differentiate between like substances, and it will report highly variable values when repeatedly run on the same sample.

BPS Pharmacotherapy Specialty Examination Content Outline

This chapter covers the following sections of the Pharmacotherapy Specialty Examination Content Outline:

1. Domain 1: Patient-Specific Pharmacotherapy

   a. Task 1: Knowledge statements: 1–7, 11–12; Task 4: Knowledge statement: 2, 5, 6

   b. Systems and Patient Care Problems

       i.   Hepatic Disease

       ii. Renal Disease

2. Domain 2: Retrieval, Generation, Interpretation and Dissemination of Knowledge in Pharmacotherapy, Task 2: Knowledge statements: 1–5

Patient Cases

1. H.R. is receiving vancomycin for methicillin-resistant *Staphylococcus aureus* bacteremia. H.R. has chronic renal failure. A 1-g intravenous dose of vancomycin is given at noon on March 21. A concentration drawn at 2:00 p.m. on March 21 is 23.8 mcg/mL. A concentration drawn at 2:00 p.m. on March 24 is 12.1 mcg/mL. If you were to give a dose at 4:00 p.m. on March 24 and your goal trough concentration was 10–15 mg/L, which would be the best time to give the next dose?

    A. 1 day after the dose on the 24th.

    B. 3 days from the dose on the 24th.

    C. 6 days from the dose on the 24th.

    D. Insufficient information to calculate when to redose.

2. After the administration of 100 mg of a drug intravenously and 200 mg of the same drug by mouth, the areas under the curves (AUCs) are 50 and 25 mg/L/hour. Which best describes the bioavailability of this drug?

    A. 25%.

    B. 37.5%.

    C. 50%.

    D. 100%.

    $$\frac{100 \cdot 25}{200 \cdot 50} = \frac{2500}{10,000}$$

3. L.B. is receiving tobramycin for resistant *Pseudomonas aeruginosa* pneumonia. L.B. has chronic renal failure. A loading dose of 160 mg is given at noon over 1 hour. A concentration is drawn at 6:00 p.m., which is 6.5 mg/L, and again at 6:00 a.m. the next day, which is 5.4 mg/L. When L.B.'s concentration is 1 mg/L, which dosage will be best to achieve a peak of 9 mg/L?

    A. 140 mg.

    B. 160 mg.

    C. 180 mg. ←

    D. 200 mg.

I. BASIC PHARMACOKINETIC RELATIONSHIPS

Table 11 contains definitions of terms.

A. Absorption $\quad F = \dfrac{\text{dose}_{iv} * \text{AUC}_{ev}}{\text{dose}_{ev} * \text{AUC}_{iv}}$

B. Distribution

   Rapid intravenous (or oral) bolus: $\quad Vd = \dfrac{F * \text{dose}}{C_0}$

   Continuous intravenous infusion at steady state: $\quad Vd = \dfrac{R_0}{k * C_{ss}}$

$F = dose \cdot auc$

$\dfrac{dose}{auc} = Cl$

$k = \dfrac{Cl}{Vd}$

$t\,{}'{}_{1/2} = \dfrac{0.693}{k}$

Continuous intravenous infusion before steady state: $Vd = \dfrac{R_0}{C*k} (1-e^{-kt_i})$ and $C = \dfrac{R_0}{V_d*k} (1-e^{-kt_i})$

Multiple intravenous bolus at steady state: $Vd = \dfrac{dose}{C_{ss\,max}*(1-e^{-k\tau})}$

Multiple intermittent intravenous infusion at steady state: $Vd = \dfrac{R_0}{k} * \dfrac{1-e^{-kt}}{C_{max} - (C_{min}*e^{-kt'})}$

$C_{ss\,max} = \dfrac{R_0*(1-e^{-kt'})}{V_d*k*(1-e^{-k\tau})}$ $C_{ss\,min} = C_{ss\,max} = * \, e^{-k(\tau-t')}$

C. Clearance

$Clearance = \dfrac{dose}{AUC}$ $k = \dfrac{Cl}{V_d}$ $k = \dfrac{(lnC_1 - lnC_2)}{(t_2 - t_1)}$ $t_{1/2} = \dfrac{0.693}{k}$

Continuous intravenous infusion at steady state: $Clearance = \dfrac{R_0}{C_{ss}}$

Continuous intravenous infusion before steady state: $Clearance = \dfrac{R_0}{C} * (1 - e^{-kti})$

Multiple intravenous (or oral) bolus at steady state: $Clearance = \dfrac{\dfrac{F*dose}{\tau}}{C_{ss,avg}}$

$K = \dfrac{Cl}{Vd}$

$\tau = \dfrac{(lnC_{max} - lnC_{min})}{k}$ $C_1 = C_0 * e^{-kt}$

$K = \dfrac{lnC - lnc}{\Delta t}$ $t'_{12} = \dfrac{0.693}{K}$

$Cl = \dfrac{dose}{auc}$

II. ABSORPTION

A. First-Pass Effect
  1. Blood that perfuses almost all the gastrointestinal (GI) tissues passes through the liver by means of the hepatic portal vein.
     a. Fifty percent of the rectal blood supply bypasses the liver (middle and inferior hemorrhoidal veins).
     b. Drugs absorbed in the buccal cavity bypass the liver.
  2. Examples of drugs with significant first-pass effect

Amitriptyline	Labetalol	Nitroglycerin
Desipramine	Lidocaine	Pentazocine
Diltiazem	Metoprolol	Propoxyphene
Doxepin	Morphine	Propranolol
Imipramine	Nicardipine	Verapamil
Isosorbide dinitrate	Nifedipine	

B. Enterohepatic Recirculation (Table 1)
1. Drugs are excreted through the bile into the duodenum, metabolized by the normal flora in the GI tract, and reabsorbed into the portal circulation.
2. Occurs with drugs that have biliary (hepatic) elimination and good oral absorption
3. Drug is concentrated in the gallbladder and expelled on sight, smell, or ingestion of food.

Table 1. Examples of Compounds Excreted in Bile and Subject to Enterohepatic Cycling

Compound	Entity in Bile
Chloramphenicol	Glucuronide conjugate
Digoxin	Parent
Estrogens	Parent
Imipramine	Parent and desmethyl metabolite
Indomethacin	Parent and glucuronide
Nafcillin	Parent
Rifampin	Parent
Sulindac	Glucuronides of parent and metabolites
Testosterone	Conjugates
Tiagabine	Glucuronide conjugate
Valproic acid	Glucuronide conjugates
Vitamin A	Conjugates

Patient Case

4. Which statement best describes P-glycoprotein?

A. It is a plasma protein that binds basic drugs.

B. It transfers drugs through the GI mucosa, increasing absorption.

C. It diminishes the effect of cytochrome P450 3A4 (CYP3A4) in the GI mucosa.

D. It is an efflux pump that decreases GI mucosal absorption.

C. P-Glycoprotein
1. P-glycoprotein is an efflux pump (located in the esophagus, stomach, and small and large intestines) that pumps drugs back into the GI lumen; it is a more important factor in drug absorption drug interactions than intestinal CYP3A4.
2. Both CYP3A4 and P-glycoprotein are located in small intestinal enterocytes and work together to decrease the absorption of xenobiotics.
3. Most CYP3A4 substrates are also P-glycoprotein substrates.
4. Many CYP3A4 inhibitors/inducers also inhibit/induce P-glycoprotein, leading to increases or decreases in bioavailability.
5. Examples of P-glycoprotein absorption drug interactions
   a. Dabigatran is affected by rifampin, St. John's wort, quinidine, ketoconazole, verapamil, amiodarone, and dronedarone.
   b. Digoxin is affected by St. John's wort, quinidine, verapamil, amiodarone, and dronedarone or dabigatran.
   c. Human immunodeficiency virus protease inhibitors are affected by rifampin and St. John's wort.

III. DISTRIBUTION

A. Definition: Apparent Vd: Proportionality constant that relates the amount of drug in the body to an observed concentration of drug

B. Protein Binding (Table 2)

Table 2. Common Proteins Involved in Drug Protein Binding

Protein	Types of Drugs Bound	Molecular Weight	Normal Concentrations	
			g/L	mcmol
Albumin	Acidic	65,000	35–50	500–700
α-1-Acid glycoprotein	Basic	44,000	0.4–1.0	9–23
Lipoprotein	Lipophilic and basic	200,000–3,400,000	Variable	Variable

C. P-Glycoprotein
   1. Functions as an efflux pump on the luminal surface of the blood-brain barrier, limiting entry to the central nervous system
   2. It may be especially important with opioids: Induction of P-glycoprotein by chronic use of opioids may decrease the opioid effect (tolerance).
   3. P-glycoprotein is also found in tumor cells, resulting in the efflux of chemotherapeutic agents from the cell and, ultimately, multidrug resistance.

IV. CLEARANCE

Table 3. Enzymes Involved in Drug Metabolism

Oxygenases	**Hydrolytic enzymes**
CYPs	Esterases
Monoamine oxygenases	Amidases
Alcohol dehydrogenases	Epoxide hydrolases
Aldehyde dehydrogenases	Dipeptidases
Xanthine dehydrogenases	
Conjugating enzymes	
Uridine diphosphate–glucuronyl transferases	
Glutathione *S*-transferase	
Acetyltransferases	
Methyltransferases	

CYP = cytochrome P450.

Table 4. Drug Transport Proteins

Transport Protein Superfamily	Transport Protein (*Gene* [Protein])	Location and Function	Drugs Affected by Transport Protein
SLC	*SLCO1A2* [OATP-A]	Hepatocyte: Bile acid uptake	Digoxin Levofloxacin Methotrexate Statins
	SLCO1B1 [OATP1B1]	Hepatocyte: Hepatic uptake of drugs	Pravastatin Rifampin Simvastatin Valsartan
	SLCO1B3 [OATP1B3]	Hepatocyte: Hepatic uptake of drugs	Digoxin Fexofenadine Rifampin Statins
	SLC22A1, SLC22A2, SLC22A6, SLC22A8 [OAT and OCT]	Hepatocyte: Hepatic uptake of drugs Renal tubule (interstitial side): Secretion of drugs	Dofetilide[b] Methotrexate[a] Organic anions and cations[b] Salicylate[a] Tetracycline[a] Zidovudine[a]
	SLCO2B1 [OATP2B1]	Hepatocyte: Hepatic uptake of drugs	Fexofenadine Glyburide Statins
	SLC15A1, SLC15A2 [PEPT1, PEPT2]	Renal tubule Intestinal enterocytes	Captopril Cephalexin Enalapril Valacyclovir
	SLC47A1, SLC47A2 [MATE1, MATE2-K]	Renal tubule	Metformin
ABC	*ABCB11* [BSEP]	Hepatocyte: Bile acid excretion into bile	Pravastatin
ABCB1 [MDR1] (P-glycoprotein) *ABCB4* [MDR3] *ABCG2* [BCRP]	*ABCC2, 3, 4,* and *5* [MRP2, 3, 4, and 5]	Hepatocyte: Excreting water-soluble drugs and metabolites into blood Renal tubule (luminal side): Secretion of drugs	Glucuronide, sulfate, and glutathione metabolites[a] Methotrexate[a] Pravastatin[a] Rifampin[a]
		Hepatocyte: See text in handout Renal tubule (luminal side): See text in handout	See text
		Hepatocyte	Digoxin Paclitaxel Vinblastine
		Hepatocyte: Biliary excretion	Daunorubicin Doxorubicin Imatinib Methotrexate Mitoxantrone Statins Topotecan

[a]Drugs affected by transport proteins in hepatocytes.

[b]Drugs affected by transport proteins in the renal tubule.

Patient Case

5. A renal transplant patient receiving cyclosporine is given a diagnosis of community-acquired pneumonia. The patient is admitted to the hospital and initiated on ceftriaxone and a macrolide. A physician asks you to choose a macrolide that will not interact with the patient's cyclosporine. Which macrolide is the best choice to meet the physician's criteria?

    A. Erythromycin.

    B. Clarithromycin.

    C. Azithromycin.

    D. Any macrolide (all macrolides inhibit CYP3A4).

A. Cytochrome P450
    1. Introduction
        a. A group of heme-containing enzymes responsible for phase 1 metabolic reactions
        b. Characteristic absorbance of light at 450 nm (hence CYP450)
        c. Located primarily in the membranes of the smooth endoplasmic reticulum in liver; small intestine; and brain, lung, and kidney
        d. Encoded by a supergene family and subfamily; separate genes code for different isoenzymes
        e. Drugs generally have a high affinity for one particular CYP, but most drugs also have secondary pathways.
        f. Nomenclature

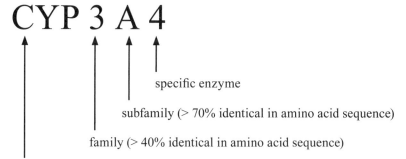

Figure 1. Nomenclature.

2. Distribution of CYP isoenzymes in human liver

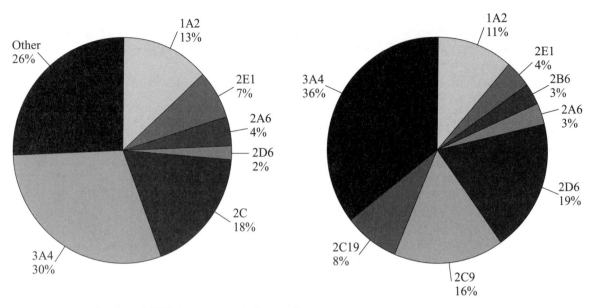

Figure 2. Distribution of CYP isoenzymes in human liver.

3. Distribution of CYP isoenzymes in human GI tract

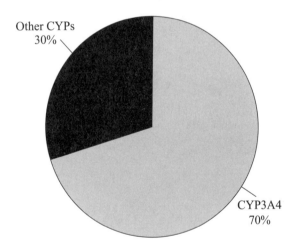

Figure 3. Distribution of CYP isoenzymes in human gastrointestinal tract.

3. Characteristics of CYP metabolism
   a. Inhibition is substrate-independent.
   b. Some substrates are metabolized by more than one CYP (e.g., tricyclic antidepressants [TCAs], selective serotonin reuptake inhibitors [SSRIs]).
   c. Enantiomers may be metabolized by a different CYP (e.g., R- vs. S-warfarin).
   d. Differences in inhibition may exist in the same class of agents (e.g., fluoroquinolones, azole anti-fungals, macrolides, calcium channel blockers, histamine-2 blockers).
   e. Substrates can also be inhibitors (e.g., erythromycin, verapamil, diltiazem).

    f.   Most inducers and some inhibitors can affect more than one isozyme (e.g., cimetidine, ritonavir, fluoxetine, erythromycin).

    g.   Inhibitors may affect different isozymes at different dosages (e.g., fluconazole inhibits CYP2C9 at dosages of 100 mg/day or greater and inhibits CYP3A4 at dosages of 400 mg/day or greater).

B. P-Glycoprotein

    1.   P-glycoprotein is an efflux pump that pumps drugs into the bile; the clinical effect of P-glycoprotein drug interactions in the bile is unknown.

    2.   P-glycoprotein pumps drugs from renal tubules into the urine; it also potentially limits the degree of reabsorption.

    3.   Examples of drug interactions: quinidine/digoxin, cyclosporine/digoxin, and propafenone/digoxin

C. Pharmacogenomics and Pharmacogenetics

    1.   Population in general is divided into poor, intermediate, extensive, and ultrarapid metabolizers; therefore, metabolism is considered polymorphic.

    2.   Definition of polymorphism: Coexistence of more than one genetic variant (alleles), which are stable components in the population (more than 1% of population)

    3.   Clear antimode results

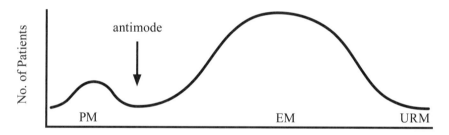

Metabolic ratio of metabolite to unchanged drug → (increasing metabolic capacity)

Figure 4. Distribution of patients in a drug that follows polymorphic metabolism.
EM = extensive metabolizer; PM = poor metabolizer; URM = ultrarapid metabolizer.

    4.   Phenotype: Expression of the trait; interaction of gene with environment

        a.   Manifestation of the trait clinically

        b.   Not necessarily constant

    5.   Genotype: Genetic makeup

Table 5. Pharmacogenetics in drug metabolism, drug transport, drug target, and adverse drug reactions.

Type	Enzyme/Target	Most Common Variant Alleles	Drug Examples
Drug metabolism	CYP2C9	CYP2C9*2 (70%–90% activity) CYP2C9*3 (10%–30% activity)	NSAIDs Phenytoin Warfarin
Drug metabolism	CYP2C19	CYP2C19*2 (poor) CYP2C19*3 (poor) CYP2C19*17 (ultrarapid) CYP2C19*4 (null variant)	Clopidogrel Diazepam Omeprazole SSRIs Tricyclic antidepressants Voriconazole
Drug metabolism	CYP2D6	CYP2D6*10 (poor) CYP2D6*17 (poor) CYP2D6*3, *4, and *5 (null)	Antiarrhythmics Antipsychotics Beta blockers Codeine, hydrocodone, oxycodone Dextromethorphan SSRIs Tamoxifen Tramadol Tricyclic antidepressants
Drug metabolism	UDP-glucuronosyltransferases	UGT1A1*6 UGT1A1*28 UGT2B7*2 UGT2B7*28	Atazanavir Irinotecan Mycophenolate NSAIDs
Drug metabolism	N-acetyltransferase	NAT2*4 NAT2*5 NAT2*6 NAT2*7	Hydralazine Isoniazid Sulfasalazine
Drug transport	SLCO1B1	SLCO1B1*1A,*1B SLCO1B1*5, *15, *17	Simvastatin
Drug target	VKOR	VKORC1*2 (increases) VKORC1*3 (decreases)	Warfarin
Adverse drug reactions	HLA-B	HLA-B*5701	Abacavir
		HLA-B*5801	Allopurinol
		HLA-B*1502	Carbamazepine, phenytoin

CYP = cytochrome P450; NSAIDs = nonsteroidal anti-inflammatory drugs; SSRIs = selective serotonin reuptake inhibitors.

6. Clinical Pharmacogenetics Implementation Consortium (CPIC)
    a. Designed to facilitate translation of pharmacogenetics information from research to clinical practice
    b. Developing guidelines for use of pharmacogenetic test results in drug dosing
    c. Focused on specific drug-gene pairs (Table 6)

Table 6. CPIC Clinical Recommendations for Drug-Gene Pairs

Drug	Gene	Recommendation
Abacavir	*HLA-B*	Avoid using because of increased incidence of hypersensitivity reactions in patients with the *HLA-B*57:01* allele
Allopurinol	*HLA-B*	Severe cutaneous adverse reactions associated with carriers of the *HLA-B*58:01* allele Avoid using allopurinol in these patients
Atazanavir	*UGT1A1*	For patients who carry 2 decreased function UGT1A1 alleles, increased risk of jaundice and subsequent nonadherence Consider alternative agents
Capecitabine/5-fluorouracil/tegafur	*DPYD*	Increased risk of serious or fatal toxicity in patients with reduced or absent dihydropyrimidine dehydrogenase activity
Carbamazepine	*HLA-B*	Avoid using because of increased incidence of severe cutaneous adverse reactions in patients with the *HLA-B*15:02* allele
Clopidogrel	*CYP2C19*	Normal dosing for ultrarapid metabolizer; alternative antiplatelet therapy in intermediate or poor metabolizers
Codeine	*CYP2D6*	Avoid using codeine because of potential toxicity or lack of efficacy in ultrarapid and poor metabolizers Specific dosing recommendations for extensive and intermediate metabolizers
Ivacaftor	*CFTR*	Recommended only for cystic fibrosis patients who are either homozygous or heterozygous for the *G551D-CFTR* variant
Peginterferon	*IFNL3*	Patients with the favorable response *IFNL3* genotype (rs12979860 CC) have greater likelihood of response to Peginterferon alpha–containing regimens
Phenytoin	*HLA-B*	Reduce initial dosage by 25% in CYP2C9 in intermediate metabolizers and 50% in poor metabolizers Severe cutaneous adverse reactions associated with carriers of the *HLA-B*58:01* allele Use an alternative anticonvulsant
Rasburicase	*G6PD*	Contraindicated in those with G6PD deficiency
Simvastatin	*SLCO1B1*	Dosing recommendations based on genotype at rs4149056 in *SLCO1B1,* including starting at lower dosages or using alternative statins
SSRIs Citalopram: 2C19 Escitalopram: 2C19 Sertraline: 2C19 Fluvoxamine: 2D6 Paroxetine: 2D6	CYP2D6, CYP2C19	Alternative drug not predominantly metabolized by CYP2C19 for CYP2C19 ultrarapid metabolizers and for CYP2C19 poor metabolizers, consider a 50% reduction of recommended starting dosage For CYP2D6 poor metabolizers, consider a 25%–50% reduction of recommended starting dosage
Tacrolimus	*CYP3A5*	Increase starting dosage by 1.5 to 2 times in CYP3A5 intermediate or extensive metabolizers (not to exceed 0.3 mg/kg/day)
Thiopurines (azathioprine, 6-mercaptopurine, thioguanine)	*TMPT*	Dosing recommendations for each drug based on *TMPT* genotype (normal/high, intermediate, and low activity)
Tricyclic antidepressants	CYP2D6, CYP2C19	Dosing recommendations for depression based on metabolizer status (ultrarapid, extensive, intermediate, poor) Limited recommendations when using for peripheral neuropathy

Table 6. CPIC Clinical Recommendations for Drug-Gene Pairs *(continued)*

Drug	Gene	Recommendation
Warfarin	VKORC1/ CYP2C9	Use available table or algorithms to initiate warfarin dosing based on *VKORC1* and *CYP2C9* genotypes
Irinotecan	*UGT1A1*	TBA
Oxycodone/tramadol	*CYP2D6*	TBA
Aripiprazole/risperidone	*CYP2D6*	TBA
Atomoxetine	*CYP2D6*	TBA
Ondansetron	*CYP2D6*	TBA
Celecoxib	*CYP2C9*	TBA
Fluoroquinolones	*G6PD*	TBA
Dapsone	*G6PD*	TBA
Trimethoprim/sulfamethoxazole	*G6PD*	TBA
Sulfasalazine	*G6PD*	TBA
Proton pump inhibitors	*CYP2C19*	TBA
Mirtazapine/venlafaxine	*CYP2D6*	TBA
Tamoxifen	*CYP2D6*	TBA
Voriconazole	*CYP2C19*	TBA

TBA = recommendations to be announced.

V. NONLINEAR PHARMACOKINETICS

Patient Case

6. C.M. is a 55-year-old man who is initiated on phenytoin after a craniotomy. His current steady-state phenytoin concentration is 6 mg/L at a dosage of 200 mg/day by mouth. If his affinity constant (Km) is calculated to be 5 mg/L, which is most likely to occur if the dosage is doubled (to 400 mg/day by mouth)?

   A. His concentration will double because phenytoin clearance is linear above the Km.

   B. His concentration will more than double because phenytoin clearance is nonlinear above the Km.

   C. His concentration will stay the same because phenytoin is an autoinducer, and clearance increases with time.

   D. His concentration will increase by only 50% because phenytoin absorption decreases significantly with dosages greater than 300 mg.

A. Michaelis-Menten Pharmacokinetics

$$velocity = \frac{V_{max} * S}{K_m + S}$$

V_{max} = capacity constant (amount/time)

K_m = affinity constant (amount/volume)

S = substrate concentration (amount/volume)

B. Nonlinear Elimination
   1. Saturation or partial saturation of the elimination pathway

$$\text{rate of elimination (dose)} = \frac{V_{max} * C}{K_m + C}$$

   V_{max} = maximum rate of elimination (amount/time)
   K_m = concentration where elimination is ½ V_{max} (affinity constant)
   C = drug concentration

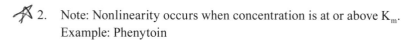

   2. Note: Nonlinearity occurs when concentration is at or above K_m.
      Example: Phenytoin
      a. V_{max} normal = 7 mg/kg/day
      b. K_m normal = 5.6 mg/L
      c. 50% variability between individuals

VI. NONCOMPARTMENTAL PHARMACOKINETICS

A. Why Noncompartmental Pharmacokinetics?
   1. Identification of the "correct" model is often impossible.
   2. A compartmental view of the body is unrealistic.
   3. Linear regression is unnecessary; it is easier to automate analysis.
   4. Requires fewer and less stringent assumptions
   5. More general methods and equations
   6. There is no need to match all data sets to the same compartmental model.

B. Definitions
   1. Zero moment concentration versus time curve
      • Area under the curve (AUC)

$$AUC = \sum \frac{(C_{n+1} + Cn)}{2} * (t_{n+1} - tn)... + \frac{C_{last}}{k}$$

   2. First moment concentration * time versus time curve
      • Area under the first moment curve (AUMC)

$$AUMC = \sum \frac{(C_{n+1} * t_{n+1} + C_n * t_n)}{2} * (t_{n+1} - tn)... + \frac{C_{last} * t_{last}}{k} + \frac{C_{last}}{k^2}$$

   3. Mean residence time (MRT)

$$MRT = \frac{AUMC}{AUC}$$

   4. Mean absorption time (MAT)

$$MAT = MRT_{ev} - MRT_{iv}$$

C. Pharmacokinetic Parameter Estimation

1. Clearance

$$\text{Clearance} = \frac{\text{dose}}{\text{AUC}}$$

2. Vd at steady state

$$V_{ss} = \frac{\text{dose} * \text{AUMC}}{\text{AUC}^2}$$

3. Elimination rate constant

$$k = \frac{1}{\text{MRT}}$$

4. Absorption rate constant

$$k_a = \frac{1}{\text{MAT}}$$

5. Bioavailability

$$F = \frac{D_{iv} * \text{AUC}_{ev}}{D_{ev} * \text{AUC}_{iv}}$$

VII. DATA COLLECTION AND ANALYSIS

Patient Case

7. R.K. is a 54-year-old woman with a history of diabetes mellitus and end-stage renal disease. She is receiving gentamicin for *P. aeruginosa* pneumonia. A gentamicin concentration is ordered after dialysis. Which is the best approach to obtaining this sample?

   A. Obtain the concentration immediately after hemodialysis.

   B. Wait a few hours to obtain the concentration because it will decrease significantly within the first few hours after hemodialysis.

   C. Wait a few hours to obtain the concentration because it will increase significantly within the first few hours after hemodialysis.

   D. Wait until the next day so that all the effects of hemodialysis will have abated.

A. Timing of Collection
1. Ensure completion of absorption and distribution phases (especially digoxin [8–12 hours] and amino-glycosides [30 minutes after infusion]).
2. Ensure completion of redistribution after dialysis (especially aminoglycosides [3–4 hours after hemodialysis]).

B. Specimen Requirements
1. Whole blood: Use anticoagulated tube. Examples: cyclosporine, amiodarone
2. Plasma: Use anticoagulated tube and centrifuge; clotting proteins and some blood cells are maintained.
3. Serum: Use red top tube, allow to clot, and centrifuge. Examples: most analyzed drugs including aminoglycosides, vancomycin, phenytoin, and digoxin

---

Patient Case

8. A drug assay is touted as having high specificity but low sensitivity. Which statement best describes what this means?
   A. The assay will not be able to distinguish the drug from like products, but it will be able to detect extremely low concentrations.
   B. The assay will not be able to distinguish the drug from like products, and it will not be able to detect extremely low concentrations.
   C. The assay will be able to distinguish the drug from like products and will be able to detect extremely low concentrations.
   D. The assay will be able to distinguish the drug from like products but will not be able to detect extremely low concentrations.

C. Assay Terminology
1. Precision (reproducibility): Closeness of agreement between the results of repeated analyses performed on the same sample
   a. Standard deviation (SD): Average difference of the individual values from the mean
   b. Coefficient of variation (CV): SD as a percentage of the mean (relative rather than absolute variation)

$$CV = \frac{SD}{Mean}$$

2. Accuracy: Closeness with which a measurement reflects the true value of an object
   • Correlation coefficient: Strength of the relationship between two variables
3. Predictive performance (measure of accuracy): Precision, expressed as the root mean squared error (RMSE)

$$MSE = \frac{1}{N}\sum_{i=1}^{N} pe_i^2 \qquad RMSE = \sqrt{mse}$$

Bias: a.k.a. mean prediction error (ME)

$$ME = \frac{1}{N}\sum_{i=1}^{N} pe_i$$

• Prediction error (*pe*) is the prediction minus the true value.

4. Sensitivity: Ability of an assay to quantitate low drug concentrations accurately; usually the lowest concentration an assay can differentiate from zero

5. Specificity (cross-reactivity): Ability of an assay to differentiate the drug in question from like substances

D. Assay Methods
   1. Immunoassays
      a. Radioimmunoassay
         i. Advantages: Extremely sensitive (picogram range)
         ii. Disadvantages: Radioimmunoassay kits have limited shelf life because of the short half-life of labels, radioactive waste, and cross-reactivity.
            • Clinical use for assaying digoxin and cyclosporine
      b. Enzyme immunoassay, e.g., enzyme multiplied immunoassay technique
         i. Advantages: Simple, automated, highly sensitive, inexpensive and stable reagents, inexpensive and widely available equipment, no radiation hazards
         ii. Disadvantages: Measuring enzyme activity more complex than radioisotopes, enzyme activity may be affected by plasma constituents, less sensitive than radioimmunoassays
      c. Fluorescence immunoassay: TDx (e.g., fluorescence polarization immunoassay): Most common therapeutic drug monitoring assay
         i. Advantages: Simple, automated, highly sensitive, inexpensive and stable reagents, inexpensive and widely available equipment, no radiation hazards
         ii. Disadvantages: Background interference attributable to endogenous serum fluorescence
   2. Assays used primarily in pharmacokinetic research studies
      a. High-pressure liquid chromatography
      b. Gas chromatography–mass spectrometry and liquid chromatography–mass spectrometry
      c. Flame photometry
      d. Bioassay

E. Population Pharmacokinetics in Therapeutic Drug Monitoring
   1. Population pharmacokinetics useful when
      a. Drug concentrations are obtained during complicated dosing regimens.
      b. Drug concentrations are obtained before steady state.
      c. Only a few drug concentrations are feasibly obtained (limited sampling strategy).
   2. Bayesian pharmacokinetics
      a. Prior population information is combined with patient-specific data to predict the most probable individual parameters.
      b. When patient-specific data are limited, there is greater influence from population parameters; when patient-specific data are extensive, there is less influence.
      c. With a small amount of individual data, Bayesian forecasting generally yields more precise results.

Patient Cases

9. K.M., an 80-year-old white woman (52 kg, 64 inches), is admitted to the hospital for pyelonephritis with sepsis. She has a history of myocardial infarction × 2, congestive heart failure, hypertension, osteoporosis, rheumatoid arthritis, and cerebrovascular accident. On admission, her BUN is 25 mg/dL, SCr is 0.92 mg/dL, and Alb is 2.9 g/dL. K.M. is initiated on the following drugs: trimethoprim/sulfamethoxazole intravenously, 240 mg of trimethoprim every 12 hours, lisinopril 10 mg/day by mouth, digoxin 0.125 mg/day by mouth, furosemide 40 mg/day by mouth, cimetidine 400 mg by mouth two times/day, acetaminophen 650 mg by mouth every 6 hours, calcium carbonate 500 mg by mouth three times/day, and carvedilol 6.25 mg by mouth two times/day. Which is the best assessment of K.M.'s renal function?

    A. Her SCr is in the normal range, and no dosage adjustments are necessary.

    B. Because of her age, K.M. will have some degree of renal dysfunction, and dosages may need to be adjusted.

    C. Because of the pyelonephritis, K.M. will have renal dysfunction, and dosages may need to be adjusted.

    D. Her SCr is in the normal range but her BUN is elevated, so dosages may need to be adjusted.

10. Which of K.M.'s drug combinations is most likely to alter her SCr concentrations?

    A. 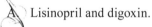 Lisinopril and digoxin.

    B. Trimethoprim/sulfamethoxazole and cimetidine.

    C. Furosemide and calcium carbonate.

    D. Acetaminophen and carvedilol.

VIII. PHARMACOKINETICS IN RENAL DISEASE

A. Estimation of Kidney Function Through Glomerular Filtration Rate (GFR) and Creatinine Clearance
    1. Creatinine production and elimination
        a. Creatine is produced in the liver.
        b. Creatinine is the product of creatine metabolism in skeletal muscle, formed at a constant rate for any one person.
        c. Creatinine is filtered at the glomerulus, where it undergoes limited secretion.
        d. CrCl is useful in approximating GFR because
            i.   At normal concentrations of creatinine, secretion is low.
            ii. The creatinine assay picks up a noncreatinine chromogen in the blood but not in the urine.

    2. CrCl calculation to estimate GFR

        •   CrCl is calculated from a 24-hour urine collection and the following equation:

$$\text{CrCl (mL/minute/1.73 m}^2) = \frac{\text{volume of urine/1440 minutes} \times \text{urine creatinine concentration}}{\text{serum creatinine concentration}}$$

        •   Normal CrCl
            Healthy young men = 125 mL/minute/1.73 m^2
            Healthy young women = 115 mL/minute/1.73 m^2

        •   After age 30, 1% of GFR is lost per year.

---

3. CrCl estimation to estimate GFR
   a. Factors affecting SCr concentrations
      i. Sex
      ii. Age
      iii. Weight/muscle mass
      iv. Renal function. Caveats: CrCl estimations worsen as renal function worsens (usually an overestimation).
   b. Jeliffe

$$\text{CrCl (mL/minute/1.73 m}^2) = \frac{98 - 0.8 \, (\text{age} - 20)}{\text{SCr}}$$

Women: Use 90% of the above equation.

- Limitations:
  SCr concentration must be stable.
  Adults 20–80 years of age
  Controversy: Rounding up SCr in patients with low concentrations (less than 0.7–1 mg/dL)

   c. Cockcroft-Gault

$$\text{CrCl(mL/min)} = \frac{(140 - \text{Age}) * (\text{weight})}{72 * \text{Scr}}$$

Women: Use 85% of the above equation.

- For "weight": Use actual body weight (ABW) in patients with body mass index (BMI) less than 18.5 kg/m2, ideal body weight (IBW) in patients with BMI 18.5–25 kg/m2, and IBW plus 40% of (ABW – IBW) in patients with BMI greater than 25 kg/m2.

  IBW (men) = 50 kg + 2.3 kg for each inch over 5 feet
  IBW (women) = 45.5 kg + 2.3 kg for each inch over 5 feet

- Generally recommended when making drug dosage adjustments in patients with renal dysfunction, because package insert recommendations generally use this formula to estimate creatinine clearance, and the use of the Modification of Diet in Renal Disease (MDRD) and Chronic Kidney Disease Epidemiology Collaboration (CKD-Epi) equations to make dosing adjustments has not been validated.

- Limitations
  SCr concentration must be stable. Developed for adults only
  Not corrected for creatinine standardization (results in lower estimations)
  Controversy: Rounding up SCr in patients with low concentrations (less than 0.7–1 mg/dL)
  Not developed in patients with obesity (see weight recommendations above)

d. MDRD study equation
Full equation

$$\text{GFR (mL/minute/1.73 m}^2\text{)} = 161.5 * (\text{SCr})^{-0.999} * (\text{age in years})^{-0.176} * 1.180 \text{ (if patient is African American)} * 0.762 \text{ (if patient is a woman)} * (\text{BUN})^{-0.170} * (\text{Alb})^{+0.318}$$

Simplified four-variable equation

$$\text{GFR (mL/minute/1.73 m}^2\text{)} = 175 * (\text{SCr})^{-1.154} * (\text{age in years})^{-0.203} * 1.212 \text{ (if patient is African American)} * 0.742 \text{ (if patient is a woman)}$$

   i. These equations directly estimate GFR (not CrCl) and were developed using standardized creatinine concentrations to stage kidney function.
   ii. These equations are recommended by the American Kidney Foundation and the European Renal Association to estimate renal function.
   iii. Not as accurate when GFR is greater than 60 mL/minute/1.73 m2
   iv. If used for drug dosing, convert value from milliliters per minute per 1.73 m2 to milliliters per minute.
   v. If used for drug dosing and significantly different from Cockcroft-Gault, use clinical judgment and optimize risk versus benefit.

e. CKD-Epi equation (Table 7)
   i. These equations directly estimate GFR (not CrCl).
   ii. These equations are more accurate than MDRD at higher GFRs (i.e., greater than 60 mL/minute/1.73 m2).

Table 7. Chronic Kidney Disease Epidemiology Collaboration Equation

Race and Sex	Serum Creatinine (mg/dL)	Equation
African American		
Female	<0.7	GFR = 166 * (SCr/0.7) – 0.329 * (0.993) Age
	>0.7	GFR = 166 * (SCr/0.7) – 1.209 * (0.993) Age
Male	<0.9	GFR = 163 * (SCr/0.9) – 0.411 * (0.993) Age
	>0.9	GFR = 163 * (SCr/0.9) – 1.209 * (0.993) Age
White or other		
Female	<0.7	GFR = 144 * (SCr/0.7) – 0.329 * (0.993) Age
	>0.7	GFR = 144 * (SCr/0.7) – 1.209 * (0.993) Age
Male	<0.9	GFR = 141 * (SCr/0.9) – 0.411 * (0.993) Age
	>0.9	GFR = 141 * (SCr/0.9) – 1.209 * (0.993) Age

GFR = glomerular filtration rate; SCr = serum creatinine.

f. Pediatric formulas (Table 8). Do not round up low SCr values in pediatric patients.

Schwartz:
$$\text{GFR (mL/minute/1.73 m}^2\text{)} = \frac{K * \text{ht (cm)}}{\text{SCr}}$$

Table 8. Schwartz Equation Constants

Age	K
Low birth weight ≤1 year	0.33
Full term ≤1 year	0.45
1–13 years	0.55
13- to 18-year-old adolescent girl	0.55
13- to 18-year-old adolescent boy	0.7

Note: $K = 0.413$ for 1–13 years old and 13- to 18-year-old adolescent girls when using standardized creatinine concentrations (other K values have not been updated); this is known as the bedside Chronic Kidney Disease in Children (CKiD) equation.

Counahan-Barratt:

$$\text{GFR (mL/minute/1.73 m}^2) = \frac{0.43 * \text{ht (cm)}}{\text{SCr}}$$

4. Factors influencing CrCl estimates
   a. Patient characteristics
      i. Age (↓ production of creatinine with age)
      ii. Female sex (↓ production of creatinine)
      iii. Race (↑ production of creatinine in African Americans)
   b. Disease states and clinical conditions
      i. Spinal cord injuries (↓ muscle mass; ↓ creatinine)
      ii. Amputations (↓ muscle mass; ↓ creatinine)
      iii. Cushing syndrome (↓ muscle mass; ↓ creatinine)
      iv. Muscular dystrophy (↓ muscle mass; ↓ creatinine)
      v. Guillain-Barré syndrome (↓ muscle mass; ↓ creatinine)
      vi. Rheumatoid arthritis (↓ muscle mass; ↓ creatinine)
      vii. Liver disease (↓ creatine; ↓ creatinine)
      viii. Glomerulopathic disease (greater amount of creatinine secretion in relation to filtration)
      ix. Hydration status (dehydration vs. fluid overload)
   c. Diet
      i. High-meat protein diets (↑ creatinine ingestion)
      ii. Vegetarians (↓ creatinine ingestion)
      iii. Protein calorie malnutrition (↓ creatinine ingestion)
   d. Drugs and endogenous substances
      i. Laboratory interaction: Kinetic alkaline picrate method
         (a) Noncreatinine chromogens: In blood but not in urine
         (b) Cephalosporins (especially cefoxitin): Chromogenic, causing false elevations that are much greater in urine than in blood
         (c) Acetoacetate (elevated in fasting patients, patients with diabetic ketoacidosis): Chromogenic, causing false elevations
      ii. Pharmacokinetic interaction: Drugs compete with creatinine for renal secretion (causing false elevations), cobicistat, trimethoprim, cimetidine, fibric acid derivatives (other than gemfibrozil), and dronedarone.

B. Drug Dosing in Renal Disease
   1. Loading dose
      a. In general, no alteration is necessary, but it should be given to hasten the achievement of therapeutic drug concentrations.
      b. Alterations in loading dose must occur if the Vd is altered secondary to renal dysfunction. Example: digoxin
   2. Maintenance dosage: Alterations should be made in either the dosage or the dosing interval.
      a. Changing the dosing interval
         i. Use when the goal is to achieve similar steady-state concentrations.
         ii. Less costly
         iii. Ideal for limited-dosage forms (i.e., oral medications)
      b. Changing the dosage
         i. Use when the goal is to maintain a steady therapeutic concentration.
         ii. More costly
      c. Changing the dosage and the dosing interval
         i. Often necessary for substantial dosage adjustment with limited-dosage forms
         ii. Often necessary for narrow therapeutic index drugs with target concentrations
            (a) If a drug is given more than once daily, then adjust the interval.
            (b) If a drug is given once daily or less often, then adjust the dosage.

Patient Case

11. S.J. is a 55-year-old man with hepatic dysfunction and fungemia caused by *Candida krusei*. He has a small amount of ascites but is not encephalopathic. He is initiated on caspofungin, and the package insert states that dosages should be decreased in patients with a Child-Pugh score of 7–9. If he has the following hepatic laboratory values, which best estimates his Child-Pugh score?

Aspartate transaminase = 85 U/L, alanine transaminase = 56 U/L, alkaline phosphatase = 190 U/L, total bilirubin = 1.8 mg/dL, Alb = 2.9 g/dL, lactic dehydrogenase = 270 U/L, prothrombin time/international normalized ratio = 14.6/1.7, γ-glutamyl transferase = 60 U/L

A. 3.

B. 5.

C. 8.

D. 11.

IX. PHARMACOKINETICS IN HEPATIC DISEASE

A. Dosage Adjustment in Hepatic Disease
   1. Clinical response is the most important factor in adjusting dosages in hepatic disease.
   2. Low–hepatic extraction ratio drugs
      a. Adjustment of maintenance dosage is necessary only when hepatic disease alters the intrinsic clearance (Cl_{int})
      b. Alterations in protein binding alone do not require alteration of maintenance dosage, even though total drug concentrations decline.
      c. Loading doses may require reduction.
      d. Examples: carbamazepine, diazepam, phenytoin, warfarin

3. High–hepatic extraction ratio drugs
   a. Intravenous administration
      i. Usually necessary to decrease maintenance dose rate as hepatic blood flow changes
      ii. Consider effect of hepatic disease on protein binding as it alters free concentrations.
   b. Oral administration: Similar to low–hepatic extraction ratio drugs; necessary to decrease mainte-nance dose rate when hepatic disease alters Cl_{int}
   c. Examples: haloperidol, morphine, metoprolol, propranolol, verapamil

B. Rules for Dosing in Hepatic Disease
   1. Hepatic elimination of high–extraction ratio drugs is more consistently affected by liver disease than hepatic elimination of low–extraction ratio drugs.
   2. The clearance of drugs that are exclusively conjugated is not substantially altered in liver disease.

Table 9. Child-Pugh Classification for Liver Disease

	Points		
	1	**2**	**3**
Encephalopathy	0	1 or 2	3 or 4
Ascites	0	+	++
Bilirubin (mg/dL)	<1.5	1.5–2.3	>2.3
Albumin (g/dL)	>3.5	2.8–3.5	<2.8
Prothrombin time (seconds over control)	0–4	4–6	>6

Pugh score: 5 = normal; 6 or 7 = mild (A); 8 or 9 = moderate (B); >9 = severe (C).

X. PHARMACODYNAMICS

Patient Case

12. Which is the most likely reason that a drug will follow clockwise hysteresis?
    A. Formation of an active metabolite.
    B. Delay in equilibrium between the blood and the site of action.
    C. Tolerance.
    D. Increased sensitivity with time.

A. Definition: Relationship Between Drug Concentrations and the Pharmacologic Response

B. Hill equation

$$E = \frac{E_{max} * C^y}{EC_{50}^{\ y} + C^y}$$

E = pharmacologic response
E_{max} = maximum drug effect
EC_{50} = concentration producing half of the maximum drug effect
γ = Hill coefficient that accommodates the shape of the curve

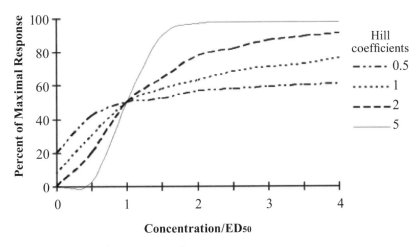

Figure 5. Concentration response plot.

    C.   Hysteresis Loops. Definition: Concentrations late after a dose produce an effect different from that produced by the same concentration soon after the dose.

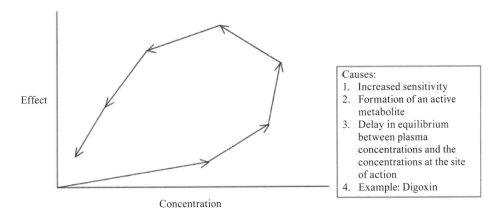

Figure 6. Counterclockwise hysteresis.

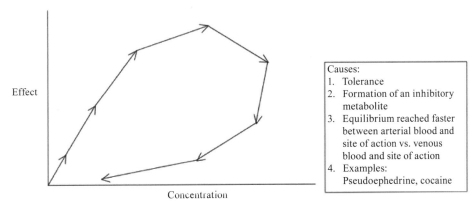

Figure 7. Clockwise hysteresis.

Patient Cases

13. P.L., a 45-year-old man with chronic renal failure, is receiving phenytoin 400 mg/day for a history of tonic-clonic seizures. His phenytoin concentration today is 13.6 mg/L, and his Alb concentration is 4.2 g/dL. Based on his current concentrations, which change should be recommended?
    A. Make no changes to his drug regimen.
    B. Keep the total daily dosage the same, but change the regimen to 200 mg two times/day.
    C. Increase the dosage for better seizure control.
    D. Decrease the dosage to prevent toxicity.

14. N.R. is a 63-year-old man with renal insufficiency who comes to the emergency department in atrial fibrillation with a ventricular rate of 120 beats/minute. Because of his history of ventricular dysfunction, it is decided to initiate him on digoxin for rate control. Which is the best dosing for this patient?
    A. The loading dose should remain the same, but the maintenance dose should be decreased.
    B. The loading dose should be decreased, and the maintenance dose should remain the same.
    C. Neither the loading dose nor the maintenance dose should be adjusted.
    D. Both the loading dose and the maintenance dose should be decrease.

15. P.P. is a 34-year-old man with a history of cerebral palsy and chronic urinary tract infections. He is admitted to the hospital with a *Pseudomonas* urinary tract infection that is resistant to all antibiotics except for aminoglycosides. He is initiated on once-daily tobramycin at 400 mg/day intravenously. Which statement best describes this high-dose, extended-interval aminoglycoside regimen?
    A. It takes advantage of the concentration-dependent killing of aminoglycoside.
    B. It is more efficacious than standard aminoglycoside dosing.
    C. It does not require the monitoring of aminoglycoside concentrations.
    D. It will not cause nephrotoxicity.

Table 10. Specific Drugs

Drug	Therapeutic Range	Sampling Issues	Comments
Aminoglycosides	Cp = 4–10 mg/L maximum Amikacin = 20–30 mg/L Cp < 2 mg/L minimum Amikacin < 10 mg/L	Duration of infusion, timing of first sample after infusion (generally should be ½–1 hour)	High-dose extended-interval ("once-daily") aminoglycoside dosing is generally recommended to decrease toxicity and improve efficacy These regimens are just as effective as traditional dosing, and meta-analyses have demonstrated less nephrotoxicity or no difference
Vancomycin	Cp = 10–15 mg/L minimum (15–20 mg/L for certain infections, including pneumonia, meningitis, and osteomyelitis)	Controversial whether to obtain peaks or concentrations altogether	Although the need for higher trough concentrations is suggested in complicated methicillin-resistant *Staphylococcus aureus* infections, those concentrations increase the risk of nephrotoxicity, with potentially limited improvement in efficacy
Phenytoin	10–20 mg/L Free: 1–2 mg/L	In general, obtain trough concentrations	Percentage free increases with renal failure and hypoalbuminemia Equations to correct: Changes in albumin: $$Cp = \frac{Cp'}{(0.9 * \frac{Alb}{4.4})} + 0.1$$ Renal failure: $$Cp = \frac{Cp'}{0.5}$$ Renal failure with change in albumin: $$Cp = \frac{Cp'}{(0.48 * 0.9 * \frac{Alb}{4.4}) + 0.1}$$ Induces liver enzymes; susceptible to metabolic drug interactions
Carbamazepine	4–12 mg/L		Autoinduction; active metabolite 10,11 epoxide
Phenobarbital	15–40 mg/L		Enzyme inducer
Valproic acid	50–100 mg/L		Saturable protein binding; percentage free increases with renal failure and hypoalbuminemia
Digoxin	0.8–2.0 mcg/L	Prolonged distribution period necessitates sampling >6–12 hours after dose	Volume of distribution decreases in renal disease; susceptible to drug interactions
Cyclosporine	100–250 mcg/L	Whole blood samples	Many drug interactions
Lithium	0.3–1.3 mmol/L	Prolonged distribution necessitates sampling 12 hours after dose	
Theophylline	10–20 mg/L		Treat as continuous infusion with sustained-release dosage forms

Cp = concentration of drug in plasma; Vd.

Table 11. Pharmacokinetic Term Definitions

AUC	Area under the curve
AUC_{ev}	Area under the curve after an extravascular dose
AUC_{iv}	Area under the curve after an intravenous dose
Cmax	Maximum concentration
Cmin	Minimum concentration
C_0	Concentration at time zero
C_{ss}	Concentration at steady state
$C_{ss\,avg}$	Average concentration at steady state
$C_{ss}\,max$	Maximum concentration at steady state
DoseEV	Dose given extravascularly
DoseIV	Dose given intravenously
F	Bioavailability
k	Elimination rate constant
R_0	Rate of infusion
τ	Dosing interval
t	Time of the infusion
ti	Time from initiation of the infusion
Vd	Volume of distribution

REFERENCES

1. Bauer LA. Applied Clinical Pharmacokinetics, 3rd ed. New York: McGraw-Hill Medical, 2014.

2. Bauer LA. Clinical pharmacokinetics and pharmacodynamics. In: DiPiro JT, Talbert RL, Yee GC, et al., eds. Pharmacotherapy: A Pathophysiologic Approach, 9th ed. New York: McGraw-Hill Medical, 2014:chap 5.

3. Burton ME, Shaw LM, Schentag JJ, eds. Applied Pharmacokinetics & Pharmacodynamics: Principles of Therapeutic Drug Monitoring, 4th ed. Baltimore: Lippincott Williams & Wilkins, 2006.

4. International Transporter Consortium. Membrane transporters in drug development. Nat Rev Drug Discov 2010;9:215-36.

5. Johnson JA. Pharmacogenetics in clinical practice: how far have we come and where are we going? Pharmacogenomics 2013;14:835-43.

6. Lee CK, Swinford RD, Cerda RD, et al. Evaluation of serum creatinine concentration–based glomerular filtration rate equations in pediatric patients with chronic kidney disease. Pharmacotherapy 2012;32:642-8.

7. Matheny CJ, Lamb MW, Brouwer KLR, et al. Pharmacokinetic and pharmacodynamic implications of P-glycoprotein modulation. Pharmacotherapy 2001;21:778-96.

8. Nyman HA, Dowling TC, Hudson JQ, et al. Comparative evaluation of the Cockcroft-Gault equation and the Modification of Diet in Renal Disease (MDRD) study equation for drug dosing: an opinion of the Nephrology Practice and Research Network of the American College of Clinical Pharmacy. Pharmacotherapy 2011;31:1130-44.

9. Winter ME. Basic Clinical Pharmacokinetics, 5th ed. Baltimore: Lippincott Williams & Wilkins, 2010.

ANSWERS AND EXPLANATIONS TO PATIENT CASES

1. Answer: C
In 6 days (2 half-lives), the concentration will decrease from 35.9 mg/L to about 9 mg/L; now is the time to redose. A 1-g dose given on March 24 will increase the concentration in the blood from 12.1 mg/L to 35.9 mg/L (12.1 + 23.8 mg/L). Given that the half-life is about 3 days, it will take longer than 1 day to reach a concentration of about 10 mg/L. In 3 days (1 half-life), the concentration will decrease from 35.9 mg/L to about 18 mg/L—still too early to redose. Redosing can be determined because plenty of information exists about how to calculate when to redose.

2. Answer: A
$F = (100 \text{ mg} * 25 \text{ mg/L/hour})/(200 \text{ mg} * 50 \text{ mg/L/hour})$.

3. Answer: C
The elimination rate constant equals (ln 6.5 mg/L − ln 5.4 mg/L)/12 hours = 0.015/hour. The concentration at the end of the infusion equals $6.5 \text{ mg/L/e} - (0.015 * 5)$ = 7 mg/L. The patient's Vd = dose/change in concentration is 160 mg/7 mg/L = 22.9 L. If you want a change in concentration from 1 mg/L to 9 mg/L (or 8 mg/L), then dose = 22.9 L * 8 mg/L = 183.2 mg. Therefore, a dose of 180 mg is appropriate.

4. Answer: D
P-glycoprotein is an efflux pump that pumps drugs back into the GI lumen. P-glycoprotein is not a plasma protein, and it does not transfer drugs through the GI mucosa; rather, it pumps drugs back into the GI lumen. In addition, P-glycoprotein acts in concert with CYP3A4 to diminish oral absorption.

5. Answer: C
Azithromycin does not inhibit CYP3A4. Erythromycin and clarithromycin are potent inhibitors of CYP3A4 and would be expected to increase cyclosporine concentrations. Cytochrome P450 inhibition is not a drug class effect.

6. Answer: B
By definition, clearance becomes nonlinear once the concentration exceeds the K_m; therefore, the concentrations will more than double. Phenytoin is not a significant autoinducer. Although phenytoin absorption decreases as the dosage is increased, it is not clinically significant until a single dose exceeds 400 mg.

7. Answer: C
The correct answer, because of redistribution, is to wait a few hours to obtain the concentration because it will increase significantly within the first few hours after hemodialysis. Waiting a full 24 hours is not necessary.

8. Answer: D
The correct answer is that the assay will be able to distinguish the drug from like products but will not be able to detect extremely low concentrations. High specificity means the assay can distinguish the drug from like products, and low sensitivity means the assay cannot detect extremely low concentrations.

9. Answer: B
Although her SCr is in the normal range, her renal function is decreased because of her age. After age 30, patients lose around 1 mL/minute/year of CrCl. Therefore, her CrCl needs to be calculated to assess drug dosing. Patients with pyelonephritis do not have a decrease in their renal function. Her elevated BUN is probably a sign of prerenal azotemia caused by dehydration associated with her infection. The BUN measurement is generally not used to assess renal function for drug dosing purposes.

10. Answer: B
Both trimethoprim/sulfamethoxazole and cimetidine compete with creatinine for secretion in the kidneys, increasing SCr concentrations. Although angiotensin-converting enzyme inhibitors may transiently increase SCr concentrations, digoxin does not affect renal function. Although furosemide may secondarily affect SCr concentrations, calcium carbonate does not affect renal function. Acetaminophen and carvedilol generally do not affect SCr concentrations.

11. Answer: C
This patient has 1 point for not being encephalopathic, 2 points for mild ascites, 2 points for the bilirubin concentration, 2 points for the Alb concentration, and 1 point for the prothrombin time value, for a total of 8 points. Normal patients have a Child-Pugh score of 5, which means no hepatic dysfunction.

12. Answer: C

Tolerance leads to a decrease in effect with time; this is clockwise hysteresis. The formation of an active metabolite, a delay in equilibrium between the blood and site of action, and the increased sensitivity with time would lead to an increase in effect with time; this is counterclockwise hysteresis.

13. Answer: D

The dosage should be decreased to prevent toxicity. In renal failure, acidic byproducts build up in the blood and compete with phenytoin for protein binding. Total concentrations must be corrected, and this correction leads to a doubling of the concentration. Therefore, the current concentration is too high, and the dosage should be decreased. Single doses of 400 mg are fine (doses higher than 400 mg should be divided).

14. Answer: D

Both the loading dose and the maintenance dose should be decreased. In general, loading doses need not be altered in renal dysfunction because they are dependent primarily on the Vd. However, the digoxin Vd is decreased in renal dysfunction. Because digoxin is eliminated renally, the maintenance dose should be decreased.

15. Answer: A

Aminoglycosides show concentration-dependent killing, and a high-dose, extended-interval aminoglycoside regimen takes advantage of this characteristic. However, it has not proved more efficacious than traditional dosing. Aminoglycoside concentrations still need to be monitored with high-dose, extended-interval therapy. In addition, high-dose, extended-interval aminoglycoside dosing can still cause nephrotoxicity (although the incidence is generally diminished).

ANSWERS AND EXPLANATIONS TO SELF-ASSESSMENT QUESTIONS

1. Answer: B
With two concentrations, there are enough data to calculate an elimination rate constant and, therefore, a half-life. In addition, the Vd can be calculated by back extrapolation to the Cmax and use of appropriate equations (because this was the first dose, and therefore it is known that the tobramycin concentration was 0 mg/L before the dose was given).

2. Answer: A
The elimination rate constant equals (ln 3.6 mg/L − ln 0.9 mg/L)/4 hours = 0.35/hour. The half-life is 0.693/0.35 = 2 hours. The concentration at the end of the infusion equals 3.6 mg/L/e − (0.35 * 1) = 5.1 mg/L. The patient's Vd = dose/change in concentration, or 110 mg/5.1 mg/L = 21.5 L.

3. Answer: B
Her clearance increased because of the improvement in renal function, which increased her elimination rate constant and decreased her half-life. The Vd would not be altered by changes in clearance (they are independent). With the diuresis and angiotensin-converting enzyme inhibitor, her Vd probably decreased, but clearance would not be altered by changes in Vd (they are independent). In addition, if her Vd decreased, her half-life would decrease, not increase.

4. Answer: C
Because the trough is too low, the interval will have to be shortened to increase the concentration. Changes in dosage will have the greatest effect on the peak concentration, and changes in interval will have the greatest effect on the trough concentration.

5. Answer: B
10To achieve flucytosine peak concentrations between 50 and 100 mcg/mL (assuming a trough concentration of 25 mcg/mL, dosing every 6 hours, and 100% bioavailability; flucytosine volume of distribution of 0.7 L/kg; half-life of 3 hours), the concentration must be changed by 25–75 mcg/mL. Using the equation ΔCp = dose/V, a dosage of 12.5 mg/kg would increase the concentration by only 17.8 mcg/mL. A dosage of 75 mg/kg would increase the concentration by 107 mcg/mL, whereas a dosage of 150 mg/kg would increase the concentration by 214 mcg/mL. The correct dosage is 37.5 mg/kg because it would increase the concentration by 53.6 mcg/mL.

6. Answer: D
Because of the patient's renal failure and low Alb, the total concentration must be corrected. The patient's corrected phenytoin concentration is 14.7 mcg/mL. Therefore, no changes should be made to the dosage.

7. Answer: C
Both of these are immunoassays. A brand name for the Abbott fluorescence polarization immunoassay is TDx, which uses a fluorescent label. The term *EMIT* stands for *enzyme multiplied immunoassay technique,* which is an immunoassay that uses an enzyme label.

8. Answer: D
The digoxin concentration was drawn too close to the 8:00 a.m. dose. The digoxin had not yet had a chance to complete its distribution phase. Once distribution is complete (generally 6–12 hours after the dose), the concentration will be lower and probably within the therapeutic range. Therefore, there is no need for the digoxin antibody, activated charcoal, or lowering of the dosage.

9. Answer: C
The correct statistical test is multiple regression. Multiple regression is used to describe the relationship between a dependent variable and two or more independent variables when both the dependent and independent variables are numeric. Analysis of variance is used to describe the relationship between a dependent variable and two or more independent variables when the dependent variable is numeric and the independent variables are nominal. Likewise, analysis of covariance is used to describe the relationship between a dependent variable and two or more independent variables when the dependent variable is numeric and the independent variables are nominal with confounding factors. Spearman rank correlation is a nonparametric test used to describe the relationship between one dependent and one independent variable when the data are ordinal or numeric and not normally distributed.

10. Answer: B

Assessing adherence and increasing her dosage, because the concentration is below the therapeutic range, is the correct answer. The valproic acid therapeutic range is 50–100 mg/L, and she is well below this concentration. Although some patients are controlled at lower concentrations, this concentration is probably too low. She definitely does not need a decrease in dosage. Although total valproic acid concentrations are affected by changes in Alb, her Alb is normal, and obtaining a free concentration is unnecessary.

11. Answer: B

Codeine's activity is due primarily to its metabolism to morphine by CYP2D6 after administration. Because this patient is a CYP2D6 poor metabolizer, less of the codeine will be metabolized to its active metabolite. Omeprazole does inhibit CYP2C19, but this enzyme does not metabolize codeine. Metoprolol is a substrate of CYP2D6 but is not an inhibitor or inducer of CYP2C9.

12. Answer: D

MDRD and CKD-Epi are actually better estimates of renal function, because they directly estimate GFR instead of creatinine clearance. Although the Cockcroft and Gault equation was developed in hospitalized patients and the MDRD and CKD-Epi equations were developed in ambulatory patients, this does not affect the setting where they can be used. Also, although the equations do have different units (mL/minute vs. mL/minute/1.73 m^2) this can easily be corrected by converting the result of the MDRD or CKD-Epi equation to mL/minute. The best reason for not using MDRD or CKD-Epi for drug dosing is that renal dosing adjustment recommendations that are published in package inserts are almost always based on creatinine clearance estimates using the Cockcroft and Gault equation.

13. Answer: A

Assays with low sensitivity will not be able to detect low drug concentrations, which may still be therapeutic. Assays that cannot differentiate between like substances have low specificity. Assays that report highly variable values when repeatedly run on the same sample have low precision. Assays that consistently over- or under-measure the true concentration have low accuracy.

Pulmonary Disorders, Gout, and Adult Immunizations

Ila M. Harris, Pharm.D., FCCP, BCPS

University of Minnesota
Minneapolis, Minnesota

PULMONARY DISORDERS, GOUT, AND ADULT IMMUNIZATIONS

ILA M. HARRIS, PHARM.D., FCCP, BCPS

UNIVERSITY OF MINNESOTA
MINNEAPOLIS, MINNESOTA

Learning Objectives

1. Accurately classify patients, assess control, and select and monitor appropriate acute and preventive treatments for pediatric and adult patients with asthma and for adult patients with chronic obstructive pulmonary disease, incorporating patient-specific factors.
2. Appropriately assess, classify, and select pharmacotherapy (acute and chronic, including nonpharmacologic therapy), and monitor, reassess, and adjust pharmacotherapy in patients with gout.
3. Determine appropriate immunizations for an adult given his or her age and medical conditions and correctly apply cautions, contraindications, and drug interactions with immunizations to adult patients.

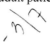

Self-Assessment Questions

Answers and explanations to these questions can be found at the end of this chapter.

1. A 20-year-old woman presents to the clinic for an asthma exacerbation. She states that she has been using her boyfriend's albuterol inhaler on a regular basis for the past 2 years. During the past few months, she has been using the inhaler throughout the day on a daily basis and sometimes at night. Which best classifies her asthma severity?

    A. Mild intermittent.
    B. Mild persistent.
    C. Moderate persistent.
    D. Severe persistent.

2. Which is the best asthma maintenance therapy for the patient in question 1?

    A. Fluticasone low dose.
    B. Montelukast.
    C. Fluticasone medium dose plus salmeterol.
    D. Fluticasone high dose.

3. Which type of measurement best classifies the number of times a short-acting β_2-agonist (SABA) is used in 1 month?

    A. Nominal.
    B. Ordinal.
    C. Interval.
    D. Ratio.

4. You are designing a study in which you will compare the percentage of patients with an asthma-related hospitalization receiving fluticasone/salmeterol with those receiving fluticasone alone. Which statistical test is best for analyzing this comparison?

    A. Analysis of variance (ANOVA).
    B. Chi-square.
    C. Mann-Whitney *U* test.
    D. Student unpaired t test.

5. A 22-year-old woman with asthma is taking an albuterol metered dose inhaler (MDI) 2 puffs as needed and fluticasone (Flovent) 110 mcg/puff MDI 2 puffs twice daily. She received the influenza vaccine during last year's influenza season, and her last tetanus vaccine (tetanus, diphtheria, and pertussis [Tdap]) was at age 17; there is no documentation of her having received a pneumococcal vaccine. Which is the best vaccine for her to receive at her next family medicine clinic appointment scheduled in July?

    A. Influenza.
    B. Pneumococcal.
    C. Td (tetanus and diphtheria).
    D. Herpes zoster.

6. A 60-year-old man with chronic obstructive pulmonary disease (COPD) has been using inhaled albuterol 2 puffs four times per day as needed. His symptoms have worsened during the past year, and now he has persistent symptoms and shortness of breath, even while walking around his one-level house. His Modified Medical Research Council (mMRC) score is 2. His spirometry shows a forced expiratory volume in 1 second (FEV_1) of 70% of predicted and an FEV_1/forced vital capacity (FEV_1/FVC) of 60% of predicted. He has had no previous COPD exacerbations. Which medication is best to initiate?

    A. Inhaled fluticasone.
    B. Inhaled tiotropium.
    C. Inhaled fluticasone/salmeterol.
    D. Oral roflumilast.

7. A patient with severe polyarticular gout and three tophi, uric acid 12.3 mg/dL, and stage 4 chronic kidney disease (CKD) (glomerular filtration rate [GFR] 25 mL/minute/1.73 m^2) needs urate-lowering therapy (ULT). Which is the most appropriate drug and starting dose?

    A. Probenecid 500 mg twice daily.

    B. Probenecid 250 mg twice daily.

    C. Allopurinol 100 mg once daily.

    D. Allopurinol 50 mg once daily.

BPS Pharmacotherapy Specialty Examination Content Outline

This chapter covers the following sections of the Pharmacotherapy Specialty Examination Content Outline:

1. Domain 1: Patient-Specific Pharmacotherapy
    a. Task 1; Knowledge 1–8, 10–15, 17
    b. Task 3; Knowledge 1–4
    c. Task 4; Knowledge 1–6
    d. Task 5; Knowledge 104
2. Domain 2: Drug Information and Evidence-Based Medicine
    a. Task 2; Knowledge 1, 2, 5, 6
3. Domain 3: System-Based Standards and Population-Based Pharmacotherapy
    a. Task 1; Knowledge 3
    b. Task 4; Knowledge 1
    c. Task 6; Knowledge 1–3

I. ASTHMA

Guidelines:

National Institutes of Health (NIH) National Heart Lung and Blood Institute (NHLBI). National Asthma Education and Prevention Program Guidelines (NAEPP). NAEPP Expert Panel Report 3. NIH Publication 08-5846. July 2007. Available at www.nhlbi.nih.gov/guidelines/asthma/. Accessed October 20, 2015. *(main guidelines presented in this chapter)*

Global Initiative for Asthma (GINA): Global Strategy for Asthma Management and Prevention 2014. Available at www.ginasthma.org/. Accessed October 20, 2015. *(for reference; these largely mirror the NHLBI guidelines)*

A. Definition: Asthma is a chronic inflammatory disorder of the airways causing recurrent episodes of wheezing, breathlessness, cough, and chest tightness, particularly at night or early in the morning. During episodes, there is variable airway obstruction, often reversible spontaneously or with treatment. There is also increased bronchial hyperresponsiveness to a variety of stimuli.

B. Diagnosis
1. Episodic symptoms of airflow obstruction are present.
2. Airway obstruction is reversible (forced expiratory volume in 1 second [FEV_1] improves by 12% or more after short-acting β_2-agonists [SABAs]).
3. Alternative diagnoses are excluded. Asthma versus chronic obstructive pulmonary disease (COPD):
   a. Cough is usually nonproductive with asthma and productive with COPD.
   b. FEV_1 is reversible with asthma but is irreversible with COPD.
   c. Cough is worse at night and early in the morning with asthma; occurs throughout the day with COPD.
   d. Asthma is often related to allergies and environmental triggers; patients with COPD have a common history of smoking or exposure to other irritants.
   e. Asthma can be reversible; lung damage from COPD is irreversible.
4. Asthma-COPD overlap syndrome (ACOS)
   a. Persistent airflow limitation with features of both asthma and COPD.
   b. If three or more features favor asthma, use diagnosis and treatment for asthma.
   c. If three or more features favor COPD, use diagnosis and treatment for COPD.
   d. If a similar number of features exist for both asthma and COPD, consider a diagnosis of ACOS (Table 1).
5. Exercise-induced bronchospasm
   a. Presents with cough, shortness of breath, chest pain or tightness, wheezing, or endurance problems during exercise.
   b. Diagnosis is made by an exercise challenge in which a 15% decrease in FEV_1 or peak expiratory flow occurs before and after exercise, measured at 5-minute intervals for 20–30 minutes.

Table 1. Syndromatic Diagnosis in Adults: Asthma vs. COPD

Feature	Asthma	COPD
Age of onset	☐ Before age 20 years	☐ After age 40 years
Pattern of symptoms	☐ Variation in symptoms over minutes, hours, or days ☐ Worse during the night or early morning ☐ Triggered by exercise, emotions, dust, or exposure to allergens	☐ Persistence of symptoms despite treatment ☐ Good and bad days but always daily symptoms and exertional dyspnea ☐ Chronic cough and sputum precede onset of dyspnea, unrelated to triggers
Lung function	☐ Record of variable airflow limitation (spirometry [Table 2] or peak flow), showing reversibility	☐ Record of persistent airflow limitation (postbronchodilator $FEV_1/FVC < 0.7$)
Lung function between symptoms	☐ Normal	☐ Abnormal
Past history or family history	☐ Previous diagnosis of asthma ☐ Family history of asthma and other allergic conditions (allergic rhinitis or eczema)	☐ Previous diagnosis of COPD, chronic bronchitis, or emphysema ☐ Heavy exposure to a risk factor: tobacco smoke, biomass fuels
Time course	☐ No worsening of symptoms over time; symptoms vary either seasonally or from year to year ☐ May improve spontaneously or have an immediate response to bronchodilators or to ICS over weeks	☐ Symptoms slowly worsen over time (progressive course over years) ☐ Rapid-acting bronchodilator provides only limited relief
Chest radiograph	☐ Normal	☐ Severe hyperinflation
ACOS Syndromatic Diagnosis Instructions		
1. Check each box in both columns that pertains to the patient. 2. Count the number of check boxes in each column. 3. If three or more boxes are checked for either asthma or COPD, that diagnosis is suggested. 4. If similar numbers of boxes are checked in each column, consider a diagnosis of ACOS.		

ACOS = asthma COPD overlap syndrome; COPD = chronic obstructive pulmonary disease; FEV_1/FVC = forced expiratory volume in 1 second/forced vital capacity; ICS = inhaled corticosteroids.

From: Global Initiative for Asthma (GINA) and Global Initiative for Chronic Obstructive Lung Disease (GOLD). Diagnosis of diseases of chronic airflow limitation: Asthma, COPD and asthma-COPD overlap syndrome (ACOS). Available at www.ginasthma.org/. Accessed October 20, 2015.

Table 2. Interpreting Spirometry

Component	What It Measures	Normal Values
FEV_1	Volume of air exhaled forcefully in the first second of maximal expiration	Normal is ≥80% In asthma, reversibility is shown by an increase in FEV_1 of ≥12% after SABA
FVC	The maximum volume of air that can be exhaled after full inspiration	Reported in liters and percentage predicted Normal adults can empty 80% of air in <6 seconds
FEV_1/FVC ratio	Differentiates between obstructive and restrictive disease	Normal: Within 5% of predicted range, which varies with age; usually 75%–80% in adults Decreased in obstructive disease (asthma, COPD) (<70%) Normal or high in restrictive disease (pulmonary fibrosis)

COPD = chronic obstructive pulmonary disease; FEV_1/FVC = forced expiratory volume in 1 second/forced vital capacity; SABA = short-acting β-agonist.

C. Classification of Asthma Severity and Control (Tables 3 and 4)

Table 3. Classification of Asthma Severity in Adults and Children[a]

Components	Age Group (years)	Intermittent	Mild Persistent	Moderate Persistent	Severe Persistent
Frequency of symptoms	All ages	≤2 days/week	>2 days/week but not daily	Daily	Throughout the day
Nighttime awakening	≥12	≤2 times/month	3 or 4 times/month	More than once weekly but not nightly	Often 7 times/week
	5–11				
	0–4	0	1 or 2 times/month	3 or 4 times/month	More than once weekly
SABA; used for symptom control	All ages	≤2 days/week	>2 days/week but not daily	Daily	Several times a day
Interference with normal activity	All ages	None	Minor limitation	Some limitations	Extremely limited
FEV$_1$/FVC[b]	≥12	Normal	Normal	Reduced 5%	Reduced >5%
	5–11	>85%	>80%	75%–80%	<75%
	0–4	N/A			
FEV$_1$ (% of normal)	≥12	>80% (normal)	>80% (normal)	>60% to <80%	<60%
	5–11				
	0–4	N/A			
Exacerbations requiring oral steroids	≥12	0 or 1/year	≥2/year	≥2/year	≥2/year
	5–11				
	0–4	0 or 1/year	≥2 in 6 months or ≥4 wheezing episodes per year[c]		
Recommended step for initiating treatment (see Table 5)	≥12	Step 1	Step 2	Step 3[d] and consider short course of oral steroids	Step 4 or 5 and consider short course of oral steroids
	5–11				Step 3[d] or 4 and consider short course of oral steroids
	0–4				Step 3 and consider short course of oral steroids

[a]The patient is classified according to the sign or symptom that is in the most severe category.

[b]Normal FEV$_1$/FVC: 8–19 years old, 85%; 20–39 years old, 80%; 40–59 years old, 75%; 60–80 years old, 70%.

[c]Episodes lasting >1 day and risk factors for persistent asthma.

[d]For ages 5–11, initial step 3 therapy should be medium-dose ICS.

FEV$_1$ = forced expiratory volume in 1 second; FVC = forced vital capacity; ICS = inhaled corticosteroid; N/A = not applicable; SABA = short-acting β-agonist.

Adapted from NIH Asthma Guidelines. National Institutes of Health National Heart, Lung, and Blood Institute. National Asthma Education and Prevention Program (NAEPP) guidelines. NAEPP Expert Panel Report 3. NIH Publication 08-5846. Available at www.nhlbi.nih.gov/guidelines/index.htm. Accessed October 20, 2015.

Table 4. Assessing Asthma Control in Adults and Children

Component	Age Group (years)	Well Controlled	Not Well Controlled	Very Poorly Controlled
Symptoms	≥12	≤2 days/week	>2 days/week	Throughout the day
	5–11	≤2 days/week but not >1 time each day	>2 days/week or >1 time/day on any day	
	0–4			
Nighttime awakenings	≥12	≤2 times/month	1–3 times/week	≥4 times/week
	5–11	≤1 time/month	≥2 times/month	≥2 times/week
	0–4		>1 time/month	>1 time/week
Interference with normal activity	All ages	None	Some limitations	Extremely limited
SABA use for symptom control[a]	All ages	≤2 days/week	>2 days/week	Several times a day
FEV_1 or peak flow	≥12	>80% of predicted/ personal best	60%–80% of predicted/ personal best	<60% of predicted/ personal best
	5–11			
	0–4	N/A	N/A	N/A
Questionnaires ACT (range 5–25)	≥12 (N/A if <12)	≥20	16–19	≤15
Exacerbations requiring oral steroids	≥12	0 or 1/year	≥2/year	≥2/year
	5–11			
	0–4		2 or 3 times/year	>3 times/year
Recommended action for treatment	All ages	Maintain current step; regular follow-up every 1–6 months; consider step-down if well controlled ≥3 months	Step-up one step Reevaluate in 2–6 weeks	Consider short course of oral steroids Step-up 1 or 2 steps Reevaluate in 2 weeks

[a]Does not include β_2-agonist used to prevent exercise-induced asthma. More than 200 doses of SABA per month is a risk factor for asthma-related death (GINA guidelines).

ACT = Asthma Control Test (Nathan et al. Allergy Clin Immunol 2004;113:59-65); FEV_1 = forced expiratory volume in 1 second; GINA = Global Initiative for Asthma; N/A = not applicable; SABA = short-acting β_2-agonist.

Adapted from NIH Asthma Guidelines. National Institutes of Health National Heart Lung and Blood Institute. National Asthma Education and Prevention Program (NAEPP) Guidelines. NAEPP Expert Panel Report 3. NIH Publication 08-5846. Available at www.nhlbi.nih.gov/guidelines/index.htm. Accessed October 25, 2015.

D. Treatment Goals
1. Minimal or no chronic symptoms day or night
2. Minimal or no exacerbations
3. No limitations on activities; no school or work missed
4. Maintain (near) normal pulmonary function
5. Minimal use of SABAs
6. Minimal or no adverse effects from medications

E. Treatment Guidelines (Table 5)

Table 5. Stepwise Pharmacologic Treatment of Asthma

Step	Age Group (years)	Long-term Control	Quick Relief
1	All ages	No controller needed	Use SABA PRN
2	≥12	Preferred: Low-dose ICS	SABA >2 times/week (excluding preexercise doses) indicates inadequate control and need to step up treatment
	5–11	Alternatives: LTM, theophylline, or cromolyn[a]	
	0–4	Preferred: Low-dose ICS Alternatives: Montelukast or cromolyn[a]	
3	≥12	Preferred: Low-dose ICS plus LABA *or* medium-dose ICS alone Alternative: Low-dose ICS plus LTM or theophylline	
	5–11	Preferred: Medium-dose ICS Alternative: Low-dose ICS plus LABA, LTM, or theophylline	
	0–4	Medium-dose ICS	
4	≥12	Preferred: Medium-dose ICS plus LABA	
	5–11	Alternative: Medium-dose ICS plus LTM or theophylline	
	0–4	Preferred: Medium-dose ICS plus LABA or montelukast Alternative: Medium-dose ICS plus other LTM or theophylline	
5	≥12	High-dose ICS plus LABA *and* consider omalizumab for patients with allergic asthma	
	5–11	Preferred: High-dose ICS plus LABA Alternative: High-dose ICS plus LTM or theophylline	
	0–4	High-dose ICS plus LABA or montelukast	
6	≥12	High-dose ICS plus LABA plus systemic corticosteroids *and* consider omalizumab for patients with allergic asthma	
	5–11	Preferred: High-dose ICS plus LABA plus systemic corticosteroids Alternative: High-dose ICS plus LTM or theophylline plus systemic corticosteroids	
	0–4	High-dose ICS plus LABA or montelukast plus systemic corticosteroids	

[a]Cromolyn and nedocromil are included in the National Asthma Education and Prevention Program guidelines. Cromolyn and nedocromil inhalers have been discontinued by the manufacturer; only generic cromolyn nebulization solution is still available.

ICS = inhaled corticosteroid; LABA = long-acting β_2-agonist; LTM = leukotriene modifier; PRN = as needed; SABA = short-acting β_2-agonist.

Adapted from NIH Asthma Guidelines. National Institutes of Health National Heart, Lung and Blood Institute. National Asthma Education and Prevention Program (NAEPP) guidelines. NAEPP Expert Panel Report 3. NIH Publication 08-5846. Available at www.nhlbi.nih.gov/guidelines/index.htm. Accessed October 20, 2015.

F. Pharmacologic Therapy for Asthma (Tables 6 and 7)

Table 6. Pharmacologic Agents Used for Asthma and COPD

Generic	Brand	Dose	Adverse Effects	Comments
Corticosteroid inhalers				
Beclomethasone MDI 40 mcg/puff 80 mcg/puff	QVAR (HFA)	See ICS dosing table	**Inhaled:** Oral candidiasis Hoarseness May slow bone growth in children but similar adult height Has a built-in spacer	ICSs are first line for persistent asthma • Use holding chambers only if needed for technique; not needed or well studied with HFA inhalers; holding chambers are only for MDIs, cannot be used for DPIs; holding chambers with a mask can be used for young children • Rinse mouth with water after inhalations • Use corticosteroid inhaler as scheduled, not as needed • Onset of improvement is 5–7 days; additional benefit may occur over several weeks • Pulmicort Respules are the only nebulized steroid available Arnuity Ellipta inhalation powder is contraindicated if severe hypersensitivity to milk proteins
Fluticasone MDI 44 mcg/puff 110 mcg/puff 220 mcg/puff	Flovent HFA			
Fluticasone DPI 50 mcg/puff 100 mcg/puff 250 mcg/puff	Flovent Diskus			
Fluticasone furoate (inhalation powder) 100 mcg/puff 200 mcg/puff	Arnuity Ellipta 1 inhalation once daily			
Mometasone DPI 220 mcg/puff	Asmanex Twisthaler Can be used once daily			
Mometasone MDI 100 mcg/puff 200 mcg/puff	Asmanex HFA			
Budesonide DPI 90 mcg/dose 180 mcg/dose 0.25-, 0.5-, and 1-mg/2-mL nebs	Pulmicort Flexhaler and Respules			
Ciclesonide MDI 80 mcg/puff 160 mcg/puff	Alvesco HFA			
Flunisolide MDI 80 mcg/puff	Aerospan HFA			

Table 6. Pharmacologic Agents Used for Asthma and COPD *(continued)*

Generic	Brand	Dose	Adverse Effects	Comments
Anticholinergics / Muscarinic antagonists: short-acting (SAMA) and long-acting (LAMA)				
Ipratropium MDI 17 mcg/puff	Atrovent HFA	2 puffs QID (up to 12 puffs/ 24 hours)	Headache Flushed skin Blurred vision Tachycardia Palpitations	SAMA Used mainly for COPD and for acute asthma exacerbations necessitating emergency treatment Duration: 2–8 hours Also available as a solution for nebulization
Tiotropium DPI 18 mcg Tiotropium mist 2.5 mcg	Spiriva Spiriva Respimat	Inhale 1 capsule/day 2 puffs once daily		LAMA Spiriva Respimat is now indicated for long-term maintenance treatment of asthma for age ≥12; all other LAMA are indicated only for COPD Long acting; not for rapid relief Duration: >24 hours
Aclidinium bromide DPI 400 mcg per puff	Tudorza Pressair	1 puff BID		LAMA for COPD Dry powder inhaler with counter; does not involve putting capsules into inhaler at each dose
Umeclidinium inhalation powder DPI 62.5 mcg/ inhalation	Incruse Ellipta	1 inhalation once daily		Once daily LAMA for COPD
β_2-Agonists (short acting): SABA				
Albuterol MDI 90 mcg/puff	Proventil HFA Ventolin HFA ProAir HFA ProAir RespiClick DPI	2 puffs every 4–6 hours PRN	Tremor Tachycardia Hypokalemia Hypomagnesemia Hyperglycemia Tachyphylaxis	Used for acute bronchospasm; regular use indicates poor control Also available as solution for nebulization Duration of effect (MDI): 3–4 hours (up to 6) RespiClick is a breath-actuated dry powder device for use in age 12 and older; cannot use with a spacer/holding chamber
Levalbuterol MDI 45 mcg/puff	Xopenex HFA	2 puffs every 4–6 hours PRN		*R*-enantiomer of albuterol Also available as a solution for nebulization Duration (MDI): 3–4 hours (up to 6)

Table 6. Pharmacologic Agents Used for Asthma and COPD *(continued)*

Generic	Brand	Dose	Adverse Effects	Comments
β_2-Agonists (long acting): LABA				
Salmeterol DPI 50 mcg/puff	Serevent Diskus	Inhale 1 blister/ puff BID	Tremor Tachycardia Electrolyte effects (rare)	Not for acute symptoms Should not be used as monotherapy for asthma Duration: 8–12 hours
Formoterol 20-mcg/2-mL nebs Arformoterol 15-mcg/2-mL nebs	Perforomist Brovana	20-mcg BID nebs 15-mcg BID nebs		Onset of action 1–3 minutes but should not be used as acute therapy Should not be used as monotherapy for asthma Duration of MDI: 8–12 hours Arformoterol is the *R,R*-isomer of racemic formoterol
Indacaterol inhalation powder 75-mcg capsule	Arcapta Neohaler	Inhale 1 capsule once daily		Indacaterol is indicated only for COPD Duration of action: 24 hours
Olodaterol inhalation spray (mist) 2.5 mcg olodaterol/spray	Striverdi Respimat	2 puffs once daily		Indicated only in COPD
Combination SABA/SAMA				
Albuterol/ ipratropium mist 100/20 mcg/puff	Combivent Respimat	1 puff QID Maximum dose 6 puffs/day		Used primarily for COPD Combivent MDI is no longer available Combination solution for nebulization is also available as DuoNeb or generic
Combination LABA/LAMA				
Umeclidinium/ vilanterol DPI 62.5/25 mcg/puff	Anoro Ellipta	1 inhalation once daily		Used once daily
Tiotropium/ olodaterol inhalation spray 2.5 mcg/2.5 mcg per spray	Stiolto Respimat	2 inhalations once daily		
Combination ICS/LABA				
Fluticasone/ salmeterol DPI 100/50, 250/50, 500/50 mcg/puff	Advair Diskus	1 puff BID		
Fluticasone/ salmeterol MDI 45/21, 115/21, 230/21 mcg/puff	Advair HFA	2 puffs BID		
Budesonide/ formoterol MDI 80/4.5, 160/4.5 mcg/puff	Symbicort (HFA)	2 puffs BID		GINA guidelines include use of low-dose ICS/formoterol as PRN in patients already taking it as a controller; not in NHLBI guidelines
Mometasone/ formoterol MDI 100/5, 200/5 mcg/ puff	Dulera (HFA)	2 puffs BID		
Fluticasone furoate/ vilanterol inhalation powder DPI 100/25 mcg	Breo Ellipta	1 inhalation once daily		• The only once-daily combination ICS/ LABA inhaler • Indicated for both asthma and COPD

Table 6. Pharmacologic Agents Used for Asthma and COPD *(continued)*

Generic	Brand	Dose	Adverse Effects	Comments
Leukotriene modifiers				
Zafirlukast 10-mg tablet 20-mg tablet	Accolate	10–20 mg BID	Hepatotoxicity (zileuton and zafirlukast only) • Zileuton: monitor LFTs (baseline, every month × 3 months, every 2–3 months for remainder of first year) • Zafirlukast: monitor symptoms, regular LFT monitoring not needed; could be considered Headache GI upset	Drug interactions: Warfarin, erythromycin, theophylline FDA approved for children ≥5 years old Bioavailability decreases with food; take 1 hour before or 2 hours after meals
Montelukast Oral 10-mg tablet Chewable 4- and 5-mg tablets Oral granules 4 mg/packet	Singulair	Dose in the evening Adults and children ≥15 years: 10 mg/day Children 6 to <15 years: 5 mg/day Children 1 to <6 years: 4 mg/day		Also indicated in exercise-induced bronchospasm and seasonal and perennial allergic rhinitis Drug interactions: Phenobarbital FDA approved for use in children ≥1 year old; used in children 6 months and older Churg-Strauss syndrome associated with tapering doses of steroids
Zileuton 600-mg CR tablet	Zyflo CR	1200 mg BID	*FDA Caution: Risk of neuropsychiatric events (behavior and mood changes: aggression, agitation, anxiousness, dream abnormalities, hallucinations, depression, insomnia, irritability, restlessness, suicidal thinking and behavior, tremor)	Drug interactions: Warfarin and theophylline Only for those ≥12 years old
Monoclonal antibody/IgE binding inhibitor				
Omalizumab	Xolair	150–375 mg SC every 2–4 weeks Dose and frequency based on baseline IgE and weight in kilograms Do not inject >150 mg per injection site	Injection site reactions • Urticaria • Thrombocytopenia (transient) • Anaphylaxis (rare) • Malignancy	September 2014: New FDA Drug Safety Communication. Slightly increased risk of cardiovascular and cerebrovascular serious adverse events, including MI, unstable angina, TIA, PE/DVT, pulmonary HTN; no increased risk of stroke or CV death Used in severe persistent allergy-related asthma Use in ≥12 years Half-life: 26 days Second-line therapy Expensive

BID = twice daily; CNS = central nervous system; COPD = chronic obstructive pulmonary disease; CR = controlled release; CV = cardiovascular; DPI = dry powder inhaler; DVT = deep vein thrombosis; FDA = U.S. Food and Drug Administration; GERD = gastroesophageal reflux disease; GI = gastrointestinal; GINA = Global Initiative for Asthma; HFA = hydrofluoroalkane; HTN = hypertension; ICS = inhaled corticosteroid; IgE = immunoglobulin E; LABA = long-acting β_2-agonist; LFT = liver function test; MDI = metered dose inhaler; MI, myocardial infarction; nebs = nebulizers; OTC = over the counter; PE = pulmonary embolism; PRN = as needed; QID = 4 times daily; SC = subcutaneously; TIA = transient ischemic attack; TID = 3 times daily.

Table 7. Inhaled Corticosteroid Daily Dosing in Children and Adults

Inhaled Corticosteroids; Available Products and Strengths (mcg unless noted)	Low Dose (mcg/day) Steps 2 and 3			Medium Dose (mcg/day) Steps 3 and 4			High Dose (mcg/day) Steps 5 and 6		
Age group (years)	0–4	5–11	≥12	0–4	5–11	≥12	0–4	5–11	≥12
Budesonide Pulmicort DPI 90, 180	N/A	180–400	180–600	N/A	>400–800	>600–1200	N/A	>800	>1200
Fluticasone Flovent HFA 44, 110, 220 Flovent DPI 50, 100, 250	176	88–176	88–264	>176–352	>176–352	>264–440	>352	>352	>440
	N/A	100–200	100–300	N/A	>200–400	>300–500	N/A	>400	>500
Fluticasone furoate Arnity Ellipta 100, 200[a,c]	N/A	N/A	100	N/A	N/A	200 (maximum dose)	N/A	N/A	N/A
Beclomethasone QVAR HFA 40, 80	N/A	80–160	80–240	N/A	>160–320	>240–480	N/A	>320	>480
Mometasone Asmanex DPI 110, 220 (delivers 100 and 200 mcg/puff)[a]	100 (age 4 only)	100	200	100 (age 4 only)	100	400	100 (age 4 only)	100	>400
Asmanex MDI 100, 200[b]	N/A	N/A	200	N/A	N/A	400	N/A	N/A	>400
Ciclesonide[c,d] Alvesco HFA 80, 160	N/A	N/A	160	N/A	N/A	320	N/A	N/A	640
Flunisolide HFA Aerospan 80	N/A	160	320	N/A	320	>320-640	N/A	≥640	>640
Budesonide suspension for nebulization Pulmicort Respules 0.25, 0.5, 1 mg	0.25–0.5 mg	0.5 mg	N/A	>0.5–1 mg	1 mg	N/A	>1 mg	2 mg	N/A

[a]Once daily.

[b]Indicated in age 12 and older

[c]Doses are estimated from package insert.

[d]Ciclesonide was not available when the National Asthma Education and Prevention Program guidelines were published. The dose ranges are estimated from the package insert.

DPI = dry powder inhaler; HFA = hydrofluoroalkane; N/A = not applicable.

Adapted from NIH Asthma Guidelines. National Institutes of Health National Heart, Lung and Blood Institute. National Asthma Education and Prevention Program (NAEPP) guidelines. NAEPP Expert Panel Report 3. NIH Publication 08-5846. Available at www.nhlbi.nih.gov/guidelines/index.htm. Accessed October 20, 2015.

Patient Cases

1. A 23-year-old woman has been coughing and wheezing about twice weekly, and she wakes up at night about three times per month. She has never received a diagnosis of asthma, and she has not been to a doctor "in years." She uses her boyfriend's albuterol inhaler, but he recently ran out of refills, so she is seeking care. Her activities are not limited by her symptoms. Spirometry is done today, and her FEV_1 is 82% of predicted. From the current NAEPP guidelines, which is the best classification of her asthma?

   A. Intermittent.

   B. Mild persistent.

   C. Moderate persistent.

   D. Severe persistent.

2. Which medication is best to recommend for her, in addition to albuterol metered dose inhaler (MDI) 1 or 2 puffs every 4–6 hours as needed?

   A. No additional therapy needed.

   B. Oral montelukast 10 mg/day.

   C. Mometasone dry powder inhaler (DPI) 220 mcg/puff 1 puff daily.

   D. Budesonide/formoterol MDI 80/4.5 mcg per puff 2 puffs twice daily.

3. At first, her symptoms were well controlled on your recommended therapy. However, when winter arrived she started having symptoms and using her albuterol about 3 or 4 days per week during the day. Which is the preferred treatment change?

   A. No change in therapy is needed.

   B. Switch to budesonide/formoterol MDI 160/4.5 mcg per puff 2 puffs twice daily.

   C. Add montelukast orally 10 mg daily.

   D. Increase mometasone DPI to 220 mcg/puff 2 puffs daily.

4. An 8-year-old boy has been having daytime asthma symptoms once or twice weekly and is awakened twice weekly at night with coughing. In addition to albuterol MDI 1 or 2 puffs every 4–6 hours as needed, which is the best initial therapy for him?

   A. Fluticasone MDI 44 mcg/puff 1 puff twice daily.

   B. Oral montelukast 10 mg/day.

   C. Fluticasone/salmeterol DPI 100/50 mcg per puff 1 puff twice daily.

   D. Fluticasone MDI 110 mcg/puff 1 puff twice daily.

G. Types of Inhalation Devices (Table 8)

Table 8. Different Types of Inhalation Devices

Type and Name[a]	Specifics	Type of Inhalation	Shake or Prime	Dose Counter	Advantages and Limitations
Metered Dose Inhalers (MDIs)					
HFA inhalers: ProAir, Ventolin, Proventil, Xopenex, Flovent, QVAR, Alvesco, Asmanex HFA, Symbicort, Dulera, Advair HFA, Atrovent	Drug is mixed with a propellant Aerospan has a built-in spacer	Press down canister at the start of a slow, deep inhalation	Prime: Yes Shake: Yes	Yes, except Proventil, Xopenex, Alvesco, Aerospan	Benefits: Slow, deep breath is easier than forceful, quick breath, Can use with a spacer or holding chamber Limitation: Requires coordination, many people have difficulty with technique
Single Dose System Dry Powder Inhalers (DPIs)					
HandiHaler (Spiriva) Neohaler (Arcapta)	Individual gelatin capsules containing drug must be inserted and pierced before each use and removed after each use	Inhalation should be a steady and deep breath, enough to hear the whirring sound of the capsule rattling. Inhalation does not need to be as forceful as some other DPIs. Can take a second inhalation if powder remains in the capsule.	Prime: No Shake: No	No But not needed	Benefit: Inhalation is easier because it does not have to be forceful Limitation: Need to load and pierce each capsule before use
Preloaded Multidose DPIs					
Pressair (Tuzorda) Twisthaler (Asmanex) Flexhaler (Pulmicort) Diskus (Advair, Flovent, Serevent)	Multiple doses are included in each device, either as a reservoir or multiunit dose; each device lasts about 1 month	Inhalation is quick, forceful and deep; more deep and forceful than single-dose systems	Prime: No, except Flexhaler Shake: No	Yes	Benefit: No need to load capsules before each inhalation Limitation: Inhalation is more difficult to do correctly because it must be quick and forceful
Newer Multidose DPI					
Ellipta (Anoro, Breo, Arnuity, Incruse)	Different multidose system; 2 separate blister strips that dispense inhalation powder Contraindicated if severe hypersensitivity to milk protein	Inhalation is deep and slow, not fast and forceful like other DPIs	Prime: No Shake: No	Yes	Benefits: Easier inhalation than other DPIs; no need to load capsules before each inhalation, once daily dosing with only 1 inhalation each time, all medications that come in the Ellipta device are 1 inhalation once daily
Breath-Actuated DPI					
ProAir RespiClick	The only DPI albuterol available Indicated only for age 12 and older Medication is automatically released on inhalation, canister is not pressed	Deep breath; not fast and forceful but with enough force for the medication to be released Cannot use with a spacer or holding chamber Contraindicated if severe hypersensitivity to milk proteins	Prime: No Shake: No	Yes	Benefit: No need to coordinate breath with actuation as with all other albuterol devices (MDIs)
Soft Mist Inhaler					
Respimat (Combivent, Spiriva, Striverdi, Stiolto)	Dose of drug is in solution and is released through a nozzle with jets of mist Lung deposition and amount of drug delivered are independent of the patient's effort	Inhalation is slow and deep	Prime: Yes Each new inhaler needs to be assembled, readied, and primed before first use; this is somewhat complicated If not used in 3 days, prime with 1 inhalation released into air Full repriming needed if not used in 21 days. Shake: No	Yes	Benefits: Ease of inhalation, consistent drug delivery Limitation: Complicated steps to ready and prime inhaler each month and after not using for 21 days

[a]For generic names and drug class, see Table 6.

DPI = dry powder inhaler; HFA = hydrofluoroalkane; MDI = metered dose inhaler.

H.   Use of long-acting muscarinic antagonist (LAMA) for asthma
   1.   Tiotropium Respimat is the only LAMA indicated for long-term treatment of asthma.
   2.   2015 GINA guidelines include tiotropium as add-on therapy in step 4 and 5 for adults with severe asthma and a history of exacerbations. (Global Initiative for Asthma [GINA]. Global strategy for asthma management and prevention. 2015. Available at www.ginasthma.org. Accessed October 20, 2015.)
   3.   Evidence shows improved lung function and increased time to severe exacerbation.

I.   Pharmacologic Treatment of Asthma-COPD Overlap Syndrome (ACOS)
   1.   If more features of asthma, use treatment strategy for asthma.
   2.   If more features of COPD, use treatment strategy for COPD.
   3.   If clinical picture suggests ACOS, start with an ICS and usually add a LABA or LAMA. (Global Initiative for Asthma [GINA]. Global strategy for asthma management and prevention. 2015. Available at: www.ginasthma.org. Accessed October 20, 2015.)

J.   Long-Acting β_2-Agonists (LABAs): According to a U.S. Food and Drug Administration (FDA) safety announcement, issued because of safety concerns with LABAs:
   1.   Use of a LABA alone without a long-term asthma control drug such as an ICS is contraindicated because of increased risk of severe worsening of asthma symptoms, leading to hospitalization and death in some children and adults.
   2.   LABAs should not be used in patients whose asthma is adequately controlled on low- or medium-dose ICSs.
   3.   LABAs should be used only as additional therapy for patients who are currently taking but not adequately controlled on a long-term asthma control agent (e.g., an ICS).
   4.   Once asthma control is achieved and maintained, patients should be assessed at regular intervals and stepped down (e.g., discontinue the LABA), if possible, and the patients should continue to be treated with a long-term asthma control agent (e.g., an ICS).
   5.   Pediatric and adolescent patients who need a LABA and an ICS should use a combination product to ensure adherence to both medications.

K.   Exercise-Induced Bronchospasm: Prevention and Treatment of Symptoms
   1.   Long-term control therapy, if otherwise appropriate (initiate or step-up)
   2.   Pretreatment with a SABA before exercise
   3.   Leukotriene modifiers (LTMs) can attenuate symptoms in 50% of patients.

L.   Monitoring
   1.   Peak flow monitoring
      a.   Symptom-based and peak flow–based monitoring have similar benefits; either is appropriate for most patients. Symptom-based monitoring is more convenient.
      b.   May consider daily home peak flow monitoring for moderate to severe persistent asthma if patient has history of severe exacerbations or has poor perception of worsening of asthma symptoms.
      c.   Personal best peak expiratory flow rate (PEFR), not predicted PEFR, should be determined if using peak flow–based asthma action plan.
         i.   Personal best PEFR is the highest number attained after daily monitoring for 2 weeks twice daily when asthma is under good control.
         ii.   Predicted PEFR is based on population norms using sex, height, and age.
   2.   Spirometry (only used if 5 years or older)
      a.   At initial assessment
      b.   After treatment is started and symptoms are stabilized
      c.   If prolonged or progressive loss of asthma control
      d.   At least every 2 years or more often depending on response to therapy

M. Asthma Action Plan (Table 9)
   1. Usually symptom based (equal benefits of symptom-based or peak flow–based monitoring)
   2. Allows home treatment of an asthma exacerbation

Table 9. Asthma Action Plan

Zone	Signs and Symptoms	Treatment
Green	Doing well; no or minimal symptoms of coughing, wheezing, or dyspnea PEFR 80%–100% of personal best	Take long-term asthma control agent only (if one is prescribed) Use 2 puffs of SABA 5–15 minutes before exercise if exercise-induced asthma and before known triggers
Yellow	Getting worse; increased frequency of symptoms (e.g., coughing, wheezing, or dyspnea) PEFR 50%–79% of personal best	Use SABA: 2–4 puffs by MDI (up to 6 puffs if needed) or 1 nebulizer treatment; may repeat in 20 minutes if needed; reassess 1 hour after initial treatment If complete response at 1 hour, contact clinician for follow-up instructions and consider OCS burst[a] If incomplete response in 1 hour (still some coughing, wheezing, or dyspnea), repeat SABA and add OCS burst; contact clinician that day for further instructions If poor response in 1 hour (e.g., marked coughing, wheezing, or dyspnea), repeat SABA immediately; add OCS burst; contact clinician immediately; proceed to the ED if the distress is severe and unresponsive to treatment; consider calling 911 May continue to use SABA every 3–4 hours regularly for 24–48 hours
Red	Medical alert (e.g., marked coughing, wheezing, or dyspnea); inability to speak more than short phrases; use of accessory respiratory muscles; drowsiness PEFR <50% of personal best	Begin treatment and consult clinician immediately Use SABA: 2–6 puffs by MDI (higher dose of 4–6 puffs usually recommended) or 1 nebulizer treatment; repeat every 20 minutes up to 3 times; add OCS burst If incomplete or poor response, repeat SABA immediately; proceed to the ED or call 911 if distress is severe and unresponsive to treatment Call 911 or go to the ED immediately if lips or fingernails are blue or gray or if there is trouble walking or talking because of shortness of breath Continue using SABA every 3–4 hours regularly for 24–48 hours

[a]OCS burst: prednisone (or equivalent) 40–60 mg/day for 5–10 days (adults) or 1–2 mg/kg/day (maximum 60 mg/day) for 3–10 days (children).

ED = emergency department; MDI = metered dose inhaler; OCS = oral corticosteroid; PEFR = peak expiratory flow rate; SABA = short-acting beta agonist.

After initial treatment, immediate medical attention is needed if patient is at high risk of a fatal attack. Risk factors: Asthma-related (history of severe attack [previous intubation or intensive care unit admission for asthma], ≥2 asthma hospitalizations for asthma in past year, ≥3 ED visits for asthma in past year, hospitalization or ED visit for asthma in past month, using >2 canisters of SABA a month, difficulty perceiving asthma symptoms), social (low socioeconomic status or inner-city residence, illicit drug use, major psychosocial problems), and comorbidities (cardiovascular disease, other chronic lung disease, chronic psychiatric disease).

N. Managing Exacerbations: Initial—Emergency Department (ED) or Hospital (Table 10)

Table 10. Classifying Severity of Asthma Exacerbations in the Urgent or Emergency Care Setting[a]

	Symptoms and Signs	**Initial PEF or FEV$_1$**[b]	**Clinical Course**
Mild	Dyspnea only with activity	≥70% of predicted or personal best	Usually cared for at home Prompt relief with an inhaled SABA Possible short course of OCS
Moderate	Dyspnea interferes with or limits usual activity	40%–69% of predicted or personal best	Usually requires office or ED visit Relief from frequently inhaled SABAs and OCS; some symptoms last for 1–2 days after treatment is begun
Severe	Dyspnea at rest; interferes with conversation	<40% of predicted or personal best	Usually requires ED visit and likely hospitalization Partial relief from frequent inhaled SABA Oral systemic corticosteroids; some symptoms last for >3 days after treatment is begun Adjunctive therapies are helpful
Life threatening	Too dyspneic to speak; perspiring	<25% of predicted or personal best	Requires ED or hospitalization, possible ICU Little or no relief from frequent inhaled SABAs IV corticosteroids Adjunctive therapies are helpful

[a]For all ages.

[b]Lung function measures (PEF or FEV$_1$) may be useful for children ≥5 years old but may not be attainable in children during an exacerbation.

ED = emergency department; FEV$_1$ = forced expiratory volume in 1 second; ICU = intensive care unit; IV = intravenous; OCS = oral corticosteroid; PEF = peak expiratory flow; SABA = short-acting β_2-agonist.

Adapted from NIH Asthma Guidelines. National Institutes of Health National Heart, Lung and Blood Institute. National Asthma Education and Prevention Program Guidelines (NAEPP). NAEPP Expert Panel Report 3. NIH Publication 08-5846. Available at www.nhlbi.nih.gov/guidelines/asthma/. Accessed October 20, 2015.

1. Mild to moderate exacerbation (FEV$_1$ of 40% or more)
   a. Oxygen to achieve oxygen saturation (Sao$_2$) of 90% or more
   b. An inhaled SABA (MDI with valved holding chamber or nebulizer) up to three doses in the first hour
      i. Adult dose: Albuterol MDI 4–8 puffs every 20 minutes for up to 4 hours, then every 1–4 hours as needed or by nebulizer 2.5–5 mg every 20 minutes for three doses, then 2.5–10 mg every 1–4 hours as needed
      ii. Pediatric dose (12 years or younger): Albuterol MDI 4–8 puffs every 20 minutes for three doses, then every 1–4 hours as needed; use holding chamber (add mask if younger than 4 years) or by nebulizer 0.15 mg/kg (minimal dose 2.5 mg) every 20 minutes for three doses, then 0.15–0.3 mg/kg up to 10 mg every 1–4 hours as needed
   c. Oral corticosteroid (OCS) if no response immediately or if patient recently took an OCS

2. Severe exacerbation (FEV$_1$ less than 40%)
   a. Oxygen to achieve Sao$_2$ of 90% or more
   b. High-dose inhaled SABA plus ipratropium by MDI plus valved holding chamber or nebulizer every 20 minutes or continuously for 1 hour
   c. Oral corticosteroids
      i. Adult dose: Prednisone 40–80 mg/day in one or two divided doses until peak expiratory flow reaches 70% of predicted
      ii. Pediatric dose (12 years or younger): 1–2 mg/kg in two divided doses (maximum 60 mg/day) until peak expiratory flow reaches 70% of predicted
   d. Consider adjunctive therapies (intravenous magnesium or heliox) if still unresponsive.
3. Impending or actual respiratory arrest
   a. Intubation and mechanical ventilation with oxygen 100%
   b. Nebulized SABA plus ipratropium
   c. Intravenous corticosteroids
   d. Consider adjunctive therapies (intravenous magnesium or heliox) if patient is still unresponsive to therapy.
   e. Admit to intensive care.

O. Managing Exacerbations: ED or Hospital After Repeat Assessment
   1. Moderate exacerbation (FEV$_1$ 40%–69%)
      a. Inhaled SABA every 60 minutes
      b. Oral corticosteroid
      c. Continue treatment for 1–3 hours if improving.
   2. Severe exacerbation (FEV$_1$ less than 40%); no improvement after initial treatment
      a. Oxygen
      b. Nebulized SABA plus ipratropium; hourly or continuous
      c. Consider adjunctive therapies.
   3. If good response to above treatment and maintained for at least 60 minutes
      a. Continue inhaled SABA.
      b. Continue OCS course.
      c. Consider initiating an ICS (if not already taking one).
      d. Discharge home.
   4. If incomplete response (FEV$_1$ 40%–69%), admit to hospital ward.
   5. If poor response (FEV$_1$ less than 40%), admit to intensive care.

Patient Case

5. A 25-year-old man presents to the ED with shortness of breath at rest. He is having trouble with conversation. He used 4 puffs of albuterol MDI at home with no resolution of symptoms. His FEV$_1$ is checked, and it is 38% of predicted. Which is the best initial therapy for him in the ED, in addition to oxygen?

   A. Oxygen alone is sufficient.

   B. Albuterol MDI 8 puffs every 20 minutes for 1 hour.

   C. Albuterol plus ipratropium by nebulizer every 20 minutes for 1 hour plus intravenous corticosteroids.

   D. Albuterol plus ipratropium by nebulizer every 20 minutes for 1 hour plus oral corticosteroids.

P. Additional Vaccines: Adults with asthma (19–64 years of age) should receive:

1. The 23-valent pneumococcal polysaccharide vaccine (PPSV23; Pneumovax) once, then follow U.S. Centers for Disease Control and Prevention (CDC) recommendations for pneumococcal vaccination at age 65 and older

2. Influenza vaccine every fall or winter

Q. Asthma in Pregnancy

1. Asthma may worsen, improve, or stay the same during pregnancy.

2. Asthma may increase the risk of perinatal mortality, hyperemesis, vaginal hemorrhage, preeclampsia, complicated labor, neonatal mortality, prematurity, and low-birth-weight infants, especially if uncontrolled. Risks are small and are not shown in all studies.

3. Medications

a. Preferred controller: Budesonide ICS (only category B ICS); however, if well controlled on other ICS before pregnancy, it may be continued.

b. Preferred rescue: Albuterol

c. LABAs are category C; less clinical experience. Use during pregnancy is reasonable if necessary for asthma control. Salmeterol is preferred LABA.

d. LTMs have limited data; most data are with montelukast (category B), and the data for montelukast are reassuring. Considered an alternative therapy.

e. Prednisone is category C; potential adverse effects in pregnancy are cleft palate, preeclampsia, gestational diabetes, low birth weight, and prematurity. However, few studies were of patients with asthma, and women might have been exposed to longer-term prednisone use. Prednisone should be used, if necessary, for acute exacerbations in pregnancy.

II. CHRONIC OBSTRUCTIVE PULMONARY DISEASE

Guidelines:

Global Initiative for Chronic Obstructive Lung Disease (GOLD). Global Strategy for Diagnosis, Management and Prevention of COPD. 2016 Update. Available at www.goldcopd.org/. Accessed January 4, 2016.

Qaseem A, Wilt TJ, Weinberger SE, et al. Diagnosis and management of stable chronic obstructive pulmonary disease: a clinical practice guideline update from the American College of Physicians, American College of Chest Physicians, American Thoracic Society, and European Respiratory Society (ACP/ACCP/ATS/ERS guidelines). Ann Intern Med 2011;155:179-91.

A. Definition: COPD is a syndrome of chronic limitation in expiratory airflow encompassing emphysema and chronic bronchitis. Airflow obstruction may be accompanied by airway hyperresponsiveness and may be not be fully reversible.

1. Chronic bronchitis consists of persistent cough plus sputum production for most days of 3 months in at least 2 consecutive years.

2. Emphysema is abnormal permanent enlargement of the airspaces distal to the terminal bronchioles, accompanied by destruction of their walls and without obvious fibrosis.

B. Diagnosis and Assessment

1. The diagnosis of COPD is based on a history of exposure to risk factors and the presence of airflow limitation that is not fully reversible, with or without the presence of symptoms.

a. Symptoms: Dyspnea (described by patients as "increased effort to breathe," "heaviness," "air hunger," or "gasping"), poor exercise tolerance, chronic cough, sputum production, wheezing

b. GOLD guidelines: Perform spirometry and consider COPD if a patient is older than 40 years and has any of the following:

  i. Dyspnea that is progressive (worsens over time), persistent (present every day), and worse with exercise or on exertion

  ii. Chronic cough that is present intermittently or every day; often present throughout the day; seldom only nocturnal. May be nonproductive

  iii. Chronic sputum production in any pattern

  iv. History of exposure to risk factors, especially tobacco smoke (most common risk factor), occupational dusts and chemicals, and smoke from home cooking and heating fuels

c. American College of Physicians, American College of Chest Physicians, American Thoracic Society, and European Respiratory Society (ACP/ACCP/ATS/ERS) guidelines: The single best predictor of airflow obstruction is the presence of all three of the following:

  i. Smoking history of more than 55 pack-years

  ii. Wheezing on auscultation

  iii. Patient self-reported wheezing

2. For the diagnosis and assessment of COPD, spirometry is the gold standard.

  a. Spirometry showing an FEV_1/FVC less than 70% of predicted is the hallmark of COPD. Bronchodilator reversibility testing is no longer recommended.

  b. Measurement of arterial blood gas tension should be considered for all patients with FEV_1 less than 50% of predicted or clinical signs suggestive of respiratory failure or right heart failure.

3. Validated symptom scales or questionnaires

  a. Modified Medical Research Council (mMRC) breathlessness scale for assessing severity of breathlessness (Bestall et al. 1999)

    i. Measures severity of shortness of breath or breathlessness

    ii. Scale of 0–4

    iii. 0 = least symptoms; breathless only with strenuous exercise

    iv. 4 = too breathless to leave house; breathless even when dressing

  b. COPD Assessment Test (CAT) measures health status impairment in COPD (www.catestonline.org).

    i. Measures not just breathlessness but also cough, sputum production, chest tightness, limitation of activities, sleep, energy level, and confidence to leave house

    ii. Scale of 5 to more than 30

    iii. 5 is upper limit of normal.

    iv. Less than 10 is low impact on life.

    v. More than 30 is high impact on life; barely can leave the house.

C. Factors Determining Severity of COPD

  1. Severity of symptoms

  2. Severity of airflow limitation (FEV_1)

  3. Frequency of exacerbations

  4. Presence of comorbidities that may restrict activity (e.g., heart failure, heart disease, musculoskeletal disorders)

D. Therapy Goals

  1. Relieve symptoms.

  2. Reduce the frequency and severity of exacerbations.

  3. Improve exercise tolerance.

  4. Improve health status.

  5. Minimize adverse effects from treatment.

E. Management of Stable COPD
1. Description of levels of evidence or grades of recommendations (Table 11)

Table 11. Grades for Strength of Recommendations for COPD Guidelines

GOLD Guidelines	
A	Randomized clinical trials Rich body of data
B	Randomized clinical trials Limited body of data
C	Nonrandomized trials Observational studies
D	Panel judgment consensus
ACP/ACCP/ATS/ERS Guidelines	
Recommendation grade	Strong (S): Benefits clearly outweigh risks and burden, or risks and burden clearly outweigh benefits
	Weak (W): Benefits finely balanced with risks and burden
Quality of evidence	High (H) – Moderate (M) – Low (L)

ACCP = American College of Chest Physicians; ACP = American College of Physicians; ATS = American Thoracic Society; COPD = obstructive pulmonary disease; ERS = European Respiratory Society; GOLD = Global Initiative for Chronic Obstructive Lung Disease.

2. Existing medications for COPD have not been shown to modify the long-term decline in lung function, the hallmark of this disease (level of evidence A). Therefore, pharmacotherapy for COPD is used to decrease symptoms, complications, or both.
3. Smoking cessation is a critical component of COPD management.
4. Bronchodilator medications are central to the symptomatic management of COPD (level of evidence A).
    a. They are given on an as-needed basis or on a regular basis to prevent or reduce symptoms.
    b. The principal bronchodilator treatments are β_2-agonists, anticholinergics, or a combination of these drugs. Theophylline is also a bronchodilator but is not recommended unless other long-term bronchodilators are unavailable or unaffordable.
    c. Inhaled therapy is preferred.
    d. The choice between a LABA, anticholinergic, theophylline, and combination therapy depends on availability and individual response in symptom relief and adverse effects.
    e. Regular treatment with a long-acting (LA) bronchodilator is more effective and convenient than regular treatment with SA bronchodilators (level of evidence A).
    f. Combining bronchodilators from different pharmacologic classes may improve efficacy with the same or fewer adverse effects compared with increasing the dose of a single bronchodilator (level of evidence A).
    g. Adding tiotropium to a LABA/ICS combination (triple therapy) improves lung function and health-related quality of life and reduces the number of exacerbations (level of evidence B). Retrospective data show decreased mortality, fewer hospital admissions, and fewer OCS bursts. All bronchodilators improve symptoms and exercise capacity.
        i. Treatment with an LA anticholinergic delays first exacerbation, reduces the overall number of COPD exacerbations and related hospitalizations, improves symptoms and health status (level of evidence A), and improves the effectiveness of pulmonary rehabilitation (level of evidence B). LA anticholinergics have no effect on the rate of decline of lung function. Initial studies with tiotropium showed elevated cardiovascular risk, but newer strong evidence shows no increase in risk. Anticholinergics may not significantly improve FEV_1.

    ii. LABAs improve health status, quality of life, and FEV_1 and decrease COPD exacerbation rate (level of evidence A). LABAs have no effect on mortality and rate of decline of lung function. Salmeterol reduces hospitalization rate (level of evidence B). Salmeterol significantly reduces the number of patients needing hospitalization and also treatment for exacerbations. Indacaterol significantly improves breathlessness, health status, and exacerbation rate (level of evidence B). Indacaterol is a LABA with a significantly greater bronchodilator effect than salmeterol and a bronchodilator effect similar to that of tiotropium (level of evidence A). LABAs do not have the same potential safety concerns as with use in asthma.

    iii. LA anticholinergic versus LABAs:

        (a) POET-COPD study: Tiotropium is more effective than salmeterol as initial LA bronchodilator therapy in moderate to very severe COPD regarding time to first exacerbation and annual number of exacerbations (Vogelmeier et al. 2011).

        (b) Cochrane review concluded that tiotropium is more effective than LABAs in preventing COPD exacerbations and COPD-related hospitalization but not in overall hospitalization or mortality. Symptom and lung function improvement were similar. However, there are only a few studies. Fewer serious adverse events and withdrawals from studies occurred with tiotropium versus LABAs (Chong et al. 2012).

5. ICSs in stable COPD

    a. ICSs improve symptoms, lung function, and quality of life and decrease the frequency of exacerbations in patients with FEV_1 less than 60% of predicted; they do not modify the progressive decline in FEV_1 or decrease mortality (level of evidence A).

    b. The dose response with ICS in COPD is unknown (in contrast to asthma treatment). Moderate to high doses have been used in COPD clinical trials.

    c. An ICS combined with a LABA is more effective than the individual components (level of evidence A). An ICS/LABA combination reduces the rate of decline of FEV_1 and reduces the exacerbation rate; the reduction in mortality compared with placebo fell just short of statistical significance (relative risk reduction 17.5%; absolute risk reduction 2.6%; adjusted p=0.052) (Calverley et al. 2007). A subsequent meta-analysis showed that ICS/LABA might reduce mortality (number needed to treat was 36) (level of evidence B) (Nannini et al. 2007).

    d. ICS use is associated with a higher incidence of pneumonia in COPD (Singh et al. 2009; Ernst et al. 2007).

    e. Long-term monotherapy with ICSs is not recommended; they are less effective than ICS/LABA combination.

    f. Long-term treatment with ICSs should not be used outside their indications because of the risk of pneumonia and possible increased risk of fractures after long-term exposure.

    g. Chronic treatment with OCSs should be avoided because of an unfavorable benefit/risk ratio (level of evidence A).

6. Patient assessment and selection of therapy

    a. GOLD guidelines combine symptoms (based on symptom scores), airflow limitation (based on postbronchodilator FEV_1), and frequency of exacerbations to determine patient risk group and recommended treatment (Tables 12 and 13).

    b. ACP/ACCP/ATS/ERS guidelines simplify treatment even further on the basis of FEV_1 in patients with COPD with symptoms. They do not provide detailed treatment guidelines (Table 14).

Table 12. GOLD Guidelines: Assessment of COPD Severity and Risk

Patient Group	Characteristic	Spirometric GOLD Classification[a]	Exacerbations per Year[a]	Symptom Score[b]
A	Low risk Fewer symptoms	GOLD 1: Mild (FEV$_1$ ≥80% of predicted) *or* GOLD 2: Moderate (50% ≤ FEV$_1$ < 80% of predicted)	≤1 and no hospitalization	mMRC 0–1 CAT <10
B	Low risk More symptoms	GOLD 1: Mild (FEV$_1$ ≥80% of predicted) *or* GOLD 2: Moderate (50% ≤ FEV$_1$ < 80% of predicted)	≤1 and no hospitalization	mMRC ≥2 CAT ≥10
C	High risk Fewer symptoms	GOLD 3: Severe (30% ≤ FEV$_1$ < 50% of predicted) *or* GOLD 4: Very severe (FEV$_1$ <30% of predicted)	≥2 or ≥1 with hospitalization	mMRC 0–1 CAT <10
D	High risk More symptoms	GOLD 3: Severe (30% ≤ FEV$_1$ < 50% of predicted) *or* GOLD 4: Very severe (FEV$_1$ < 30% of predicted)	≥2 or ≥1 with hospitalization	mMRC ≥2 CAT ≥10

[a]Postbronchodilator FEV$_1$ should be used. To determine the risk of exacerbation, either the spirometric GOLD classification or the number of exacerbations per year can be used. If they are both used and the patient would fall into 2 different categories, always assign patient to the category with the highest risk and symptoms.

[b]CAT score is preferred, but any can be used.

CAT = COPD Assessment Test (validated questionnaire); COPD = chronic obstructive pulmonary disease; FEV$_1$ = forced expiratory volume in 1 second; GOLD = Global Initiative for Chronic Obstructive Lung Disease; mMRC = Modified Medical Research Council breathlessness scale (validated questionnaire).

Adapted from: Global Initiative for Chronic Obstructive Lung Disease (GOLD). Global Strategy for Diagnosis, Management and Prevention of COPD. 2016 Update. Available at www.goldcopd.org/. Accessed January 4, 2016.

Table 13. GOLD Guidelines: Pharmacotherapy for Stable COPD

Patient Group	Recommended First Choice	Alternative Choice	Other Possible Treatments[a]
A	SA anticholinergic PRN *or* SABA PRN	LA anticholinergic *or* LABA *or* SABA + SA anticholinergic	Theophylline[b]
B	LA anticholinergic *or* LABA	LA anticholinergic + LABA	SABA *and/or* SA anticholinergic Theophylline[b]
C	ICS + LABA *or* LA anticholinergic	LA anticholinergic + LABA *or* LA anticholinergic + PDE-4 inhibitor[c] *or* LABA + PDE-4 inhibitor[c]	SABA *and/or* SA anticholinergic Theophylline[b]
D	ICS + LABA *and/or* LA anticholinergic	ICS + LABA + LA anticholinergic *or* ICS + LABA + PDE-4 inhibitor[c] *or* LA anticholinergic + LABA *or* LA anticholinergic + PDE-4 inhibitor[c]	N-acetylcysteine SABA *and/or* SA anticholinergic Theophylline[b]

Note: All medication choices are listed in alphabetical order and are not necessarily in order of preference.

[a]Medications listed as other possible treatments can be used alone or in combination with first- and alternative-choice columns.

[b]Theophylline is not recommended unless other long-term bronchodilators are unavailable or unaffordable.

[c]If patient has chronic bronchitis.

COPD = chronic obstructive pulmonary disease; GOLD = Global Initiative for Chronic Obstructive Lung Disease; ICS = inhaled corticosteroid; LA = long-acting; LABA = long-acting β$_2$-agonist; PDE-4 = phosphodiesterase type-4; PRN = as needed; SA = short-acting; SABA = short-acting β$_2$-agonist.

Adapted from: Global Initiative for Chronic Obstructive Lung Disease (GOLD). Global Strategy for Diagnosis, Management and Prevention of COPD. 2016 Update. Available at www.goldcopd.org/. Accessed January 4, 2016.

Table 14. ACP/ACCP/ATS/ERS Guidelines: Treatment Recommendations for Stable COPD

- For patients with respiratory symptoms and FEV_1 between 60% and 80% of predicted, treatment with LA inhaled bronchodilators is suggested.

  (Grade W, level of evidence L)

- For patients with respiratory symptoms and FEV_1 <60% of predicted, treatment with LA inhaled bronchodilators is recommended.

  (Grade S, level of evidence M)

- Monotherapy using either LA inhaled anticholinergics or LABAs is recommended for symptomatic patients with FEV_1 <60% of predicted. The choice of specific monotherapy should be based on patient preference, cost, and adverse effect profile.

  (Grade S, level of evidence M)

- Combination inhaled therapies (LA inhaled anticholinergics, LABAs, or ICS) may be used for symptomatic patients with FEV_1 <60% of predicted.

  (Grade W, level of evidence M)

COPD = chronic obstructive pulmonary disease; FEV_1 = forced expiratory volume in 1 second; ICS = inhaled corticosteroid; LA = long-acting; LABA = long-acting β-agonist.

Qaseem A et al. ACP/ACCP/ATS/ERS COPD guidelines. Ann Intern Med 2011;155:179-91.

7. Other pharmacologic treatments
    a. Phosphodiesterase-4 inhibitor: Roflumilast (Daliresp)
        i.   Indication: As a daily treatment to reduce the risk of COPD exacerbations in patients with severe COPD (FEV_1 less than 50% of predicted) associated with chronic bronchitis and a history of frequent exacerbations. In these patients, studies show a reduction in exacerbations and a reduction in the composite end point of moderate exacerbations treated with oral or systemic corticosteroids or severe exacerbations necessitating hospitalization or causing death (level of evidence B). These effects also occur when roflumilast is added to LA bronchodilators (level of evidence B). No trials have assessed the effects of roflumilast on COPD exacerbations when added to an ICS/LA bronchodilator combination. No comparison of adding roflumilast versus ICS to LA bronchodilators is available (currently being studied).
        ii. Mechanism: Reduces inflammation through inhibition of the breakdown of intracellular cyclic adenosine monophosphate; no direct bronchodilator activity
        iii. Dose: 500 mcg orally once daily
        iv. Contraindications: Moderate to severe liver impairment; use in nursing mothers
        v.   Precautions: Weight loss (monitor); psychiatric events including suicidality (monitor; weigh risk/benefit ratio in patients with preexisting psychiatric illness). Twenty percent of patients studied had weight loss of 5%–10% of body weight, compared with 7% with placebo; average weight loss was 2 kg.
        vi. Adverse reactions: Diarrhea, weight loss or decreased appetite, nausea, headache, back pain, influenza, insomnia, and dizziness
        vii. Drug interactions: Use with strong cytochrome P450 (CYP) enzyme inducers is not recommended (e.g., rifampin, phenobarbital, carbamazepine, phenytoin); use with CYP3A4 inhibitors or dual inhibitors of CYP3A4 and CYP1A2 (e.g., erythromycin, ketoconazole, fluvoxamine) increases roflumilast exposure and adverse effects (risk/benefit ratio must be weighed).
    b. Smoking cessation therapy (essential for all patient groups A–D)
    c. Influenza vaccine annually (essential for all patient groups A–D)

    d.   The 23-valent pneumococcal polysaccharide vaccine (PPSV23; Pneumovax) once before age 65, then follow CDC recommendations for pneumococcal vaccination at age 65 and older.

    e. α_1-Antitrypsin augmentation therapy (level of evidence C)

        i.   A once-weekly intravenous therapy of α_1 proteinase inhibitor (Prolastin)

        ii.   For young patients with severe hereditary α_1-antitrypsin deficiency and established emphysema, but an expensive treatment

        iii.   Patients with α_1-antitrypsin deficiency usually are white, usually develop COPD at a young age (younger than 45 years), and have a strong family history. It may be worthwhile to screen such patients.

Patient Cases

6. A 62-year-old man was recently diagnosed with COPD. Spirometry shows he has an FEV_1/FVC 60%, pre-bronchodilator FEV_1 70% of predicted, and postbronchodilator FEV_1 72% of predicted. His symptoms are very bothersome. He reports walking more slowly than others because of shortness of breath and having to stop to catch his breath every so often when walking on level ground (mMRC grade 2). He had one exacerbation in the past year. Which is the most appropriate patient group classification for him, according to the GOLD guidelines?

    A. Group A.

    B. Group B.

    C. Group C.

    D. Group D.

7. In addition to albuterol HFA 2 puffs every 4–6 hours as needed, which pharmacotherapy option is most appropriate to initiate?

    A. No additional therapy needed.

    B. Formoterol: Inhale contents of 1 capsule twice daily.

    C. Salmeterol/fluticasone 50/500 1 puff twice daily.

    D. Salmeterol/fluticasone 50/500 1 puff twice daily plus roflumilast 500 mcg orally once daily.

8. A 52-year-old woman with COPD reports a gradual worsening in shortness of breath during the past few years. Spirometry shows FEV_1/FVC 55% and FEV_1 63% of predicted. Her CAT score is 10. She has not had a COPD exacerbation or received systemic corticosteroids in the past 2 years. Her current COPD medications are tiotropium inhaler once daily and albuterol HFA as needed. According to the GOLD guidelines, which is the most appropriate course of action?

    A. Add salmeterol 1 puff twice daily.

    B. Add long-term azithromycin 250 mg once daily.

    C. Add fluticasone 110 mcg 2 puffs twice daily.

    D. Discontinue tiotropium and initiate salmeterol/fluticasone 250/50 1 puff twice daily.

8. Nonpharmacologic therapy
    a. Home oxygen therapy
        i. Recommended in patients who have a Pao_2 of 55 mm Hg or less (or 55–60 mm Hg if pulmonary hypertension, peripheral edema, or polycythemia [level of evidence D]) or Sao_2 of 88% or less, with or without hypercapnia, confirmed twice during a 3-week period (level of evidence B)
        ii. Long-term (more than 15 hours/day) use in patients with chronic respiratory failure improves survival.
    b. Pulmonary rehabilitation (essential for patient groups B–D; level of evidence A)
        i. Includes exercise training, nutrition counseling, and education
        ii. Recommended for stage II–IV COPD. Patients should be referred when they have moderate (stage II) COPD; do not wait until it is more severe.
        iii. Improves many outcomes in COPD, including quality of life and survival
9. Newer data in COPD
    a. Chronic azithromycin for prevention of COPD exacerbations (Albert et al. 2011)
        i. Compared with placebo, daily azithromycin significantly lengthened time to first exacerbation, decreased rate of exacerbations, and improved quality of life in patients with COPD at increased risk of exacerbations, at the expense of risk of hearing decrements and increasing macrolide-resistant organism colonization.
        ii. Number needed to treat to prevent one acute exacerbation of COPD is 2.86; number needed to harm for hearing decrements is 20.
        iii. There is little evidence of a treatment effect in smokers.
        iv. The GOLD guidelines state that the role of treatment with daily antibiotics is unclear and that treatment is currently not recommended because of an unfavorable balance between benefits and adverse effects.
    b. β-Blockers
        i. Observational data suggest that long-term treatment with β-blockers reduces risk of exacerbations and improves survival, even in patients without overt cardiovascular disease (Rutten et al. 2010).
        ii. More than half of the patients studied had cardiovascular risk factors or coronary artery disease. Mostly cardioselective β-blockers were used.
        iii. It is too early to recommend β-blockers for the treatment of COPD, but β-blockers should not be withheld in patients with COPD who also have heart disease, chronic heart failure, or other cardiovascular conditions in which β-blockers are beneficial (Salpeter et al. 2002, update 2005, reviewed 2008)
        iv. Mechanism for benefit in COPD is unknown, but β-blockers can upregulate $β_2$-receptors in the lungs, which may improve the effectiveness of inhaled β-agonists.

F. Management of Acute Exacerbations of Chronic COPD
    1. A COPD exacerbation is an acute worsening of a patient's baseline respiratory symptoms (e.g., dyspnea, cough, and/or an increase in quantity or purulence of sputum) that is worse than normal day-to-day variation and results in a change in medication. Diagnosis is based purely on clinical presentation.
    2. Common precipitating factors include infection of tracheobronchial tree and viral upper respiratory tract infections (most common) and air pollution. However, the cause of one-third of exacerbations cannot be determined.
    3. Spirometry is not accurate during an exacerbation and is not recommended.

4. Pulse oximetry can be used to determine the need for supplemental oxygen, which should be given in severe exacerbations. In exacerbations necessitating hospitalization, an arterial blood gas measurement should be performed.

5. Inhaled bronchodilators (inhaled SABAs with or without short-acting anticholinergics) are the preferred treatment of COPD exacerbations (level of evidence C).
   a. Usual doses of albuterol are 2.5 mg via nebulizer every 1–4 hours as needed or 4–8 puffs by MDI with holding chamber every 1–4 hours as needed.
   b. Short-acting anticholinergics (ipratropium) are generally added for acute exacerbation.

6. Systemic corticosteroids are effective, and they shorten recovery time, improve FEV_1, and improve hypoxemia (level of evidence A). They also lower the risk of treatment failure, early relapse rate, and length of hospital stay. Systemic corticosteroids should be used in most exacerbations. OCS dose for outpatient treatment: 40 mg of oral prednisone once daily for 5 days is recommended in the GOLD guidelines (level of evidence B), but insufficient data are available to provide strong conclusions about the optimal duration.
   a. Higher daily doses or oral prednisone/prednisolone may be used (e.g., 50–60 mg daily).
   b. A recent study showed that in patients with a COPD exacerbation presenting to the hospital, a shorter course of systemic corticosteroids (5 days) was noninferior to a longer (14 days) course with respect to re-exacerbation within 6 months (Leuppi et al. 2013).

7. Antibiotic treatment should be initiated for exacerbations if the criteria below are met. The most common pathogens in COPD exacerbations: *Streptococcus pneumoniae, Haemophilus influenzae,* and *Moraxella catarrhalis.* In patients with GOLD 3 and 4 severity, *Pseudomonas aeruginosa* infection becomes an important pathogen.
   a. The three cardinal symptoms in COPD exacerbations are increased dyspnea, increased sputum volume, and increased sputum purulence.
      i. Antibiotics should be given if all three cardinal symptoms are present (level of evidence B).
      ii. Antibiotics should be given if two of the three cardinal symptoms are present and if increased sputum purulence is one of the symptoms (level of evidence C).
      iii. Antibiotics should be given to patients with a severe exacerbation requiring mechanical ventilation (level of evidence B).
   b. Recommended duration of antibiotic treatment is usually 5–10 days (level of evidence D).
   c. Recommended antibiotics
      i. Optimal antibiotic therapy has not been determined but should be based on local resistance patterns.
      ii. If recent (less than 3 months) antibiotics, use alternative class.
      iii. Usual initial antibiotics for uncomplicated COPD include azithromycin, clarithromycin, doxycycline, trimethoprim/sulfamethoxazole, and amoxicillin, with or without clavulanate.
      iv. In complicated COPD with risk factors: Amoxicillin/clavulanate, levofloxacin, moxifloxacin. Risk factors: Comorbid diseases, severe COPD (FEV_1 less than 50% of predicted), more than 3 exacerbations/year, antibiotic use in past 3 months
      v. If at risk of *Pseudomonas* infection: High-dose levofloxacin (750 mg) or ciprofloxacin; obtain sputum culture. Risk factors: Four or more courses of antibiotics in past year, recent hospitalization (past 90 days), isolation of *Pseudomonas* during past hospitalization, severe COPD (FEV_1 less than 50% of predicted)
      vi. If exacerbation does not respond to initial antibiotic, sputum culture and sensitivity should be performed.

G. Vaccinations
   1. All patients with COPD should receive the influenza vaccine yearly
   2. All patients with COPD should receive the pneumococcal polysaccharide vaccine (PPSV23) once before age 65; then follow U.S. Centers for Disease Control and Prevention (CDC) recommendations for pneumococcal vaccination at age 65 and older

---

Patient Case

9. A 64-year-old woman with COPD in GOLD patient group A presents for a clinic visit. In the past few days, she has had a worsening in shortness of breath and a productive cough with more "cloudy" and more copious sputum than usual. Pulse oximetry is 95% on room air. She has a nebulizer at home. In addition to regular use of albuterol plus ipratropium by nebulizer every 1–4 hours, which is the best course of action?

   A. No additional therapy is necessary.

   B. Add oral prednisone 40 mg once daily for 5 days

   C. Add trimethoprim/sulfamethoxazole double-strength 1 tablet twice daily for 7 days.

   D. Add oral prednisone 40 mg once daily for 5 days and trimethoprim/sulfamethoxazole double strength 1 tablet twice daily for 7 days.

III. GOUT

Guidelines:

Khanna D, Fitzgerald JD, Khanna PP, et al. 2012 American College of Rheumatology Guidelines for Management of Gout. Part 1. Systematic nonpharmacologic and pharmacologic therapeutic approaches to hyperuricemia. Arthritis Care Res 2012;64:1431-46.

Khanna D, Khanna PP, Fitzgerald JD, et al. 2012 American College of Rheumatology Guidelines for Management of Gout. Part 2. Therapy and antiinflammatory prophylaxis of acute gouty arthritis. Arthritis Care Res 2012;64:1447-61.

A. Definition: A spectrum of clinical and pathologic features caused by hyperuricemia (serum urate level more than 6.8 mg/dL), resulting in tissue deposition of monosodium urate monohydrate crystals in the extracellular fluid of joints and other sites. Most common rheumatic disease of adults; prevalence estimated at 3.9% of adults (around 8.3 million people)

B. Diagnosis
   1. Typically presents as acute episodic arthritis.
   2. Can also present as chronic arthritis of one or more joints.
   3. Tophi may be present: Detected by physical examination or imaging and pathology.
   4. Renal manifestations include urolithiasis.
   5. Features of acute gouty attack
      a. Severe pain, redness, swelling; maximum severity in 12–24 hours; may continue for a few days to several weeks.
      b. Most often occurs in the lower extremities and in a single joint.
         i. Most common joint: First metatarsophalangeal joint (podagra) or knee
         ii. May occur in many other joints, including upper extremity
         iii. May be polyarticular at first presentation (less than 20% of cases)

6. Ideally, definitive diagnosis should be made by visualization of monosodium urate crystals by polarized compensated light microscopy in fluid aspirated from the affected joint during an acute gouty attack.
   a. For diagnosis of gout, monosodium urate crystals are negatively birefringent (needle-shaped or rods).
   b. In pseudogout, crystals are calcium pyrophosphate dihydrate and are weakly positively birefringent (rods or rhomboidal).
   c. Diagnosis by joint aspiration is difficult because patients are in severe pain and often refuse joint aspiration during an acute attack. In this case, a provisional diagnosis may be made according to clinical data.
7. If diagnosis by joint aspiration is not possible, a tentative diagnosis may be made by a combination of presentation or clinical picture and elevated uric acid. Use of hyperuricemia as one of the criteria for diagnosing gout may be difficult during an initial acute attack because serum uric acid may be low during flares. Best time to check uric acid is 2 weeks after a flare.

C. Predisposing Factors (Singh et al. 2011)
   1. Dietary: High meat and seafood consumption, fatty foods, dietary overindulgence, high intake of beer and spirits in men (not wine), sugar-sweetened soft drinks, high-fructose foods
   2. Drugs: Xanthine oxidase inhibitors (XOIs) and uricosuric agents (with initial therapy), thiazides and loop diuretics, niacin, calcineurin inhibitors, low-dose aspirin (325 mg/day or less)
   3. Medical conditions and other factors: Obesity, diabetes, hypertension, dyslipidemia, renal insufficiency, early menopause, trauma, surgery, starvation, dehydration

D. Classification
   1. Three stages of gout:
      a. Acute gouty arthritis
      b. Intercritical gout (intervals between attacks)
      c. Chronic recurrent gout
   2. Severities of chronic tophaceous gouty arthropathy (CTGA)
      a. Mild: One joint, stable disease
      b. Moderate: Two to four joints, stable disease
      c. Severe
         i. Chronic CTGA of more than four joints *or*
         ii. One or more unstable, complicated, severe articular tophi
   3. Size of joints
      a. Large joints (e.g., knee, ankle, wrist, elbow, hip, shoulder)
      b. Medium joints (e.g., wrist, ankle, elbow)
      c. Small joints (e.g., interphalangeal)

E. Treatment Goals
   1. Serum urate target: Less than 6 mg/dL
   2. Serum urate target of less than 5 mg/dL may be needed to improve gout signs and symptoms. Consider goal of less than 5 mg/dL if tophi present.
   3. Decrease frequency of acute gouty attacks.

F.   Nonpharmacologic Therapy (Table 15)

Table 15. Nonpharmacologic Therapy for Gout

Lifestyle and General Health		
Weight loss if obese Healthy overall diet Exercise Smoking cessation Proper hydration		
Food and Drink to Avoid	**Food and Drink to Limit**	**Food and Drink to Encourage**

Organ meats high in purine (e.g., liver, kidney, sweetbreads)	Serving sizes of:
	   Beef, lamb, pork
	   Seafood with high purine content
	   (e.g., sardines, shellfish)
		Low-fat or nonfat dairy products

High-fructose corn syrup–sweetened sodas, beverages, and foods	Servings of naturally sweet fruit juices Table sugar, sweetened beverages, desserts Table salt	Vegetables
Alcohol overuse (>2 per day for men and >1 per day for women) in all patients Any alcohol use during times of frequent gouty attacks or advanced gout under poor control	Alcohol (particularly beer but also wine and spirits)	

Adapted from: Khanna D, Fitzgerald JD, Khanna PP, et al. 2012 American College of Rheumatology Guidelines for Management of Gout. Part 1. Systematic nonpharmacologic and pharmacologic therapeutic approaches to hyperuricemia. Arthritis Care Res 2012;64:1431-46.

G.   Pharmacologic Treatment of Hyperuricemia
   1.   Consider discontinuing nonessential medications that cause hyperuricemia.
   2.   Indications for urate-lowering therapy (ULT)
      a.   Tophi by clinical examination or imaging study
      b.   Two or more acute gouty attacks per year
      c.   CKD stage 2 or worse
      d.   Past urolithiasis
   3.   ULT can be initiated during an acute gouty attack as long as concomitant anti-inflammatory therapy is given.
   4.   First-line ULT
      a.   XOI: Allopurinol or febuxostat
      b.   Can switch to alternative XOI if patient is intolerant of or refractory to first XOI.
   5.   Alternative first-line ULT (uricosuric): Probenecid (if at least one XOI is contraindicated or not tolerated). History of urolithiasis and CrCl less than 50 mL/minute contraindicates first-line use of probenecid.

6. Initiate anti-inflammatory prophylaxis for acute gout concomitantly with or just before ULT in all patients.
    a. Early increase in acute gouty attacks during initiation of ULT
        i.   May be caused by rapid decrease in urate concentrations, resulting in remodeling of articular urate crystal deposits
        ii. Often leads to nonadherence to ULT; patient education is critical.
    b. Oral low-dose colchicine is first-line option.
    c. Other first-line option is low-dose nonsteroidal anti-inflammatory drugs (NSAIDs) (lower evidence grade than colchicine). Add concomitant proton pump inhibitor or other agent for suppression of peptic ulcer disease when indicated.
    d. OCS is an alternative for anti-inflammatory gouty attack prophylaxis (level of evidence C).
        i.   If colchicine and NSAIDs are contraindicated, not tolerated, or ineffective
        ii. Because of risks associated with prolonged use of OCSs, the risk/benefit ratio of this strategy should be considered and reevaluated with continued ULT therapy because the risk of acute gout decreases in time.
    e. Anti-inflammatory prophylaxis of acute gout should continue for the greater of:
        i.   6 months (level of evidence A)
        ii.   3 months after achieving target serum urate level if no tophi (level of evidence B)
        iii. 6 months after achieving target serum urate level if tophi were previously present but are now resolved (level of evidence C)
        iv.   However, continue anti-inflammatory prophylaxis if any clinical evidence of gout disease activity is present (tophi, recent acute gouty attacks, chronic gouty arthritis).
7. Monitor serum urate every 2–5 weeks. After goal is achieved, continue monitoring every 6 months. If serum urate goals are not achieved:
    a. Titrate single-agent XOI to maximum appropriate dose.
    b. Next, add uricosuric to XOI (probenecid, losartan, or fenofibrate). Probenecid is first-line uricosuric; losartan and fenofibrate are off-label but recommended second-line uricosurics.
    c. If goal serum urate still not achieved, add pegloticase only if severe gout disease burden *and* patient is refractory to or intolerant of other ULT options. Pegloticase is not recommended for first-line therapy in any case.
8. Indefinite duration of ULT is recommended.
9. Allopurinol hypersensitivity syndrome (AHS)
    a. Risk of severe morbidity and hospitalization
    b. Mortality rate of 20%–25% in AHS
    c. Manifestations of AHS: Stevens-Johnson syndrome, toxic epidermal necrolysis, clinical constellation of symptoms: eosinophilia, rash, vasculitis, major end-organ disease
    d. Highest risk is during the first few months of therapy.
    e. Risk factors: Concomitant thiazide diuretics, renal impairment, people of Han Chinese or Thai descent (irrespective of renal function), people of Korean descent with stage 3 or worse CKD. Consider testing for *HLA-B*5801* in these ethnic groups (if positive, higher risk of AHS).

H. Treatment of Acute Gout
1. Assess severity of gouty attack (Table 16) and select treatment according to severity.
2. Initiate pharmacologic treatment within 24 hours of onset of acute gouty attack (Table 17). Colchicine is appropriate only if initiated within 36 hours of attack onset.
3. Continue established ULT without interruption during acute gouty attack (do not discontinue ULT).

Table 16. Severity, Duration, and Extent of Acute Gouty Attacks

Severity (self-reported; based on visual analog scale; 0–10)	
Mild	≤4
Moderate	5–6
Severe	≥7
Duration Since Onset	
Early	<12 hours after attack onset
Well established	12–36 hours after attack onset
Late	>36 hours after attack onset
Extent	
One or a few small joints	
One or two large joints	Large joints: Ankle, knee, wrist, elbow, hip, shoulder
Polyarticular	Four or more joints involving >1 region (regions: forefoot, midfoot, ankle or hindfoot, knee, hip, fingers, wrist, elbow, shoulder) Three separate large joints

a. For mild to moderate pain affecting one or a few small joints or one or two large joints, use monotherapy.
b. For severe pain or polyarticular attack, or if multiple large joints are affected, use initial combination therapy.
   i. Monotherapy: NSAID *or* OCSs *or* colchicine (level of evidence A for all choices), supplemented with topical ice (adjunctive therapy) as needed
      (a) No preference for one choice over another; select treatment according to gout flare presentation, comorbidities, previous response, and patient preference.
         (1) Consider intra-articular corticosteroids if one or two large joints; use OCSs for all other presentations; may consider single-dose intramuscular triamcinolone followed by an OCS.
         (2) Concomitant use of colchicine with P-glycoprotein (Pgp) inhibitors or strong CYP3A4 inhibitors is contraindicated in renal or hepatic impairment (fatal toxicity has occurred).
         (3) Colchicine dose should be reduced if normal renal or hepatic function and concomitant use of Pgp inhibitors or moderate to strong CYP3A4 inhibitors.
         (4) If the patient has received acute gout treatment with colchicine in the past 2 weeks, use alternative therapy.
         (5) Colchicine should not be used to treat gouty attacks in patients with renal or hepatic impairment who are taking prophylactic colchicine, according to labeling.

(b) Celecoxib is an option in certain patients with contraindications or intolerance to NSAIDs; risk-benefit ratio unclear.

(c) Adrenocorticotropic hormone 20–40 international units subcutaneously is an option if patient is unable to take medication by mouth.

ii. Initial combination therapy: Can use full doses of both agents or, when appropriate, full dose of one agent and prophylactic dose of another agent

(a) Colchicine plus an NSAID

(b) OCSs plus colchicine

(c) Intra-articular steroids with all other modalities

(d) Combination of an NSAID and systemic corticosteroids has synergistic GI toxicity.

iii. Continue acute treatment until the gouty attack has resolved.

4. If inadequate response to initial treatment of acute gouty attack:

a. Inadequate response defined as either less than 20% improvement in pain score in 24 hours or less than 50% improvement in 24 hours or more after starting drug therapy for acute attack.

b. If inadequate response, switch to a different monotherapy (level of evidence C) or add a second agent (level of evidence C).

c. Biologic agents that inhibit interleukin-1 (anakinra and canakinumab) are considered investigational for the treatment of acute gout but can be considered when gout flares are frequent and resistant to all other therapies.

5. Educate patients and provide a prescription so that patients can initiate treatment for acute gouty attacks on their own.

Table 17. Medication Dosing for Gout

Drug	Dose	Comments
Acute Gouty Attack Treatment		
Colchicine (Colcrys)	1.2 mg, then 0.6 mg 1 hour later, then 0.6 mg once or twice daily until attack resolves CrCl 30–80 mL/minute: Monitor for adverse effects; dose adjustment not necessary CrCl <30 mL/minute: Dose adjustment not necessary but may be considered; do not repeat course of treatment more than every 2 weeks Dialysis: 0.6-mg single dose; do not repeat course of treatment more than every 2 weeks Severe hepatic impairment: Dose reduction not necessary but may be considered; do not repeat course of treatment more frequently than every 2 weeks	Concomitant use of colchicine with Pgp inhibitors or strong CYP3A4 inhibitors is contraindicated in renal or hepatic impairment (fatal toxicity has occurred) Colchicine dose should be reduced if renal and hepatic function is normal and if used concomitantly with Pgp inhibitors or moderate to strong CYP3A4 inhibitors
NSAIDs	Naproxen: 750 mg initially, followed by 250 mg every 8 hours Naproxen ER: 1000–1500 mg once daily, followed by 1000 mg once daily Indomethacin: 50 mg 3 times daily until pain tolerable, then reduce dose until attack resolves Sulindac: 200 mg twice daily Use at anti-inflammatory or analgesic doses of other NSAIDs, same as for treatment of acute pain or inflammation	Only FDA-approved NSAIDs are naproxen, indomethacin, and sulindac; however, other NSAIDs may be as effective Continue full dose until attack completely resolves Can taper dose if comorbidities or renal or hepatic impairment is present
Celecoxib (Celebrex)	800 mg once, followed by 400 mg on day 1, then 400 mg twice daily for 1 week	Only in certain patients when NSAIDs are contraindicated or not tolerated
Corticosteroids	OCSs for all cases of gout (level of evidence B) Prednisone 0.5 mg/kg per day for 5–10 days (level of evidence A) *or* Prednisone 0.5 mg/kg per day for 2–5 days, then taper for 7–10 days, then discontinue (level of evidence C) *or* Methylprednisolone dose pack (level of evidence C) Option for 1 or 2 large joints: Intra-articular corticosteroids (level of evidence B) Dose based on the size of the joint (e.g., triamcinolone 40 mg for large joint, 30 mg for medium joint, 10 mg for small joint or equivalent) IM triamcinolone followed by OCS (level of evidence C) 60 mg IM, followed by OCS (dosed as above)	Intra-articular corticosteroids can be used in combination with OCSs, NSAIDs, or colchicine (level of evidence B)

Table 17. Medication Dosing for Gout *(continued)*

Drug	Dose	Comments
Urate-Lowering Therapy		
Allopurinol (Zyloprim)[a]	Starting dose: 100 mg daily (50 mg daily in stage 4 CKD) Gradually titrate dose every 2–5 weeks to appropriate maximum dose (800 mg daily with normal renal function) or until goal urate level reached Maintenance dose can be higher than 300 mg daily, even in CKD, as long as patient is educated and regular monitoring occurs for hypersensitivity, rash, pruritus, elevated hepatic enzymes, and eosinophilia	XOI Low starting dose reduces early gout flares and risk of hypersensitivity syndrome Consider keeping dose lower in CKD and not increasing to maximum dose; data with dosing >300 mg/day in CKD are limited Dose reduction algorithms in CKD have been developed but are not evidence based; the ACR guidelines do not recommend following them
Febuxostat (Uloric)[a]	Starting dose: 40 mg once daily May increase dose to 80 mg once daily if goal serum urate not reached CrCl <30 mL/minute: Use caution; insufficient data	XOI More expensive than allopurinol; no generic available
Probenecid (generic only)[a]	Starting dose: 250 mg twice daily May increase weekly in 500-mg/day increments to maximum dose of 1 g twice daily if needed Avoid if CrCl < 30 mL/minute	Uricosuric; first-line According to the guidelines, not recommended for first-line or alternative first-line treatment if CrCl < 50 mL/minute or history of urolithiasis Do baseline and periodic urine uric acid; elevated urine uric acid level (uric acid overproduction) is contraindication When initiating, increase fluid intake and consider urine alkalinization (e.g., potassium citrate)
Losartan	Dose according to other indications and as tolerated	Uricosuric; second-line Off-label use
Fenofibrate	Dose according to other indications and as tolerated	Uricosuric; second line Off-label use
Pegloticase (Krystexxa)[a]	8 mg intravenously every 2 weeks No dosage adjustment for CKD	Use only if severe gout disease burden *and* refractory to or intolerant of other ULT options All other antihyperuricemic agents must be discontinued before initiating pegloticase; do not administer concomitantly Premedicate with antihistamines and corticosteroids

Table 17. Medication Dosing for Gout *(continued)*

Drug	Dose	Comments
Gouty Attack Prophylaxis		
Colchicine (Colcrys)	0.6 mg once or twice daily CrCl 30–80 mL/minute: Monitor for adverse effects; dose adjustment not necessary CrCl <30 mL/minute: Initial dose 0.3 mg/day; use caution and monitor if dose titrated further Dialysis: 0.3 mg twice weekly; monitor for adverse effects Severe hepatic impairment: Dose reduction not necessary but may be considered; do not repeat course of treatment more often than every 2 weeks	First-line Concomitant use of colchicine with Pgp inhibitors or strong CYP3A4 inhibitors is contraindicated in renal or hepatic impairment (fatal toxicity has occurred) Colchicine dose should be reduced if renal and hepatic function is normal and if used concomitantly with Pgp inhibitors or moderate to strong CYP3A4 inhibitors
NSAIDs	Lower doses than used for acute attacks (e.g., naproxen 250 mg twice daily, indomethacin 25 mg twice daily)	Alternative first line; less strong evidence than with colchicine Consider concomitant proton pump inhibitor or other agent for suppression of PUD when indicated
OCSs	Prednisone or prednisolone ≤10 mg daily	Alternative Only if colchicine and NSAIDs are both contraindicated, ineffective, or not tolerated

[a]Always initiate concomitant prophylactic therapy.

ACR = American College of Rheumatology; CKD = chronic kidney disease; CrCl = creatinine clearance; CYP = cytochrome P450; ER = extended release; FDA = U.S. Food and Drug Administration; IM = intramuscular(ly); NSAID = nonsteroidal anti-inflammatory drug; OCS = oral corticosteroid; Pgp = P-glycoprotein; PUD = peptic ulcer disease; ULT = urate-lowering therapy; XOI = xanthine oxidase inhibitor.

Patient Cases

10. A 60-year-old man presents with his third gouty attack in the past year. His last attack was 10 days ago, for which he took colchicine with good response. His pain is in his left knee and in the third and fourth proximal interphalangeal joints on his left hand. The pain started about 10 hours ago. He rates his pain as 6/10. He has COPD and dyslipidemia, his renal function is normal, and his weight is 80 kg. His uric acid level from 1 month ago is 10 mg/day. He has no tophi. His only medications are inhaled tiotropium, albuterol, and simvastatin. Which is most appropriate for treatment of this acute gouty attack?

    A. Naproxen 750 mg, then 250 mg every 8 hours.

    B. Colchicine 1.2 mg, then 0.6 mg in 1 hour, then 0.6 mg every 12 hours.

    C. Intra-articular triamcinolone injection of all affected joints.

    D. Prednisone 40 mg daily plus naproxen 750 mg, then 250 mg every 8 hours.

11. Which is most appropriate regarding ULT in this patient?

    A. Probenecid should be started, but treatment should be delayed until after the acute attack is resolved.

    B. Probenecid should be started and can be initiated during the acute attack.

    C. Oral allopurinol should be started, but treatment should be delayed after the acute attack has resolved.

    D. Oral allopurinol should be started and can be initiated during the acute attack.

Patient Cases *(continued)*

12. Which regimen for anti-inflammatory prophylaxis with ULT therapy is most appropriate in this patient, once the acute attack has resolved?

   A. Colchicine orally 0.6 mg once daily.

   B. Prednisone 10 mg daily.

   C. Colchicine 0.6 mg once daily plus naproxen 250 mg twice daily.

   D. Pegloticase 8 mg intravenously every 2 weeks.

13. What is the initial goal uric acid level and duration of anti-inflammatory prophylaxis in this patient?

   A. Goal <6 mg/dL; continue for a total of 6 months.

   B. Goal <6 mg/dL; continue for 3 months after achieving goal serum urate for at least 6 months total.

   C. Goal <5 mg/dL; continue for a total of 6 months.

   D. Goal <5 mg/dL; continue for 3 months after achieving goal serum urate for at least 6 months total.

IV. ADULT IMMUNIZATIONS

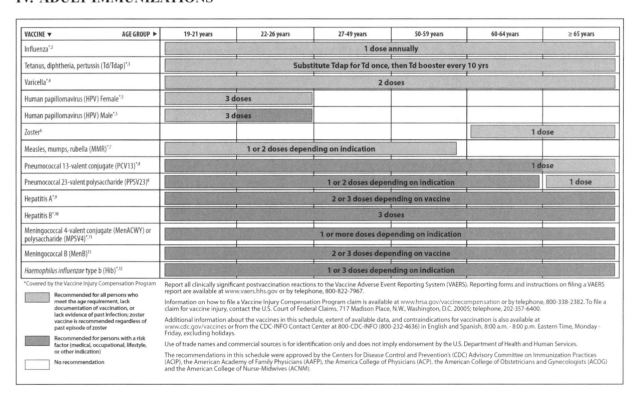

Figure 1. Recommended adult immunization schedule, by vaccine and age group,[1] United States, 2016.

Centers for Disease Control and Prevention (CDC). Advisory Committee on Immunization Practices (ACIP). Recommended Immunization Schedule for Adults Aged 19 Years and Older: United States, 2016. Available at www.cdc.gov/vaccines/schedules/downloads/adult/adult-combined-schedule.pdf.

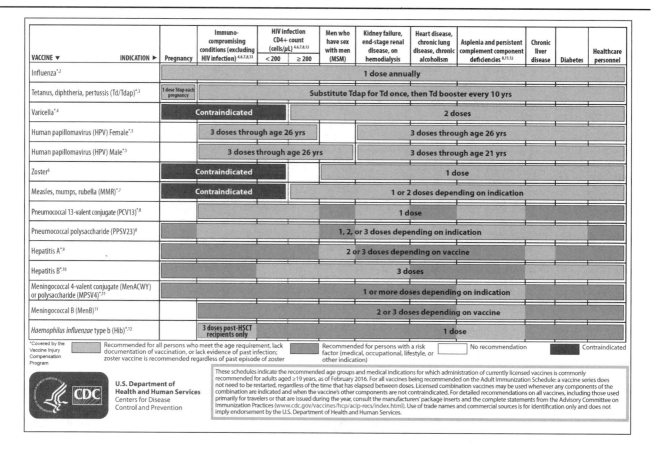

Figure 2. Vaccines that might be indicated for adults, based on medical and other indications,[1,a] United States, 2016.

[a]The above recommendations must be read together with the footnotes on the following pages of this schedule.

Centers for Disease Control and Prevention (CDC). Advisory Committee on Immunization Practices (ACIP). Recommended Immunization Schedule for Adults Aged 19 Years and Older: United States, 2016. Available at www.cdc.gov/vaccines/schedules/downloads/adult/adult-combined-schedule.pdf

Footnotes—Recommended Immunization Schedule for Adults Aged 19 Years or Older: United States, 2016

1. **Additional information**
   - Additional guidance for the use of the vaccines described in this supplement can be found in the ACIP Recommendations.
   - Information on vaccination recommendations when vaccination status is unknown and other general immunization information can be found in the General Recommendations on Immunization.
   - Information on travel vaccine (e.g., for hepatitis A and B, meningococcal, and other vaccines) can be found in travel vaccine requirements and recommendations.
   - Additional information and resources regarding pregnant women can be found in vaccination of pregnant women.

2. **Influenza vaccination**
   - Annual vaccination against influenza is recommended for all persons aged ·6 months. A list of currently available influenza vaccines can be found atwww.cdc.gov/flu/protect/vaccine/vaccines.htm.
   - Persons aged ·6 months, including pregnant women, can receive the inactivated influenza vaccine (IIV). An age-appropriate IIV formulation should be used.
   - Intradermal IIV is an option for persons aged 18 through 64 years.
   - High-dose IIV is an option for persons aged ·65 years.
   - Live attenuated influenza vaccine (LAIV [FluMist]) is an option for healthy, non-pregnant persons aged 2 through 49 years.
   - Recombinant influenza vaccine (RIV [Flublok]) is approved for persons aged ·18 years.
   - RIV, which does not contain any egg protein, may be administered to persons aged ·18 years with egg allergy of any severity; IIV may be used with additional safety measures for persons with hives-only allergy to eggs.
   - Health care personnel who care for severely immunocompromised persons who require care in a protected environment should receive IIV or RIV; health care personnel who receive LAIV should avoid providing care for severely immunosuppressed persons for 7 days after vaccination.

3. **Tetanus, diphtheria, and acellular pertussis (Td/Tdap) vaccination**
   - Administer 1 dose of Tdap vaccine to pregnant women during each pregnancy (preferably during 27-36 weeks' gestation) regardless of interval since prior Td or Tdap vaccination.
   - Persons aged ·11 years who have not received Tdap vaccine or for whom vaccine status is unknown should receive a dose of Tdap followed by tetanus and diphtheria toxoids (Td) booster doses every 10 years thereafter. Tdap can be administered regardless of interval since the most recent tetanus or diphtheria-toxoid containing vaccine.
   - Adults with an unknown or incomplete history of completing a 3-dose primary vaccination series with Td-containing vaccines should begin or complete a primary vaccination series including a Tdap dose.
   - For unvaccinated adults, administer the first 2 doses at least 4 weeks apart and the third dose 6-12 months after the second.
   - For incompletely vaccinated (i.e., less than 3 doses) adults, administer remaining doses.
   - Refer to the ACIP statement for recommendations for administering Td/Tdap as prophylaxis in wound management (see footnote 1).

4. **Varicella vaccination**
   - All adults without evidence of immunity to varicella (as defined below) should receive 2 doses of single-antigen varicella vaccine or a second dose if they have received only 1 dose.
   - Vaccination should be emphasized for those who have close contact with persons at high risk for severe disease (e.g., health care personnel and family contacts of persons with immunocompromising conditions) or are at high risk for exposure or transmission (e.g., teachers; child care employees; residents and staff members of institutional settings, including correctional institutions; college students; military personnel; adolescents and adults living in households with children; nonpregnant women of childbearing age; and international travelers).
   - Pregnant women should be assessed for evidence of varicella immunity. Women who do not have evidence of immunity should receive the first dose of varicella vaccine upon completion or termination of pregnancy and before discharge from the health care facility. The second dose should be administered 4-8 weeks after the first dose.

   - Evidence of immunity to varicella in adults includes any of the following:
     - documentation of 2 doses of varicella vaccine at least 4 weeks apart;
     - U.S.-born before 1980, except health care personnel and pregnant women;
     - history of varicella based on diagnosis or verification of varicella disease by a health care provider;
     - history of herpes zoster based on diagnosis or verification of herpes zoster disease by a health care provider; or
     - laboratory evidence of immunity or laboratory confirmation of disease.

5. **Human papillomavirus (HPV) vaccination**
   - Three HPV vaccines are licensed for use in females (bivalent HPV vaccine [2vHPV], quadrivalent HPV vaccine [4vHPV], and 9-valent HPV vaccine [9vHPV]) and two HPV vaccines are licensed for use in males (4vHPV and 9vHPV).
   - For females, 2vHPV, 4vHPV, or 9vHPV is recommended in a 3-dose series for routine vaccination at age 11 or 12 years and for those aged 13 through 26 years, if not previously vaccinated.
   - For males, 4vHPV or 9vHPV is recommended in a 3-dose series for routine vaccination at age 11 or 12 years and for those aged 13 through 21 years, if not previously vaccinated. Males aged 22 through 26 years may be vaccinated.
   - HPV vaccination is recommended for men who have sex with men through age 26 years who did not get any or all doses when they were younger.
   - Vaccination is recommended for immunocompromised persons (including those with HIV infection) through age 26 years for those who did not get any or all doses when they were younger.
   - A complete HPV vaccination series consists of 3 doses. The second dose should be administered 4-8 weeks (minimum interval of 4 weeks) after the first dose; the third dose should be administered 24 weeks after the first dose and 16 weeks after the second dose (minimum interval of at least 12 weeks).
   - HPV vaccines are not recommended for use in pregnant women. However, pregnancy testing is not needed before vaccination. If a woman is found to be pregnant after initiating the vaccination series, no intervention is needed; the remainder of the 3-dose series should be delayed until completion or termination of pregnancy.

6. **Zoster vaccination**
   - A single dose of zoster vaccine is recommended for adults aged ·60 years regardless of whether they report a prior episode of herpes zoster. Although the vaccine is licensed by the U.S. Food and Drug Administration for use among and can be administered to persons aged ·50 years, ACIP recommends that vaccination begin at age 60 years.
   - Persons aged ·60 years with chronic medical conditions may be vaccinated unless their condition constitutes a contraindication, such as pregnancy or severe immunodeficiency.

7. **Measles, mumps, rubella (MMR) vaccination**
   - Adults born before 1957 are generally considered immune to measles and mumps. All adults born in 1957 or later should have documentation of 1 or more doses of MMR vaccine unless they have a medical contraindication to the vaccine or laboratory evidence of immunity to each of the three diseases. Documentation of provider-diagnosed disease is not considered acceptable evidence of immunity for measles, mumps, or rubella.

   Measles component:
   - A routine second dose of MMR vaccine, administered a minimum of 28 days after the first dose, is recommended for adults who:
     - are students in postsecondary educational institutions,
     - work in a health care facility, or
     - plan to travel internationally.
   - Persons who received inactivated (killed) measles vaccine or measles vaccine of unknown type during 1963-1967 should be revaccinated with 2 doses of MMR vaccine.

   Mumps component:
   - A routine second dose of MMR vaccine, administered a minimum of 28 days after the first dose, is recommended for adults who:
     - are students in a postsecondary educational institution,
     - work in a health care facility, or
     - plan to travel internationally.

Footnotes—Recommended Immunization Schedule for Adults Aged 19 Years or Older: United States, 2016

- Persons vaccinated before 1979 with either killed mumps vaccine or mumps vaccine of unknown type who are at high risk for mumps infection (e.g., persons who are working in a health care facility) should be considered for revaccination with 2 doses of MMR vaccine.

  Rubella component:
- For women of childbearing age, regardless of birth year, rubella immunity should be determined. If there is no evidence of immunity, women who are not pregnant should be vaccinated. Pregnant women who do not have evidence of immunity should receive MMR vaccine upon completion or termination of pregnancy and before discharge from the health care facility.

  Health care personnel born before 1957:
- For unvaccinated health care personnel born before 1957 who lack laboratory evidence of measles, mumps, and/or rubella immunity or laboratory confirmation of disease, health care facilities should consider vaccinating personnel with 2 doses of MMR vaccine at the appropriate interval for measles and mumps or 1 dose of MMR vaccine for rubella.

8. **Pneumococcal vaccination**
   - General information
     - Adults are recommended to receive 1 dose of 13-valent pneumococcal conjugate vaccine (PCV13) and 1, 2, or 3 doses (depending on indication) of 23-valent pneumococcal polysaccharide vaccine (PPSV23).
     - PCV13 should be administered at least 1 year after PPSV23.
     - PPSV23 should be administered at least 1 year after PCV13, except among adults with immunocompromising conditions, anatomical or functional asplenia, cerebrospinal fluid leak, or cochlear implant, for whom the interval should be at least 8 weeks; the interval between PPSV23 doses should be at least 5 years.
     - No additional dose of PPSV23 is indicated for adults vaccinated with PPSV23 at age ·65 years.
     - When both PCV13 and PPSV23 are indicated, PCV13 should be administered first; PCV13 and PPSV23 should not be administered during the same visit.
     - When indicated, PCV13 and PPSV23 should be administered to adults whose pneumococcal vaccination history is incomplete or unknown.
   - Adults aged ·65 years (immunocompetent) who:
     - have not received PCV13 or PPSV23: administer PCV13 followed by PPSV23 at least 1 year after PCV13.
     - have not received PCV13 but have received a dose of PPSV23 at age ·65 years: administer PCV13 at least 1 year after PPSV23.
     - have not received PCV13 but have received 1 or more doses of PPSV23 at age <65 years: administer PCV13 at least 1 year after the most recent dose of PPSV23. Administer a dose of PPSV23 at least 1 year after PCV13 and at least 5 years after the most recent dose of PPSV23.
     - have received PCV13 but not PPSV23 at age <65 years: administer PPSV23 at least 1 year after PCV13.
     - have received PCV13 and 1 or more doses of PPSV23 at age <65 years: administer PPSV23 at least 1 year after PCV13 and at least 5 years after the most recent dose of PPSV23.
   - Adults aged ·19 years with immunocompromising conditions or anatomical or functional asplenia (defined below) who:
     - have not received PCV13 or PPSV23: administer PCV13 followed by PPSV23 at least 8 weeks after PCV13. Administer a second dose of PPSV23 at least 5 years after the first dose of PPSV23.
     - have not received PCV13 but have received 1 dose of PPSV23: administer PCV13 at least 1 year after the PPSV23. Administer a second dose of PPSV23 at least 8 weeks after PCV13 and at least 5 years after the first dose of PPSV23.
     - have not received PCV13 but have received 2 doses of PPSV23: administer PCV13 at least 1 year after the most recent dose of PPSV23.
     - have received PCV13 but not PPSV23: administer PPSV23 at least 8 weeks after PCV13. Administer a second dose of PPSV23 at least 5 years after the first dose of PPSV23.
     - have received PCV13 and 1 dose of PPSV23: administer a second dose of PPSV23 at least 8 weeks after PCV13 and at least 5 years after the first dose of PPSV23.

- If the most recent dose of PPSV23 was administered at age <65 years, at age ·65 years, administer a dose of PPSV23 at least 8 weeks after PCV13 and at least 5 years after the last dose of PPSV23.
- Immunocompromising conditions that are indications for pneumococcal vaccination are: congenital or acquired immunodeficiency (including B- or T-lymphocyte deficiency, complement deficiencies, and phagocytic disorders excluding chronic granulomatous disease), HIV infection, chronic renal failure, nephrotic syndrome, leukemia, lymphoma, Hodgkin disease, generalized malignancy, multiple myeloma, solid organ transplant, and iatrogenic immunosuppression (including long-term systemic corticosteroids and radiation therapy).
- Anatomical or functional asplenia that are indications for pneumococcal vaccination are: sickle cell disease and other hemoglobinopathies, congenital or acquired asplenia, splenic dysfunction, and splenectomy. Administer pneumococcal vaccines at least 2 weeks before immunosuppressive therapy or an elective splenectomy, and as soon as possible to adults who are newly diagnosed with asymptomatic or symptomatic HIV infection.

- Adults aged ·19 years with cerebrospinal fluid leaks or cochlear implants: administer PCV13 followed by PPSV23 at least 8 weeks after PCV13; no additional dose of PPSV23 is indicated if aged <65 years. If PPSV23 was administered at age ·65 years, at age ·65 years, administer another dose of PPSV23 at least 5 years after the last dose of PPSV23.
- Adults aged 19 through 64 years with chronic heart disease (including congestive heart failure and cardiomyopathies, excluding hypertension), chronic lung disease (including chronic obstructive lung disease, emphysema, and asthma), chronic liver disease (including cirrhosis), alcoholism, or diabetes mellitus, or who smoke cigarettes: administer PPSV23. At age ·65 years, administer PCV13 at least 1 year after PPSV23, followed by another dose of PPSV23 at least 1 year after PCV13 and at least 5 years after the last dose of PPSV23.
- Routine pneumococcal vaccination is not recommended for American Indian/Alaska Native or other adults unless they have the indications as above; however, public health authorities may consider recommending the use of pneumococcal vaccines for American Indians/Alaska Natives or other adults who live in areas with increased risk for invasive pneumococcal disease.

9. **Hepatitis A vaccination**
   - Vaccinate any person seeking protection from hepatitis A virus (HAV) infection and persons with any of the following indications:
     - men who have sex with men;
     - persons who use injection or noninjection illicit drugs;
     - persons working with HAV-infected primates or with HAV in a research laboratory setting;
     - persons with chronic liver disease and persons who receive clotting factor concentrates;
     - persons traveling to or working in countries that have high or intermediate endemicity of hepatitis A (see footnote 1); and
     - unvaccinated persons who anticipate close personal contact (e.g., household or regular babysitting) with an international adoptee during the first 60 days after arrival in the United States from a country with high or intermediate endemicity for hepatitis A (see footnote 1). The first dose of the 2-dose hepatitis A vaccine series should be administered as soon as adoption is planned, ideally 2 or more weeks before the arrival of the adoptee.
   - Single-antigen vaccine formulations should be administered in a 2-dose schedule at either 0 and 6-12 months (Havrix), or 0 and 6-18 months (Vaqta). If the combined hepatitis A and hepatitis B vaccine (Twinrix) is used, administer 3 doses at 0, 1, and 6 months; alternatively, a 4-dose schedule may be used, administered on days 0, 7, and 21-30, followed by a booster dose at 12 months.

10. **Hepatitis B vaccination**
    - Vaccinate any person seeking protection from hepatitis B virus (HBV) infection and persons with any of the following indications:
      - sexually active persons who are not in a long-term, mutually monogamous relationship (e.g., persons with more than 1 sex partner during the previous 6 months); persons seeking evaluation or treatment for a sexually transmitted disease (STD); current or recent injection drug users; and men who have sex with men;

Footnotes—Recommended Immunization Schedule for Adults Aged 19 Years or Older: United States, 2016

- health care personnel and public safety workers who are potentially exposed to blood or other infectious body fluids;
- persons who are aged <60 years with diabetes as soon as feasible after diagnosis; persons with diabetes who are aged ·60 years at the discretion of the treating clinician based on the likelihood of acquiring HBV infection, including the risk posed by an increased need for assisted blood glucose monitoring in long-term care facilities, the likelihood of experiencing chronic sequelae if infected with HBV, and the likelihood of immune response to vaccination;
- persons with end-stage renal disease (including patients receiving hemodialysis), persons with HIV infection, and persons with chronic liver disease;
- household contacts and sex partners of hepatitis B surface antigen-positive persons, clients and staff members of institutions for persons with developmental disabilities, and international travelers to regions with high or intermediate levels of endemic HBV infection (see footnote 1); and
- all adults in the following settings: STD treatment facilities, HIV testing and treatment facilities, facilities providing drug abuse treatment and prevention services, health care settings targeting services to injection drug users or men who have sex with men, correctional facilities, end-stage renal disease programs and facilities for chronic hemodialysis patients, and institutions and nonresidential day care facilities for persons with developmental disabilities.
- Administer missing doses to complete a 3-dose series of hepatitis B vaccine to those persons not vaccinated or not completely vaccinated. The second dose should be administered at least 1 month after the first dose; the third dose should be administered at least 2 months after the second dose (and at least 4 months after the first dose). If the combined hepatitis A and hepatitis B vaccine (Twinrix) is used, give 3 doses at 0, 1, and 6 months; alternatively, a 4-dose Twinrix schedule may be used, administered on days 0, 7, and 21–30, followed by a booster dose at 12 months.
- Adult patients receiving hemodialysis or with other immunocompromising conditions should receive 1 dose of 40 mcg/mL (Recombivax HB) administered on a 3-dose schedule at 0, 1, and 6 months or 2 doses of 20 mcg/mL (Engerix-B) administered simultaneously on a 4-dose schedule at 0, 1, 2, and 6 months.

11. Meningococcal vaccination
- General Information
  - Serogroup A, C, W, and Y meningococcal vaccine is available as a conjugate (MenACWY [Menactra, Menveo]) or a polysaccharide (MPSV4 [Menomune]) vaccine.
  - Serogroup B meningococcal (MenB) vaccine is available as a 2-dose series of MenB-4C vaccine (Bexsero) administered at least 1 month apart or a 3-dose series of MenB-FHbp (Trumenba) vaccine administered at 0, 2, and 6 months; the two MenB vaccines are not interchangeable, i.e., the same MenB vaccine product must be used for all doses.
  - MenACWY vaccine is preferred for adults with serogroup A, C, W, and Y meningococcal vaccine indications who are aged ·55 years, and for adults aged ·56 years: 1) who were vaccinated previously with MenACWY vaccine and are recommended for revaccination or 2) for whom multiple doses of vaccine are anticipated; MPSV4 vaccine is preferred for adults aged ·56 years who have not received MenACWY vaccine previously and who require a single dose only (e.g., persons at risk because of an outbreak).
  - Revaccination with MenACWY vaccine every 5 years is recommended for adults previously vaccinated with MenACWY or MPSV4 vaccine who remain at increased risk for infection

(e.g., adults with anatomical or functional asplenia or persistent complement component deficiencies, or microbiologists who are routinely exposed to isolates of Neisseria meningitidis).

MenB vaccine is approved for use in persons aged 10 through 25 years; however, because there is no theoretical difference in safety for persons aged >25 years compared to those aged 10 through 25 years, MenB vaccine is recommended for routine use in persons aged ·10 years who are at increased risk for serogroup B meningococcal disease.
  - There is no recommendation for MenB revaccination at this time.
  - MenB vaccine may be administered concomitantly with MenACWY vaccine but at a different anatomic site, if feasible.
  - HIV infection is not an indication for routine vaccination with MenACWY or MenB vaccine; if an HIV-infected person of any age is to be vaccinated, administer 2 doses of MenACWY vaccine at least 2 months apart.
- Adults with anatomical or functional asplenia or persistent complement component deficiencies: administer 2 doses of MenACWY vaccine at least 2 months apart and revaccinate every 5 years. Also administer a series of MenB vaccine.
- Microbiologists who are routinely exposed to isolates of Neisseria meningitidis: administer a single dose of MenACWY vaccine; revaccinate with MenACWY vaccine every 5 years if remain at increased risk for infection. Also administer a series of MenB vaccine.
- Persons at risk because of a meningococcal disease outbreak: if the outbreak is attributable to serogroup A, C, W, or Y, administer a single dose of MenACWY vaccine; if the outbreak is attributable to serogroup B, administer a series of MenB vaccine.
- Persons who travel to or live in countries in which meningococcal disease is hyperendemic or epidemic: administer a single dose of MenACWY vaccine and revaccinate with MenACWY vaccine every 5 years if the increased risk for infection remains (see footnote 1); MenB vaccine is not recommended because meningococcal disease in these countries is generally not caused by serogroup B.
- Military recruits: administer a single dose of MenACWY vaccine.
- First-year college students aged ·21 years who live in residence halls: administer a single dose of MenACWY vaccine if they have not received a dose on or after their 16th birthday.
- Young adults aged 16 through 23 years (preferred age range is 16 through 18 years): may be vaccinated with a series of MenB vaccine to provide short-term protection against most strains of serogroup B meningococcal disease.

12. Haemophilus influenzae type b (Hib) vaccination
- One dose of Hib vaccine should be administered to persons who have anatomical or functional asplenia or sickle cell disease or are undergoing elective splenectomy if they have not previously received Hib vaccine. Hib vaccination 14 or more days before splenectomy is suggested.
- Recipients of a hematopoietic stem cell transplant (HSCT) should be vaccinated with a 3-dose regimen 6-12 months after a successful transplant, regardless of vaccination history; at least 4 weeks should separate doses.
- Hib vaccine is not recommended for adults with HIV infection since their risk for Hib infection is low.

13. Immunocompromising conditions
- Inactivated vaccines (e.g., pneumococcal, meningococcal, and inactivated influenza vaccine) generally are acceptable and live vaccines generally should be avoided in persons with immune deficiencies or immunocompromising conditions. See ACIP Recommendations for information on specific conditions.

Figure 3. Footnotes from adult immunization schedule, United States, 2016.

Centers for Disease Control and Prevention (CDC). Advisory Committee on Immunization Practices (ACIP). Recommended Immunization Schedule for Adults Aged 19 Years and Older: United States, 2016. Available at www.cdc.gov/vaccines/schedules/downloads/adult/adult-combined-schedule.pdf.

Table 18. Contraindications and Precautions to Commonly Used Vaccines in Adults: United States, 2016

Vaccine	Contraindications	Precautions
Influenza, inactivated (IIV)[2]	Severe allergic reaction (e.g., anaphylaxis) after previous dose of any influenza vaccine; or to a vaccine component, including egg protein	• Moderate or severe acute illness with or without fever • History of Guillain-Barré Syndrome within 6 weeks of previous influenza vaccination • Adults with egg allergy of any severity may receive RIV; adults with hives-only allergy to eggs may receive IIV with additional safety measures.[2]
Influenza, recombinant (RIV)	Severe allergic reaction (e.g., anaphylaxis) after previous dose of RIV or to a vaccine component. RIV does not contain any egg protein.[2]	• Moderate or severe acute illness with or without fever. • History of Guillian-Barré Syndrome within 6 weeks of previous influenza vaccination.

Influenza, live attenuated (LAIV)[2, 3]	• Severe allergic reaction (e.g., anaphylaxis) to any component of the vaccine, or to a previous dose of any influenza vaccine
	• In addition, ACIP recommends that LAIV not be used in the following populations:
	  ▪ pregnant women
	  ▪ immunosuppressed adults
	  ▪ adults with egg allergy of any severity
	  ▪ adults who have taken influenza antiviral medications (amantadine, rimantadine, zanamivir, or oseltamivir) within the previous 48 hours; avoid use of these antiviral drugs for 14 days after vaccination
		• Moderate or severe acute illness with or without fever.
		• History of Guillain-Barré Syndrome within 6 weeks of previous influenza vaccination
		• Asthma in persons aged 5 years and older
		• Other chronic medical conditions, e.g., other chronic lung diseases, chronic cardiovascular disease (excluding isolated hypertension), diabetes, chronic renal or hepatic disease, hematologic disease, neurologic disease, and metabolic disorders

Tetanus, diphtheria, pertussis (Tdap); tetanus, diphtheria (Td)	• Severe allergic reaction (e.g., anaphylaxis) after a previous dose or to a vaccine component • For pertussis-containing vaccines: encephalopathy (e.g., coma, decreased level of consciousness, or prolonged seizures) not attributable to another identifiable cause within 7 days of administration of a previous dose of Tdap, diphtheria and tetanus toxoids and pertussis (DTP), or diphtheria and tetanus toxoids and acellular pertussis (DTaP) vaccine	• Moderate or severe acute illness with or without fever • Guillain-Barré Syndrome within 6 weeks after a previous dose of tetanus toxoid-containing vaccine • History of Arthus-type hypersensitivity reactions after a previous dose of tetanus or diphtheria toxoid-containing vaccine; defer vaccination until at least 10 years have elapsed since the last tetanus toxoid-containing vaccine • For pertussis-containing vaccines: progressive or unstable neurologic disorder, uncontrolled seizures, or progressive encephalopathy until a treatment regimen has been established and the condition has stabilized
Varicella[3]	• Severe allergic reaction (e.g., anaphylaxis) after a previous dose or to a vaccine component • Known severe immunodeficiency (e.g., from hematologic and solid tumors, receipt of chemotherapy, congenital immunodeficiency, or long-term immunosuppressive therapy,[4] or patients with human immunodeficiency virus [HIV] infection who are severely immunocompromised) • Pregnancy	• Recent (within 11 months) receipt of antibody-containing blood product (specific interval depends on product)[5] • Moderate or severe acute illness with or without fever • Receipt of specific antivirals (i.e., acyclovir, famciclovir, or valacyclovir) 24 hours before vaccination; avoid use of these antiviral drugs for 14 days after vaccination
Human papillomavirus (HPV)	Severe allergic reaction (e.g., anaphylaxis) after a previous dose or to a vaccine component.	• Moderate or severe acute illness with or without fever • Pregnancy
Zoster[3]	• Severe allergic reaction (e.g., anaphylaxis) to a vaccine component • Known severe immunodeficiency (e.g., from hematologic and solid tumors, receipt of chemotherapy, or long-term immunosuppressive therapy,[4] or patients with HIV infection who are severely immunocompromised) • Pregnancy	• Moderate or severe acute illness with or without fever • Receipt of specific antivirals (i.e., acyclovir, famciclovir, or valacyclovir) 24 hours before vaccination; avoid use of these antiviral drugs for 14 days after vaccination

Table 18. Contraindications and Precautions to Commonly Used Vaccines in Adults: United States, 2016 *(cont'd)*

Vaccine	Contraindications	Precautions
Measles, mumps, rubella (MMR)[3]	• Severe allergic reaction (e.g., anaphylaxis) after a previous dose or to a vaccine component • Known severe immunodeficiency (e.g., from hematologic and solid tumors, receipt of chemotherapy, congenital immunodeficiency, or long-term immunosuppressive therapy,[4] or patients with HIV infection who are severely immunocompromised) • Pregnancy	• Moderate or severe acute illness with or without fever • Recent (within 11 months) receipt of antibody-containing blood product (specific interval depends on product)[5] • History of thrombocytopenia or thrombocytopenic purpura • Need for tuberculin skin testing[6]
Pneumococcal conjugate (PCV13)	Severe allergic reaction (e.g., anaphylaxis) after a previous dose or to a vaccine component, including to any vaccine containing diphtheria toxoid.	• Moderate or severe acute illness with or without fever.
Pneumococcal polysaccharide (PPSV23)	Severe allergic reaction (e.g., anaphylaxis) after a previous dose or to a vaccine component.	• Moderate or severe acute illness with or without fever.
Hepatitis A	Severe allergic reaction (e.g., anaphylaxis) after a previous dose or to a vaccine component.	• Moderate or severe acute illness with or without fever.
Hepatitis B	Severe allergic reaction (e.g., anaphylaxis) after a previous dose or to a vaccine component.	• Moderate or severe acute illness with or without fever.
Meningococcal, conjugate (MenACWY); meningococcal, polysaccharide (MPSV4)	Severe allergic reaction (e.g., anaphylaxis) after a previous dose or to a vaccine component.	• Moderate or severe acute illness with or without fever.
Meningococcal serogroup B (MenB)	Severe allergic reaction (e.g., anaphylaxis) after a previous dose or to a vaccine component.	• Moderate or severe acute illness with or without fever.
Haemophilus influenzae **Type b (Hib)**	Severe allergic reaction (e.g., anaphylaxis) after a previous dose or to a vaccine component.	• Moderate or severe acute illness with or without fever.

Vaccine package inserts and the full ACIP recommendations for these vaccines should be consulted for additional information on vaccine-related contraindications and precautions and for more information on vaccine excipients. Events or conditions listed as precautions should be reviewed carefully. Benefits of and risks for administering a specific vaccine to a person under these circumstances should be considered. If the risk from the vaccine is believed to outweigh the benefit, the vaccine should not be administered. If the benefit of vaccination is believed to outweigh the risk, the vaccine should be administered. A contraindication is a condition in a recipient that increases the chance of a serious adverse reaction. Therefore, a vaccine should not be administered when a contraindication is present.

1. For more information on use of influenza vaccines among persons with egg allergies and a complete list of conditions that CDC considers to be reasons to avoid receiving LAIV, see CDC. Prevention and control of seasonal influenza with vaccines: recommendations of the Advisory Committee on Immunization Practices (ACIP) — United States, 2015–16 Influenza Season. *MMWR* 2015;64(30):818-25.
2. LAIV, MMR, varicella, or zoster vaccines can be administered on the same day. If not administered on the same day, live vaccines should be separated by at least 28 days.
3. Immunosuppressive steroid dose is considered to be ≥2 weeks of daily receipt of 20 mg of prednisone or the equivalent. Vaccination should be deferred for at least 1 month after discontinuation of such therapy. Providers should consult ACIP recommendations for complete information on the use of specific live vaccines among persons on immune-suppressing medications or with immunosuppression because of other reasons.
4. Vaccine should be deferred for the appropriate interval if replacement immune globulin products are being administered. See CDC. General recommendations on immunization: recommendations of the Advisory Committee on Immunization Practices (ACIP). *MMWR* 2011;60(No. RR-2).
5. Measles vaccination might suppress tuberculin reactivity temporarily. Measles-containing vaccine may be administered on the same day as tuberculin skin testing. If testing cannot be performed until after the day of MMR vaccination, the test should be postponed for at least 4 weeks after the vaccination. If an urgent need exists to skin test, do so with the understanding that reactivity might be reduced by the vaccine.

†Regarding latex allergy, consult the package insert for any vaccine administered.

Adapted from CDC. General recommendations on immunization: recommendations of the Advisory Committee on Immunization Practices (ACIP). *MMWR* 2011;60(No. RR-2):40-1 (Table 6. Contraindications and precautions to commonly used vaccines) and from Hamborsky J, Kroger A, Wolfe C, eds. Epidemiology and prevention of vaccine preventable diseases. 13th ed. Appendix A. Washington, DC: Public Health Foundation, 2015.

Centers for Disease Control and Prevention (CDC). Advisory Committee on Immunization Practices (ACIP). Recommended Immunization Schedule for Adults Aged 19 Years and Older: United States, 2016. Available at www.cdc.gov/vaccines/schedules/downloads/adult/adult-combined-schedule.pdf.

A. Major Changes in the 2016 Adult Immunization Schedule from the 2015 Schedule

1. MenB (serogroup B meningococcal vaccine) is a meningococcal vaccine now available for use in persons age 10 years and older at increased risk for serogroup B meningococcal disease. The CDC offers no recommendations for MenB vaccine at this time. The other available meningococcal vaccines (MenACWY and MPSV4) are serogroup A, C, W and Y. Both MenB and MenACWY or MPSV4 can be administered at the same time at different sites.

2. Nine-valent human papillomavirus vaccine (9vHPV) is now available and can be used for routine HPV vaccination of both females and males. For females, either bivalent, quadrivalent or nine-valent can be used; for males, either quadrivalent or nine-valent can be used.

3. 23-valent pneumococcal polysaccharide vaccine (PPSV23) is no longer recommended in people aged 19-64 who reside in nursing homes or long-term care facilities.

B. Recent Changes Regarding Pneumococcal Vaccination

1. 13-valent pneumococcal conjugate vaccine (PCV13) [Prevnar] should now be used for adult pneumococcal vaccination in people age 65 years and older, in addition to PPSV23 [Pneumovax].

2. In pneumococcal vaccine–naive patients 65 years or older: PCV13 at age 65 years or older, followed by PPSV23 at least 1 year later.

3. In patients who previously received PPSV23 at age 65 years or older: Vaccinate with PCV13 1 year or more after PPSV23.

4. In patients who previously received PPSV23 before age 65 years who are now aged 65 years or older: Vaccinate with PCV13 1 year or more after receipt of PPSV23 and revaccinate with PPSV23 at least 1 year after PCV13, as long as 5 or more years has passed since the previous PPSV23.

5. The interval between PCV13 and PPSV23 is at least 8 weeks for people with immunocompromising conditions, anatomical or functional asplenia, cerebrospinal fluid leaks, or cochlear implants.

C. Egg Allergy and Influenza Vaccination

1. If an adult has any severity of egg allergy, he or she may receive recombinant influenza vaccine (RIV), which does not contain any egg protein.

2. If an adult has experienced only hives after eating eggs or egg-containing foods, he or she can receive inactivated influenza vaccine (IIV), with additional safety measures. Avoid live attenuated influenza vaccine (LAIV) nasal spray.

3. Some people who report egg allergies may not actually be allergic to eggs. Those who are able to eat lightly cooked egg (e.g., scrambled egg) without a reaction are not likely to be allergic and can receive any influenza vaccine.

D. Current Issues with Herpes Zoster Vaccine (HZV): The HZV package insert states not to give HZV and PPSV concurrently but to separate them by at least 4 weeks because of decreased immunologic response to HZV. Their conclusion is based on a Merck-sponsored, unpublished study. The ACIP states that the clinical relevance of this recommendation is unknown, and a subsequent study showed no compromise in HZV efficacy. The Advisory Committee on Immunization Practices/Centers for Disease Control and Prevention (ACIP/CDC), which reviewed the data, continues to recommend that HZV and PPSV be administered at the same visit if the person is eligible for both vaccines.

Patient Cases

14. A 71-year-old woman with COPD is taking tiotropium (Spiriva) inhaled 1 capsule/day. She received the influenza vaccine last October, her last tetanus and diphtheria (Td) vaccine was at age 65, and her PPSV23 was given at age 60. She has not previously received the zoster vaccine, but she had an episode of severe zoster infection 5 years ago. Which is the most appropriate choice of vaccines that should be given at her October internal medicine clinic appointment?

    A. Only the influenza vaccine should be given.

    B. Influenza and PCV13 vaccines should be given.

    C. Influenza, PCV13, and zoster vaccines should be given.

    D. Influenza, PCV13, zoster, and tetanus, diphtheria, and pertussis (Tdap) vaccines should be given.

15. A 20-year-old woman who is going away to college presents for a physical examination in July. She will be living in the dormitory. She smokes 1/2 pack/day but has no other medical conditions. She is up to date with all of her routine childhood vaccines, but she has not received any vaccines in the past 11 years. She is not sexually active. Which is the most appropriate choice for vaccines that should be given today?

    A. Td and human papillomavirus (HPV) vaccines.

    B. Tdap, quadrivalent meningococcal conjugate vaccine (MenACWY), and HPV vaccines.

    C. MenACWY, PPSV23, and Td vaccines.

    D. MenACWY, PPSV23, Tdap, and HPV vaccines.

16. A 21-year-old man with type 1 diabetes presents for an influenza vaccine. He has an egg allergy and has experienced angioedema and difficulty breathing after eating eggs. Which is the most appropriate regarding influenza vaccination in this patient?

    A. Either IIV, RIV, or LAIV can be used; observe patient for 30 minutes.

    B. Either IIV or RIV can be used; observe patient for 30 minutes.

    C. Only RIV should be used.

    D. He should not receive any type of influenza vaccine.

REFERENCES

Asthma

1. Agency for Healthcare Research and Quality. Module 4: measuring quality of care for asthma. Available at www.ahrq.gov/qual/asthmacare/asthmod4.htm. Accessed September 1, 2014.

2. Global Initiative for Asthma (GINA). Global Strategy for Asthma Management and Prevention 2015. Available at www.ginasthma.org. Accessed October 20, 2015.

3. Global Initiative for Asthma (GINA) and Global Initiative for Chronic Obstructive Lung Disease (GOLD). Diagnosis of diseases of chronic airflow limitation: asthma, COPD and asthma-COPD overlap syndrome (ACOS). Available at www.ginasthma.org. Accessed October 20, 2015.

4. Martinez FD, Chinchilli VM, Morgan WJ, et al. Use of beclomethasone dipropionate as rescue treatment for children with mild persistent asthma (TREXA): a randomized, double-blind, placebo-controlled trial. Lancet 2011;377:650-7.

5. National Institutes of Health National Heart, Lung and Blood Institute. National Asthma Education and Prevention Program (NAEPP) guidelines. NAEPP Expert Panel Report 3. NIH Publication 08-5846. July 2007. Available at www.nhlbi.nih.gov/guidelines/index.htm. Accessed October 20, 2015.

6. Nelson HS, Weiss ST, Bleecker ER, et al. The Salmeterol Multicenter Asthma Research Trial (SMART): a comparison of usual pharmacotherapy for asthma or usual pharmacotherapy plus salmeterol. Chest 2006;129:15-26.

7. Perera BJ. Salmeterol Multicentre Asthma Research Trial (SMART): interim analysis shows increased risk of asthma-related deaths. Ceylon Med J 2003;48:99.

8. Peters SP, Kunselman SJ, Icitovic N, et al. Tiotropium bromide step-up therapy for adults with uncontrolled asthma (TALC study). N Engl J Med 2010;363:1715-26.

9. Price D, Musgrave SD, Shepstone L, et al. Leukotriene antagonists as first-line or add-on asthma-controller therapy. N Engl J Med 2011;364:1695-707.

Chronic Obstructive Pulmonary Disease

1. Albert RK, Connett J, Bailey WC, et al. Azithromycin for prevention of exacerbations of COPD. N Engl J Med 2011;365:689-98.

2. Bestall JC, Paul EA, Garrod R, et al. Usefulness of the Medical Research Council (MRC) dyspnea scale as a measure of disability in patients with chronic obstructive pulmonary disease. Thorax 1999;54:581-6.

3. Calverley PMA, Anderson JA, Celli B, et al. Salmeterol and fluticasone propionate and survival in chronic obstructive pulmonary disease (the TORCH study). N Engl J Med 2007;356:775-89.

4. Chong J, Karner C, Poole P. Tiotropium versus long-acting beta-agonists for stable chronic obstructive pulmonary disease. Cochrane Database Syst Rev 2012;9:CD009157.

5. Ernst P, Gonzalez AP, Brassard P, et al. Inhaled corticosteroid use in chronic obstructive pulmonary disease and the risk of hospitalization for pneumonia. Am J Respir Crit Care Med 2007;176:162-6.

6. Fiore MC, Jaen CR, Baker TB, et al. Treating Tobacco Use and Dependence: 2008 Update. Rockville, MD: U.S. Department of Health and Human Services, Public Health Service, 2008. Available at www.ncbi.nlm.nih.gov/bookshelf/br.fcgi?book=hsahcpr&part=A28163. Accessed September 26, 2011.

7. Global Initiative for Chronic Obstructive Lung Disease Workshop Executive Summary: Global Strategy for the Diagnosis, Management, and Prevention of Chronic Obstructive Pulmonary Disease, 2015 Update. Available at www.goldcopd.org. Accessed October 20, 2015.

8. Global Initiative for Asthma (GINA) and Global Initiative for Chronic Obstructive Lung Disease (GOLD). Diagnosis of diseases of chronic airflow limitation: asthma, COPD and asthma-COPD overlap syndrome (ACOS). Available at www.ginasthma.org. Accessed October 20, 2015.

9. Heffner JE, Mularski RA, Calverley PM. COPD performance measures: missing opportunities for improving care. Chest 2010;137:1181-9.

10. Leuppi JD, Schuetz P, Bingisser R, et al. Short-term vs conventional glucocorticoid therapy in acute exacerbations of chronic obstructive pulmonary disease: the REDUCE randomized clinical trial. JAMA 2013;309:2223-31.

11. McEvoy CE, Neiwoehner DE. Adverse effects of corticosteroid therapy for COPD: a critical review. Chest 1997;111:732-43.

12. Nannini LJ, Cates CJ, Lasserson TJ, et al. Combined corticosteroid and long-acting beta-agonist in one inhaler versus placebo for chronic obstructive pulmonary disease. Cochrane Database Syst Rev 2007;4:CD003794.

13. Rutten FH, Zuithoff NP, Hak E, et al. Beta-blockers may reduce mortality and risk of exacerbations in patients with chronic obstructive pulmonary disease. Arch Intern Med 2010;170:880-7.

14. Salpeter SR, Ormiston T, Salpeter E, et al. Cardioselective beta-blockers for chronic obstructive pulmonary disease [review]. Cochrane Database Syst Rev 2002;2:CD003566. Update in: Cochrane Database Syst Rev 2005;4:CD003566.

15. Singh S, Amin AV, Loke YK. Long-term use of inhaled corticosteroids and the risk of pneumonia in chronic obstructive pulmonary disease. Arch Intern Med 2009;169:219-29.

16. VanDerMolen T, Willemse BW, Schokker S, et al. Development, validity and responsiveness of the Clinical COPD Questionnaire. Health Qual Life Outcomes 2003;1:13.

17. van Grunsven PM, van Schayck CP, Dereene JP, et al. Long-term effects of inhaled corticosteroids in chronic obstructive pulmonary disease: a meta-analysis. Thorax 1999;54:7-14.

18. Vogelmeier C, Hederer B, Glaab T, et al. Tiotropium versus salmeterol for the prevention of exacerbations of COPD (POET-COPD study). N Engl J Med 2011;364:1093-103.

19. Welte T, Miravitlles M, Hernandez P, et al. Efficacy and tolerability of budesonide/formoterol added to tiotropium in patients with chronic obstructive pulmonary disease. Am J Respir Crit Care Med 2009;180:741-50.

Gout

1. Khanna D, Fitzgerald JD, Khanna PP, et al. 2012 American College of Rheumatology Guidelines for Management of Gout. Part 1. Systematic non-pharmacologic and pharmacologic therapeutic approaches to hyperuricemia. Arthritis Care Res 2012;64:1431-46.

2. Khanna D, Khanna PP, Fitzgerald JD, et al. 2012 American College of Rheumatology Guidelines for Management of Gout. Part 2. Therapy and antiinflammatory prophylaxis of acute gouty arthritis. Arthritis Care Res 2012;64:1447-61.

3. Singh JA, Reddy SG, Kundukulam J. Risk factors for gout and prevention: a systematic review of the literature. Curr Opin Rheumatol 2011;23:192-202.

Immunizations

1. Centers for Disease Control and Prevention (CDC). Advisory Committee on Immunization Practices (ACIP). Recommended Immunization Schedule for Adults Aged 19 Years and Older: United States, 2016. Available at www.cdc.gov/vaccines/schedules/downloads/adult/adult-combined-schedule.pdf.

2. Use of 13-valent pneumococcal conjugate vaccine and 23-valent pneumococcal polysaccharide vaccine among adults aged $\geq$ 65 years: Recommendations of the Advisory Committee on Immunization Practices (ACIP). MMWR Morb Mortal Wkly Rep 2014;63(37):822–5. Available at www.cdc/gov/mmwr/preview/mmwrhtml/mm6337a4.htm. Accessed October 20, 2015.

ANSWERS AND EXPLANATIONS TO PATIENT CASES

1. Answer: B

Her symptom frequency of twice weekly, her FEV_1 of more than 80% of predicted (normal), and the lack of interference with activity are consistent with intermittent asthma. However, her night awakenings for asthma symptoms occur three times per month, which is consistent with mild persistent asthma. In addition, mild persistent asthma still has normal spirometry. The specific level of persistent asthma is based on the most severe category met, so even though only one of her signs and symptoms falls under mild persistent and the rest under intermittent, she would be categorized as mild persistent.

2. Answer: C

Because she has mild persistent asthma, step 2 is recommended for initial treatment. In addition to an inhaled SABA as needed, she would need to use a low-dose ICS (preferred treatment); mometasone 220 mcg once daily is a low-dose ICS. Montelukast is an alternative therapy (not first line) for step 2. Budesonide/formoterol, in the dose listed, is a low-dose ICS plus a LABA, which is a step 3 therapy.

3. Answer: D

Her asthma is not well controlled because the frequency of her daytime symptoms, and albuterol use is greater than 2 days/week. Recommended action for treatment is to step up to step 3: a low-dose ICS plus a LABA or a medium-dose ICS alone. The budesonide/formoterol MDI is incorrect because it is a medium-dose ICS plus a LABA (a step 4 treatment). Adding montelukast to low-dose ICS is an alternative therapy.

4. Answer: D

This patient has moderate persistent asthma because of his nighttime symptoms twice weekly and needs step 3 therapy. A medium-dose ICS alone is preferred as initial therapy in this age group (5–11 years). Fluticasone 44 mcg 1 puff twice daily is a low-dose ICS for this age group. Montelukast is not recommended as monotherapy for moderate persistent asthma in this age group; montelukast is recommended only in combination with a low-dose ICS. Fluticasone/salmeterol 100/50 twice daily is a medium-dose ICS plus a LABA, which is step 4 in this age group.

5. Answer: D

Because he is experiencing shortness of breath at rest, has trouble with conversation, and has an FEV_1 less than 40%, his asthma exacerbation is classified as severe. For severe asthma exacerbations in the ED setting, the recommended treatment is oxygen to achieve an Sao_2 of 90% or greater, high-dose inhaled SABA plus ipratropium by either nebulizer or MDI with valved holding chamber every 20 minutes for 1 hour or continuously, and OCSs.

6. Answer: B

He is in GOLD guidelines patient group B because his postbronchodilator FEV_1 is between 50% and 80%, he has had 1 or no exacerbations in the past year, and his mMRC score is 2 or more. If the CAT were being used, the score would be 10 or greater.

7. Answer: B

According to the GOLD guidelines, the recommended treatment for patient group B is regular treatment with an LA bronchodilator (either a LABA or LA anticholinergic), in addition to an SA bronchodilator as needed. Inhaled corticosteroids are recommended only in groups C and D. Roflumilast is recommended only if FEV_1 is less than 50% of predicted with chronic bronchitis and the patient has a history of frequent exacerbations.

8. Answer: A

This patient is in GOLD risk group B, according to spirometry and CAT score, and is on the first-choice therapy. Because her control is worsening, she should go to the second-choice therapy, for which combined LA bronchodilators can be used. Inhaled corticosteroids are recommended only in risk groups C and D. Although a recent study showed benefits with chronic azithromycin, the guidelines do not recommend regular treatment with long-term antibiotics. In addition, the study showing the benefits of azithromycin included only patients at a higher risk of exacerbations (on continuous oxygen therapy or using systemic corticosteroids, plus a history of exacerbation necessitating an ED visit or hospitalization). She does not meet these criteria.

9. Answer: D

According to the latest GOLD guidelines, OCSs are indicated in most exacerbations. The recommended dose is oral prednisone 40 mg daily for 5 days. Antibiotic treatment is also indicated because the patient has all three cardinal symptoms of airway infection: increased sputum purulence, increased sputum volume, and increased dyspnea. Trimethoprim/sulfamethoxazole is one of the recommended antibiotics.

10. Answer: A

NSAIDs (in anti-inflammatory or acute pain doses), colchicine, or corticosteroids are all appropriate for first-line therapy for acute gout. However, colchicine would not be recommended for this patient because he took acute colchicine doses in the past 2 weeks. Intra-articular corticosteroids are recommended only if only one or two large joints are affected. This patient is having an acute gouty attack of moderate severity. Combination therapy is recommended for initial therapy only if the patient has a severe attack. Oral prednisone alone would also be appropriate; however, this was not a choice.

11. Answer: D

Urate-lowering therapy is indicated in this patient because he has had two or more attacks in the past year. Allopurinol and febuxostat (XOIs) are first-line ULTs; probenecid is an alternative first-line ULT only if XOIs are contraindicated or not tolerated. Urate-lowering therapy can be initiated during an acute gouty attack, according to the American College of Rheumatology guidelines, as long as anti-inflammatory prophylaxis is instituted.

12. Answer: A

Oral corticosteroids are associated with significant risks in long-term therapy; they should not be used for anti-inflammatory prophylaxis unless both colchicine and NSAIDs are contraindicated, not tolerated, or ineffective. Combination therapy is not recommended for anti-inflammatory prophylaxis. Pegloticase is ULT, not anti-inflammatory prophylaxis.

13. Answer: B

If no tophi are present, the initial goal serum urate is less than 6 mg/dL; if gouty signs and symptoms are still present, then a secondary goal urate is less than 5 mg/dL. Anti-inflammatory prophylaxis if no tophi are present should continue for 3 months after goal serum urate is achieved, as long as the total duration is at least 6 months.

14. Answer: D

The CDC recommends that the influenza vaccine be given every year to every person 6 months and older. People 65 years and older should be vaccinated with PCV13, either for their first pneumococcal vaccination or if they were vaccinated 5 or more years previously and were younger than 65 years at the time of first pneumococcal vaccination. This patient should receive a second PPSV23 at least 1 year after the PCV13 vaccination today. Zoster vaccination is recommended in all adults 60 years and older, regardless of previous zoster infection. The Tdap vaccine is recommended in all people, now including those 65 years and older.

15. Answer: D

First-year college students up to age 21 who live in dormitories, if not previously vaccinated on or after age 16, should receive the meningococcal vaccine (MenACWY; Menactra, Menevo). The PPSV23 is recommended for smokers 19–64 years of age, and this patient is a smoker. The Td vaccine should be given every 10 years. In adults younger than 65, a one-time dose of Tdap should be given, regardless of the time interval since the most recent tetanus vaccination. The HPV vaccine is for girls and women 11–26 years of age. Ideally, it should be given before the start of sexual activity, but it should still be administered to sexually active girls and women.

16. Answer: C

In people with a severe egg allergy, only RIV can be used.

ANSWERS AND EXPLANATIONS TO SELF-ASSESSMENT QUESTIONS

1. Answer: D
That she uses the inhaler throughout the day, every day, and sometimes at night indicates she has daily symptoms. "Severe persistent" means that frequency of symptoms is throughout the day, nighttime symptoms are often 7 times/week, a SABA several times a day, normal activity is extremely limited, FEV_1 is less than 60% of predicted, and FEV_1/FVC is reduced more than 5%.

2. Answer: C
"Severe persistent" initial treatment is step 4 or 5. Step 4 preferred treatment is inhaled steroid (medium dose) plus an LABA. Step 5 preferred treatment is inhaled steroid (high dose) plus an LABA.

3. Answer: D
Ratio data are ranked in a specific order with a consistent level of magnitude difference between units, with an absolute zero.

4. Answer: B
The percentage of patients receiving fluticasone/salmeterol who have an asthma-related hospitalization will be compared with the percentage of patients receiving fluticasone who have an asthma-related hospitalization. We assume that these two groups are normally distributed. These data are considered nominal. Chi-square test is appropriate to analyze nominal or categoric data. Analysis of variance is appropriate when there are more than two treatment groups. The Student unpaired t test is used for continuous data that are normally distributed. The Mann-Whitney U test is appropriate when continuous data are not normally distributed.

5. Answer: B
Pneumococcal vaccine is recommended in people 19–64 years of age with asthma. This patient falls into this category. Influenza vaccine is recommended in people with chronic cardiovascular or pulmonary diseases such as asthma. However, usually the influenza vaccine is given in the fall or early winter to offer protection when the risk of infection is highest. The tetanus booster (Td) is recommended every 10 years, and it has not been 10 years since this patient's last Td, which was given as Tdap. The HZV (Zostavax) is recommended at 60 years and older by the CDC; however, it is indicated at 50 years and older in the manufacturer's package insert.

6. Answer: B
This patient is in GOLD patient group B. A single LA bronchodilator is first choice for medication treatment. Tiotropium is an LA bronchodilator (anticholinergic) that would be appropriate to initiate in this patient. An LABA would also be appropriate, but it was not one of the choices. Roflumilast is only indicated in severe COPD (FEV_1 less than 50% of predicted) associated with chronic bronchitis and a history of frequent exacerbations. An ICS is recommended only in patient group C or D and should never be used as monotherapy in COPD.

7. Answer: D
The starting allopurinol dose is 50 mg/day in stage 4 (GFR 15–29 mL/minute/1.73 m^2) or worse CKD; the dose should be gradually titrated every 2–5 weeks. Probenecid is not recommended as first-line ULT if CrCl is less than 50 mL/minute.